The LITTLE
BLACK BOOK
of NEUROLOGY

The LITTLE BLACK BOOK of NEUROLOGY

SIXTH EDITION

Osama O. Zaidat, MD, MS, FSVIN
Vascular and Interventional Neurologist
Professor, North East Ohio Medical University (NeoMed);
Neuroscience and Stroke Director
Bon Secours Mercy Health St Vincent Hospital
Toledo, OH

J. Douglas Miles, MD, PhD
Assistant Professor
Department of Medicine
University of Hawaii John A. Burns School of Medicine;
Director, Neuroscience Education
Neuroscience Institute
The Queen's Medical Center
Honolulu, HI

Alan J. Lerner, MD
Professor
Neurology
Case Western Reserve University;
Director
Brain Health and Memory Center
University Hospitals Cleveland Medical Center
Cleveland, OH

ELSEVIER

Elsevier
1600 John F. Kennedy Blvd.
Ste 1600
Philadelphia, PA 19103-2899

THE LITTLE BLACK BOOK OF NEUROLOGY,
SIXTH EDITION
ISBN: 978-0-323-52979-2

Previous editions copyrighted 2008, 2002, and 1995.

Library of Congress Control Number: 2019936492

Content Strategist: Marybeth Thiel
Content Development Specialist: Meghan B. Andress
Publishing Services Manager: Deepthi Unni
Project Manager: Beula Christopher
Design Direction: Bridget Hoette

Printed in the United States of America.

Last digit is the print number: 9 8 7 6 5 4 3 2 1

Working together
to grow libraries in
developing countries

www.elsevier.com • www.bookaid.org

To

Our Families

To

Our Mentor, Professor Robert Daroff

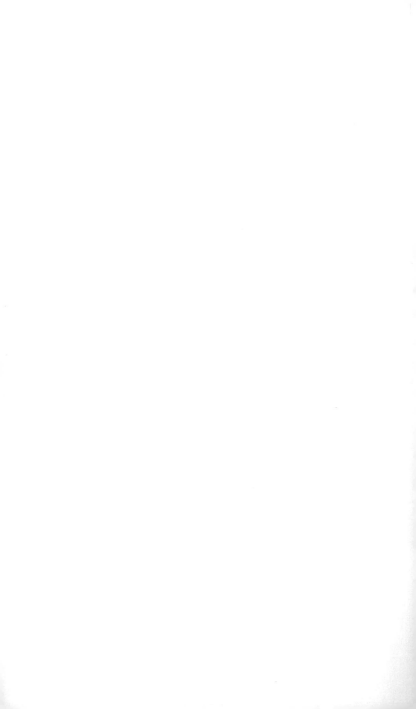

Contributors

Samer Abdulkareem, MD
Rafeed Alkawadri, MD
Ali Al Balushi, MD, MRCP(UK)
Sami Al Kasab, MD
Ayham Alkhachroum, MD
Syeda Laila Alqadri, MD
Joelle Ballone, DO
Luke K. Barr, MD
Michael J. Bradshaw, MD
Pola Alida Chojecka, MD
Jason Chua, MD, PhD
Nikita Dedhia, MD
Salman Farooq, MD
Mary Hollist, DO
Luis Antonio Sanchez Iglesias, MD
Cigdem Isitan, MD
Mohammad W. Kassem, MD, MBA
Ehtesham Khalid, MD, MRCP (UK), FCPS (PAK)
William A. Kilgo, MD
Erik Krause, DO
Alain Lekoubou Looti, MD, MS
Alan J. Lerner, MD
A. Sebastian Lopez-Chiriboga, MD
Supriya Mahajan, BA, MD
J. Douglas Miles, MD, PhD
Fábio A. Nascimento, MD
Elizabeth A. Ng, MD
Jerris-Stephanie Okonkwo, MD
Fausto E. Ordonez, MD
Diana OYoung-Oliver, DO, MS
Umera Paracha, MD
Amanda C. Peltier, MD, MS
Lauren Peruski, DO
Suraj Rajan, MSc, MD
Sujan T. Reddy, MD, MPH
James Rini, MD, MPH
Daniel I. Ro, MD
Junaid Siddiqui, MD, MRCP
Lauren Tardo, MD
Philip Tipton, BS, MD
Igor B. Títoff, DO, MA

Melanie Truong-Le, DO, OD
Israr Ul Haq, MD
Emily J. Volger, PharmD, BCACP, MSCR
Han Wang, MD, MPH
Kevin Wilson, MD
Ting Wu, MD
Kyan Younes, MD
Derek Y. Yuan, MD, MS
Osama O. Zaidat, MD, MS, FSVIN
Jonathan L. Zande, MD
Rabia Zubair, MD

Preface

The Little Black Book of Neurology returns after a several-year hiatus, incorporating changes in neurologic practice as well as changes in book publishing. However, it remains true to the original vision of Robert Daroff, MD of an easy-to-access guide, with topics arranged in alphabetical order and written primarily by neurology residents.

The sixth edition differs in two important ways from previous editions. The first is that previous editions were generated by neurology residents at Case Western Reserve University, and reflected neurology as practiced in Cleveland, OH. In this edition, we reached out to neurology program directors and residents throughout the United States, in essentially all neurology programs. This is important since it broadens the diversity of views contained in the various chapters to reflect differences in practice in different locations.

The second major change relates to technological advances in book publishing and how content is accessed to maximal effect. The concept of a comprehensive, authoritative book in a pocket format has also run up against a bewildering explosion of new treatments, treatment guidelines and algorithms, and evidence-based recommendations. The sixth edition gladly embraces the e-book revolution. It will also become a platform for incorporating even newer advances in neurology, linking neurologists and other medical professionals to the latest changes in knowledge and practice.

The Little Black Book of Neurology has been a success for 30 years, and many of the features will be familiar. We include tables with guidelines and treatment algorithms. Second, because of career moves, our focus has moved beyond the residency program at University Hospitals of Cleveland and Case Western Reserve University, which had provided authorship for previous editions.

The majority of the chapters have been updated or rewritten, with new tables and references added. At least one new suggested reading or reference of a landmark study or review article is provided at the end of most chapters, and we recommend that readers take note of those excellent references.

We have updated the Neurologic Emergency and Therapeutic appendices at the back of the book. The Neurologic Emergency Appendix provides in short monograph, table, or algorithm format approaches to areas such as acute ischemic stroke, meningitis, myasthenia crisis, headache, hemorrhagic stroke, intracranial pressure, pain, quadriplegia, spinal cord injury, and status epilepticus. Topics covered in the Therapeutic Appendix include dementia, epilepsy, headache, insomnia, multiple sclerosis, myasthenia gravis, pain management, Parkinson disease, and stroke.

We have also included the American Academy of Neurology (AAN) Guideline Summaries. These guidelines are important in our daily practice to provide better care of our patients and for Neurology Board Recertification. We conclude the appendices with a comprehensive scales index.

The new LBBN-6e is still the neurology pocket book of choice providing a concise, up-to-date, and easy-to-read practical overview of neurologic topics large and small. This work will be very useful for neurologists, neurosurgeons, internists, family practitioners, physical medicine and rehabilitation staff, neuroradiologists, residents, medical students, nurses, physician assistants, and nurse practitioners, or any health care providers caring for neurologic patients. Our greatest satisfaction will be when the LBBN-6e is helpful in providing optimal patient care in the hands of health care providers.

I would like to thank our publisher, Elsevier, including Jim Merritt, Marybeth Thiel, Meghan Andress, Beula Christopher and the whole production team for their endless efforts and hard work to provide an excellent well-organized volume to our readers. This book extends our patient-centric focus we learned from our mentors and colleagues, including many of the giants of modern neurology, Joseph Foley, Robert Daroff, Dennis Landis, Anthony Furlan, Hans Luders, David Preston, Bashar Katirji, Peter Whitehouse, Robert Friedland, and countless others throughout the United States and across the globe. I also would like to thank my co-editors, Osama Zaidat and J. Douglas Miles, and especially all of our contributors throughout the United States for their extraordinary hard work and patience during the long hours spent updating and editing the chapters.

Alan J. Lerner
Cleveland, OH

Contents

A

ABSCESS, BRAIN

Brain abscess is a focal pyogenic infection of the brain parenchyma. They constitute less than 2% of intracranial masses and develop mainly in four clinical situations, although 15% to 20% are cryptogenic.

I. *Contiguous spread* (45%–50% of all cases) via direct extension from local neighboring infection sites—frontal or ethmoid sinusitis or dental infection (frontal lobe abscess), middle ear or mastoid air cell infection (temporal lobe and cerebellar abscess), spread by local osteomyelitis or by septic thrombophlebitis of emissary vein.

II. *Hematogenous spread* from distant sites of infection (25%), usually multiple and multiloculated, often in the middle cerebral artery distribution. Common sources of metastatic brain abscesses are pulmonary or abdominopelvic infections, cyanotic heart disease, congenital heart malformations with right-to-left shunts (oral bacterial flora after dental procedures), or bacterial endocarditis.

III. *Trauma* including penetrating head injury or neurosurgical procedures (10%)—compound depressed skull fractures, basal skull fractures with cerebrospinal fluid (CSF) fistulae/leak, and previous craniotomy can lead to brain abscess, sometimes months or years after the acute event. Postneurosurgic abscesses may occur, especially when surgery involves paranasal air sinuses.

IV. *Immunosuppression.* People with acquired immune deficiency syndrome (AIDS) or with other causes of immunosuppression (e.g., neoplasms, steroid use) are susceptible to bacterial infections or infections associated with decreased T-cell immunity such as mycobacteria, fungi, or *Toxoplasmosis*.

Pathogens isolated from abscesses are related to the site of origin, as follows (organisms are listed in order of significance; many abscesses are polymicrobial):

I. Middle ear infection: streptococci (aerobic and anaerobic), *Bacteroides fragilis,* and Enterobacteriaceae (Proteus).

II. Sinusitis: same as middle ear infections, plus *Staphylococcus aureus, Haemophilus* species, and mucormycosis (also seen with orbital cellulitis).

III. Penetrating head trauma: *S. aureus*, streptococci, Enterobacteriaceae, *Clostridium* species, and *Pseudomonas aeruginosa*.

IV. AIDS/immunocompromised: *Toxoplasma, Mycobacterium, Listeria* species infection, *Listeria monocytogenes, Nocardia*, and *Cryptococcus neoformans.*

CLINICAL FEATURES

Clinical features usually resemble those of other space-occupying lesions (focal signs, seizures in 25%–35% of patients) with most symptoms related to increased intracranial pressure (ICP) (headache, nausea, vomiting, lethargy, and stupor). Fever occurs in only 50% of cases.

HISTOPATHOLOGIC STAGES

Days 1 to 3: Early cerebritis produces a local inflammatory response (usually within white matter or at the gray-white matter junction) around a necrotic center.

Days 4 to 9: Late cerebritis is characterized by increased necrosis and inflammation, with initial fibroblastic formation of the collagen capsule.

Days 10 to 13: Early encapsulation stage shows further development of the collagen capsule, which is typically thinner on the less vascular ventricular side.

Days 14 and later: Late capsular stage shows five distinct histologic layers—the necrotic center, inflammatory cells and fibroblasts, collagen capsule, neovascular layer, and surrounding reactive gliosis and edema.

WORK-UP

I. Blood cultures should be drawn (positive in 15% of cases) and empiric parenteral antibiotic therapy must be initiated before computed tomography (CT) scan or magnetic resonance imaging (MRI). Lumbar puncture may be considered if mass effect is not prominent. However, the diagnostic yield is low and the risk of herniation is greater with abscess than with other mass lesions.

II. CT scans correlate well with the histopathologic stages. In the cerebritis stage, CT without contrast shows the necrotic center as a hypodensity. Ring enhancement begins in the later stages of cerebritis. In capsular stages the capsule becomes visible on CT without contrast as a faint hyperdense ring that produces ring-enhancing lesion with contrast, which is thinner on the ventricular side.

III. MRI appearance is bright on diffusion-weighted images (DWIs): T_1 delineates the abscess capsule as hyperintense/isointense and hypointense center and surrounding edema; T_2 demonstrates the hyperintense edema and center and hypointense capsule, enhances with gadolinium.

IV. MR spectroscopy (MRS) can differentiate between abscess, necrotizing tumor, or granuloma. The main finding of MRS in abscesses is elevation of metabolites of bacterial origin, including acetate, lactate, succinate, and amino acids versus necrotic brain tumors with elevated choline and decreased N-acetylaspartate (NAA). The MRS pattern may monitor effectiveness of medical treatment of a brain abscess, showing a decline of the metabolites after a positive response to therapy.

V. Other studies include electroencephalogram (EEG) which may show nonspecific findings such as focal slowing, seizure activity, and evidence of encephalopathy. Cerebral angiography may show avascular mass and luxury perfusion.

TREATMENT

A combination of broad-spectrum antimicrobials, management of raised ICP, neurosurgical drainage or excision, and eradication of the primary infectious focus is indicated. If CT shows only cerebritis or abscess less than 2.5 cm and the patient is neurologically stable, antibiotics without surgery may suffice. Neurologic deterioration usually mandates surgery.

Excision or aspiration is performed for abscesses greater than 2.5 cm in diameter. Aspiration has become the procedure of choice because it is equally effective and less invasive than excision. Empiric antibiotics should be given based on the expected etiologic agents, presumed route and source of infection, predisposing factors, and adjusted based on the cultures. When the cause is unknown, the patient should receive a third- or fourth-generation cephalosporin, for example, ceftazidime 2 g IV q 8 hr (or ceftriaxone 2 g IV q 12 hr) or penicillin (PCN) G 5 MU IV q 6 hr, and metronidazole 500 mg IV q 6 hr. For paranasal sinus sources, administer PCN and metronidazole. In treatment of posttraumatic cases, administer nafcillin 2 g IV q 2 hr (or vancomycin 1 g IV q 12 hr, if methicillin-resistant *S. aureus* is suspected) and a third-generation cephalosporin such as ceftazidime 2 g IV q 8 hr. Treatment should be given for 6 to 8 weeks, often followed by additional 2 to 6 months of oral therapy or until the resolution of neuroimaging findings. Three to 4 weeks may be adequate in patients treated with surgical drainage. In human immunodeficiency virus (HIV)-positive patients, coverage should be added for toxoplasmosis with pyrimethamine plus sulfadiazine or clindamycin. Mucormycosis is treated with amphotericin B. Antiepileptic drugs may be given for up to 3 months. Routine corticosteroid administration is controversial and should be used only when mental status is significantly depressed and substantial mass effect can be demonstrated on imaging, and therapy should be of short duration.

A

ABSCESS, BRAIN

PROGNOSIS

Mortality rates range from 5% to 15%. Poor prognosis is associated with very young or old age; anaerobic pathogens; large, multiple, deep, cerebellar, or multiloculated abscesses; acute clinical presentation with stupor/coma; intraventricular or subarachnoid rupture; concomitant pulmonary infection or sepsis; and specific organisms (i.e., *Aspergillus* and *Pseudomonas* species, fungal). Long-term sequelae include cognitive deficits (developmental delay in children), seizures, and focal deficits.

REFERENCES

Brook, I. (2017). Microbiology and treatment of brain abscess. *J Clin Neurosci, 38*, 8–12. https://doi.org/10.1016/j.jocn.2016.12.035.

Brouwer, M. C., Tunkel, A. R., McKhann, G. M., et al. (2014). Brain abscess. *N Engl J Med, 31*, 447–456.

ABSCESS, EPIDURAL

EPIDEMIOLOGY

Spinal epidural abscess (SEA) is an uncommon condition with an estimated incidence of 0.2 to 2.0/10,000 hospital admissions and a peak incidence in the sixth and seventh decades of life. Conditions commonly associated with SEA include diabetes mellitus, intravenous drug misuse, chronic renal failure, alcoholism, and cancer.

ETIOLOGY

The majority of SEAs are thought to result from the hematogenous spread of bacteria usually from a cutaneous or mucosal source with spread to the posterior aspect of the spinal canal. Direct spread from an adjacent source is less common and typically presents within the anterior aspect of the canal. The most common causative organisms are *Staphylococcus aureus* (57%–73%), *Mycobacterium tuberculosis* (25%), other gram-positive cocci (10%), gram-negative organisms 18%, and anaerobes 2%.

CLINICAL FEATURES

The initial manifestations of SEA are often nonspecific and include fever and malaise. The classical diagnostic triad consists of fever, spinal pain, and neurologic deficits. However, over time, an untreated abscess may progress from focal back pain, to radicular pain, to neurologic deficits (motor weakness, sensory changes, and bladder or bowel dysfunction), and then paralysis. Once paralysis develops, it may quickly become irreversible. Thus urgent intervention may be required if progression of weakness or other neurologic findings are detected.

TREATMENT

Surgical decompression and drainage with systemic antibiotic therapy is the treatment of choice. Empirical antimicrobial must be started early and be delivered intravenously in high doses and immediately following the collection of two sets of blood cultures. Appropriate empiric parenteral regimens include: vancomycin (15–20 mg/kg IV every 8–12 hours. Trough levels should be drawn 30 minutes prior to the next dose) for empiric coverage of methicillin resistant Staphylococcus aureus (MRSA) plus either ceftriaxone (2 g IV q 12 hr) or cefepime (2 g IV q 8 hr) or ceftazidime (2 g IV q 8 hr). Treatment should be continued for at least 4 weeks but may be prolonged for 8 weeks or longer if vertebral osteomyelitis is suspected.

PROGNOSIS

Overall prognosis is poor; 5% die due to uncontrolled sepsis or other complications, irreversible paraplegia occurs in 4% to 22%, and residual motor weakness in 37%.

REFERENCES

Arko, L., Quach, E., Nguyen, V., Chang, D., Sukul, V., & Kim, B. S. (2014). Medical and surgical management of spinal epidural abscess: a systematic review. *Neurosurg Focus, 37*(2), E4.

Bond, A., & Manian, F. A. (2016). Spinal epidural abscess: a review with special emphasis on earlier diagnosis. *Biomed Res Int, 2016*, 1614328.

ACALCULIA

Acalculia refers to an acquired computational disability (as opposed to developmental dyscalculia which occurs in 5% of school-age children and is usually associated with dyslexia). The ability to perform mathematical calculations is complex as it requires not only an arithmetic brain center, but also intact attention, language processing, spatial orientation, memory, body knowledge, and executive function.

Acalculia may be classified as either primary or secondary. Primary acalculia (anarithmetia), an acquired isolated defect in comprehending numerical systems, is rare. Notable secondary types due to other cognitive defects are: aphasic, an inability to read or write numbers, usually occurring with left posterior parietal lesions; spatial, a mental misalignment of numbers usually due to right posterior hemispheric lesions; and frontal, due to impaired attention, perseveration, and executive dysfunction.

Acalculia can be part of Gerstmann syndrome (acalculia, agraphia, right-left disorientation, and finger agnosia) due to left angular gyrus lesions. Common causes of acalculia include epilepsy, metabolic or genetic disorders, focal lesions (e.g., stroke, tumor, trauma, or abscess), or commonly as part of a neurodegenerative disease (e.g., dementia). Rehabilitation is treatment of choice, with variable results. Spontaneous recovery is seen in many stroke and trauma patients.

REFERENCES

Ardila, A., & Rosselli, M. (2002). Acalculia and dyscalculia. *Neuropsychol Rev, 12*(4), 179–231.

Rapin, I. (2016). Dyscalculia and the calculating brain. *Pediat Neurol, 61*, 11–20.

ACID-BASE DISTURBANCES

RESPIRATORY ALKALOSIS

This condition is most frequently observed in patients with hepatic cirrhosis, bronchial asthma, salicylate intoxication, hypoxia, sepsis, pneumonia, and acute anxiety (hyperventilation syndrome). Acute respiratory alkalosis constricts cerebral arterioles and decreases cerebral blood flow. Confusion accompanied by a slow electroencephalogram (EEG) may develop. Symptoms of milder respiratory alkalosis include paresthesias, dizziness, cramps as a result of coexistent tetany, hyperreflexia, and muscle weakness. More severe alkalosis (pH 7.52–7.65) in patients with respiratory insufficiency and hypoxia may result in a symptom complex of hypotension, seizures, asterixis, myoclonus, and coma. Treatment is to correct the underlying cause.

RESPIRATORY ACIDOSIS

Acute respiratory acidosis is a condition of low pH and high CO_2 concentration, occurring as a result of impairment of the rate of alveolar ventilation. Causes of acute respiratory acidosis include sedative drugs, brainstem injury, neuromuscular disorders, chest injury, airway obstruction, and acute pulmonary disease. Lethargy and confusion occur as the PCO_2 rises above 55 mm Hg. Seizures, stupor, or coma may occur with levels greater than 70 mm Hg. The serum bicarbonate level is either normal or high, depending on how rapidly the respiratory failure developed. Neurologic manifestations resulting from cerebral vasodilation include headache, increased intracranial pressure, and papilledema. Hyperreflexia or hyporeflexia and myoclonus may also occur.

Chronic respiratory acidosis generally occurs in patients with chronic obstructive pulmonary disease (COPD), restrictive lung disease (e.g., severe kyphoscoliosis), or extreme obesity (Pickwickian syndrome). It is most often symptomatic with acute exacerbations of disease. Compensatory polycythemia often results from chronic hypercapnic states. Hypoventilation or Pickwickian syndrome may manifest as excessive daytime somnolence.

Therapy of respiratory acidosis involves ventilatory support and treating the underlying disorder. The possibility of sedative or narcotic drug ingestion must be suspected in otherwise healthy patients who suddenly develop acute respiratory depression.

METABOLIC ALKALOSIS

Metabolic alkalosis may result from either excessive ingestion of base or excessive loss of acid. Causes of hypokalemic metabolic alkalosis include Cushing syndrome, vomiting or gastric drainage, diuretic therapy, and primary aldosteronism. Neurologic manifestations include paresthesias, cramps (due to tetany), muscle weakness (due to associated hypokalemia), and hyporeflexia. Severe metabolic alkalosis produces a blunted, confused state rather than stupor or coma and may result in cardiac arrhythmias and severe compensatory hypoventilation.

Treatment depends on the underlying cause.

METABOLIC ACIDOSIS

Metabolic acidosis occurs when a decrease in plasma bicarbonate level lowers pH. Cardinal features are hyperventilation and, when severe, *Kussmaul* respirations. In chronic metabolic acidosis, hyperventilation may be difficult to detect on clinical examination. The most common causes of metabolic acidosis sufficient to produce coma and hyperpnea include uremia, diabetes, lactic acidosis, and ingestion of acidic poisons. Ketoacidosis occasionally develops in severe alcoholics after prolonged drinking episodes. In diabetics treated with oral hypoglycemic agents, lactic acidosis and diabetic ketoacidosis must be considered.

The presence of neurologic symptoms depends on various factors, including the type of systemic metabolic defect, whether the fall in systemic pH affects the pH of the brain and cerebrospinal fluid (CSF), the rate at which acidosis develops, and the specific anion causing the metabolic disorder. All forms of metabolic acidosis produce hyperpnea as the first neurologic symptom. Other manifestations include lethargy, drowsiness, confusion, and mild, diffuse skeletal muscle hypertonus. Extensor plantar responses occur at a later stage. Stupor, coma, or seizures generally develop only preterminally. Because metabolic acidosis is a manifestation of a variety of different diseases, the treatment varies depending on the underlying process and on the acuteness and severity of the acidosis.

REFERENCE

Yee, A. H., & Rabinstein, A. A. (2010). Neurologic presentations of acid-base imbalance, electrolyte abnormalities, and endocrine emergencies. *Neurology Clinics*, 28(1), 1–16.

ADEM DISEASE

ACUTE DISSEMINATED ENCEPHALOMYELITIS

Acute disseminated encephalomyelitis (ADEM) is a monophasic multifocal demyelinating disorder of the CNS, often following infection or vaccination. ADEM is more frequent in children; however, it may occur at any age. The most frequent preceding infections are flulike illnesses, nonspecific upper respiratory tract infections, and gastroenteritis. Although viral etiologies are most common, it can also follow a bacterial infections and, in rare cases, parasitic infections. Postvaccination ADEM is seen in approximately 10% of cases and is most common after measles, mumps, and rubella.

CLINICAL PRESENTATION

Initial presentation may include meningoencephalitis, fever, encephalopathy, seizures, headache, and meningismus. Focal motor or sensory deficits, ataxia, cranial neuropathies, or brain stem pathology may also be seen.

A more severe presentation known as acute hemorrhagic encephalomyelitis may develop.

DIAGNOSIS
MRI

MRI shows multifocal demyelinating lesions in CNS white matter, with increased signal in T2-weighted and FLAIR images. Lesions may be large, with poorly defined margins, and are often asymmetric. Lesions may enhance with contrast depending on the time of onset. Lesions that are hypointense on T1 argue against the diagnosis.

CSF

Lymphocytic pleocytosis and elevated protein are commonly seen; however, CSF studies can be normal.

TREATMENT

High-dose intravenous steroids are used based on their efficacy in treating MS relapses. The aim of steroid treatment is primarily to reduce the CNS inflammatory reaction and accelerate clinical recovery.

Methylprednisolone 20 to 30 mg/kg/day in children and 1 g/day in adults for 3 to 5 days, followed by oral prednisolone 1 to 2 mg/kg/day for 1 to 2 weeks, with subsequent tapering over 2 to 6 weeks. The exact duration of steroid taper is not known; however, early discontinuation may convey a higher risk of relapse. IVIG and sometimes PLEX are used as a second line treatment in patients who do not respond to steroids.

PROGNOSIS

In children, ADEM has a favorable prognosis in 60% to 80% of cases. Most children have functional recovery, and severe disability is rarely seen. Mortality is $\leq$5%. Adults have a less favorable prognosis compared with children. Functional recovery is the outcome in 45% to 65% of adult patients. Mortality can be as high as 15%.

REFERENCES

Kamm, C., & Zettl, U. K. (2012). Autoimmune disorders affecting both the central and peripheral nervous system. *Autoimmun Rev, 11*(3), 196–202.

Marchioni, E., Ravaglia, S., Montomoli, C., et al. (2013). Postinfectious neurologic syndromes: a prospective cohort study. *Neurology, 80*(10), 882–889.

AGNOSIA

This rare condition is characterized by impaired recognition of objects, people, and sounds despite intact primary visual, auditory, and tactile senses. An agnosic patient will be able to sense the presence of an object, but will not be able to apply meaning to the previously recognized object and thus fails to recognize it. Agnosia is seen in a variety of neurologic insults including stroke, tumor, neurodegenerative conditions, and trauma. It is important to demonstrate intact vision, hearing, and sensation modalities before diagnosing agnosia. It is also important to rule out anomic aphasia prior to diagnosing any visual agnosia. In both visual agnosia and anomic aphasia, a patient will not be able to name an object. However, a patient with anomic aphasia will recognize the object.

There are three forms of agnosia:

I. Visual agnosia refers to inability to visually recognize familiar objects. There are two main forms of visual agnosia.
   A. The apperceptive type is a deficit of visual processing in which abnormal visual percepts are formed and may occur after bilateral injury to the primary visual cortex. Patients are unable to copy or match visually presented items.

B. The associative type occurs when the deficit occurs after percept formation but before meaning has been associated. Patients may be able to copy objects, but will not recognize them. The majority of these patients have associated achromatopsia.

Object agnosia (inability to recognize objects), prosopagnosia (loss of recognition of specific members of a generic group; distinguishing and recognizing faces, cars, houses, etc.), and achromatopsia (inability to perceive color) are associative visual agnosias occurring with bilateral occipito-temporal lesions. Simultanagnosia is a visual agnosia in which the patient will be able to recognize individual parts of an object or single objects but not a scene as whole. This is seen as part of Balint syndrome of simultanagnosia, optic ataxia, and ocular motor apraxia usually due to bilateral occipito-parietal lesions.

The image in Fig. 1 may be used to detect simultanagnosia. A patient is presented with the image and asked to describe the scene. A normal patient will be able to describe the actions occurring in the scene; however, a patient with simultanagnosia may be able to recognize a few individual objects, but not their relationship to each other.

II. Auditory agnosia refers to an inability to recognize sounds that cannot be attributed to a hearing defect. It may be restricted to nonspeech sounds (selective auditory agnosia) or speech sounds (pure word deafness), or may involve both (generalized auditory agnosia). Thus, a patient may be able to hear a bird chirping, but not recognize that the sound is originating from a bird.

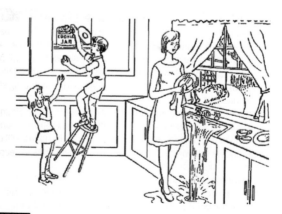

FIGURE 1

Simultagnosia test.

Simultagnosia is characterized by the inability to recognize two or more things at the same time.

III. Tactile agnosia refers to the inability to recognize objects by the tactile sense, despite intact primary sensation sense (light touch, temperature, pinprick, etc.). The patient usually can visually recognize the object. Astereognosis, an inability to recognize objects placed in the hand, is not well characterized due to the difficulty of separating it from primary sensory loss.

There is also a rare agnosia called anosagnosia that refers to a denial of illness. This may be seen as part of a neglect syndrome with right hemispheric damage. The patient may not recognize a body part, such as an arm, as belonging to the self.

REFERENCE

Corrow, S. L., Dalrymple, K. A., & Barton, J. J. (2016). Prosopagnosia: current perspectives. *Eye Brain*, *8*, 165–175.

AGRAPHIA

Agraphia is a neurologic sign resulting in the inability to communicate through writing. The existence of a writing center remains controversial; writing involves multiple functional systems, visual or auditory input processing, language analysis, spatial organization of hand gestures, gesture planning, and highly specific hand movements.

Neuropsychologists and linguists have defined two systems of writing. The phonological system decodes speech sounds (phonemes) into letters. In phonological agraphia, produced by lesions of supramarginal gyrus or the insula medial to it, the patient is unable to spell nonsense words but is capable of spelling familiar words. The lexical system retrieves visual word images when spelling. Lexical agraphia is marked by errors in spelling irregular words, but these errors are phonologically correct (rough spelled as ruf). Lexical agraphia occurs with lesions at the junction of the posterior angular gyrus and parieto-occipital lobule.

Agraphia, "aphasia of writing," occurs in five clinical forms:

I. Pure agraphia (no other language abnormality present) is rarely seen in pure form. It occurs with lesions of the second frontal convolution (Exner area), superior parietal lobule, and the posterior sylvian region.

II. Aphasic agraphia is the writing disturbance of aphasics that usually resembles their spoken speech.

III. Agraphia with alexia is produced by a dominant angular gyrus lesion. Alexia without agraphia occurs with dominant hemisphere lesions affecting the parieto-occipital region and the splenium of the corpus callosum.

IV. Apractic agraphia, in which production of letters and words is abnormal, usually occurs with a dominant superior parietal lobule lesion.

V. Spatial agraphia with abnormalities of spacing letters and maintaining a horizontal line is usually produced by nondominant parietal lesions.

REFERENCES

Lubrano, V., Roux, F. E., & Démonet, J. F. (2004). Writing-specific sites in frontal areas: a cortical stimulation study. *J Neurosurg, 101*(5), 787–798.

Mesulam, M. M. (2000). *Principles of behavioral and cognitive neurology.* New York: Oxford University Press.

AIDS

DEFINITION

Acquired immunodeficiency syndrome (AIDS) is caused by the human immunodeficiency virus (HIV), a retrovirus. Neurologic manifestations can occur at any level of the neuraxis at any stage of infection and can be a result of direct HIV infection, HIV-induced immune dysregulation, opportunistic diseases, or pharmacologic therapy for the disease and its complications. Specific syndromes tend to occur more frequently during particular phases of HIV infection (but can appear at almost any point during the course), and virtually all have been described as the initial presenting feature of HIV infection. Coexistent systemic infections are common and should be specifically sought and treated concomitantly. The standard method for diagnosing HIV infection is measurement of antibody by enzyme-linked immunosorbent assay (ELISA) followed by Western blot for confirmation of ELISA-positive samples. Prior to host antibody response ("window period"), HIV antigen tests (e.g., p24 protein antigen) and nucleic acid (RNA, proviral DNA) tests are more sensitive. Rate of disease progression is directly related to HIV RNA levels (viral load).

MAJOR HIV-ASSOCIATED CENTRAL NERVOUS SYSTEM (CNS) DISORDERS CLASSIFIED BY NEUROANATOMIC LOCALIZATION

Meninges

  I. Aseptic HIV meningitis

  II. Cryptococcal meningitis

  III. Tuberculous meningitis

  IV. Syphilitic meningitis

  V. *Listeria monocytogenes* meningitis

  VI. Lymphomatous meningitis

Brain (Predominantly Nonfocal)

  I. HIV-associated dementia (HAD)

  II. HIV-associated mild cognitive dysfunction (MCMD)

  III. Toxoplasma encephalitis

  IV. Cytomegalovirus (CMV) encephalitis

  V. Aspergillus encephalitis

  VI. Herpes encephalitis

  VII. Metabolic encephalopathy (alone or concomitantly)

Brain (Predominantly Focal)

I. Cerebral toxoplasmosis
II. Primary CNS lymphoma (PCNSL)
III. Progressive multifocal leukoencephalopathy (PML)
IV. Cryptococcoma
V. Tuberculoma
VI. Varicella-zoster virus (VZV) encephalitis
VII. Stroke

Spinal Cord

I. Vacuolar myelopathy (VM)
II. CMV myeloradiculopathy
III. VZV myelitis
IV. Spinal epidural or intradural lymphoma (metastatic)
V. Human T-cell lymphotropic virus (HTLV)-1-associated myelopathy

CLASSIFICATION OF HIV-ASSOCIATED NEUROMUSCULAR DISORDERS

Peripheral Neuropathies

I. Early stages (immune dysregulation)
   A. Acute inflammatory demyelinating polyneuropathy (AIDP)
   B. Chronic inflammatory demyelinating polyneuropathy (CIDP)
   C. Vasculitic myelopathy
   D. Brachial plexopathy
   E. Lumbosacral plexopathy
   F. Cranial mononeuropathy
   G. Multiple mononeuropathies
II. Midstage and late stage (HIV-replication driven)
   A. Distal sensory polyneuropathy
   B. Autonomic neuropathy
III. Late stages (opportunistic infection, malignancy)
   A. CMV polyradiculomyelitis
   B. Syphilitic polyradiculomyelitis
   C. Tuberculous polyradiculomyelitis
   D. Lymphomatous polyradiculopathy
   E. Zoster ganglionitis
   F. CMV mononeuritis multiplex
   G. Nutritional neuropathy (vitamins B_{12}, B_6)
   H. AIDS-cachexia neuropathy
   I. Amyotrophic lateral sclerosis (ALS)-like motor neuropathy
IV. All stages (toxic neuropathy)
   A. Nucleoside reverse transcriptase inhibitors (didanosine, zalcitabine, Stavudine)
   B. Other drugs (vincristine, isoniazid, ethambutol, thalidomide)

Myopathies
I. Polymyositis
II. Pyomyositis
III. Inclusion body myositis
IV. Toxic (zidovudine) myopathy
V. AIDS-cachexia myopathy

NEUROLOGIC EVENTS IN HIV INFECTION
Early HIV Infection
Initial HIV infection usually manifests as a nonspecific viral syndrome of fever, arthralgias, myalgias, and malaise lasting several days. Formed antibodies to HIV proteins take 6 months to appear. Prior to seroconversion, standard anti-HIV antibody assays are negative, and diagnosis can be made only by means of Western blot assay for viral antigen. Several syndromes can be associated with this early phase of infection, and their association with HIV may be discerned only if Western blot is obtained.

I. HIV meningoencephalitis—a viral meningitis can accompany the syndrome of initial infection. In a few patients, this affects the brain parenchyma as well, resulting in a self-limited encephalopathy.
II. Transverse myelitis rarely accompanies acute HIV infection.
III. AIDP, also called Guillain-Barré syndrome (GBS), can occur upon or shortly after initial infection. In cases associated with HIV, there may be a mild CSF pleocytosis; however, this is not always the case. A case series by Thornton et al. found a higher incidence of HIV infection among people with GBS, thus HIV testing of patients with GBS should be considered. Course and treatment of HIV-related GBS are similar to those for idiopathic GBS.
IV. Sensory ganglioneuropathy.
V. Brachial plexitis.
VI. Rhabdomyolysis can accompany initial infection. Steroids can be beneficial.

Midstage HIV Infection (CD4 Count 200–500/µL)
I. HIV meningitis can recur at any point and may remain asymptomatic. The resulting elevated CSF protein and pleocytosis significantly complicates work-up for other infections.
II. CIDP is the chronic form of AIDP. Patients can benefit from intravenous immunoglobulin or plasmapheresis.
III. Mononeuritis multiplex, when apparent in early or midstage HIV infection, is often self-limited.
IV. Nucleoside antiviral polyneuropathy—didanosine, zalcitabine, and stavudine—can all cause a dysesthetic sensory neuropathy, especially at higher doses. Often of subacute onset over weeks, it gradually improves after change of offending agent; both features help to distinguish this from HIV-related distal sensory neuropathy.

V. Inflammatory myopathy presents as proximal muscle weakness and sometimes myalgia. Biopsy shows inflammation. Steroids are beneficial, if immune status permits.

VI. Zidovudine (AZT) myopathy occurs because AZT is a mitochondrial toxin. Presentation is similar to inflammatory myopathy. Biopsy suggests mitochondrial dysfunction but may also show inflammation. Clinical improvement after AZT withdrawal is the best means of diagnosis.

Late HIV Infection (CD4 Count <200/µL)

I. Focal brain lesions

A. Cerebral toxoplasmosis—caused by intracerebral reactivation of infection with the parasite *Toxoplasma gondii*, this syndrome is usually manifested in fever, headache, confusion, seizures, and focal neurologic signs, although any or all of these can be lacking. Neuroimaging typically reveals multiple ring-enhancing lesions. Antibiotics are usually quite effective.

B. PCNSL occurs in 2% of AIDS patients. PCNSL is the second most common cause of ring-enhancing lesions on computerized tomography/magnetic resonance imaging (CT/MRI) and is usually unifocal. It can be distinguished from *T. gondii* by single-photon emission CT (SPECT) or positron emission tomography (PET). Any patient with ring-enhancing lesions that are atypical for toxoplasmosis or do not respond to several weeks of anti-Toxoplasma therapy must undergo biopsy. Mean survival is 1 month from diagnosis without whole-brain radiotherapy and 4 to 6 months with it.

C. Progressive multifocal leukoencephalopathy (PML) results from reactivation of John Cunningham (JC) virus, an infection generally of no consequence to the immunocompetent. Reactivation in oligodendroglia leads to demyelinating white matter disease, focal neurologic deficits, and non–ring-enhancing white matter lesions on scan. Mean survival is 2 to 4 months. Ten percent of patients have enhancing lesions, which may be associated with increased survival. No specific therapy is known, although occasional patients have responded to treatment with cytarabine or cidofovir.

D. Stroke is not a complication of HIV per se, but 4% of AIDS patients have a symptomatic stroke during their lives. Ischemic stroke may be caused by AIDS-related bacterial endocarditis, viral-associated vasculitis, or perivascular infection, or it may be a result of more traditional risk factors such as hypertension and hyperlipidemia; intracranial hemorrhage can complicate PCNSL, metastatic Kaposi sarcoma, or (rarely) toxoplasmosis.

E. Focal brain lesions in AIDS patients can be due to any of the previously mentioned conditions, plus cysticercosis, fungal abscess (due to Candida infection, Aspergillus infection, mucormycosis, coccidioidomycosis, etc.), bacterial abscess (caused by mycobacteria, *T. pallidum, Nocardia, Listeria*, etc.), or other tumors (glioma, Kaposi sarcoma, other metastases). The usual approach in a patient with typical imaging findings such as a ring-enhancing lesion and positive toxoplasma serologic test is to treat empirically for toxoplasmosis and proceed to biopsy if repeat scan shows no improvement. Those with negative serologic findings or atypical scan should undergo biopsy immediately.

II. Cryptococcal meningitis develops in 10%. It often presents as a combination of cognitive impairment, personality change, lethargy, cranial neuropathies, and increased intracranial pressure, with or without typical signs and symptoms of meningismus. Fungal CSF culture is the "gold standard," but results take weeks; CSF cryptococcal antigen is rapid and highly sensitive and specific. India ink smear is also rapid and increases sensitivity. Initial treatment should be amphotericin B with flucytosine. Unfortunately, response can be as low as 40%, and recurrence is common; however, in those surviving the initial infection, long-term suppression with daily fluconazole can be effective.

III. Syphilitic meningitis and meningovasculitis frequently complicate HIV infection, because *T. pallidum* shares some risk factors with HIV. Findings include meningismus, cranial neuropathies, and with chronic infections, classic tertiary syphilis. Diagnosis depends on a combination of serologic testing and clinical suspicion. Treatment is with penicillin.

IV. Tuberculous meningitis is more common in AIDS patients than in those who are not immunosuppressed. Tuberculomas may also rarely occur. CSF polymerase chain reaction (PCR) can complement culture.

V. HIV encephalopathy (AIDS dementia complex, HAD) is a subcortical dementia of unclear pathogenesis characterized by cognitive slowing, emotional blunting, and motor impairment. Prevalence estimates vary widely (5%–60%); in the pediatric population, the prevalence is much higher (90%). Work-up consists of ruling out treatable infections (cryptococcus, syphilis, CMV encephalitis) and medical conditions (hypothyroidism, vitamin B_{12} deficiency). No specific treatment beyond antiviral therapy is known.

VI. VM is present in up to 55% on autopsy but symptomatic in far fewer. It is of uncertain pathogenesis, and pathologic findings include vacuolization in the dorsal and lateral columns of the spinal cord. Symptoms, which develop late, include constipation, urinary disturbances, ataxia, and spastic paraparesis. There is no treatment. The process is painless and slowly progressive; pain or rapid progression should prompt evaluation for other causes, such as viral myelitis, metastatic cord compression, or epidural abscess. Other subacute myelopathies sometimes associated with AIDS include syphilis and vitamin B_{12} deficiency.

VII. Mononeuritis multiplex in late HIV infection is often due to CMV and benefits from ganciclovir. CMV can also cause encephalitis, meningitis, retinitis, myelitis, or polyradiculitis. CSF PCR for central nervous system CMV infections has approximately 90% sensitivity.

VIII. VZV can cause encephalitis, Ramsay-Hunt syndrome, myelitis, vasculitis, and segmental zoster rashes (shingles). Herpes simplex virus (HSV) can cause encephalitis or myelitis. Both HSV and VZV are treated with acyclovir.

IX. Distal symmetric polyneuropathy is an axonal, predominantly sensory neuropathy with impairment of all sensory modalities, often with paresthesias, which can be painful. Tricyclic antidepressants and anticonvulsants can help dysesthetic symptoms, but some patients may require opiates. Capsaicin may also help.

All Stages

I. HIV-related meningitis: aseptic (acute or recurrent) or chronic
II. Asymptomatic CSF abnormalities: elevated protein, lymphocytic pleocytosis, normal glucose
III. Nucleoside neuropathy and zidovudine myopathy
IV. Inflammatory myopathy

FOR MORE INFORMATION

www.cdcnpin.org (epidemiologic data)
www.cc.nih.gov/phar/hiv-mgt. (consensus panel reports on treatment of HIV infection)

REFERENCES

Bhatia, N. S., & Chow, F. C. (2016). Neurologic complications in treated HIV-1 infection. *Curr Neurol Neurosci Rep*, *16*(7), 62.
Bradley, W. G., Daroff, R. B., Fenichel, G. M., & Jankovic, J. (2004). *Neurology in clinical practice*, ed 4. Philadelphia: Butterworth-Heinemann.

ALCOHOL

Neurologic effects of alcohol are due to a combination of its direct neurotoxic effects, its metabolites, nutritional factors, and genetic predisposition.
Neurologic complications associated with alcohol abuse can be conceptually divided into the following five categories (Table 1):

I. **Intoxication:** Acute intoxication with alcohol correlates roughly with blood concentrations. Cognitive dysfunction tends to occur early, and cerebellar, autonomic, and vestibular symptoms tend to occur at higher blood levels. Positional vertigo may result from alcohol diffusing into the cupula when the recumbent position is assumed. As the alcohol concentration rises to a certain level, the intoxication is greater than when it falls to the same level. Blackouts are periods of amnesia, usually during binge drinking, and occur in persons with and without alcohol dependence.

II. **Withdrawal syndromes:** These occur in individuals with alcohol dependency resulting from either decreased intake or abrupt cessation of

TABLE 1	
NEUROLOGIC COMPLICATIONS ASSOCIATED WITH ALCOHOL ABUSE	
Causes	Complications
Direct effects of alcohol	Acute intoxication
	Fetal alcohol syndrome
Alcohol withdrawal	Delirium tremens
	Seizure
Nutritional deficiency	Wernicke encephalopathy
	Korsakoff syndrome
Other related syndromes	Cerebellar degeneration
	Peripheral neuropathy
	Optic neuropathy
	Myopathy
Disease of uncertain pathogenesis	Central pontine myelinolysis
	Marchiafava-Bignami disease
	Cortical atrophy

A

ALCOHOL

drinking. The syndromes may be early or late. Most common are the early symptoms, which begin 12 to 24 hours after decreased intake. Tremulousness is common and may be accompanied by nausea, vomiting, insomnia, and hallucinations (visual, tactile, or auditory). *Treatment* consists of benzodiazepines. Auditory hallucinations may persist, necessitating the use of neuroleptics.

Withdrawal seizures are always generalized tonic-clonic and begin within the first 24 hours but may occur after several days. Focal seizures should not be attributed to alcohol withdrawal and should warrant further investigation including computed tomography (CT) of head to rule out any structural abnormality.

Treatment of withdrawal seizures is controversial because they are usually self-limited. Initial loading with phenytoin and slowly tapering off after several days is one approach. Thiamine is routinely given and hypomagnesemia, if present, is treated.

Delirium tremens is the most severe, deadly complication of withdrawal and has a peak incidence 72 to 96 hours after decreased alcohol intake. Confusion, agitation, vivid hallucinations, tremors, and increased autonomic activity (tachycardia, fever, sweating, and hypertension or orthostatic hypotension) are characteristic. These symptoms can last 1 to 3 days and can be fatal ($\sim$10%). *Treatment* consists of sedation with benzodiazepines, hydration with intravenous (IV) fluids, and administration of thiamine, multivitamins, and magnesium (if indicated). Autonomic hyperactivity should be treated aggressively if present.

III. **Wernicke-Korsakoff syndrome:** This is the most common deficiency syndrome due to chronic alcoholism. Wernicke syndrome, or Wernicke encephalopathy, is reversible and represents the acute phase presentation with the triad of encephalopathy, ataxia, and oculomotor disturbance (nystagmus, ophthalmoplegia, and gaze palsy). However, a complete triad of signs is often not present. Atrophy of the mammillary bodies is common. Korsakoff syndrome, which is irreversible, is a more chronic condition and includes anterograde amnesia (the inability to incorporate ongoing experience into memory) leading to confabulation. Both syndromes are attributed to thiamine deficiency and can also be seen in non-alcoholic malnutrition states, although much less commonly. *Treatment* consists of IV thiamine 500 mg three times daily for two days, then 250 mg intravenous (IV) or intramuscular (IM) for five days, then oral thiamine indefinitely. IV glucose should never be given without thiamine to a chronic alcoholic because of the risk of precipitating Wernicke encephalopathy. As with most alcohol-related syndromes, supplemental vitamins and magnesium may be beneficial.

IV. **Other alcohol-related syndromes:** These include cerebellar degeneration, peripheral neuropathy, optic neuropathy, and myopathy.

Cerebellar degeneration invariably involves the anterior and superior cerebellar vermis and paravermian regions with resultant truncal and gait ataxia. Limb ataxia, if present, is much milder than truncal ataxia and more severe in the legs than in the arms.

Chronic peripheral neuropathy, which can involve both sensory and motor nerves, is usually heralded by complaints of numb, burning feet involving distal limbs symmetrically. Minor motor signs may evolve. Pathogenesis seems to involve both toxic alcohol effects as well as poor nutrition status. Abstinence from alcohol is paramount for treatment success.

Nutritional amblyopia (previously called tobacco-alcohol amblyopia) consists of gradual visual loss over a period of several weeks and is caused by selective lesion of the optic nerves secondary to poor nutrition and is not a direct toxic effect of alcohol. Treatment with a combination of adequate diet and B vitamins, despite the continuation of drinking and smoking, results in visual recovery.

Alcoholic myopathy is believed to be caused by the toxic effects of alcohol and improves with abstinence. It may occur as an acute necrotizing disorder with muscle pain and rhabdomyolysis, or as a more slowly progressive disease with proximal weakness. The combination of thiamine, multivitamins, and abstinence is the treatment of choice for these syndromes.

V. **Conditions of somewhat uncertain etiology:** Additional syndromes occurring in chronic alcoholics include central pontine myelinolysis, Marchiafava-Bignami syndrome, and cortical atrophy.

Central pontine myelinolysis is a rare cerebral white matter disorder, associated with basis pontis lesions with resultant progressive quadriparesis, horizontal gaze palsy, and obtundation leading to coma. It occurs with excessively rapid correction of hyponatremia.

Marchiafava-Bignami syndrome is a rare demyelinating disease of the corpus callosum and adjacent subcortical white matter, sometimes associated with excessive consumption of crude red wine. Patients can have cognitive impairment that resembles a frontal lobe or dementia syndrome, spasticity, dysarthria, and impaired gait. The CT scan appearance of "atrophy" or "parenchymal volume loss" is probably related to fluid shifts in the brain and may reverse with abstinence.

Alcoholics have an increased incidence of stroke related to a variety of factors, including rebound thrombocytosis, altered cerebral blood flow, and hyperlipidemia.

REFERENCES

Bradley, W. G., Daroff, R. B., et al. (2004). *Neurology in clinical practice*, ed 4. Philadelphia: Butterworth-Heinemann.

Keil, V. C., Greschus, S., Schneider, C., Hadizadeh, D. R., & Schild, H. H. (2015). The whole spectrum of alcohol-related changes in the CNS: practical MR And CT imaging guidelines for daily clinical use. *Rofo, 187*(12), 1073–1083.

ALEXIA

Alexia denotes a group of acquired disorders of reading, which helps to distinguish it from the more common syndrome of dyslexia. Reading uses neural networks, including the occipital cortex for perception of visual language, and the heteromodal association cortex of the angular gyrus for processing into auditory language.

Alexia occurs in three main forms:

Alexia without agraphia (pure alexia). This form was described first by Dejerine in 1892. As if blindfolded, the patient loses the ability to read but can still write. This is seen with left occipital lesions (e.g., left posterior cerebral artery (PCA) infarct, tumors, abscess), usually affecting the splenium of the corpus callosum. All visual information must be processed by the right occipital lobe because the left is damaged (Fig. 2). However, this information cannot pass from the right visual area to the left language centers due to injury of the splenium. As such, there is associated right hemianopia or superior quadrantanopia and impaired color naming (achromatopsia). Further deficits involve short-term memory for visual language elements or an inability to process multiple letters at once (simultagnosia).

Alexia with agraphia. The patient loses the ability to read and write. This is seen most often with left middle cerebral artery (MCA) stroke or mass lesion affecting the left inferior parietal lobule, especially the angular gyrus. In addition to alexia with agraphia, the patient may also display the entire Gerstmann syndrome of agraphia, acalculia, left-right disorientation, and finger agnosia. There may also be a right homonymous hemianopia, and mild receptive Wernicke-type aphasia.

Aphasic alexia. This form of alexia is secondary to underlying severe aphasia (language processing) including Broca or Wernicke aphasia. Depending on the subtype of aphasic alexia, different components of reading and language processing will be affected. The four main subtypes include "letter-by-letter" (equivalent to pure alexia), "deep dyslexia" (reading/recognizing only familiar words like concrete nouns and verbs, independent of

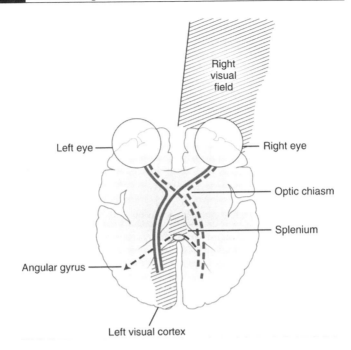

FIGURE 2

Horizontal brain diagram of pure alexia without agraphia. From Kirshner, H. S.: Aphasia and aphasic syndromes. In Daroff, R. B., Jankovic, J., Mazziotta, J. C., & Pomeroy, S. L. (Eds.), (2016). *Bradley's neurology in clinical practice*, ed 7. Philadelphia: Elsevier, pp 128–144.e2. Figure 13-6.

length; commonly with severe aphasia), "phonological dyslexia" (reading/ recognizing familiar words, with failure of comprehension), and "surface dyslexia" (able to piece together nonsense syllables to make words but unable to simply recognize words at a glance; cannot process words with silent letters).

REFERENCE

Daroff, R. B., Jankovic, J., Mazziotta, J. C., & Pomeroy, S. L. (Eds.), (2016). *Bradley's neurology in clinical practice*, ed 7. Philadelphia: Elsevier.

AMAUROSIS FUGAX

Amaurosis fugax (AFx) refers to a transient loss of vision in one or both eyes. The term "amaurosis fugax" has classically been used to imply a vascular cause for the vision loss, but the term continues to be used to describe transient visual loss from any origin. Ischemia is the most common cause of transient monocular vision loss. Other causes include ocular disease including papilledema, optic neuropathy, and increased intraocular pressure. Migraine is the most common cause of bilateral transient visual loss. Other causes include visual seizures and vertebrobasilar ischemia. AFx due to ischemia has a short duration (seconds to minutes) and usually consists of negative symptoms (blackness or graying of the visual field) with an occasional positive phenomenon (scintillating scotomas or points of light). Funduscopic examination may show the cholesterol emboli (Hollenhorst plaques). Embolization from the internal carotid artery, aorta, or heart may be the cause (Table 2).

Treatment of classical AFx depends on the underlying cause. Aspirin and warfarin may be indicated, or endarterectomy may be necessary in cases of severe internal carotid artery stenosis. AFx due to vasospasm (i.e., particularly in young adults) may respond to calcium channel blockers nifedipine or verapamil.

A

AMAUROSIS FUGAX

TABLE 2

CAUSES OF TRANSIENT MONOCULAR BLINDNESS

I. Embolic
  A. Carotid embolism
  B. Cardiac and aortic embolism
  C. Embolism related to intravenous drug abuse

II. Hemodynamic
  A. Hypoperfusion
  B. Vasospasm
  C. Inflammatory arteritides such as temporal arteritis, Takayasu syndrome, and polyarteritis nodosa
  D. Severe atherosclerotic occlusive disease of internal carotid or ophthalmic artery
  E. Carotid dissection
  F. Hypertensive crises

III. Ocular
  A. Anterior ischemic optic neuropathy
  B. Central retinal vein occlusion
  C. Intraocular causes such as hemorrhage, tumor, and glaucoma
  D. Drusen

IV. Neurologic disorders
  A. Disease of the vestibular or oculomotor system
  B. Optic neuritis (mainly demyelinating diseases)
  C. Optic nerve or optic chiasmal compression
  D. Increased intracranial pressure
  E. Migraine

V. Psychogenic

VI. Idiopathic

From Bernstein EF. *Amaurosis fugax*, Springer-Verlag, New York, 1987, p 286. Adapted from Amaurosis Fugax Study Group. (1990). Current management of amaurosis fugax. *Stroke, 21*, 201–208.

REFERENCES

Amaurosis Fugax Study Group. (1990). *Stroke*, *21*, 201–208.
Winterkorn, J. M., & Beckman, R. L. (1995). *J Neuroophthalmol*, *15*, 209–211.

ANEURYSMAL SUBARACHNOID HEMORRHAGE

Subarachnoid hemorrhage (SAH) accounts for 50% of hemorrhagic strokes with the other half being caused by intracerebral hemorrhage. Most SAHs are caused by ruptured aneurysm. Risk factors include female gender, smoking, alcohol, hypertension, cocaine drug abuse, and use of sympathomimetic drugs. The risk of rupture primarily depends on aneurysm size and location, with higher risk associated with larger aneurysms and posterior circulation location.

CLINICAL PRESENTATION

The most common presentation of aneurysmal SAH is sudden, severe ("thunderclap") headache (97% of cases). Other symptoms include nausea, vomiting, meningismus, and altered mental status. Seizures occur the first 24 hours in less than 10% of cases. Hunt and Hess (HH) grading is commonly used to grade the severity of SAH (I, headache; II, severe headache with cranial nerve palsy; III, drowsiness with neurologic deficit; IV, stupor; and V, coma).

DIAGNOSIS

Non-contrast head computed tomography (CT) is the cornerstone for SAH diagnosis. CT scan has 92% sensitivity if done within 24 hours. A lumbar puncture (LP) is mandated with a negative CT and a high clinical suspicion of SAH. Elevated opening pressure and markedly elevated red blood cell (RBC) count with no decrease in RBCs between tubes 1 and 4 are the classic findings in SAH. The presence of xanthochromia (yellow color) from RBC degradation in the cerebrospinal fluid (CSF) indicates that blood has been in the CSF for at least 2 hours. Conventional angiography remains the gold standard for identifying the aneurysm, although modern magnetic resonance imaging and CT angiography may reliably detect aneurysms as small as 3 to 5 mm.

MANAGEMENT

All patients with aneurysmal SAH should be admitted to the neurological intensive care unit for neurologic and hemodynamic monitoring. Patients with Glasgow Coma Scale < 8, elevated intracranial pressure, hypoventilation, and hemodynamic instability should be intubated. Deep vein thrombosis (DVT) prophylaxis with SQ heparin is started after the aneurysm is secured. Ventriculostomy device is placed in patients with evidence of hydrocephalus on CT of the head or World Federation of Neurological Surgeons ≥ 3 (Table 3). Nimodipine (40 mg PO q 6 hr for 21 days) may reduce morbidity risk from symptomatic vasospasm, although it may induce undesired hypotension. Euvolemia and normal blood pressure should be maintained.

TABLE 3

WORLD FEDERATION OF NEUROLOGICAL SURGEONS SUBARACHNOID
HEMORRHAGE GRADING SCALE

Grade	GCS	Motor deficit
1	15	Absent
2	13–14	Absent
3	13–14	Present
4	7–12	Present or absent
5	3–6	Present or absent

GCS, Glasgow Coma Scale.

Definitive treatment should occur at the earliest available opportunity to avoid aneurysm re-rupture. The International Subarachnoid Aneurysm Trial study showed superiority for coiling in patients with SAH thought by surgeon and interventionalist to be suitable for either coiling or clipping (31% morbidity and mortality rates with clipping versus 24% with coiling). Indications for delayed treatment (i.e., on SAH days 10–14) may include subacute presentation (worse outcome associated with surgical clipping performed between SAH days 2 and 10) and poor clinical grade (HH grade 4, 5) at presentation (early treatment may not alter ultimate outcome). These results were replicated in the US-based randomized clinical trial comparing clipping versus coiling showing superiority of coiling over clipping.

Vasospasm typically occurs between SAH days 3 and 10, with peak incidence at days 7 to 10. The Fisher scale is widely used as an index of vasospasm risk (I, no blood; II, diffuse deposition of blood less than 1 mm thick; III, localized clots or blood $\geq$ 1 mm thickness; IV, intracerebral or intraventricular clots). Neurologic deterioration necessitates a stat head CT to rule out intracranial hemorrhage, hydrocephalus, or rehemorrhage; if none are present, vasospasm is assumed. Initial treatment is with "triple H therapy": hypertension (mean arterial pressure [MAP] > 100), hypervolemia (central venous pressure > 8), hemodilution (HTC 28%–30%). If there is no improvement, cerebral angiography with potential angioplasty or local intra-arterial papaverine or calcium channel blocker infusion is considered.

Treat other complications of SAH: Correct hyponatremia (cerebral salt wasting vs. syndrome of inappropriate ADH secretion), dobutamine for neurogenic pulmonary edema, monitor cardiac abnormalities including myocardial infarction, vasopressin for diabetes insipidus, and external ventriculostomy or serial LPs for hydrocephalus.

OUTCOME

Outcome is poor; the 30-day mortality rate is 40% to 50% for those admitted to a hospital, and 15% die prior to reaching medical care. Only one third of surviving patients return to their baseline lifestyle, and one third remain moderately to severely disabled.

See also Endovascular Treatment of Cerebral Aneurysm.

REFERENCES

Spetzler, R. F., McDougall, C. G., Zabramski, J. M., Albuquerque, F. C., et al. (2015). The Barrow Ruptured Aneurysm Trial: 6-year results. *J Neurosurg, 123*, 609–617.

ISAT study. *Lancet* 361:431, 2003, and 366:809–817, *Lancet* 2005 and *Lancet* 2015;385:691–697.

ANGELMAN SYNDROME

Angelman syndrome is a genetic disorder associated with aberrations of imprinted genes—specifically, maternal deletions of the 15q11.2q13.1 gene with lack of expression of the UBE3A gene.

Angelman syndrome affects approximately 1:40,000 children and constitutes about 6% of all children with severe intellectual disability and epilepsy. Paternally derived deletions of this chromosomal section cause Prader-Willi syndrome.

Individuals with Angelman syndrome are best known for behavioral features such as happy demeanor, severe language and speech impairment, frequent laughter and smiling, hand flapping, water fascination, hyperactivity, sleep disturbances, and short attention span. Affected individuals frequently have severe intellectual disability (Intelligence Quotient [IQ] levels 20–40) and developmental delay. Physical prototype includes acquired microcephaly (deceleration of head growth during the first year), flat neck, fair complexion and hair, open mouth with tongue protrusion, prognathism, and wide-spaced teeth. Other features include epilepsy (present in 90% and usually in patients younger than 3 years of age), movement disorder (ataxic gait, tremulous movements of limbs), and hyperactive tendon reflexes. Magnetic resonance imaging (MRI) shows microcephaly with slight hemispheric asymmetries. Electroencephalography (EEG) shows high amplitude 2 to 3 Hz delta activity with intermittent spike and slow wave discharges maximal in the occipital region and sleep-activated generalized epileptiform discharges. Seizure treatment includes valproate and benzodiazepines. Sedation should be avoided, as it may increase seizure activity.

REFERENCES

Daroff, R. B., Jankovic, J., Mazziotta, J. C., & Pomeroy, S. L. (Eds.). (2016). *Bradley's neurology in clinical practice,* ed 7. Philadelphia: Elsevier.

Dulac, O., Lassonde, M., & Sarnat, H. B. (Eds.), (2013). *Handbook of clinical neurology: vol. 111/112/113. Pediatric neurology, Part I/II/III*, ed 1. New York: Elsevier.

ANGIOGRAPHY

Conventional cerebral angiography combines continuous fluoroscopy with injection of radiopaque contrast material directly into the arterial system of interest. This is done by advancing a catheter (usually through the femoral artery in the groin) into the aortic arch or selectively into the carotid or vertebrobasilar systems. Computerized digital subtraction techniques remove the bone density, improving visualization of the blood vessels. Angiography also provides evaluation of blood flow hemodynamics by following the movement/distribution of contrast agent through the blood vessels in real time. Indications for angiography include the evaluation of suspected vascular malformations, aneurysms, vasculopathies, stenotic or ulcerative vascular lesions, preoperative delineation of vascular anatomy, and blood supply to tumors, serving as a platform for endovascular procedures. Advances with high-resolution machines and 3D angiography technology, along with the use of smaller catheters and less ionic contrast material, made it more useful and safer.

The most common complication following angiography is a hematoma developing at the femoral arterial puncture site; this typically responds to local pressure. Uncommonly, a persistent arterial pseudoaneurysm develops, requiring ultrasound-guided thrombin injection. Acute stroke complicates less than 1% of procedures, with permanent neurologic deficit occurring in fewer than 0.5%. Elderly patients and those with preexisting carotid stenosis are at slightly higher risk. Allergic contrast reaction is rare, ranging from hives to anaphylaxis; a previous history of any contrast reaction obligates pretreatment with steroids. Patients with decreased renal function are at risk of developing contrast nephropathy; this risk may be reduced with adequate hydration before and after angiography, and pretreatment with N-acetylcysteine (Mucomyst) 600 mg PO q 12 hr 48 to 72 hours prior to angiography and sodium bicarbonate solution 1 hour before and 4 to 6 hours after.

Angiographic anatomy is depicted in Figs. 3 and 4.

ANGIOMAS

Angiomas are abnormalities involving small blood vessels. Majority of angiomas found intracranially can be grouped under one of three subtypes: (1) cavernous angiomas, (2) venous angiomas or developmental venous anomalies (DVAs), and (3) telangiectasia. All three subtypes are considered to be low-flow vascular malformations.

Cavernous angiomas, also known as cavernous malformation, cavernous hemangioma, and cavernoma, are collections of enlarged capillary cavities with surrounding hemosiderin ("leaky") but *without normal brain parenchyma* in the interim. Based on magnetic resonance imaging (MRI) and autopsy studies, prevalence is estimated at 0.1% to 0.5% of the population and encompasses 5% to 15% of all cerebral vascular malformations. These can be sporadic or familial, which is inherited in an autosomal dominant (AD) fashion with incomplete penetrance and typically presents with multiple lesions that may enlarge over time. Mutations in three genes have been identified: KRIT1 on 7q21-q22 (CCM1), MGC4067 on 7p13 (CCM2), and PDCD10 on 3q26-q27 (CCM3). Commonly these become symptomatic around age 30 with

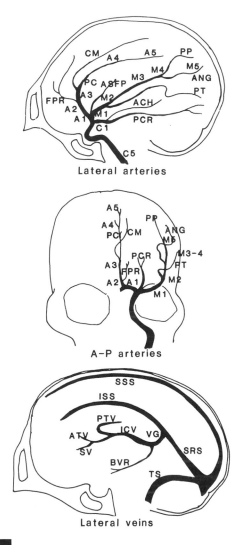

FIGURE 3

Internal carotid circulation.

A_1–A, Segments of anterior cerebral artery; ACH, anterior choroidal artery; ANG, angular artery; ASFP, ascending frontoparietal artery; ATV, anterior terminal vein; BVR, basal vein of Rosenthal; CM, callosomarginal artery; C_1–C_5, segments of internal carotid artery; FPR, frontopolar artery; ICV, internal cerebral vein; ISS, inferior sagittal sinus; M_1–M_5, segments of middle cerebral artery; PC, pericallosal artery; PCR, posterior cerebral artery; PP, posterior parietal artery; PTV, posterior terminal vein; SRS, straight sinus; SSS, superior sagittal sinus; SV, septal vein; TS, transverse sinus; VG, great cerebral vein of Galen.

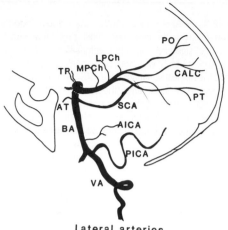

Lateral arteries

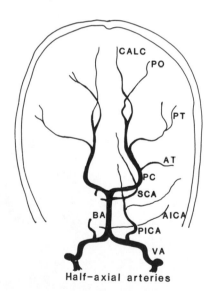

Half-axial arteries

FIGURE 4

Vertebrobasilar circulation.

AICA, Anterior inferior cerebellar artery; *AT,* anterior temporal artery (branch of PC); *BA,* basilar artery; *CALC,* calcarine artery (branch of PC); *LPCh,* lateral posterior choroidal artery; *MPCh,* medial posterior choroidal artery; *PC,* posterior cerebral artery; *PICA,* posterior inferior cerebellar artery; *PO,* parieto-occipital artery (branch of PC); *PT,* posterior temporal artery (branch of PC); *SCA,* superior cerebellar artery; *TP,* thalamoperforate artery; *VA,* vertebral artery.

hemorrhage (32%–59%) or seizure (40%–70%), and a majority (up to 80%) are supratentorial. MRI is the preferred imaging modality with the classic "popcorn" or "berry" sign and ring of hypointensity on FLAIR and T2 weighted images though susceptibility weighted sequences and gradient echo sequences have the highest sensitivity (Fig. 5C). When symptomatic, complete surgical resection can be considered, though recent literature has suggested higher risk of intracranial hemorrhage or new focal deficit following resection.

Venous angiomas, also known as congenital DVA, are characterized by abnormally thickened veins that may be considered a variant of physiological venous drainage system. Usually asymptomatic and found incidentally, these rarely can present with hemorrhage or seizures when associated with cavernous malformation, which can occur in 20% to 30% of patients. Even more rare, there can be thrombosis resulting in focal edema. These may appear on post contrast computed tomography (CT), MRI, and venous phase angiography as finger-like, projecting from a main vein (the caput medusae sign, see Fig. 5B). In general, intervention is neither necessary nor recommended.

Telangiectasia arise from arterioles and develop as clusters of pencil-like vessels, specifically favoring pons, cerebellum, and spinal cord. Most are asymptomatic and found incidentally. Notable exceptions are when these occur as part of **Osler-Weber-Rendu syndrome** (AD), in which case they may present with spontaneous rupture and intracranial hemorrhage. MRI is the preferred imaging modality. No treatment is necessary.

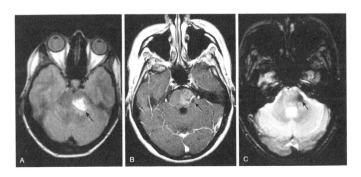

FIGURE 5

(A) Subacute pontine hemorrhage on noncontrast T1 weighted MR image. (B) Caput medusa sign on T1 with gadolinium injection on follow up image after hematoma resorption. (C) With associated cavernous malformation which appear as hypointense lesion on T2* weighted image. (From Stapf, C. (2016). Arteriovenous malformations and other vascular anomalies. In J. C. Grotta, et al. (Eds.), 2016. *Stroke: pathophysiology, diagnosis, and management*, ed 6 (p. P547, Figure 30-9). Philadelphia: Elsevier.

REFERENCES

Kim, H., Pawlikowska, L., Su, H., & Young, W. L. (2016). Genetics and vascular biology of angiogenesis and vascular malformations. In J. C. Grotta, et al. (Eds.), *Stroke: pathophysiology, diagnosis, and management,* ed 6 (pp. P149–P162). Amsterdam, Netherlands: Elsevier.

Stapf, C. (2016). Arteriovenous malformations and other vascular anomalies. In J. C. Grotta, et al. (Eds.), *Stroke: pathophysiology, diagnosis, and management,* ed 6 (pp. P537–P549). Amsterdam, Netherlands: Elsevier.

ANTIBODY TESTING IN NEUROMUSCULAR DISEASE

Immune-mediated neuromuscular disease is an important focus of diagnosis, as these disorders are frequently immunologically mediated and may respond to immunomodulatory therapy. In myasthenia gravis (MG), the pathogenic role of antibodies has been conclusively demonstrated. In many other conditions, associations with antibodies have been described, but the pathogenic role is unclear. The same antibody may be present in more than one condition, leading to poor specificity. In general, antibody testing should be performed to answer specific clinical questions. Table 4 summarizes some of the more established antibody associations.

MULTIFOCAL MOTOR NEUROPATHY

Multifocal motor neuropathy (MMN) is a rare treatable cause of neuropathy. It is more frequent in men than women, and presents between 20 and 50 years of age. Patients usually have slowly progressive asymmetrical weakness in the distribution of named peripheral nerves with no sensory loss; early onset of

TABLE 4

NEUROPATHY SYNDROMES ASSOCIATED WITH AUTOANTIBODIES

Condition	Antigen	Antibody	% Positive
GANGLIOSIDE ANTIBODIES			
Multifocal motor neuropathy	GM1	Poly IgM	30–80
Distal lower motor neuron syndromes	GM1	Poly IgM	30–65
AMAN variant of Guillain-Barré syndrome	GM1, GD1a	Poly IgG, IgM	20–30
Miller-Fisher syndrome	GQ1b	Poly IgG	~95
GLYCOPROTEIN ANTIBODIES			
Monoclonal IgM to MAG	MAG	Mono IgM	50
RNA-BINDING PROTEIN ANTIBODIES			
Paraneoplastic sensory neuronopathy	Hu	IgG	>95
GLYCOSPHINGOLIPID ANTIBODIES			
Chronic sensory neuropathy	Sulfatide	Mono IgM	—
		Poly IgM, IgG	—

AMAN, Acute motor axonal neuropathy; *MAG,* myelin-associated glycoprotein.

A

ANTIBODY TESTING IN NEUROMUSCULAR DISEASE

diffuse weakness excludes the diagnosis of MMN. No spasticity, extensor plantar responses, clonus, or pseudobulbar palsy should be present. Electrodiagnostic studies are crucial to the diagnosis of MMN, typically showing conduction block of motor nerves (outside normal entrapment sites), with normal sensory nerve responses. High titers of immunoglobulin M (IgM) antibody to GM1 and other glycolipids, including asialo-GM1, GD1a, and GM2, may occur. Reported rates of anti-GM1 IgM range from 30% to 80%. Anti-GM1 antibodies also occur in other dysimmune neuropathies, as well as 5% of amyotrophic lateral sclerosis (ALS) patients. If anti-GM1 titers are very high ($>$1:6400), then specificity for MMN or a lower motor neuron syndrome is high, but levels this high occur in only 20% of MMN patients. The anti-GM1 antibodies' role is not clear; hence diagnostic criteria for MMN published by the AANEM include no role for anti-GM1 antibody testing. In practice, if MMN cannot be differentiated from motor neuron disease, a trial of intravenous gamma globulin (IVIG) is appropriate, even if anti-GM1 antibodies are absent. MMN can develop in lymphoma patients and following treatment with tumor necrosis factor-α antagonists, but this is a rare clinical scenario.

AMYOTROPHIC LATERAL SCLEROSIS

Although detectable serum levels of anti-GM1 have been reported in ALS, titers are usually low compared with MMN. The frequency of a detectable positive anti-GM1 titer in ALS has been reported to be as high as 50%. In the setting of classical ALS, there is no current utility for autoantibody testing.

GUILLAIN-BARRÉ SYNDROME

A high proportion of GBS patients, particularly those with *Campylobacter jejuni* infection, have a high titer of IgG and/or IgM antibodies to GM1. The presence of anti-GM1b antibodies appears to be associated with the acute motor axonal neuropathy (AMAN) form of GBS. There is some evidence that IgG antibodies are more linked to an axonal variant than are IgM antibodies. Other antibodies linked to the AMAN presentation of GBS are anti-GM1b, anti-GD1a, and anti-GalNAc-GD1a IgG antibodies. Similar antibody associations have been found in acute motor and sensory neuropathy (AMSAN) presentation as well, suggesting that AMAN and AMSAN are related entities.

ANTI-GANGLIOSIDE GQ1B AND MILLER-FISHER SYNDROME

Miller-Fisher syndrome (MFS) is the most common variant of GBS and accounts for 5% to 10% of GBS cases. It presents with a triad of ataxia, ophthalmoparesis, and areflexia. MFS provides a compelling example of a disorder in which ganglioside autoimmunity is believed to play a pathogenic role. More than 90% of patients with MFS have IgG antibodies to GQ1b, while these antibodies are absent in other conditions and in control populations. GQ1b is a ganglioside enriched in myelin and specifically present in the paranodal myelin of oculomotor, trochlear, and abducens nerves, but not the other cranial nerves. This finding appears to explain the ophthalmoplegia seen in MFS. GQ1b epitopes can be found on some strains of *C. jejuni*, and some patients report an antecedent infection. IgG antibodies to GQ1b are also markers for GBS variants with acute ophthalmoplegia that do not meet full MFS criteria.

Up to 60% of patients with Bickerstaff brainstem encephalitis have anti-GQ1b IgG antibodies Conversely, GBS patients without ophthalmoplegia are invariably anti-GQ1b negative. The high sensitivity and specificity of this antibody for MFS and ophthalmoplegic variants of GBS make this test clinically useful to rule out other causes of acute and subacute ophthalmoparesis.

ANTI-MYELIN-ASSOCIATED GLYCOPROTEIN AND ASSOCIATED NEUROPATHIES

Monoclonal gammopathy of undetermined significance (MGUS) is frequently associated with neuropathy, although the true prevalence is unclear. Approximately half of MGUS-associated neuropathies have IgM antibody activity directed against myelin-associated glycoprotein (MAG). IgM gammopathy with anti-MAG antibodies is not frequent in normal individuals, such that IgM anti-MAG antibodies are usually not an incidental finding. MAG is a membrane glycoprotein located in peripheral and central myelin. The pathogenesis of the neuropathy is not well understood; animal models of anti-MAG neuropathy suggest the antibodies are pathogenic and along with complement deposition mediate damage to the myelin sheath.

Anti-MAG neuropathy is the best characterized of the antinerve antibody syndromes. There is insidious onset of sensory gait ataxia and progressive symmetrical ascending numbness with progression over months to years. Motor involvement is much less pronounced, and early on the clinical picture may resemble a sensory neuronopathy (SN). Eventually, clinical motor involvement occurs in the majority of patients. Peripheral nerves may be thickened and palpable. EMG studies show prolongation of distal latencies and dispersion of motor potentials, even when weakness is not evident. Sensory responses are frequently absent or attenuated. Spinal fluid often shows a protein of 100 mg/dL.

Compared with chronic inflammatory demyelinating polyneuropathy (CIDP) without IgM paraproteinemia, anti-MAG polyneuropathy is less responsive to steroids, plasmapheresis, and IVIG. Oral cyclophosphamide or intravenous cyclophosphamide with steroids may be effective.

ANTISULFATIDE ANTIBODIES AND SENSORIMOTOR NEUROPATHY

Polyneuropathies associated with serum IgM antisulfatide antibodies have been described. These neuropathies are usually more sensory than motor, with distal, symmetrical sensory loss, and pain is common. Tremor and gait ataxia have been reported. In patients with an associated M protein and MGUS, EMG may show demyelination. In patients without an M protein EMG shows axonal loss. At this time there is no established diagnostic role for these antibodies in the routine evaluation of sensory or sensory-predominant peripheral neuropathy.

A

ANTIBODY TESTING IN NEUROMUSCULAR DISEASE

PARANEOPLASTIC NEUROMUSCULAR SYNDROMES

Many neurologic syndromes result from paraneoplastic causes (Table 5). This discussion is concerned with the neuromuscular syndromes only, although antibodies associated with non-neuromuscular syndromes are summarized in Table 5.

I. Paraneoplastic sensory neuronopathy (PSN) is the classic paraneoplastic neuropathy whose neurologic symptoms classically precede tumor discovery by months. The neuropathy is painful, subacute in onset, often initially asymmetrical, and evolves into a complete loss of proprioception with prominent sensory ataxia and pseudoathetosis of the hands. SN has a limited differential diagnosis other than paraneoplastic causes that includes chemotherapy with platinum-containing agents, pyridoxine (vitamin B_6) intoxication, and Sjögren syndrome. This condition is rare, but dramatic, affecting less than 1% of patients with small-cell lung carcinoma (SCLC) and rarely seen in other neoplasms. Anti-amphiphysin, ANNA 3, and anti-CV2 antibodies have also been associated with this syndrome, again usually with SCLC. Patients with anti-Hu may have more widespread disease that may include cerebellar degeneration and limbic or brainstem encephalitis (paraneoplastic encephalomyelitis (PEM)/ SN). In the setting of a SN, a positive anti-Hu is diagnostic of paraneoplastic etiology (specificity of 99% and a sensitivity of 82%), emphasizing the importance of a thorough evaluation for lung cancer. If no cancer is found, periodic screening should be performed, as cancer is eventually found in 80% to 90% of patients with anti-Hu. In general, recovery of sensation following treatment of the underlying cancer is poor, but the associated cancer is often limited and responds to treatment.

II. Sensorimotor polyneuropathy may also be associated with anti-Hu or anti-CV2. The possibility of a paraneoplastic syndrome is often overlooked, as patients with cancer may have multiple potential causes for a sensorimotor polyneuropathy.

III. Subacute autonomic neuropathy. Paraneoplastic neuropathy may also present as a severe dysautonomia with anti-Hu antibodies.

IV. Lambert-Eaton myasthenic syndrome (LEMS) is a presynaptic neuromuscular junction disorder associated with underlying cancer in about 60% of cases, usually SCLC but sometimes lymphoma. LEMS presents with proximal leg weakness and less frequently arm weakness. Although progressive augmentation of muscle strength may occur initially with exercise, the dominant symptom is fatigable weakness, as in MG. Ocular symptoms are much less frequent than in MG. Characteristically EMG studies of LEMS show low motor CMAP amplitudes with an increment in amplitude following brief exercise of greater than 100%. The prevalence of LEMS in patients with known SCLC is around 3%. Antivoltage gated calcium channels are almost always present in LEMS, but do not differentiate between paraneoplastic and nonparaneoplastic causes. The presentation of LEMS may precede the diagnosis of the cancer by many months, and repeated screening is recommended.

V. Myasthenia Gravis is considered elsewhere in this book.

TABLE 5

AUTOANTIBODIES IN NEUROLOGIC PARANEOPLASTIC SYNDROMES

Syndrome	Antibody for Diagnosis	Antibody for Paraneoplastic Etiology	Associated Cancer (Most Frequent)
Subacute sensory neuropathy		Anti-Hu	SCLC
		Anti-amphiphysin	SCLC
		ANNA-3	SCLC
		Anti-CRMP5/CV2	SCLC, thymoma
Sensory-motor peripheral neuropathy		Anti-Hu	SCLC
		Anti-amphiphysin	SCLC
		Anti-CRMP5/CV2	SCLC, thymoma
Stiff-man/person syndrome	Anti-GAD	Ant -amphiphysin	Breast
Myelitis		Anti-Hu	SCLC
Lambert-Eaton myasthenic syndrome	Anti-VGCC	Not available	SCLC
Myasthenia gravis	Anti-AchR, Anti-MUSK	Anti-titin	Thymoma
Dermatomyositis	Anti- Mi2, Anti-synthetase Ab, Anti-TIFγ, NXP2, MDA5	Ovarian, lung, pancreas	
Subacute cerebellar degeneration		Anti-Hu	SCLC
		Anti-PCA-2	SCLC
		ANNA-3	SCLC
		Anti-CRMP5/CV2	SCLC, thymoma
		Anti-Yo	Ovary, breast
		Anti-Ta/Ma2	Testis
		Anti-Ma	Multiple
		Anti-Ri	Breast

Continued

A

ANTIBODY TESTING IN NEUROMUSCULAR DISEASE

TABLE 5

AUTOANTIBODIES IN NEUROLOGIC PARANEOPLASTIC SYNDROMES—CONT'D

Syndrome	Antibody for Diagnosis	Antibody for Paraneoplastic Etiology	Associated Cancer (Most Frequent)
Opsoclonus/myoclonus (child)		Anti-Tr	Hodgkin's lymphoma
Opsoclonus/myoclonus (adult)		Anti-Hu	Neuroblastoma
		Anti-Ri	Breast
		Anti-Hu	SCLC
		Anti-Ma	Multiple
		Anti-Ta/Ma2	Testis
Limbic encephalitis		Anti-Hu	SCLC
		Anti-Ta/Ma2	Testicular
		ANNA-3	SCLC
		Anti-CRMP5/CV2	SCLC, thymoma
Retinopathy		Anti-recoverin, Anti-retinal	Lung
		Anti-Hu	SCLC
		Anti-Hu	SCLC
Extrapyramidal syndromes		Anti-Ta/Ma2	Testis
		Anti-Ma	Multiple
		Anti-CRMP5/CV2	SCLC, thymoma

SCLC, Small-cell lung carcinoma

VI. Dermatomyositis represents a paraneoplastic syndrome in approximately 30% of patients. Frequently associated tumors are ovarian, lung, pancreatic, stomach, colon, rectum, and non-Hodgkin lymphoma. There are multiple antibodies with variable predictive value for the presence of underlying malignancy—positive in up to 60% to 70% of patients with dermatomyositis. Polymyositis is less frequently associated with a paraneoplastic form.

VII. Stiff-person syndrome is characterized by chronic rigidity of axial musculature and spasms believed to arise from a functional deficit of GABA in the central nervous system. Antibodies to glutamic acid decarboxylase (anti-GAD) are present in serum and CSF in about 70% of patients. Stiff-person syndrome is associated with other autoimmune conditions such as diabetes, autoimmune thyroiditis, pernicious anemia, and vitiligo. Epilepsy occurs in 10% of patients. In 5% of patients, stiff-man syndrome is associated with cancer, particularly breast cancer. Antiamphiphysin antibodies are found in the paraneoplastic stiff-man syndrome.

REFERENCES

Pourmand, R. (2004). *Neurol Clin*, *22*, 703–717.
Willison, H. J., & Yuki, N. (2002). *Brain*, *125*, 2591–2625.

ANTIDEPRESSANTS

Antidepressants encompass several groups of compounds belonging to several generations. The first generation of these drugs, the monoamine oxidase inhibitors, inhibit metabolism of monoamines like dopamine (DA), norepinephrine (NE) and 5-hydroxytryptamine (5-HT), making more of these neurotransmitters available for secretion. Examples include phenelzine and tranylcypromine. Tricyclic antidepressants (TCAs) inhibit NE and 5-HT reuptake and include well-known drugs like imipramine, doxepin, and amitriptyline. These earlier antidepressants, owing to their food and drug interactions, were slowly supplanted by second-generation drugs comprising selective serotonin reuptake inhibitors (SSRIs). The SSRIs (e.g., sertraline, paroxetine) were created by structurally modifying TCAs, and they selectively inhibit the reuptake of serotonin into the presynaptic terminals, making serotonin available for neurotransmission. The serotonin-norepinephrine reuptake inhibitors (SNRIs), such as venlafaxine, duloxetine, and milnacipran, enhance serotonergic and noradrenergic effects at synapses. Antagonism at the 5-HT$_2$ subgroup of serotonin receptors makes drugs like trazodone and mirtazapine effective antidepressants but more frequently used for their sedative effects in insomnia. Relatively SNRIs like maprotiline and reboxetine are the newest members of the antidepressant family. Bupropion exerts its antidepressant effect by inhibiting NE, DA, and the vesicular monoamine transporters, enhancing the effects of NE and DA.

Table 6 summarizes the relative side effects of common antidepressants. TCAs have notable anticholinergic side effects including blurred vision, dry constipation, urinary retention, memory dysfunction, and exacerbation of

TABLE 6

FREQUENCY OF SIDE EFFECTS OF ANTIDEPRESSANT MEDICATIONS

Medication	Sedation	Agitation	Anticholinergic Effects[a]	Postural Hypotension	Gastrointestinal Upset	Sexual Dysfunction	Weight Gain	Weight Loss
Serotonin and norepinephrine reuptake inhibitors								
Venlafaxine	0	0/+	0	0	+++	+++	0	Not available
Tricyclics (tertiary amines)								
Amitriptyline	++++	0	++++	+++	+	+	++	0
Doxepin	++++	0	++++	+++	+	+	+	0
Imipramine	++++	0	++++	+++	+	+	+	0
Tricyclics (secondary amines)								
Desipramine	+++	0	+++	++	+	+	+	0
Nortriptyline	+++	0	+++	++	+	+	+	0
Bicyclic								
Venlafaxine	++	+	++	0	+++	++	0	+
Selective serotonin reuptake inhibitors								
Citalopram	0	0	+	0	++	+	+	+
Fluoxetine	+	++	+	0	++	++	+	+
Paroxetine	++	0	+	0	++	++	+	+
Sertraline	+	+	+	0	++	++	+	+
Serotonin antagonist								
Mirtazapine	+++	0	++	+	0	0	++	0
Norepinephrine and dopamine reuptake inhibitor								
Bupropion	+	++	++	0	++	0	+	++
Serotonin antagonists and reuptake inhibitors								
Nefazodone	++	0	++	+	+	0	0	0
Trazodone	++++	0	++	+	+	0	+	+

0, None; +, minimal (>5% of patients); ++, low frequency (5%–20%); +++, moderate frequency (21%–40%); ++++, high frequency (>40%).

[a]Side effects may include dry mouth, dry eyes, blurred vision, constipation, urinary retention, tachycardia, or confusion.

Adapted from Whooley M.A., Simon G.E. (2000). Managing depression in medical outpatients. *N Engl J Med.* 343(26):1942–1950.

TABLE 7

THE EFFECT OF BLOCKING OR STIMULATING CERTAIN CNS RECEPTORS

Receptor Type	Potential Side Effect
α1 adrenergic receptor blocker	Orthostatic hypotension, reflex tachycardia
H1 histamine receptors blockers	Sedation, weight gain
M1 muscarine receptors blockers	Urinary retention, dry mouth, confusion, tachycardia
Serotonin 5-HT1 receptor stimulation	Antidepressant, anxiolytic effect, hypophagia
Serotonin 5-HT2 receptor stimulation	Sexual dysfunction, decreased libido or impotence, agitation, insomnia
Serotonin 5-HT3 receptor stimulation	Gastrointestinal side effects

H1, Histamine; *5-HT*, 5-hydroxytryptamine; *M1*, muscarine.

narrow-angle glaucoma. Patients with dementia and concomitant depression may worsen as a result of anticholinergic effects, whereas patients with Parkinson disease may improve (e.g., MAO-B selective inhibitors, selegiline, and rasagiline). Patients with migraine or chronic pain may benefit from antidepressants with a relatively high affinity for serotonin receptors (e.g., amitriptyline, duloxetine). SSRIs (fluoxetine, sertraline, citalopram, and paroxetine) may cause headache. Choice of antidepressant must be based on assessment of the patient's clinical state, especially cardiac conduction and ability to tolerate orthostatic hypotension, as well as the specific drug's side effect profile. Suicide risk should be assessed in all depressed patients, because TCA overdose is commonly fatal. A possible association between SSRI use and suicides in the early phase treatments of children and adolescents has prompted a "black box" warning from the U.S. Food and Drug Administration (FDA). Tables 7 and 8 summarize the side effects of blocking or stimulating certain central nervous system (CNS) receptors and epileptogenicity of selected antidepressants.

REFERENCES

Morrissette, D. A., & Stahl, S. M. (2014). Modulating the serotonin system in the treatment of major depressive disorder. *CNS Spectr*, *19*(S1), 54–68.

O'Donnell, J. M., & Shelton, R. C. (2014). Drug therapy of depression and anxiety disorders. In Brunton, et al. (Eds.), *Goodman & Gilman's: the pharmacological basis of therapeutics*, ed 12. New York: McGraw-Hill.

APHASIA

Aphasia is a language disorder acquired as a result of brain damage; it is distinct from congenital or developmental language disorders, disorders of speech (e.g. dysphonia, dysarthria, stuttering, and speech apraxia), and disorders of thought. Approximately 70% to 95% of all people have left hemispheric specialization of language "dominance," although more left-handed people have bilateral language function. Recent data, including functional MRI (fMRI) studies, demonstrate greater variation in patterns of language lateralization that may be independent of handedness.

TABLE 8

EPILEPTOGENIC POTENTIAL OF ANTIDEPRESSANT DRUGS AND THEIR RECEPTOR SPECIFICATIONS

Drug	Action on receptor:						Seizures/Epilepsy
	H1	M1	NA	5-HT1	5-HT2	5-HT3	
Imipramine	-	-	+	+	+	+	0.1%–4%, in overdose 3.8%–8%
Paroxetine	0	0	0	+	+	+	Prolonged seizures during electroconvulsive therapy. In overdose: no seizures in 15 patients with maximum dose 850 mg
Sertraline	0	0	0	+	+	+	Rare, secondary to SIADH. In overdose: no seizures in 40 patients up to 8000 mg
Fluoxetine	0	0	0	+	+	+	<0.1%
Citalopram	0	0	0	+	+	+	No worsening of epilepsy in 16 patients. In overdose: 100–1.9 g 18%–49%
Reboxetine	0	0/-	+	0	0	0	0.13%
Venlafaxine	0	0	+	+	+	+	0.18% In overdose: seizures in dosages over 1 g
Nefazodone	0	0	0	+	-	+	No seizures in premarketing trials, since then rare reports of convulsions
Mirtazapine	-	0	+	+	-	-	<0.1%

0, No or negligible effect; +, stimulation; -, blockade; H1, histamine; 5-HT1, 5-HT2, 5-HT3, serotonin receptors; M1, muscarine; NA, noradrenaline; SIADH, syndrome of inappropriate secretion of ADH.

TABLE 9

APHASIAS

Aphasia	Fluency	Comprehension	Repetition	Associated Signs	Localization
Broca	**Impaired**	Intact	Impaired	Right hemiparesis, hemianesthesia, apraxia	Posterior inferior frontal gyrus (Brodmann 44, 45)
Wernicke	Intact	**Impaired**	Impaired	+/- Right hemianopsia	Posterior superior temporal gyrus (Brodmann 22)
Conduction	Intact	Intact	**Impaired**	Left limb apraxia, mild right hemiparesis, hemianesthesia, hemianopsia	Arcuate fasciculus[a]
Global	**Impaired**	**Impaired**	**Impaired**	Right hemiparesis, hemianesthesia, hemianopsia	Large, including inferior frontal and superior temporal

Localizations refer to typically affected areas in the dominant hemisphere.

[a]It has been debated that the arcuate fasciculus might not be involved in repetition, and that conduction aphasia may be related to deficits in auditory immediate memory from lesions in the supramarginal gyrus.

A

APHASIA

Language cannot be adequately assessed during casual conversation alone. A bedside language assessment of six parts was popularized by Benson and Geschwind. (1) Fluency: Spontaneous speech assessment to evaluate fluency, phrase length, prosody (melodic intonation), phonation/volume. (2) Naming: Name several objects and their parts, colors, individuals, and body parts. (3) Auditory comprehension: Follow axial and appendicular, one-, two-, and three-step commands. Multiple language functions can be screened with a single command—for example, "Touch your left earlobe with your right index finger." (4) Repetition: Complex sentences are most sensitive—for example, "The orchestra played the concert and the audience applauded" or a sentence with grammatical complexity such as "No ifs, ands, or buts about it." (5) Reading: Comprehension should be tested; premorbid abilities must be considered. (6) Writing: Spontaneous writing, such as why the patient has presented may be the most sensitive test of mild aphasia.

In clinical practice, most patients do not present with pure classical aphasia syndromes. Fluency, comprehension, and repetition are the most readily localizable (Table 9). Transcortical motor aphasia is an analogue of Broca's aphasia with fluent repetition that localizes to areas supplied by the anterior cerebral artery (frontal lobe, anterior to Broca area, deep frontal white matter, medial frontal region/near supplementary motor area). Transcortical sensory aphasia is analogous to Wernicke aphasia with preserved repetition and is relatively uncommon. Subcortical aphasia occurs from lesions in the basal ganglia or deep cerebral white matter and can mimic the more classical aphasia syndromes. For example, lesions in the thalamus (typically paramedian or anterior nuclei) tend to produce a syndrome similar to Wernicke aphasia, but they do so with less impaired comprehension and may include a fluctuating level of alertness.

The Gerstmann syndrome includes (AAAD): Agraphia, Acalculia, Agnosia to the fingers, and Disorientation to right versus left, and localizes to the angular gyrus and is seen more commonly with brain tumors.

Alexia without agraphia localizes to the right primary visual cortex and the splenium of the corpus callosum.

REFERENCES

Kirshner, H. (2016). In R. B. Daroff, et al. (Eds.), (2016). *Bradley's neurology in clinical practice,* ed 7. Philadelphia: Elsevier.

Mazoyer, B., Zago, L., Jobard, G., et al. (2014). Gaussian mixture modeling of hemispheric lateralization for language in a large sample of healthy individuals balanced for handedness. *PLoS One, 9,* e101165.

APRAXIA

Apraxia is the inability to perform a previously learned skilled movement in the presence of intact motor, sensory, coordination, and comprehension systems. The terminology of apraxia is complex, and several main types have been found to be clinically relevant. Apraxia occurs in a variety of settings, and despite the shared name "apraxia," it is unclear if the underlying neurobiology is similar between clinical phenotypes. *Speech apraxia* may be developmental or acquired, as seen in right hemisphere presentations of frontotemporal dementia.

Testing for apraxia includes asking the patient to follow simple commands (such as "close your eyes" or "lick your lips"), to perform tasks with left and right extremities (for instance, comb hair, brush teeth, hammer a nail, or blow a kiss), and to use objects (as in lighting a match or using the telephone). Patients with ideomotor apraxia are usually self-sufficient because they can manipulate objects correctly on their own, whereas patients with ideational apraxia are often unable to care for themselves. Mild apraxia may appear with use of "body part as object," such as extending a finger and moving it between the teeth when asked to show how one brushes their teeth. *Apraxia of eyelid opening* is an example of a specific spontaneous movement that may occur with brainstem disorders.

Ideomotor apraxia is the inability to voluntarily complete an act in response to a verbal command. However, the same act can be performed spontaneously. It may involve buccofacial, limb, or truncal musculature. It is often associated with lesion in the left hemisphere and often complicates Broca aphasia. A lesion in the arcuate fasciculus may result in bilateral apraxia and conduction aphasia.

Limb-kinetic apraxia refers to loss of fine skilled movement following a premotor lesion. The patient is often clumsy and slow in executing motor tasks. One common situation corresponding to limb-kinetic apraxia is seen when the amplitude of rapid alternating movements is small, and the movements irregular.

Ideational apraxia (apraxia for object use) is the inability to perform sequential movements to use common objects in a proper manner despite the retained ability in performing the individual movements.

Constructional apraxia occurs in two-thirds of patients with right parietal lobe lesions. The patient is unable to copy or spontaneously draw figures and construct or mentally manipulate three-dimensional structures.

Callosal apraxia results from a lesion in the anterior corpus callosum and manifests as a disconnection syndrome with left-sided apraxia and intact right-sided praxis.

Oculomotor apraxia occurs as part of Balint syndrome and is seen with bilateral occipito-parietal lesion. *Gait apraxia* occurs with frontal lesions and patients have trouble initiating steppage. It may occur with normal pressure hydrocephalus and is seen with advancing dementia such as in Trisomy 21. *Dressing apraxia* occurs with right parietal syndromes, and may not be a true apraxia as it is task limited.

REFERENCE

Bieńkiewicz, M. M., Brandi, M. L., Goldenberg, G., et al. (2014). The tool in the brain: apraxia in ADL. Behavioral and neurological correlates of apraxia in daily living. *Front Psychol, 5*, 353.

ARTERIOVENOUS MALFORMATIONS

Arteriovenous malformations (AVMs) are characterized by a tortuous collection (nidus) of dilated arteries that drain into deep or superficial veins. The nidus lacks capillaries and is considered to be a high flow, low pressure vascular system.

Pathogenesis is unclear. Historically, AVMs are considered to be developmental abnormalities arising from the embryonic vascular system. However, this teaching is being questioned. No cases have been detected on prenatal patients in the United States. Furthermore, de novo lesions in adulthood, and their ability to grow or regress after treatment (especially after radiotherapy performed in childhood), are not consistent with the developmental theory. Ongoing studies are working to identify associated candidate genes.

Prevalence is between 10 to 18 per 100,000 adults and accounts for 1% to 2% of all strokes, including the majority of hemorrhagic strokes in children and young adults. One known association is Hereditary Hemorrhagic Telangiectasia, in which the AVMs tend to be smaller, more numerous, and more likely to be cortical. Familial cases are extremely rare. There is 10% association with aneurysms.

AVMs present between 10 and 40 years of age. The annual rate of hemorrhage is 3%, with an initial rate of 2% and re rupture rate of 4.5%; there is an increased risk of hemorrhage (6%–18%) in the first year after initial rupture. Risk of bleeding increases with a history of prior hemorrhage, deep location, exclusive deep venous drainage, and associated aneurysms. There is no increased risk associated with pregnancy. Intraparenchymal hemorrhage (50% of cases, occasionally with subarachnoid hemorrhage) and seizures (30% of cases, more likely in frontal and frontoparietal location) are the most common presentation. Less common presentations are headaches (usually nondescript) and progressive hemiparesis or focal neurological deficit, which may be due to compression of a neighboring structure. The compression may result from a mass effect or a phenomenon termed "intracerebral steal," where blood is shunted from the vicinity via the greatly dilated vascular channels.

The gold standard for diagnosis is an angiogram, which is also valuable for evaluating flow dynamics. AVMs may also be detected by computed tomography angiography, magnetic resonance imaging, and magnetic resonance angiography (Fig. 6). A bruit may be detected on a physical exam in the neck or behind the eyeball with moderate to large lesions; these can be exacerbated with repetitive squatting exercises.

There are three modalities for treatment and their use is guided by the Spetzler Martin grading system for surgical risk stratification (Table 10).

The three modalities of an AVM are surgical resection of the nidus, embolization of feeder arteries, and radiotherapy (delayed obliteration after 18–24 months). Table 11 represents an updated version of the grading system as proposed by Spetzler-Ponce. For class A lesions, the surgical morbidity range is between 1% and 2.5%. Class B lesions comprise a heterogeneous group, and a multimodality approach is recommended; morbidity and mortality

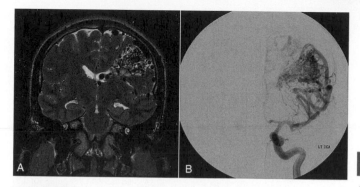

FIGURE 6

MRI (A) and angio (B) findings in cAVM with flow void signals of feeding arteries and draining veins on MRI and nidus appearance on angio and MRI.

TABLE 10

SPETZLER-MARTIN GRADING SYSTEM

AVM characteristic		Score
Size	<3 cm	1
	3–6 cm	2
	>6 cm	3
Location		
	Non-eloquent	0
	Eloquent	1
Venous Drainage	Superficial	0
	Deep	1

Total calculated score constitutes the AVM grade.

AVM, Arteriovenous malformation.

Adapted from Russin, J., & Spetzler, R. F. (2016). Surgical management of cranial and spinal arteriovenous malformations. In J. C. Grotta, et al. (Eds.), 2016. *Stroke: pathophysiology, diagnosis, and management*, ed 6 (pp. P1158–1170). Philadelphia: Elsevier.

TABLE 11

MODIFIED SPETZLER-PONCE GRADING SYSTEM WITH TREATMENT RECOMMENDATIONS

Class	Grade	Treatment Recommendation
A	I & II	Microsurgical resection with preoperative embolization
B	III	Multimodality
C	IV & V	Multimodality to conservative

Adapted from Russin, J., & Spetzler, R. F. (2016). Surgical management of cranial and spinal arteriovenous malformations. In J. C. Grotta, et al. (Eds.), 2016. *Stroke: pathophysiology, diagnosis, and management*, ed 6 (pp. P1158–1170). Philadelphia: Elsevier.

can vary significantly with the specific size, location, and venous drainage of a given AVM. For class C lesions, a conservative approach is generally favored as surgical morbidity and mortality rates range from at least 20% to 30%.

The management of unruptured AVMs remains controversial. The ARUBA (A Randomized Trial of Unruptured Brain Arteriovenous Malformations) trial was the first randomized controlled trial to compare intervention and medical management of unruptured AVMs, yet study design challenges, selection bias, and incomplete reporting have called the validity and generalizability of its conclusions into question. Results from subsequent studies, for example, suggest that microsurgery may be associated with less disability than reported in the ARUBA trial.

REFERENCES

Stapf, C. (2016). Arteriovenous malformations and other vascular anomalies. In J. C. Grotta, et al. (Eds.), 2016. *Stroke: pathophysiology, diagnosis, and management,* ed 6 (pp. P537–P549). Philadelphia: Elsevier.

Wong, J., Slomovic, A., Ibrahim, G., et al. (2017). Microsurgery for ARUBA trial-eligible unruptured brain arteriovenous malformations. *Stroke, 48,* 136–144.

ASTERIXIS

DEFINITION

Asterixis, also known as "negative myoclonus," is a sudden brief loss of postural tone, secondary to involuntary interruption in muscle contraction, typically seen in the setting of metabolic or systemic disturbances such as hepatic encephalopathy, respiratory failure, uremia, drug intoxication, or infection, and can also be associated with structural lesions or the result of a medication side effect. Asterixis usually manifests as the inability to hold the wrists in forced dorsiflexion with arms extended; however, it can affect all four limbs, the trunk, and the face.

PRESENTATION

Typically sudden wrist flexion is followed by rapid correction to the original dorsiflexed position, resulting in a characteristic flapping tremor. The loss of postural tone can also be evident during tongue protrusion or forced eye closure.

Electrophysiologic studies reveal an electrically silent period on electromyography (EMG) corresponding to the lapse of posture, which can be preceded by electroencephalogram (EEG) transients by 20 to 40 ms, suggesting a possible cortical generator of this phenomenon.

NEUROLOGIC EXAM

To evaluate for asterixis, the patient should adopt a posture extending the arms, pronated, at 90° to the body and extending the wrists with the fingers spread; straight leg raising with dorsiflexion at the ankle is helpful to evaluate the lower extremity.

ETIOLOGY

Once thought to be pathognomonic of hepatic encephalopathy (hence the term "liver flap"), it can be seen in many other toxic-metabolic conditions. When asterixis is unilateral, however, ischemic or hemorrhagic cerebral lesions, especially in the thalamus, are the most common cause.

DRUGS ASSOCIATED WITH ASTERIXIS

Medications associated with asterixis include opiates, levodopa, anticholinergics, lithium, benzodiazepines, gabapentin, phenytoin, valproate, and carbamazepine.

TREATMENT

Treatment depends on the underlying cause generating the metabolic disturbance. Treatment should focus on correcting the identified metabolic abnormalities and removal of any offending iatrogenic agents.

REFERENCES

Ellul, M. A., Cross, T. J., et al. (2017). *Asterixis Pract Neurol, 17*(1), 60–62.

ATAXIA, SPINOCEREBELLAR DEGENERATION

Usually the hallmark of cerebellar dysfunction, ataxia is an abnormality of movement characterized by errors in rate, range, direction, timing, and force ("coordination") of motor activity. Patients report being clumsy, slow with movements, or unsteady when walking. Speech and vision may also become symptomatic. Elements of ataxia include:

I. Asynergia—Decomposition of smooth movement into uncoordinated component parts.
II. Dysmetria—Poorly controlled speed, force, or distance of movement; includes past pointing, abnormal checking response, excessive rebound phenomenon.
III. Dysdiadochokinesia—Impairment of rapid alternating movements.

Ataxia may involve limbs, trunk, eyes, or bulbar musculature, and may be due to disease of the cerebellum, brainstem, spinal cord, or motor or sensory nerves. It results from defective timing of sequential contractions of agonist and antagonist muscles. Cerebellar hemispheric disease commonly produces limb ataxia, whereas midline cerebellar disease manifests as truncal and gait ataxia. Patients classically develop a broad-based gait to compensate for truncal instability. Owing to the double-crossing of the cerebellar pathways, ataxia is ipsilateral to cerebellar lesions.

Not all causes of ataxia are due to cerebellar lesions. Lesions of the afferent or efferent cerebellar pathways can result in ataxia as well, seen in some lacunar strokes and known as ataxic hemiparesis. Pontine lesions sparing the cerebellum often result in ataxia as well. Sensory disturbances resulting in loss of proprioception can also create the appearance of ataxia.

Cerebellar ataxia is frequently accompanied by other findings:

I. Tremor, which classically becomes worse near the target
II. Dysarthria—slurring, aprosody, scanning
III. Nystagmus, which can produce blurring or vertigo
IV. Saccadic dysmetria—over/undershooting on saccades

Tremor in cerebellar disease may be an action or intention tremor (disease of dentate nucleus or superior cerebellar peduncle) or more coarse ("rubral tremor"). Titubation, a nodding-head tremor, is seen with midline cerebellar disease and may involve the trunk. Ataxic speech has abnormal variability of volume, rate, and phonation, and may be slow and slurred or have alternating loudness and quietness. Gait ataxia may accompany vertigo in vestibular dysfunction.

Impaired proprioception resulting from disorders such as tabes dorsalis, hereditary disease, or dorsal root ganglionopathies may lead to sensory ataxia with impaired gait and presence of Romberg sign. Worsening of the ataxia with eyes closed and absence of dysarthria and ocular symptoms suggest sensory rather than cerebellar involvement. Cerebellar ataxia normally persists despite visual clues.

ACUTE ONSET ATAXIA

This form often results from cerebellar hemorrhage or infarction. Hemorrhage is usually associated with headache. Acute ataxia accompanied by other cranial nerve abnormalities should raise immediate concern for vertebrobasilar stroke. Multiple sclerosis, neuromyelitis optica, transverse myelitis, toxic disorders, and basilar migraine can also be acute causes. Viral cerebellitis causes an acute, reversible ataxia in children 2 to 10 years of age and is most common after chickenpox.

SUBACUTE ATAXIA

Hydrocephalus, foramen magnum compression, posterior fossa tumor, abscess, or parasitic infection in any age group can produce subacute ataxia. Other causes are infections (Human immunodeficiency virus, Creutzfeldt-Jakob disease, brainstem encephalitis), alcohol, vitamin deficiency (vitamin B_{12}, thiamine, vitamin E), celiac sprue (gliadin antibodies) and anti-glutamic acid decarboxylase antibodies, drugs (antiepileptics, lithium, chemotherapy, solvents, metals [mercury, manganese, bismuth, thallium]), and paraneoplastic syndromes in association with bronchogenic or ovarian carcinoma.

ATAXIA WITH EPISODIC COURSE

Ataxia with episodic course may be encountered in the following conditions: multiple sclerosis, neuromyelitis optica, vertebrobasilar transient ischemic attacks, foramen magnum compression, intermittent obstruction of ventricular system due to colloid cyst and dominantly inherited, acetazolamide responsive episodic ataxia. In children, metabolic causes including inherited defects of the urea cycle, aminoaciduria, Leigh disease, and mitochondrial encephalomyopathies should be considered.

ATAXIA WITH CHRONIC PROGRESSIVE COURSE

Chronic alcoholism with progressive cerebellar degeneration is common. Structural lesions such as posterior fossa tumors, foramen magnum compression, or hydrocephalus must be excluded first. Rarely, infectious agents such as chronic panencephalitis due to rubella in children can have a chronic progressive course. Primary progressive multiple sclerosis can manifest as chronic deterioration. Genetic diseases and other metabolic derangements can produce chronic ataxia as part of the clinical picture (see the next section).

SPINOCEREBELLAR DEGENERATION

Spinocerebellar degeneration refers to a large group of disorders that produce ataxia as a primary symptom, often early in life (except for the dominant ataxias). Most are very rare. Autosomal recessive causes include Friedreich ataxia, ataxia-telangiectasia, ataxia with isolated vitamin E deficiency, ataxia with oculomotor apraxia, abetalipoproteinemia, Unverricht-Lundborg disease, and others. Progressive ataxias are caused by leukodystrophies, xeroderma pigmentosum, coenzyme Q deficiency, vanishing white matter disease, GM2 gangliosidoses, Ramsay-Hunt syndrome, ceroid lipofuscinosis, sialidosis, sphingomyelin storage diseases, Wilson disease, Leigh disease, Refsum disease, and hexosaminidase deficiency (Tay-Sachs). Mitochondrial diseases such as MELAS, MERRF, and Kearns-Sayre produce progressive ataxias along with many other typical symptoms. Abnormal metabolism such as disorders of urea metabolism, aminoacidurias (Hartnup, branched chain), and various disorders of pyruvate/lactate metabolism can cause ataxia, sometimes intermittently. There is a large group of autosomal dominant ataxias that typically present after age 20 (see spinocerebellar ataxia).

Friedreich ataxia is the most common type of spinocerebellar degeneration. It is caused by a triple nucleotide repeat (GAA) expansion at chromosome 9 that encodes the protein frataxin. Symptoms develop from 18 months to 24 years of age and consist of progressive limb and truncal ataxia, dysarthria, and areflexia in the lower extremities. Pyramidal signs and loss of position and vibration sense evolve gradually. There is degeneration of cranial nerves VIII, X, and XII, the cerebellar hemispheres and tracts, and large myelinated nerves throughout the body. Skeletal deformities (kyphoscoliosis and pes cavus) and cardiomyopathy are seen in more than two thirds of patients. Systemic involvement manifests by increased incidence of diabetes, blindness, and deafness. Ambulation is usually lost by age 25, and death frequently occurs in the 4th or 5th decade of life. Treatment is aimed at symptomatic management of the skeletal deformities, diabetes, and the cardiac disorders. Investigational therapies targeting mitochondrial iron accumulation with idabenone and iron chelation with deferiprone have not improved neurologic outcomes thus far in clinical trials, though idabenone has shown modest benefit in the cardiac manifestations of Freidreich ataxia. Early-onset cerebellar ataxia with retained reflexes is often a variant with the frataxin mutation, but sometimes has unknown causes.

Ataxia-telangiectasia is characterized by progressive ataxia, neuropathy, choreoathetosis, areflexia, ocular telangiectasias (dilated capillaries in the conjunctiva), and frequent infections.

Ataxia sometimes occurs sporadically later in life with no identifiable cause. This condition is sometimes due to a degenerative condition known as olivopontocerebellar atrophy (OPCA). OPCA can progress to multisystem atrophy, which carries a very poor prognosis.

EVALUATION AND TREATMENT

Evaluation of a patient with progressive ataxia requires careful attention to disease progression, associated systemic and neurologic signs, and family history. Testing to rule out treatable secondary causes should include MRI, TSH, vitamin E, vitamin B_{12}, RPR, paraneoplastic antibodies (Yo, Hu, Ri, Ta, Ma, CV2 antiglutamate), autoimmune markers (anti-TPO, anti-GAD, and anti-gliadin antibodies), and CSF with cytology. The rare Miller-Fisher variant of Guillain-Barré syndrome (anti-GQ1b, anti-GM1 antibodies) should be considered as well in patients with ophthalmoplegia and areflexia in addition to ataxia. In younger patients, specialized metabolic tests may be needed, and diagnosis can be challenging. DNA testing for most of the inherited disorders is commercially available. Treatment for autoimmune and inflammatory etiologies includes high-dose glucocorticoids, intravenous immunoglobulin, and plasma exchange, in addition to more aggressive immunomodulatory treatments if deemed necessary. Treatment for the inherited ataxias at this time is largely investigational.

REFERENCES

Curr Opin Neurol. 28(4):413–22, 2015. doi: 10.1097/WCO.0000000000000227. http://www.emedicine.com/neuro/topic556.htm.

Pandolfo M, et al. Ann Neurol 76(4):509–521, 2014. doi: 10.1002/ana.24248. Epub 2014 Aug 30.

ATHETOSIS (SEE ALSO CHOREA)

Athetosis, derived from the Greek word *"athetos,"* meaning "without position," is the *involuntary, slow, continuous, irregular, and writhing movement of any muscle group*; it is usually most prominent in the distal extremities. It frequently coexists with other abnormal movements, particularly chorea and dystonia. Like those movements, athetosis is associated with *lesions in the basal ganglia*. The key difference between athetosis and chorea is that the same regions of the body are constantly involved in athetosis. Athetosis differs from dystonia by the lack of sustained postures; however, as it is often superimposed with dystonia, it can be difficult to distinguish in clinical practice. Electromyography (EMG) *study* reveals loss of reciprocation between muscle agonists and antagonists. *Etiology:* In adults, athetosis usually involves only one side of the body and is most often associated with strokes. In contrast, in children, athetosis involves both sides of the body ("double athetosis") and is often seen in cerebral palsy and postkernicterus. Athetosis can also be drug-induced (e.g., levodopa-induced dyskinesias). Athetosis may be seen in many hereditary and metabolic diseases, such as Huntington disease, Wilson disease, Lesch-Nyhan syndrome, glutaric acidemia, sulfite oxidase deficiency, Niemann-Pick disease, Fahr disease (idiopathic calcification of the basal ganglia), and Pantothenate kinase-associated neurodegeneration, formerly known as Hallervorden-Spatz disease.

Treatment may include Xenazine (12.5 mg p.o. daily increased 1 week later to BID with maximum daily dose of 50 mg in total in divided doses BID or TID). Other medications include benzodiazepine and Artane.

REFERENCE

Waln, O., & Jankovic, J. (2015). Paroxysmal movement disorders. *Neurol Clin*, *33*(1), 137–152.

ATTENTION-DEFICIT HYPERACTIVITY DISORDER

EPIDEMIOLOGY

Attention-deficit hyperactivity disorder (ADHD) is estimated to affect up to 20% of school-age children, with a prevalence of 5% among children and 2.5% among adults in most cultures. It occurs approximately twice as often in males than in females. However, females are more likely to present primarily with inattentive features that may be harder to detect. It has a substantial genetic component with reported heritability ranging from 0.7 to 0.88 in twins and occurring in one-fourth of the first-degree relatives of a child proband with ADHD. Comorbid neurobehavioral disorders include Tourette syndrome, obsessive-compulsive disorder, anxiety, and learning disabilities (with approximately 35% of patients having academic disorders). Oppositional defiant disorder and conduct disorder are the most frequently associated behavioral problems and occur in approximately 40% of children and adolescents with ADHD. There is a high frequency of co-occurrence in preterm infants (about 20%) and in epilepsy patients (30% in children with benign childhood epilepsy with centrotemporal spikes).

Dopamine is the primary neurotransmitter involved in ADHD, with dopamine D4 receptor being the most well studied and prevalent in the basal ganglia-frontal networks implicated in the pathophysiology of ADHD. It is postulated that hypodopaminergic states result in decreased activities of the inhibitory areas of the prefrontal cortex, striatum, caudate, and thalamic nuclei, which lead to an inability of the affected children to control their attention, impulses, and motor activity.

CLINICAL PRESENTATIONS

Table 12 lists the criteria for the diagnosis of attention deficit hyperactivity disorder.

TABLE 12

CRITERIA FOR THE DIAGNOSIS OF ATTENTION-DEFICIT HYPERACTIVITY DISORDER

People with ADHD show a persistent pattern of inattention and/or hyperactivity/impulsivity that interferes with functioning or development:

1. Inattention: Six or more symptoms of inattention for children up to age 16, or five or more for adolescents aged 17 and older and adults; symptoms of inattention have been present for at least 6 months, and they are inappropriate for developmental level:
   - Often fails to give close attention to details or makes careless mistakes in schoolwork, at work, or with other activities.
   - Often has trouble in holding attention on tasks or play activities.
   - Often does not seem to listen when spoken to directly.
   - Often does not follow through on instructions and fails to finish schoolwork, chores, or duties in the workplace (e.g., loses focus, side-tracked).
   - Often has trouble organizing tasks and activities.
   - Often avoids, dislikes, or is reluctant to do tasks that require mental effort over a long period of time (such as schoolwork or homework).
   - Often loses things necessary for tasks and activities (e.g., school materials, pencils, books, tools, wallets, keys, paperwork, eyeglasses, mobile telephones).
   - Is often easily distracted.
   - Is often forgetful in daily activities.

2. Hyperactivity and impulsivity: Six or more symptoms of hyperactivity-impulsivity for children up to age 16, or five or more for adolescents 17 and older and adults; symptoms of hyperactivity-impulsivity have been present for at least 6 months to an extent that is disruptive and inappropriate for the person's developmental level:
   - Often fidgets with or taps hands or feet, or squirms in seat.
   - Often leaves seat in situations when remaining seated is expected.
   - Often runs about or climbs in situations where it is not appropriate (adolescents or adults may be limited to feeling restless).
   - Often unable to play or take part in leisure activities quietly.
   - Is often "on the go" acting as if "driven by a motor."
   - Often talks excessively.
   - Often blurts out an answer before a question has been completed.
   - Often has trouble waiting his/her turn.
   - Often interrupts or intrudes on others (e.g., butts into conversations or games).
   - In addition, the following conditions must be met:
   - Several inattentive or hyperactive-impulsive symptoms were present before age 12 years.
   - Several symptoms are present in two or more settings, (e.g., at home, school or work; with friends or relatives; in other activities).
   - There is clear evidence that the symptoms interfere with, or reduce the quality of, social, school, or work functioning.
   - The symptoms do not happen only during the course of schizophrenia or another psychotic disorder. The symptoms are not better explained by another mental disorder (e.g., mood disorder, anxiety disorder, dissociative disorder, or a personality disorder).

Continued

TABLE 12

CRITERIA FOR THE DIAGNOSIS OF ATTENTION-DEFICIT HYPERACTIVITY DISORDER—CONT'D

Based on the types of symptoms, three kinds (presentations) of ADHD can occur:

Combined presentation: if enough symptoms of both criteria inattention and hyperactivity-impulsivity were present for the past 6 months.

Predominantly inattentive presentation: if enough symptoms of inattention, but not hyperactivity-impulsivity, were present for the past 6 months.

Predominantly hyperactive-impulsive presentation: if enough symptoms of hyperactivity-impulsivity but not inattention were present for the past 6 months.

Because symptoms can change over time, the presentation may change over time as well.

Reprinted with permission from American Psychiatric Association. (2013). *Diagnostic and statistical manual of mental disorders*, ed 5. Washington DC: American Psychiatric Association.

A

ATTENTION-DEFICIT HYPERACTIVITY DISORDER

MANAGEMENT

I. Children and adolescents
- A. Stimulant medications are the mainstay of treatment for ADHD (approximately 75% of children respond to stimulants initially) and work better than behavioral modification alone, as shown by - Multimodal Treatment Study of ADHD sponsored by the National Institutes of Health. Fig. 7 shows an algorithm for the psychopharmacological treatment of ADHD.
- B. Children with comorbid anxiety or oppositional behavior do best with the combination of medication and behavioral management.
- C. Pharmacological treatment of attention deficit hyperactivity disorder (Table 13).
- D. The development of time-released medications (e.g., Concerta, Adderall XR) has helped with compliance and with preventing attention from waning due to short-acting medication (immediate-release methylphenidate typically lasts about four hours). It allows children to avoid the stigma of receiving medication from school nurses.
- E. Side effects of stimulants, such as weight loss, rebound depression, flat affect, insomnia, decreased appetite, irritability, headache, stomachache, growth suppression, and cardiovascular effects, can limit the treatment effectiveness. Some children may take drug holidays, such as summer vacation, when attentional needs are relaxed.
- F. Tourette's disorder and tics are not a contraindication to stimulant use in ADHD although stimulants may unmask tics.
- G. Non-stimulants are used in children who fail to respond to or cannot tolerate the stimulants and in those with significant comorbid conditions such as anxiety, depression, tics, aggression, or substance abuse.
- H. In addition to medication, treatment should also focus on behavioral modifications (setting goals, defining progress, determining incentives), parents' skill training, educational accommodations (preferential seating, extended time/separate testing site for testing, organizational supports), cognitive behavioral therapy, and social skills training.

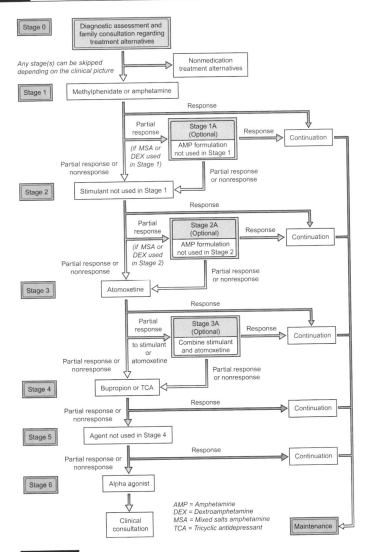

FIGURE 7

Algorithm for the psychopharmacological treatment of attention-deficit hyperactivity disorder. (From Pliszka, S. R., Crismon, M. L., Hughes, C. W., et al. 2006. The Texas Children's Medication Algorithm Project: revision of the algorithm for pharmacotherapy of attention-deficit/hyperactivity disorder. *J Am Acad Child Adolesc Psychiatry 45*, 642–657.)

TABLE 13	
PHARMACOLOGIC TREATMENT OF ATTENTION-DEFICIT HYPERACTIVITY DISORDER	
Stimulants	Methylphenidate (Ritalin, Focalin, Concerta, Daytrana), dextroamphetamine (Dexedrine, Adderall, Vyvanse)
α-Agonists	Clonidine (Catapres), guanfacine (Tenex), Intuniv
Antidepressants	SSRIs; tricyclic antidepressants; bupropion (Wellbutrin); trazodone; SSNRIs (venlafaxine [Effexor], duloxetine [Cymbalta]); MAOIs (selegiline [Deprenyl])
Antimanic	Lithium carbonate (Lithium)
Mood stabilizers	Carbamazepine (Tegretol), divalproex sodium (Depakote), gabapentin (Neurontin), topiramate (Topamax)
Beta-blockers	Propranolol (Inderal), atenolol (Tenormin)
Anxiolytics	Buspirone (BuSpar); clonazepam (Klonopin), SSRIs
Atypical neuroleptics	Risperidone (Risperdal, Zyprexa) and others
Nonstimulants	Atomoxetine (Strattera), modafinil (Provigil)

MAOI, Monoamine oxidase inhibitor; *SSNRI*, selective serotonin and norepinephrine reuptake inhibitor; *SSRI*, selective serotonin reuptake inhibitor.

Data from Biederman, J., & Faraone, V. (2005). ADHD. *Lancet, 366*, 237–245; Dopheide, J. A., & Pliszka, S. R. (2009). Attention-deficit-hyperactivity disorder: an update. *Pharmacotherapy, 29*, 66–79; and Swanson, J. M., Greenhill, L. L., Lopez, F. A., et al. (2006). Modafinil film-coated tablets in children and adolescents with attention-deficit/hyperactivity disorder: results of a randomized, double-blind, placebo-controlled, fixed-dose study followed by abrupt discontinuation. *J Clin Psychiatry, 67*, 137–147.

II. Adults
  A. ADHD is being increasingly recognized in adulthood, but the diagnosis requires obligate onset in childhood, even if it was not diagnosed as such. The presentation is similar, but they are of the primarily inattentive subtype.
  B. Thirty percent of ADHD patients diagnosed in childhood will outgrow their symptoms, 40% will continue to display significant symptoms often accompanied by depression and anxiety, and 30% will decline with the development of additional psychopathologies such as alcoholism, substance abuse, or antisocial personality disorders. Thus 60% to 70% of people with ADHD in childhood will continue to be symptomatic into adulthood where it often impacts social or occupational functioning.
  C. Many patients may discontinue medication in early adulthood, only to find that tasks such as college coursework or job-related functions are difficult because of the lack of ability to organize and attend to details.
  D. Differential diagnosis includes adult-onset attentional disorders (e.g., hypothyroidism, HIV, traumatic brain injury, dementia, focal lesions, medication effects), substance abuse, and mood disorders.
  E. The treatments for adults is the same as that for children. However, the stimulants often are dosed by weight, and higher dosages may be required for efficacy in adults.

REFERENCES

Daroff, R. B., Jankovic, J., Mazziotta, J. C., & Pomeroy, S. L. (Eds.), (2016). *Bradley's neurology in clinical practice*, ed 7. Philadelphia: Elsevier.

Dulac, O., Lassonde, M., & Sarnat, H. B. (Eds.), (2013). *Handbook of Clinical Neurology: vol. 111/112/113. Pediatric neurology, Part I/II/III*, ed 1. New York: Elsevier.

AUTISM

I. Autism Spectrum Disorders

Autism spectrum disorders (ASD) are a group of neurodevelopmental disorders characterized by impairments in two areas: (1) deficits in social communication and social interactions and (2) restricted and repetitive patterns of behavior, interests, and activities. There is a significant increase in the prevalence of ASD since the 1990s with a reported prevalence rate of 14.7 per 1000 (1 in 68) among 8-year-olds.

Normal early milestones are followed by regression at the age of 1 to 3 years in approximately one-third of children with ASD. Language regression is estimated in 25%, and both language and social regression are present in 38%. Approximately 55% of individuals with autism have intellectual disabilities (IQ < 70). One-third of patients with autism develop epilepsy.

The DSM-V Criteria for Autistic Spectrum Disorder requires an individual to exhibit three deficits in social communication and at least two symptoms in the category of the restricted range of activities/repetitive behavior. See Table 14: DSM-V Criteria for an Autistic Spectrum Disorder.

Long-term prognosis correlates with language skills at 5 to 6 years of age with those having conversational language doing significantly better than children with little or no language.

Diagnostic evaluation should include clinical history, observation, screening questionnaires and formal audiological assessment. Electroencephalography should be performed if there are seizures or history of developmental regression. Imaging is rarely indicated. Treatment consists of special education, behavior modification programs and medications targeted at specific behaviors. See Table 15: Medications for Autism Spectrum Disorders.

II. Syndromes with prominent autistic features

A. Fragile X syndrome: the second most common cause of mental retardation; dysmorphic facies, macro-orchidism after puberty, hyperactive; one-third of female heterozygotes are mildly retarded.

B. Angelman's syndrome ("happy puppet" syndrome): maternal 15q deletion; infantile feeding problems, severe retardation, microcephaly, autism, jerky puppet-like ataxia, paroxysmal laughter, protruding

TABLE 14

DSM-V CRITERIA FOR AN AUTISTIC SPECTRUM DISORDER

DIAGNOSTIC CRITERIA FOR 299.00 AUTISM SPECTRUM DISORDER

A. Persistent deficits in social communication and social interaction across multiple contexts, as manifested by the following, currently or by history (examples are illustrative, not exhaustive):

1. Deficits in social-emotional reciprocity, ranging, for example, from abnormal social approach and failure of normal back-and-forth conversation; to reduced sharing of interests, emotions, or affect; to failure to initiate or respond to social interactions.

2. Deficits in nonverbal communicative behaviors used for social interaction, ranging, for example, from poorly integrated verbal and nonverbal communication; to abnormalities in eye contact and body language or deficits in understanding and use of gestures; to a total lack of facial expressions and nonverbal communication.

3. Deficits in developing, maintaining, and understanding relationships, ranging, for example, from difficulties adjusting behavior to suit various social contexts; to difficulties in sharing imaginative play or in making friends; to absence of interest in peers.

Specify current severity:

Severity is based on social communication impairments and restricted, repetitive patterns of behavior.

B. Restricted, repetitive patterns of behavior, interests, or activities, as manifested by at least two of the following, currently or by history (examples are illustrative, not exhaustive):

1. Stereotyped or repetitive motor movements, use of objects, or speech (e.g., simple motor stereotypes, lining up toys or flipping objects, echolalia, idiosyncratic phrases).

2. Insistence on sameness, inflexible adherence to routines, or ritualized patterns of verbal or nonverbal behavior (e.g., extreme distress at small changes, difficulties with transitions, rigid thinking patterns, greeting rituals, need to take same route or eat same food every day).

3. Highly restricted, fixated interests that are abnormal in intensity or focus (e.g., strong attachment to or preoccupation with unusual objects, excessively circumscribed or perseverative interests).

4. Hyper- or hyporeactivity to sensory input or unusual interest in sensory aspects of the environment (e.g. apparent indifference to pain/temperature, adverse response to specific sounds or textures, excessive smelling or touching of objects, visual fascination with lights or movement).

Specify current severity:

Severity is based on social communication impairments and restricted, repetitive patterns of behavior.

C. Symptoms must be present in the early developmental period (but may not become fully manifest until social demands exceed limited capacities, or may be masked by learned strategies in later life).

D. Symptoms cause clinically significant impairment in social, occupational, or other important areas of current functioning.

Continued

TABLE 14
DSM-V CRITERIA FOR AN AUTISTIC SPECTRUM DISORDER—CONT'D

E. These disturbances are not better explained by intellectual disability (intellectual developmental disorder) or global developmental delay. Intellectual disability and autism spectrum disorder frequently co-occur; to make comorbid diagnoses of autism spectrum disorder and intellectual disability, social communication should be below that expected for general developmental level.

Note: Individuals with a well-established DSM-IV diagnosis of autistic disorder, Asperger disorder, or pervasive developmental disorder not otherwise specified should be given the diagnosis of autism spectrum disorder. Individuals who have marked deficits in social communication, but whose symptoms do not otherwise meet criteria for autism spectrum disorder, should be evaluated for social (pragmatic) communication disorder.

Specify if:

With or without accompanying intellectual impairment

With or without accompanying language impairment

Associated with a known medical or genetic condition or environmental factor

Associated with another neurodevelopmental, mental, or behavioral disorder

With catatonia (refer to the criteria for catatonia associated with another mental disorder)

Adapted from American Psychiatric Association. (2013). *Diagnostic and statistical manual of mental disorders*, ed 5. Washington DC: American Psychiatric Association; and https://www.cdc.gov/ncbddd/autism/hcp-dsm.html.

TABLE 15
MEDICATIONS FOR AUTISM SPECTRUM DISORDERS

Hyperactivity and inattention	Psychostimulants (methylphenidate; dextroamphetamine); α-agonists (clonidine, tenex, intuniv, kapvay)
Obsessive-compulsive behaviors and anxiety	Selective serotonin reuptake inhibitors: fluoxetine (Prozac), sertraline (Zoloft), paroxetine (Paxil), fluvoxamine (Luvox), citalopram (Celexa)
	Anxiolytics: Buspirone (BuSpar)
	Tricyclics: clomipramine (Anafranil)
Aggressive and impulsive behaviors	Atypical neuroleptics: risperidone (Risperdal), olanzapine (Zyprexa), ziprasidone (Geodon), aripiprazole (Abilify)
	α-agonists: clonidine (Catapres), guanfacine (Tenex), Intuniv, Kapvay
	Beta-blockers: propranolol (Inderal)
	Mood stabilizers: carbamazepine (Tegretol), divalproex sodium (Depakote), gabapentin (Neurontin), topiramate (Topamax), lithium (Lithium)
Tics/stereotypies	Clonidine, Tenex, clonazepam (Klonopin), pimozide (Orap), haloperidol (Haldol), risperidone (Risperdal), baclofen (Lioresal), deep brain stimulation
Self-mutilation	Naloxone (Narcan), propranolol, fluoxetine, clomipramine, lithium
Psychosis	Neuroleptics: Haloperidol, risperidone, olanzapine, ziprasidone
Seizures	Depakote, Lamictal, Trileptal, Tegretol, Topamax

Modified from Soorya, L., Kiarashi, J., Hollander, E. (2008). Psychopharmacologic interventions for repetitive behaviors in autism spectrum disorders. *Child Adolesc Psychiatr Clin N Am, 17*, 753–771.

tongue. By contrast, Prader-Willi syndrome (paternal 15q deletion) presents with hypotonia at birth; dysmorphism, mental retardation; and later, hyperphagia, hypogonadism, Pickwickian syndrome.

C. Rett's syndrome: girls develop normally until 6 to 12 months of age; thereafter, regression with acquired microcephaly, ataxia, and autistic-like behavior; repetitive hand-wringing or hand-wetting movements; irregular breathing.

D. Tuberous sclerosis; hypomelanosis of Ito.

E. Metabolic disorders with autistic features include phenylketonuria, hyperammonemia/urea cycle defects, creatinine synthesis/creatinine transporter defects, lysosomal disorders, Lemli-Opitz syndrome, purine and Pyrimidine abnormalities.

REFERENCES

Daroff, R. B., Jankovic, J., Mazziotta, J. C., & Pomeroy, S. L. (Eds.), (2016). *Bradley's neurology in clinical practice*, ed 7. Philadelphia: Elsevier.

Dulac, O., Lassonde, M., & Sarnat, H. B. (Eds.), (2013). *Handbook of clinical neurology: vol. 111/112/113. Pediatric neurology, Part I/II/III*, ed 1. New York: Elsevier.

AUTONOMIC DYSFUNCTION

CLASSIFICATION

Autonomic failure occurs either as an isolated syndrome or in association with spinocerebellar or parkinsonian features. Autonomic dysreflexia can occur in the context of spinal cord lesions above the T6 level. This is mediated by an interruption in the brain's ability to dilate the splanchnic vascular bed and manifests as a marked rise in blood pressure, along with headache, goose flesh, diaphoresis, flushing, or chills; it affects half to three-quarters of the population. Acute pandysautonomia may occur as a variant of Guillain-Barré syndrome or may complicate more typical cases of Guillain-Barré syndrome. Several hereditary, acquired, or peripheral small fiber neuropathies can have autonomic features. A neurologist comes across these patients frequently with questions of how to differentiate between the cardiogenic and neurogenic etiology of syncopal events (Table 16). Disorders marked by autonomic dysfunction are given in Table 17.

DIAGNOSIS

Autonomic dysfunction is suspected in the presence of orthostatic hypotension or other derangements of cardiovascular regulation, decreased sweating, bladder or bowel dysfunction, impotence, or pupillary abnormalities. The following screening tests can be performed at the bedside:

I. Orthostatic blood pressure and heart rate (HR): An estimate is made of the time typically required to produce symptoms while standing. After 20 minutes of inactivity, baseline supine HR and blood pressure are

A

AUTONOMIC DYSFUNCTION

FEATURES THAT DISTINGUISH NEUROGENIC AND NON-NEUROGENIC OH

	Non-neurogenic OH	Neurogenic OH
Frequency	Frequent	Less frequent
Onset	Variable	Usually chronic (Acute in immune-mediated neuropathies and ganglionopathies)
Causes	Intravascular volume loss Inadequate vasoconstriction Heart failure Physical deconditioning Medications	Failure to increase in sympathetic activity upon standing due to defective norepinephrine release (Sympathetic activity can be normal in MSA, but would not be as elevated as in POTS, same with the increase in norepinephrine)
Outcome	Resolves when the underlying cause is corrected	Chronic disorder
Sympathetic activity	Elevated	Low or absent
Increase in heart rate upon standing	Pronounced	Mild or absent
Blood pressure overshoot (phase 4) in Valsalva	Present	Absent
Increase in norepinephrine upon standing	Normal or enhanced	Blunted or absent
Additional symptoms of autonomic failure	No	Constipation Erectile dysfunction Urinary abnormalities Sweating abnormalities
Concurrent neurological findings	None	Parkinsonism Cerebellar symptoms Cognitive issues Neuropathy

Modified from Kaufmann, H., Norcliffe-Kaufmann, L., Palma, J. A. (2015). Droxidopa in neurogenic orthostatic hypotension. *Expert Rev Cardiovasc Ther, 13*(8), 875–891.

recorded. The standing measurements are taken at 3 minutes or after the estimated time interval that it takes the patient to become symptomatic. The cuff on the arm is kept at the level of the heart at all times. Orthostatic hypotension is defined as a reduction in systolic blood pressure of at least 20 mm Hg or a reduction in diastolic blood pressure of at least 10 mm Hg within 3 minutes of standing. HR normally increases by 11 to 29 beats/min immediately on standing. If the patient has had electrocardiogram (ECG) leads placed prior to testing, the ratio between the longest R-R interval (slowest rate), which occurs about 30 beats after standing, divided by the shortest R-R interval, which occurs at about 15 beats, is called the 30:15

TABLE 17

CLASSIFICATION OF AUTONOMIC DISORDERS

I. Diseases affecting the central nervous system
  A. Progressive autonomic failure (PAF), idiopathic orthostatic hypotension
    1. Pure PAF
    2. PAF with multiple-system atrophy (Shy-Drager syndrome)
      a. With parkinsonian features
      b. With spinocerebellar degeneration
  B. Parkinson's disease
  C. Spinal cord lesions
  D. Wernicke encephalopathy
  E. Miscellaneous diseases
    1. Cerebrovascular disease
    2. Brainstem tumors
    3. Multiple sclerosis
    4. Adie's syndrome
    5. Tabes dorsalis
II. Diseases affecting the peripheral autonomic nervous system
  A. Disorders with no associated sensory-motor peripheral neuropathy
    1. Acute and subacute autonomic neuropathy
      a. Pandysautonomia
      b. Cholinergic dysautonomia
    2. Botulism
  B. Diseases associated with sensory-motor peripheral neuropathy in which autonomic dysfunction is clinically important
    1. Diabetes
    2. Amyloidosis
    3. Guillain-Barré syndrome
    4. Acute intermittent porphyria
    5. Familial dysautonomia (Riley-Day syndrome: hereditary motor-sensory neuropathy [HMSN III])
    6. Chronic sensory and autonomic neuropathy
  C. Disorders in which autonomic dysfunction is usually clinically unimportant
    1. Alcohol-induced neuropathy
    2. Toxic neuropathies (caused by vincristine sulfate, acrylamide, heavy metals, perhexiline maleate, or organic solvents)
    3. HMSNs I, II and V
    4. Malignancy
    5. Vitamin B12 deficiency
    6. Rheumatoid arthritis
    7. Chronic renal failure
    8. Systemic lupus erythematosus
    9. Mixed connective tissue disease
    10. Fabry's disease
    11. Chronic inflammatory neuropathy

Modified from McLeod, J. G., & Tuck, R. R. (1987). Disorders of the autonomic nervous system: Part 1. Pathophysiology and clinical features. *Ann Neurol, 21*(5), 419–430.

A

AUTONOMIC DYSFUNCTION

ratio. Normal 30:15 ratio is above 1.04 with slight age-related variation. Orthostatic BP assesses sympathetic adrenergic efferents, and the HR tests assess parasympathetic cholinergic (cardiovagal) efferents; both assess baroreceptor and CN IX and X integrity. Of note, HR may not change on standing if the patient is on beta blockers.

II. Respiratory-HR variation: The patient breathes deeply at 6 breaths/min, and the inspiration and expiration time are noted on the ECG tracing. HR difference between inspiration and expiration of less than 10 beats/min, or an expiration-to-inspiration ratio of R-R intervals of less than 1:2, is abnormal in individuals under the age of 40. Normally, the increase in HR during inspiration (respiratory sinus arrhythmia) is due to decreased cardiovagal activity. This is the single best cardiovagal test, although the effect decreases with the increase in age.

III. Tests of pupillary function: Installation of dilute 0.1% epinephrine into the conjunctival sac has no effect on normal pupil but dilates a pupil with postganglionic sympathetic innervation lesion; this reaction is due to denervation supersensitivity. Similarly, dilute 0.125% pilocarpine causes little or no constriction in normal pupils but causes miosis if abnormal parasympathetic innervation is present. Pharmacological tests are distorted by corneal trauma (e.g., contact lenses, corneal reflex testing) within 24 hours of administering the eye drops.

IV. Valsalva maneuver: Normally, a decrease in an inter-beat interval during a fall in BP with BP overshoot will cause the HR to increase at the end of the procedure.

V. Other tests: More extensive autonomic testing includes measurement of plasma norepinephrine levels and determination of denervation supersensitivity and tilt-table testing, baroreflex sensitivity testing, thermal sweat testing, quantitative sudomotor axon reflex testing, and skin blood flow measurements.

TREATMENT (FIG. 8)

Management of orthostatic hypotension begins with supportive measures:

I. Avoid or optimize drugs that cause orthostasis (e.g., diuretics, antihypertensives, and psychotropic agents).

II. Recommend avoiding sudden standing, straining during urination or defecation, excessive heat, high carbohydrate meals, and alcohol. Additionally, elevate the head of the bed to reduce nocturnal volume loss and increase salt intake, unless there is congestive heart failure.

III. Treat medical conditions that exacerbate hypotension, including anemia, heart failure, etc. Waist-high elastic garments may be helpful but are cumbersome.

PHARMACOLOGIC THERAPY

1. Fludrocortisone—Start at 0.1 mg/day and increase up to 0.4 to 0.6 mg/day based on response (max 1 mg/day). Complications: supine hypertension, peripheral edema, hypokalemia, and congestive heart failure.

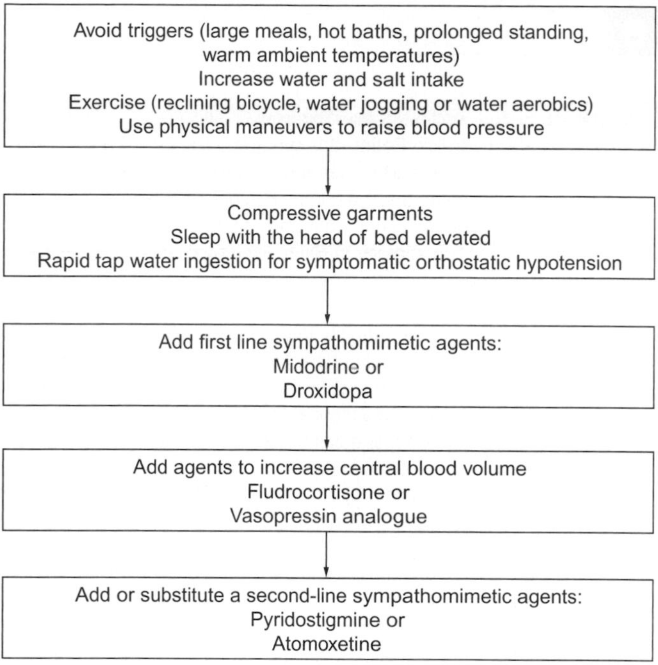

A

AUTONOMIC DYSFUNCTION

Avoid triggers (large meals, hot baths, prolonged standing,
warm ambient temperatures)
Increase water and salt intake
Exercise (reclining bicycle, water jogging or water aerobics)
Use physical maneuvers to raise blood pressure

Compressive garments
Sleep with the head of bed elevated
Rapid tap water ingestion for symptomatic orthostatic hypotension

Add first line sympathomimetic agents:
Midodrine or
Droxidopa

Add agents to increase central blood volume
Fludrocortisone or
Vasopressin analogue

Add or substitute a second-line sympathomimetic agents:
Pyridostigmine or
Atomoxetine

FIGURE 8

The Treatment Algorithm for Neurogenic Orthostatic. Hypotension Nonpharmacological
and pharmacological interventions to treat neurogenic orthostatic hypotension. (From
Freeman, et al. (2018). Orthostatic Hypotension: JACC State-of-the-Art Review. 72(11)).

2. Midodrine—Start at 5 mg TID; it can be titrated to 10 mg TID. It should not
be taken after mid-afternoon to avoid supine hypertension.
3. Mestinon—Start with 30 mg BID; it can be titrated to 60 mg TID. It has
synergistic effect with midodrine without causing supine hypertension.
4. Droxidopa—100 mg PO TID initially, not to exceed 600 mg TID.

REFERENCES

Figueroa, J. J. (2010). Preventing and treating orthostatic hypotension: As easy as
A, B, C. Cleve Clin J Med, 77(5), 298–306.
Kaufmann, H. (2015). Droxidopa in neurogenic orthostatic hypotension. Expert Rev
Cardiovasc Ther, 13(8), 875–891.

B

BALINT SYNDROME

Described in 1909 by Reszö Balint, this syndrome consists of a rare triad of simultagnosia, optic ataxia, and ocular apraxia owing to bilateral parietal lesions. As a result, patients present complex visual disturbances, or seem as if blind—unable to integrate visual input from their surroundings—despite preservation of vision. The etiology of Balint syndrome may include stroke, tumor, trauma, neurodegenerative diseases (e.g., Creutzfeldt-Jakob or Alzheimer disease), and HIV infection.

I. *Simultagnosia* refers to the inability to see the totality of a scene, despite being able to see the individual characteristics of the whole. A diagram showing a familiar scene with people and objects (e.g., the "Boston Cookie Theft," frequently used in the National Institutes of Health (NIH) stroke scale) can be used to test for simultagnosia. Unlike a normal patient able to describe actions of the objects and people in relationship to each other, someone with simultagnosia may only be able to describe parts of the scene or only parts of objects, but not their relationships to each other. Lesion to the temporo-parietal junction is typically responsible.

II. *Ocular ataxia* refers to difficulty reaching for objects under visual guidance despite normal limb strength and intact joint position sense. Though typical of *bilateral* lesions to the parietal lobe, it has been described in unilateral superior parietal lobule lesions independently of Balint syndrome patients.

III. *Optic apraxia*, described originally as "psychic paralysis of gaze," refers to an inability to shift gaze voluntarily toward objects of interest despite unrestricted eye movements. This is due to impairment in saccade planning arising from bilateral parietal lesions.

While traditionally Balint syndrome arises from bilateral occipitoparietal lesions, comprehensive reviews suggest that different combinations of lesions in areas deriving from the parietal lobe can yield this presentation. For example, bifrontal lesions resulting in attentional impairment or right hemispheric lesions can produce a neglect syndrome that may mimic Balint syndrome.

REFERENCES

Chechlacz, M., & Humphreys, G. (2014). The enigma of Bálint's syndrome: neural substrates and cognitive deficits. *J Frontiers in Human Neurosci*, *8*, 1–3.

Rizzo, M., & Vecera, S. P. (2002). Psychoanatomical substrates of Bálint's syndrome. *J Neurol Neurosurg Psychiatry*, *72*, 162–178.

BENZODIAZEPINES

Benzodiazepines are used in the treatment of anxiety, insomnia, epilepsy, catatonia, vertigo, and certain movement disorders in addition to management of ethanol withdrawal. Non-parenteral formulations are well known in the acute treatment of epileptic seizures, and intranasal and intramuscular injections are being developed. Prolonged use of any drug in this class may cause physical dependence, particularly in patients with a history of alcohol or substance abuse. Benzodiazepines are one of the top three classes of drugs responsible for death from overdose. Therefore, only the lowest effective doses should be used for the shortest possible period. Side effects include sedation, suppression of rapid eye movement (REM) sleep, amnesia, agitation, and gait disorder. Withdrawal symptoms may occur after 4 to 6 weeks of use and include flulike symptoms, rebound insomnia, irritability, seizures, nausea, headache, tremor, and muscle cramps. In those at risk for withdrawal, the dose should be tapered over several weeks. Acute intoxication with depressed mental status may be reversed with the benzodiazepine receptor antagonist flumazenil, starting at 0.2 mg IV over 30 seconds with a risk of precipitating seizures in the predisposed individual. Failure to respond to a total dose of 5 mg makes it unlikely that sedation is due to benzodiazepines.

REFERENCES

Mula, M. (2017). New non-intravenous routes for benzodiazepines in epilepsy: a clinician perspective. *CNS Drugs*, *31*(1), 11–17. https://doi.org/10.1007/s40263-016-0398-4.

Rasmussen, S. A., Mazurek, M. F., & Rosebush, P. I. (2016). Catatonia: our current understanding of its diagnosis, treatment and pathophysiology. *World J Psychiatry*, 6(4), 391–398. https://doi.org/10.5498/wjp.v6.i4.391.

BLADDER

Normal bladder function is controlled by bladder stretch receptors (generating sympathetic input to the spinal cord), the bladder wall detrusor muscle (activated by parasympathetic outflow), the internal sphincter (smooth muscle), and the external sphincter (striated muscle under voluntary control). Neural control is mediated by cerebral hemispheric centers (orbitofrontal cortex), the pontine micturition left, the sacral micturition left, and the hypogastric, pelvic, and pudendal nerves (Fig. 9). These centers and nerves work together to achieve: (1) storage of urine without leaking, (2) adequate perception of increased intravesical pressure, (3) release of cortical inhibition of emptying in appropriate circumstances, (4) proper synergy of urinary tract muscular structures, and (5) complete bladder emptying.

Disorders of bladder control can be caused by local factors, such as previous childbirth, pelvic surgery, or urinary tract infection, or disorders of the upper or lower motor neuron (Table 18).

Detrusor hyperreflexia, resulting from cerebral cortical dysfunction, is a deficit of normal inhibitory mechanisms that occurs when the micturition reflex is intact and the lesion is above the pontine micturition left. Symptoms include frequency, urgency, and urge incontinence. Common neurologic disorders leading to uninhibited bladder contraction include stroke, mass lesion, and hydrocephalus.

Bladder dyssynergia, due to suprasacral spinal cord lesions, leads to loss of detrusor-sphincter coordination. Simultaneous contraction of detrusor and

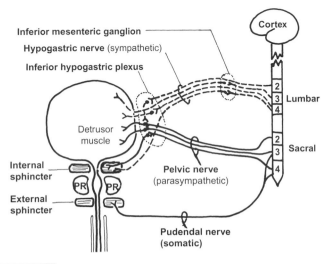

Neuroanatomy of bladder control.

sphincter can lead to increased intravesical pressures and upper urinary tract damage. Multiple sclerosis, a spinal cord tumor or trauma, vascular malformation, and herniated intervertebral disc are common causes.

Detrusor areflexia is caused by lesions of the sacral micturition left or its connections to the bladder. Sphincter function is preserved but detrusor contraction is not activated, commonly resulting in overflow incontinence. Causes include myelopathy resulting from a herniated disc or tumor and interruption of the reflex arc as a result of pelvic or pudendal nerve injury following trauma or operation.

Autonomic dysreflexia occurs after spinal cord lesions above the region of major sympathetic outflow (T5–L2). Splanchnic sympathetic outflow is no longer moderated by supraspinal centers, and bladder distention, catheterization, or other manipulation may cause an acute syndrome of severe hypertension, anxiety, diaphoresis, headache, and bradycardia. Prompt recognition and treatment, including blood pressure control and treatment of local bladder problems, are essential.

Table 19 includes agents traditionally used in the pharmacologic management of upper and lower motor neuron bladder dysfunction. Tolterodine (Detrol) is a nonselective antimuscarinic agent which can be used for treatment of detrusor hyperreflexia (symptoms of frequency, urgency, urge incontinence). Its efficacy is equivalent to that of oxybutynin, and it offers the advantages of twice-daily dosing and fewer anticholinergic side effects.

TABLE 18

BLADDER DYSFUNCTION

	Upper Motor Neuron	Lower Motor Neuron
Characteristic Feature	Decreased capacity for storage	Decreased emptying ability
Cause	Injury to cerebral hemisphere or to spinal cord above T12 (trauma, multiple sclerosis, stroke, tumor)	1. Sensory: diabetes mellitus, tabes dorsalis 2. Motor: amyotrophic lateral sclerosis 3. Mixed sensory and motor: spinal dysraphism (meningomyelocele), tumor or trauma of lower cord, conus, or cauda
History	Urge incontinence with dry intervals Wet at night	Overflow incontinence Urinary retention Straining to void Wet or dry at night
Bulbocavernosus Reflex	Present	Absent
Cystometrogram	Hyperreflexic bladder Small bladder capacity Small residual volumes Vesicoureteral reflux (and upper urinary tract damage) may occur at peak pressures.	Flaccid bladder Large bladder capacity Large residual volumes Vesicoureteral reflux (and upper urinary tract damage) can occur with persisting urinary retention.

B

BLADDER

TABLE 19	
TREATMENT OF BLADDER DYSFUNCTION	
Upper Motor Neuron	**Lower Motor Neuron**
Treatment goal: increase storage capacity Treatment	Increase bladder tone; avoid storage of large urinary volumes; promote bladder emptying

Oxybutynin (Ditropan) anticholinergic dose:
    Child: 2.5 mg PO bid–tid
 	
    Adult: 5 mg PO tid–qid
	Bethanechol (Urecholine) cholinergic dose:
	    Child: 5 mg/day, increase as below for adult
	    Adult: 2.5–10 mg SC tid–qid, or 5–50 mg PO tid–qid

Side effects: dry mouth, blurred vision	Contraindicated asthma, hyperthyroidism, coronary artery disease, ulcer disease

Propantheline bromide (Pro-Banthine) antimuscarinic agent
Dose:
    Child: not currently approved for use (USA)
    Adult: 15–30 mg PO tid–qid
	Phenoxybenzamine (Dibenzyline) anti-adrenergic
	Dose:
	    Child: 0.3–0.5 mg/kg/day
	    Adult: 10–30 mg/day
	Side effects: retrograde ejaculation, drowsiness, orthostatic hypotension

Side effects: dry mouth, blurred vision
Imipramine (Tofranil) mixed anticholinergic and adrenergic
Dose:
    Child: 1.5–2 mg/kg qid
    Adult: 25 mg PO qid
Side effects: dry mouth, blurred vision, constipation, tachycardia, sweating, fatigue, tremor	

Intermittent self-catheterization	Intermittent self-catheterization or Credé maneuver

REFERENCES

Fowler, C. J., & O'Malley, K. J. (2003). Investigation and management of neurogenic bladder dysfunction. *J Neurol Neurosurg Psychiatry, 74*, iv27–iv31.

Groen, J., et al. (2016). Summary of European Association of Urology (EAU) Guidelines on Neuro-Urology. *Eur Urol, 69*(2).

BOTULINUM TOXIN

Botulinum toxin is produced by the bacterium *Clostridium botulinum.* There are seven different known serotypes: A, B, C1, D, E, F, and G. One of the most potent toxins known to man, botulinum toxin's first clinical use was in 1981, when it was shown to be an effective strabismus treatment. Since then, the clinical literature has exploded with new uses for this drug. To date, the Food and Drug Administration (FDA) has given approval for its use in treatment of strabismus, cervical dystonia, blepharospasm, hemifacial spasm, axillary hyperhidrosis, and cosmetic treatment of frown lines.

Botulinum toxin is injected locally, at the site of the muscle whose action is to be inhibited. Onset of action is approximately 2 days after injection. The treatment should be effective for about 3 months, at which time the injections must be repeated.

Adverse reactions depend on the site of injection. For treatment of blepharospasm, ptosis, dry eyes, and punctate keratitis are common side effects, whereas injection of neck muscles in treatment of cervical dystonia can result in dysphagia, upper respiratory infection, neck pain, and headache. Hypersensitivity reactions can occur. Botulinum toxin resistance after repeated injections may be due to the formation of antibodies. Development of neutralizing antibodies appears to be minimized with smaller doses of botulinum toxin and when at least 2 to 3 months elapse between doses.

Once injected, botulinum toxin inhibits the release of acetylcholine from presynaptic neurons, causing chemo denervation. It therefore affects not only the neuromuscular junction, but potentially cholinergic synapses in the autonomic nervous system.

Other potential uses for botulinum toxin include treatment of spasticity (e.g., in cerebral palsy, stroke, multiple sclerosis), headache, pain, dystonia, tics, stuttering, constipation, anal fissures, and other neurologic and non-neurologic ailments.

REFERENCES

Dutta, S. R., Passi, D., Singh, M., Singh, P., Sharma, S., & Sharma, A. (2016). Botulinum toxin the poison that heals: a brief review. *Nat J Maxillofacial Surg, 7*, 10–16.

Mehanna, R., & Jankovic, J. (2014). Botulinum neurotoxins as therapeutics. In K. Richard (Ed.), *Handbook of neurotoxicity* (pp. 553–590). New York: Springer Science+Business Media.

BRACHIAL PLEXUS

The brachial plexus (Fig. 10) comprises the anastomoses derived from the anterior primary rami of vertebral segments C5 to T1. The plexus may be divided conceptually into the supraclavicular plexus (proximal to the division), and the infraclavicular plexus (distal to the division). The supraclavicular plexus has upper (C5 and C6 roots and upper trunk), middle (C7 root and middle trunk), and lower (C8) parts. Injuries to the supraclavicular plexus clinically resemble root injuries while those to the infraclavicular plexus clinically resemble terminal nerve injuries. Injuries to the supraclavicular plexus are more frequent, usually more severe, and usually have a less

B

BRACHIAL PLEXUS

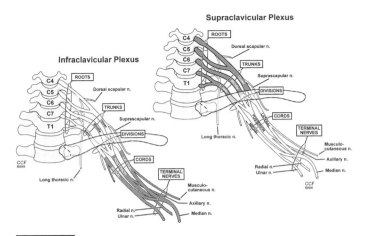

Supraclavicular Plexus

Infraclavicular Plexus

FIGURE 10

Brachial plexus. (From Wilbourn, A. J. (2007). Plexopathies. *Neurol Clin, 25*(1), 139–171.)

favorable outcome. Injuries to the upper part of the supraclavicular plexus tend to recover more completely as these lesions are more commonly demyelinating, located closer to the muscles they innervate, and extraforaminal (i.e., surgically accessible). Causes of injury are also different between the two sites. Owing to its relative lack of protection, the supraclavicular plexus is more frequently damaged than the infraclavicular plexus.

CLINICAL PRESENTATION

Upper trunk lesions result in weakness of shoulder abduction, external rotation, forearm flexion and supination, and variable amounts of triceps weakness with sensory loss in the deltoid region, the external aspect of the upper arm, and the radial side of the forearm. Lower trunk lesions result in weakness of the intrinsic hand muscles, thenar muscles, long finger flexors, and finger extensors with sensory loss in the medial arm, medial forearm, and the ulnar hand. Infraclavicular plexopathies' clinical presentation mimics those of single or multiple peripheral nerve lesions. Lateral cord lesions result in weakness of forearm flexion and pronation and wrist flexion with sensory loss in the radial forearm and the first three digits of the hand. Posterior cord lesions result in complete radial nerve palsies with additional weakness of shoulder abduction and adduction. Sensory loss involves the lateral arm, posterior arm and forearm, and the radial dorsal hand. Medial cord lesions result in a presentation that is almost identical to a lower trunk lesion, except that finger extensors are spared. Sensory loss again involves the medial arm, forearm, and ulnar hand.

ETIOLOGIES

Trauma is the most common cause of damage to the supraclavicular brachial plexus with the most severe traction injuries resulting in root avulsions (which usually result in severe pain and irreversible loss of function) and less severe traction injury resulting in demyelination or axonal loss in either the upper or lower trunks. Chronic pressure on the shoulder may result in upper trunk injury (Pack palsy). Obstetric paralysis due to shoulder dystocia can damage either the upper trunk (Erb palsy) or the lower trunk (Klumpke palsy). Other causes of supraclavicular plexus injury include rucksack paralysis, burner syndrome, postmedian sternotomy lesions, true neurogenic thoracic outlet syndrome, classic postoperative paralysis, and neoplastic invasion. Infraclavicular plexopathies' etiologies have less site predilection. Lesions at the cord level include radiation plexopathies, mostly in women after radiation therapy for breast cancer. Symptoms usually begin 12 to 20 months after radiation therapy. If present, myokymia (a spontaneous discharge pattern on electromyography) is highly suggestive of radiation plexopathy. At the terminal nerve level, the median nerve and the radial nerve (with crutch palsies) are the most affected. The musculocutaneous nerve is more affected by surgical procedures. Neuralgic amyotrophy (Parsonage-Turner syndrome, idiopathic brachial plexitis) is a common non-site-specific brachial plexopathy with clinical presentation that includes severe shoulder pain followed about a week later by weakness affecting preferentially the anterior interosseous, posterior interosseous, long thoracic, suprascapular, and axillary nerves.

REFERENCES

Ferrante, M. A. (2004). Brachial plexopathies: classification, causes, and consequences. *Muscle Nerve, 30*(5), 547–568.
Katirji, B., et al. (Eds.), (2014). *Neuromuscular disorders*, ed 2. New York: Springer.

BRAIN DEATH

Brain death is the irreversible loss of all clinical brain functions, including the brainstem, and consists of irreversible coma, absent brainstem reflexes, and apnea. Brain death is accepted as a definition of death in the United States, although some criteria vary by state and institution. In an effort to standardize the diagnosis and improve consistency, the American Academy of Neurology has published and updated their practice parameter on the determination of brain death in adults. In practice, there remain inconsistency and poor adherence to an appropriate, structured determination of brain death.

DIAGNOSIS OF BRAIN DEATH
Prerequisites
An irreversible and proximate cause of coma must be identified. It is critical to exclude with complete certainty all possible confounders. A normal core temperature ($>36°C$) and normal systolic blood pressure (ideally $\geq$ 100 mm Hg) must be achieved. Exclude lingering effects of drugs. Five to seven half-lives should pass prior to brain death evaluation. When possible, serum levels of drugs should be checked and be below therapeutic levels. Drugs with long elimination half-lives include phenobarbital (100 hours), diazepam (40 hours), amitriptyline (24 hours), and lorazepam (15 hours). Ethanol levels should be below 0.08%. The use of therapeutic hypothermia significantly prolongs the metabolism and elimination of drugs, necessitating additional caution.

THE CLINICAL EXAMINATION
Coma consists of no response to noxious stimulation, including eye movements/opening, and no motor response other than spinally mediated reflexes (e.g., reproducible/stereotyped triple flexion, finger flexion or extension, head turning, and slow arm lifting; these do not include decorticate or decerebrate posturing, which imply intact brainstem circuitry).

Absence of All Brainstem Functions
The brainstem is resilient and often among the last areas to lose function. The pupils should be unreactive to light (mid-position or dilated most often; constriction suggests medication effect). Corneal reflexes should be absent (sterile saline drops, sterile cotton). No response to oculocephalic and oculovestibular testing should be observed (elevate head of bed to 30 degrees, infuse 50 mL ice water into the external ear canal; no eye movements should be seen over 2 minutes; wait several minutes before contralateral testing). The gag reflex (jiggle endotracheal tube/move the uvula with a tongue depressor) and cough reflex should be absent (deep bronchial suctioning with at least two passes). No breathing effort should be apparent.

Apnea Testing
Apneic oxygenation diffusion to determine apnea is safe; however there is insufficient evidence comparing the safety of different methods of apnea testing. Prerequisites: (1) normotension, (2) normothermia, (3) euvolemia, (4) eucapnia ($PaCO_2$ 35–45 mm Hg), (5) no hypoxia, and (6) no prior evidence of CO_2 retention. Abort apnea testing if systolic blood pressure decreases to less than 90 mm Hg.
1. Prior to testing, preoxygenate with 100% FiO_2 for at least 10 min to PaO_2 greater than 200 mm Hg.
2. Reduce ventilator rate to 10 breaths/min. Reduce PEEP to 5 cm H_2O. Obtain baseline blood gas if pulse oximetry remains greater than 95%. Disconnect the patient from the ventilator, and thread a small catheter

through the endotracheal tube to supply 100% FiO_2 at 6 L/minute of oxygen. Do not obstruct the endotracheal tube.

3. Observe for any evidence of respiratory effort during apneic oxygenation for 8 to 10 minutes. If no respiratory effort is observed, repeat blood gas. The test supports a diagnosis of brain death if the PCO_2 rises to 60 mm Hg or more or increases at least 20 mm Hg above the patient's baseline.

Ancillary Testing

Ancillary tests such as electroencephalogram (EEG) (electrical silence), transcranial Doppler ultrasound (TCD) (to and fro pattern), angiogram (no intracranial flow), or positron emission tomography (PET) scan (empty vault sign) should not in any way replace the clinical assessment and have considerable inaccuracies. They are used in less than 5% of brain death cases in the United States and should generally be avoided but may be used for supplemental information when clinical examination cannot be fully performed due to patient factors or if the apnea test cannot be performed (e.g., due to hemodynamic instability, poor oxygenation, or chronic carbon dioxide retention).

Determining Brain Death in Children and Infants

The fundamentals of determining brain death in children and infants are the same as in adults with a few additional recommendations. Minimum observation periods of 24 hours for neonates (37 weeks gestation to term infants 30 days of age) and 12 hours for infants and children (>30 days to 18 years) are recommended. Two different attending physicians should perform two separate and complete examinations, including apnea testing. If apnea testing cannot be performed because of hemodynamic instability, desaturation to less than 85% or an inability to reach a $PaCO_2$ of $\geq$ 60 mm Hg, ancillary testing is suggested but cannot replace the clinical examination.

REFERENCES

Nakagawa, T. A., Ashwal, S., Mathur, M., et al. (2011). Guidelines for the determination of brain death in infants and children: an update of the 1987 Task Force recommendations. *Crit Care Med*, *39*, 2139–2155.

Wijdicks, E. F. (2015). Determining brain death. *Continuum (Minneap Minn)*, *21*, 1411–1424.

BULBAR PALSY

"Bulbar" refers to the "bulb," an archaic term for the medulla. Bulbar palsy refers to the clinical picture of weakness or paralysis of muscles supplied by those cranial nerves which have motor nuclei in the medulla: IX, X, XI, and XII. The weakness may be due to lesions of the nuclei or nerves. Involved muscles include those of the pharynx, larynx, sternocleidomastoid, upper trapezius, and tongue.

CLINICAL PRESENTATION

Clinical features include dysarthria, hoarseness, nasal voice, dysphagia, palatal deviation, diminished gag reflex, or weakness of the sternocleidomastoid, upper trapezius, or tongue muscles. Atrophy and fasciculation may be present.

ETIOLOGY

Degenerative: motor neuron disease variant (e.g., progressive bulbar palsy); see genetic syndromes below.

Infections: meningitis, encephalitis, herpes zoster, poliomyelitis, diphtheria, West Nile virus.

Inflammatory/Autoimmune: myasthenia gravis (MG), granulomatous disease, bone lesions (e.g., platybasia, Paget disease), and postirradiation changes, Guillain-Barré syndrome (GBS), Miller-Fisher syndrome, pharyngeal-cervical-brachial, poliomyelitis, Lyme disease, multiple sclerosis, neuromyelitis optica spectrum disorder.

Neoplastic: intra- and extramedullary posterior fossa tumors.

Vascular: cerebrovascular lesions of the brainstem; ischemic stroke, arteriovenous malformation (AVM), and aneurysms (uncommon).

Trauma/congenital: syringobulbia which may be associated with syringomyelia.

Genetic: riboflavin transporter deficiency neuronopathy which is similar if not identical to Brown-Vialetto-Van Laere syndrome (also known as pontobulbar palsy with deafness), Fazio-Londe syndrome (which lacks CN VIII involvement), and Kennedy disease (X-linked spinal and bulbar muscular atrophy associated with androgen insensitivity).

Peripheral nervous system disorder: GBS, may present with bulbar symptoms. MG and other neuromuscular disorders (e.g., polymyositis, West Nile virus infection, high-voltage electrical injury) must be considered in the differential diagnosis. Bulbar palsy must be differentiated from pseudobulbar palsy, which affects the pathways descending from the cortex to the cranial nerve motor nuclei due to upper motor neuron lesions.

REFERENCES

Albers, J. W., et al. (1983). Juvenile progressive bulbar palsy. *Arch Neurol, 40,* 351–353.

Kim, J., et al. (2016). Acute bulbar palsy as a variant of Guillain-Barré syndrome. *Neurology, 86*(8), 742–747. https://doi.org/10.1212/WNL.0000000000002256. Epub 2015 Dec 30.

C

CADASIL

Cerebral autosomal dominant arteriopathy with subcortical infarcts and leukoencephalopathy (CADASIL) is the most common and recognized genetic form of small vessel disease. In its advanced form, it leads to vascular dementia. CADASIL is caused by mutations in the NOTCH3 gene; NOTCH3 protein is expressed in vascular smooth muscle cells, whose degeneration results in progressively impaired cerebrovascular autoregulation, hypoperfusion, and ischemia.

Migraine—often beginning around age 30—is the most common initial symptom in CADASIL and is reported in up to half of CADASIL patients (but is less common in Asian patients). About 80% of CADASIL patients with migraine have migraine with aura.

Transient ischemic attacks and stroke are reported in approximately 85% of symptomatic individuals. Mean age at onset of ischemic episodes is 45 to 50 years but the range at onset is throughout adulthood. Ischemic episodes typically present as a lacunar syndrome, but strokes may occur in the brainstem, in the hemispheres, or may be lacunar syndromes. Large vessel strokes have also been reported. Stroke volume burden is associated with the manifestations of the vascular dementia which often includes gait disturbance, urinary incontinence, pseudobulbar palsy, and cognitive impairment.

Encephalopathy, cognitive impairment, and psychiatric disturbances are common in CADASIL. An acute encephalopathy evolving from a migraine attack may be a presenting symptom in about 10% of patients. It is commonly mistaken for encephalitis or other causes of acute delirium. Cognitive deficits often begin with executive dysfunction, although memory is eventually affected; cortical signs are less common and cortical infarcts can occur. Psychiatric symptoms of apathy and depression are also common.

The diagnosis of CADASIL is often suspected from the clinical presentation coupled with a brain MRI showing extensive white matter changes, with frequent involvement of the anterior temporal pole and external capsule. No abnormality is pathognomonic, but confluent bilateral anterior temporal pole T2-hyperintensities are highly suggestive. Definitive diagnosis is via genetic testing for NOTCH3 mutations. An autosomal recessive variant—cerebral autosomal recessive arteriopathy with subcortical infarcts and leukoencephalopathy (CARASIL)—has been described, mainly in Japanese families, presenting with extensive white matter changes, dementia, alopecia, and low back pain due to mutations in the serine protease HTRA1.

There are no specific treatments for CADASIL although aspirin is often used, as in typical cerebral small vessel disease. A study of Donepezil yielded no clear cognitive benefit.

REFERENCE

DiDonato, I., Bianchi, S., De Stefano, N., et al. (2017). Cerebral Autosomal Dominant Arteriopathy with Subcortical Infarcts and Leukoencephalopathy (CADASIL) as a model of small vessel disease: update on clinical, diagnostic, and management aspects. *BMC Med*, *15*, 41. https://doi.org/10.1186/s12916-017-0778-8.

CALORIC TESTING

Caloric testing is a method of assessing the integrity of the vestibulo-ocular reflex (VOR), particularly in comatose patients. The presence of nystagmus indicates that both vestibular and cortical inputs are intact.

Water that is colder or warmer than body temperature, when applied to the tympanic membrane, changes the firing rate of the ipsilateral vestibular nerve, causing ocular deviation and nystagmus. Cold water normally induces a slow ipsilateral deviation with contralateral "corrective" fast phases. Warm water induces a slow contralateral deviation and ipsilateral fast phases. Because the direction of nystagmus is conventionally described as the direction of the fast phase, the mnemonic *cold opposite, warm same* indicates the direction of caloric nystagmus for cold and warm stimuli. Bilateral irrigation induces vertical nystagmus; the mnemonic *cold up, warm down* refers to the fast phases.

Caloric testing may be done qualitatively at the bedside or quantitatively in a laboratory. Quantitative caloric testing is used to evaluate vestibular function. Bedside caloric testing is used (1) to establish the integrity of the ocular motor system in patients with an apparent gaze paresis, and (2) to evaluate altered states of consciousness. Caloric stimulation may be used to elicit vestibular eye movements if oculocephalic maneuvers (see VOR) have negative results or when a cervical injury is suspected.

Bedside caloric testing is performed after the external auditory canal has been examined, cerumen removed, and the patency of the tympanic membrane verified. The head is elevated 30 degrees from horizontal, aligning the lateral semicircular canal in the horizontal plane and maximizing amplitude of lateral horizontal nystagmus, if elicited. Water is gently injected with a syringe through a soft catheter inserted in the external auditory canal. Usually 1 mL of ice water is sufficient in alert patients and minimizes discomfort. Up to 100 mL of ice water can be used in unresponsive patients, and several minutes should be allowed for a response. Irrigation is repeated in the opposite ear after waiting at least 5 minutes for vestibular equilibration. Warm water (44°C) may also be used. Because of the risk of thermal injury, hot water should never be used.

Eye movements elicited by vestibular stimuli, whether with passive head rotation or caloric stimulation, may allow localization of lesions within the ocular motor system. Impaired movement of both eyes to one side occurs with lesions of the ipsilateral paramedian pontine reticular formation. Impaired abduction in one eye suggests a palsy of CN VI. Impaired adduction is seen in third-nerve palsies and in the eye ipsilateral to a medial longitudinal fasciculus lesion (internuclear ophthalmoplegia). Bilateral internuclear ophthalmoplegias cause, in addition to bilateral adduction weakness, impaired vertical vestibular eye movements. Eye deviation may occur in aberrant directions in patients with drug intoxication or structural disease of central vestibular connections.

As consciousness declines, the caloric stimulus-induced eye movements relate to the integrity of brainstem structures. Tonic eye deviation indicates integrity of brainstem function but impaired cortical inputs. Asymmetrical horizontal responses are interpreted as previously described and may give localizing information. Lack of any response may result from lesions of VOR pathways in the medulla or pons, the eighth CN, or the labyrinth or from drug intoxications, such as those resulting from vestibular suppressants (barbiturates, phenytoin, tricyclic antidepressants, or major tranquilizers) and neuromuscular blockers. The presence of caloric-induced nystagmus in an unresponsive patient suggests a psychogenic etiology.

REFERENCE
Gonçalves, D. U., Felipe, L., & Lima, T. M. (2008). Interpretation and use of caloric testing. *Braz J Otorhinolaryngol*, *74*, 440–446.

C

CARDIOPULMONARY ARREST (See also BRAIN DEATH, COMA)

The outcome for patients with cardiac arrest remains poor despite improved resuscitation practices. Accurate prediction of neurologic outcome in comatose patients following cardiac arrest is of great importance not only to help families with decision-making but also to avoid prolonged use of health care resources in patients with invariable poor outcome.

The 2006 American Academy of Neurology (AAN) practice parameters for prediction of outcome in comatose survivors after cardiopulmonary resuscitation (CPR) provide very useful prognostication guidelines. However, these guidelines were based on studies done before the widespread use of hypothermia, and neurologists should be cautious when providing prognostication in such patients. Delay in making decisions about prognostication might be appropriate in patients undergoing hypothermia.

According to AAN practice guidelines, prognosis cannot be made based on circumstances of CPR or elevated body temperature alone. There is not enough evidence to make clinical decisions based on abnormal S100 levels, or that creatine kinase brain isoenzyme predicts poor outcome. Similarly, there is also not enough evidence that abnormal brain imaging accurately predicts poor recovery.

The prognosis is invariably poor in comatose patients with absent pupillary or corneal reflexes, or absent extensor motor responses at 3 days after cardiac arrest. Patients with myoclonic status epilepticus within the first day after cardiac arrest have a poor prognosis. There is good evidence that absent N20 component of the somatosensory evoked potential within 1 to 3 days after CPR accurately predicts poor recovery from coma.

REFERENCE
Wijdicks, E. F. (2006). Practice parameter: prediction of outcome in comatose survivors after cardiopulmonary resuscitation (an evidence-based review): report of the Quality Standards Subcommittee of the American Academy of Neurology. *Neurology*, *67*(2), 203–210.

CARDIOPULMONARY ARREST

CAROTID-CAVERNOUS FISTULA

DEFINITION

A carotid-cavernous fistula (CCF) is an abnormal shunt between the carotid artery or its branches and the cavernous sinus (CS).

CLASSIFICATION

Classification is based on etiology (traumatic vs. spontaneous), flow rate (high vs. low flow) or vessel architecture (direct vs. indirect). Barrow classification of CCF defines four types based on arterial supply:

Type A (most common type): direct fistula from internal carotid artery (ICA) to CS. Usually high-flow and traumatic; 20% to 30% are spontaneous, mainly in older women.

Type B and C are supplied only by dural branches of the ICA and external carotid artery (ECA) respectively.

Type D: supplied by meningeal branches of both ICA and ECA.

CLINICAL FEATURES

Dandy's clinical triad of pulsatile exophthalmos, chemosis, and orbital pain is common in direct, high-flow CCF. Cranial nerve (V, IV, III, and VI) deficits are common, especially double vision. Resultant ipsilateral venous hypertension may result in vision loss, and intracerebral or subarachnoid hemorrhages. Massive, even life-threatening epistaxis may also occur in 1% to 2% of cases. Indirect CCFs manifest as chronic conjunctival injection and are usually caused by sinus thrombosis.

DIAGNOSIS

Computed tomography angiography and magnetic resonance angiogram are used for workup, but conventional digital subtraction angiography (DSA) (Fig. 11) is essential for diagnosis, classification, and treatment planning.

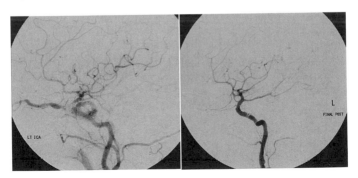

FIGURE 11

Pre- *(left)* and post- *(right)* treatment.
Note retrograde flow in superior ophthalmic vein and inferior venous drainage pre-treatment *(left)*.

TREATMENT

Symptomatic high-flow direct CCFs are considered emergencies. First-line treatment is endovascular (stent-assisted coil embolization or flow diversion), although surgery, radiosurgery, or ICA sacrifice can be done in refractory cases. Low-flow indirect CCFs are usually treated medically, and many resolve spontaneously.

REFERENCE

Ellis, J. A., Goldstein, H., Connolly, E. S., Jr., & Meyers, P. M. (2012). Carotid-cavernous fistulas. *Neurosurg Focus*, *32*(5), E9.

C

CAROTID STENOSIS (See also ISCHEMIA)

CAROTID STENOSIS

EPIDEMIOLOGY

As many as 20% to 30% of strokes are due to carotid artery disease. The clinical presentation of cerebral ischemia is explained in the discussion of stroke under "Ischemia." Briefly, a stroke or transient ischemic attack (TIA) has to be related to the territory of the stenosed artery to be symptomatic, as confirmed by a neurologist. Amaurosis fugax, as well as middle cerebral artery and/or anterior cerebral artery TIAs/minor or major strokes, are common.

DIAGNOSIS

The gold standard is a diagnostic cerebral angiogram, followed by a computed tomography angiogram, magnetic resonance angiogram, and carotid ultrasound (its reliability in routine daily practice is not as effective as has been shown in clinical studies). However, a carotid ultrasound is routinely used for surveillance of asymptomatic carotid stenosis due to its cost-efficient and non-invasive nature.

TREATMENT

Approaches to therapy include surgery and stenting in appropriate settings, but medical therapy is a critical component of managing carotid artery disease. Ideal medical therapy for carotid stenosis includes antiplatelet therapy with daily aspirin, angiotensin-converting enzyme inhibitor, and statin (regardless of lipid panel status). Smoking cessation and intensive treatment of diabetes are crucial aspects of therapy as well. Four randomized studies treating symptomatic carotid stenosis comparing carotid endarterectomy (CEA) to aspirin showed that patients with symptomatic severe stenosis (50%–70%) benefited from revascularization, with an absolute risk reduction of 17% over 2 years and with numbers needed to treat to achieve a benefit of 3 to 6. Patients with asymptomatic carotid stenosis less than 50% are best managed medically. Combined surgeon and surgical center perioperative morbidity and mortality rates should be below 3% in order for surgical intervention to be favorable for asymptomatic patients.

Carotid angioplasty and stenting are currently indicated for high-risk surgical patients; the most common indications are as follows:

I. Anatomic indication: infraclavicular lesions in the chest, high lesion (at the angle of jaw/C2 or higher), tandem lesion with 50% or higher diameter stenosis

II. Prior radiation to the neck

III. Prior neck surgery and dissection

IV. Prior CEA

V. Contralateral high-grade stenosis or occlusion

VI. Contralateral cranial nerve palsy and hoarseness from neck surgery or nerve injury

VII. Co-morbidities, coronary artery disease, congestive heart failure, ejection fraction less than or equal to 30%, severe chronic obstructive pulmonary disease, poorly controlled diabetes mellitus, end-stage renal disease

VIII. Patients older than 75 years of age

For low surgical risk group, it has been shown to be equivalent to CEA in the Carotid Revascularization Endarterectomy vs. Stenting Trial; however, patients younger than 70 years of age tend to do better with stenting and those older than 70 years of age tend to do better with CEA in this low surgical group. Well-trained and experienced neurointerventionalists who can address potential procedural complications, as well as surgeons experienced in CEA, are critical in achieving good procedural and surgical outcomes over medical therapy alone. The use of a distal embolic protection device is recommended.

REFERENCE

Chaturvedi, S., & Bhattacharya, P. (2014). Large artery atherosclerosis: carotid stenosis, vertebral artery disease, and intracranial atherosclerosis. *Continuum (Minneap Minn)*, *20*, 323–334.

CARPAL TUNNEL SYNDROME

Carpal tunnel syndrome (CTS) occurs as a result of compression of the median nerve as it courses beneath the transverse carpal ligament (Fig. 12). Occupational trauma from repetitive motion is a common cause. Inflammatory and infiltrative conditions like arthritis and tenosynovitis; structural lesions like ganglion and neuroma; systemic diseases like hypothyroidism, amyloidosis, and mucopolysaccharidoses; and fluid-overload states such as pregnancy and obesity can be associated with CTS. Often, no apparent cause is identified (idiopathic). Half of the cases are bilateral, and the dominant hand is affected more. Causes other than idiopathic should be considered if CTS is worse in the nondominant hand. CTS prevalence is about 276 per 100,000 person-years. More than 80% of patients are over 40 years old, and 65% to 75% are women.

Patients characteristically complain of nocturnal numbness and paresthesia or burning pain in the median distribution (but which may radiate to the forearm, elbow, or shoulder). Weakness and atrophy of the opponens

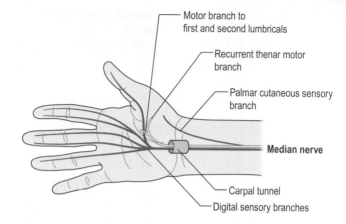

Motor branch to
first and second lumbricals

Recurrent thenar motor
branch

Palmar cutaneous sensory
branch

Median nerve

Carpal tunnel

Digital sensory branches

FIGURE 12

Distal motor and sensory branches of the median nerve. (From Preston, D. C., & Shapiro, B. E.
(2013). Median neuropathy at the wrist. In *Electromyography and neuromuscular disorders*,
ed 3. London: Elsevier, pp. 267–288. Chapter 17, Fig. 17.3.)

pollicis, abductor pollicis brevis, and first two lumbricals and loss of two-point
discrimination are late signs of long-term involvement. The symptoms may be
reproduced by tapping over the median nerve at the carpal tunnel *(Tinel's sign)*
or by maximum flexion of the wrist for 60 seconds *(Phalen's sign)*. Awakening
from sleep and needing to shake the affected hand is characteristic. Nerve
conduction studies show prolongation of distal median sensory and motor
latencies across the wrist. A difference in latencies of ≥ 0.4 ms between the
distal median and ulnar nerves measured by "palmar mixed comparison study"
is the most sensitive electrodiagnostic feature (Table 20). Ultrasound of
median nerve or magnetic resonance imaging of wrist can reveal structural
lesions.

Differential diagnosis includes degenerative arthritis at the wrist, more
proximal median neuropathies, mononeuritis multiplex, C6 or C7
radiculopathy, brachial plexopathy, thoracic outlet syndrome, and
polyneuropathies. Evaluation for underlying causes is dependent on clinical
presentation and should be individualized.

Treatment consists of avoiding activities that precipitate symptoms and
wearing a wrist extension splint at night. Local steroid injections with or
without lidocaine may provide limited relief but may worsen symptoms.
Indications for surgery are weakness, atrophy, or electromyography evidence
of denervation. Surgical treatment, which can be done by either open or
endoscopic approach, is usually not necessary during pregnancy as symptoms
resolve spontaneously.

TABLE 20

ELECTRODIAGNOSTIC FEATURES OF CARPAL TUNNEL SYNDROME

Study	Stimulation Site	Recording Site	Findings	Significance
Median nerve sensory	Wrist	Index finger	Slowing of conduction (prolonged latency or reduced CV), reduced SNAP amplitudes	Compression at the wrist causing demyelination and/or axonal loss
Median nerve motor	Wrist and elbow	APB at the ball of the thumb	Slowing of conduction (prolonged latency or reduced CV), reduced CMAP amplitudes	Compression at the wrist causing demyelination and/or axonal loss
Median F-waves	Wrist	APB muscle	Prolonged minimum F-waves	Slowing or blocking of F-waves at the wrist
Ulnar sensory	Wrist	Little finger	Normal	Ulnar nerve is unaffected at wrist
Ulnar motor	Wrist	ADM muscle	Normal	Ulnar nerve is unaffected at wrist
Ulnar F-waves	Wrist	ADM muscle	Normal	Ulnar nerve is unaffected at wrist
Median-ulnar palmar comparison	8 cm from wrist in the palm along the ulnar sensory distribution and median sensory distribution	Wrist, over the ulnar and median sides of the wrist	Difference of ≥ 4 ms between median and ulnar peak latencies	Median conduction through the wrist is slower than that of ulnar

Note: Coexisting ulnar nerve neuropathy can affect these studies and should be interpreted in its context. Axonal neuropathies such as in diabetes can also confound these studies. Additional nerves are studied in cases of suspected polyneuropathy.

ADM, Abductor digiti minimi; *APB,* abductor pollicis brevis; *CMAP,* compound muscle action potential; *CV,* conduction velocity; *SNAP,* sensory nerve action potential.

REFERENCES

Ghasemi-rad, M., Nosair, E., Vegh, A., et al. (2014). A handy review of carpal tunnel syndrome: from anatomy to diagnosis and treatment. *World J Radiol*, 6(6), 284–300.

Preston, D. C., & Shapiro, B. E. (2013). Median neuropathy at the wrist. In *Electromyography and neuromuscular disorders: clinical-electrophysiologic correlations* (pp. 267–288). London: Elsevier.

CATAMENIAL EPILEPSY

Catamenial epilepsy is a resistant form of epilepsy during which a woman is more likely to have seizures during a particular phase of her menstrual cycle. Seizures or seizure clusters tend to occur during or immediately before menses, or around ovulation. Metabolites of steroid hormones such as progesterone enhance gamma amino butyric acid-A (GABA-A) receptor function. Fluctuation of these hormones during the menstrual cycle is thought to lead to an increase in seizure susceptibility, and a reduction in the therapeutic effect of commonly prescribed anticonvulsants.

Estimates of prevalence among women with epilepsy range from 12.5% to 78%. Three patterns have been identified (Fig. 13):

- Perimenstrual (C1), with more seizures during days −3 to +3 compared with other phases. Perimenstrual is the most common form of catamenial epilepsy.
- Periovulatory (C2), with greater than average daily seizure frequency during days 10 to −13 in normal cycles.

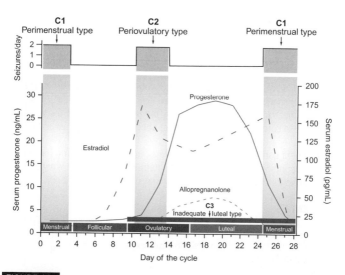

FIGURE 13

The three subtypes of catamenial epilepsy.

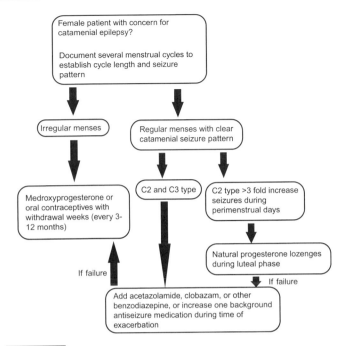

FIGURE 14

Treatment algorithm for catamenial epilepsy. (From Navis, A., & Harden, C. (2016). A treatment approach to catamenial epilepsy. *Curr Treat Options Neurol, 18*(7), 30.)

- Luteal (C3), marked by frequent seizures within 14 days before menstruation during inadequate luteal phase cycles.

To diagnose catamenial epilepsy, ask the patient to keep a diary that tracks seizures in relation to menses; check progesterone level during seizures.

Treatment consists of antiepileptic drugs, acetazolamide, and hormonal therapy depending upon the subtype of catamenial pattern. Be wary of giving progesterone to those interested in becoming pregnant. Refer to Fig. 14.

REFERENCES

Navis, A., & Harden, C. A. (2016). Treatment approach to catamenial epilepsy. *Curr Treat Options Neurol, 18*(7), 30.

Reddy, D. S. (2017). The neuroendocrine basis of sex differences in epilepsy. *Pharmacol Biochem Behav, 152*, 97–104.

CAUDA EQUINA AND CONUS MEDULLARIS

Clinical features of cauda equina and conus medullaris syndromes are summarized in Table 21.

TABLE 21

CLINICAL DIFFERENTIATION OF CAUDA EQUINA AND CONUS MEDULLARIS SYNDROMES

Feature	Conus Medullaris (Lower Sacral Cord)	Cauda Equina (Lumbosacral Roots)
Sensory deficit	Saddle distribution	Saddle distribution
	Bilateral, symmetrical	Asymmetrical
	Sensory dissociation present	Sensory dissociation absent
	Presents early	Presents relatively later
Pain	Uncommon	Prominent, early
	Relatively mild	Severe
	Bilateral, symmetrical	Asymmetrical
	Perineum and thighs	Radicular
Motor deficit	Symmetrical	Asymmetrical
	Mild	Moderate to severe
	Atrophy absent	Atrophy more prominent
Reflexes	Achilles reflex absent	Reflexes variable involved
	Patellar reflex normal	
Sphincter dysfunction	Early, severe	Late, less severe
	Absent anal and bulbocavernosus reflex	Reflex abnormalities less common
Sexual dysfunction	Erection and ejaculation impaired	Less common

Modified from DeJong, R. N. (1979). *The neurologic examination*, ed 4. New York: Harper & Row.

CEREBELLUM

General anatomy: The cerebellum makes up 10% of the brain's total weight and volume, but contains approximately 50% of all brain neurons.

The anterior lobe, rostral to the primary fissure, is made up of the paravermian cortex and the anterosuperior vermis which receives proprioceptive information from muscle and tendons via the dorsal spinocerebellar tracts (from lower limb) and ventral spinocerebellar tracts (upper limb) to modulate posture and muscle tone.

The posterior lobe, caudal to the primary fissure, contains the middle vermis and its lateral extensions. Inputs from the cerebral cortex via the pontine nuclei and brachium pontis are processed to modulate coordination.

The flocculonodular lobe, inferiorly separated from the main cerebellum by the posterolateral fissure, receives proprioceptive input from the vestibular nuclei for control of equilibrium.

C

CEREBELLUM

The cerebellum may also be divided into longitudinal zones which project to the deep nuclei of the cerebellum. The vermis projects to the fastigial nuclei, intermediate zone to the interpositus nuclei and lateral zone to the dentate nucleus. Refer to Fig. 15A and B.

DEEP CEREBELLAR NUCLEI
The dentate nucleus receives afferent from the premotor and supplementary motor cortex via pontocerebellar system and sends efferents to the contralateral ventrolateral thalamus which projects to the motor cortex for the initiation of volitional movements.

The interpositus nucleus receives input from the pontocerebellar system as well as the spinocerebellar system (Golgi tendon organs, muscle spindles,

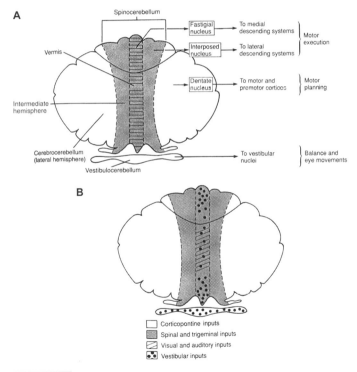

FIGURE 15

The cerebellum has three functional components (vestibulocerebellum, spinocerebellum, and cerebrocerebellum) with different outputs (A) and inputs (B).

cutaneous afferents, and spinal cord interneurons) to fine tune movement and is involved in control of physiological tremor.

The fastigial nucleus sends output to the bilateral vestibular nuclei and reticular formation as well as alpha and gamma motor neurons in the spinal cord to maintain antigravity and modulate standing and walking synergies.

Cellular anatomy: The cerebellar cortex is composed of three layers and five types of neurons.

The outermost molecular layer contains two types of inhibitory cells, stellate and basket, which are scattered among dendrites of Purkinje cells.

The middle layer is composed of Purkinje cell bodies, which as the primary output of the cerebellum, sends inhibitory signals to the deep cerebellar nuclei.

The innermost granular layer contains densely packed granule cells and larger Golgi interneurons. Axons of granule cells send excitatory output to the Purkinje cells and are the only neurons to send excitatory signals among all five cell types.

Mossy fibers carry input from axons of spinocerebellar tracts, pons, vestibular and reticular nuclei to send excitatory signals to the granule layer. Their primary neurotransmitter is aspartate.

Climbing fibers receive afferent from the crossed inferior olivary nuclei and send excitatory signal on to Purkinje as well as stellate and basket cells.

C

CEREBELLUM

CLINICAL PRESENTATION OF CEREBELLUM LESIONS

Cerebellum lesions disturb the rate, range, and force of an action to cause undershooting or overshooting and fragmentation of smooth movements into irregular jerks. Often the velocity and force of an action is affected. Common signs seen in testing include ataxia of volitional movement, dysdiadochokinesis, and a type of intentional tremor which is composed of (increasing) horizontal oscillations when approaching target (e.g., finger to nose testing). With acute lesions, muscle tone tends to be diminished. When deep nuclei or cerebellar peduncles are affected, especially if dentate or the superior cerebellar peduncle, the clinical picture may mimic that of an extensive cerebellar hemispheric lesion. Lesion of the cerebellar cortex and subcortical white matter, on the other hand, may cause minimal if any clinical signs.

Gait: With lesion of the anterior vermis, the patient may walk with uneven steps and lurch due to misaligned foot placement. Midline anterior cerebellar lesions may present solely as gait disturbance without any other associated features, so anyone suspected of a cerebellar lesion should have gait tested if possible.

Speech: Cerebellar dysarthria is characterized by slow scanning disrupted speech, a breakdown of words into syllables, and explosive speech with various changes in intonation.

Eyes: Testing of extraocular movements may demonstrate loss of smooth pursuit with rapid repetitive saccades. Periodic alternating nystagmus is one of the few lesions associated with cerebellar lesions, in this case of the flocculonodular lobe.

Causes of cerebellar dysfunction include congenital lesions, childhood tumors (e.g., medulloblastoma), multiple sclerosis, paraneoplastic syndromes (e.g., anti-Purkinje cell antibodies), stroke and hemorrhage, metastatic lesions, medication and drug effects (e.g., alcohol, ARA-C chemotherapy, Dilantin toxicity), and Arnold-Chiari malformations and other developmental abnormalities. Cerebellar-type lesions can be caused by focal dysfunction in afferent and efferent structures and pathways in the brainstem, vestibular nuclei, and thalamus.

REFERENCE

Ropper, A. H., Samuels, M. A., & Klein, J. P. (2014). Ataxia and disorders of cerebellar function. In A. H. Ropper, M. A. Samuels, & J. P. Klein (Eds.), *Adam and Victor's principles of neurology,* ed 10 (pp. 81–91). China: McGraw-Hill Education.

CEREBRAL ANEURYSMS

EPIDEMIOLOGY

Cerebral aneurysms occur in approximately 5% of the general population (9% in first-degree relatives). The ratio of ruptured to unruptured is approximately 1:1, although the number of incidentally discovered aneurysms may be increasing with the widespread use of magnetic resonance imaging and computed tomography angiography. Most are believed to be acquired, with only 2% occurring during childhood. An increased incidence of cerebral aneurysms is associated with various collagen synthesis disorders, such as Ehlers-Danlos syndrome, Marfan syndrome, autosomal dominant polycystic kidney disease (15%), α_1-antitrypsin deficiency, and neurofibromatosis type 1.

PATHOLOGY

Saccular aneurysms are responsible for most subarachnoid hemorrhages. Fusiform aneurysms and mycotic aneurysms are less common. Fusiform aneurysms consist of dilation of the entire involved vessel. Atherosclerosis can lead to fusiform aneurysm. Mycotic aneurysm is formed as a result of infected embolus usually due to ineffective endocarditis. Saccular aneurysms occur along bends in the artery, or at arterial branch points, in direct line with the blood flow. The underlying defect appears to be fragmentation of the internal elastic lamina and absent muscularis at the aneurysm neck; the aneurysm wall is composed of a thin adventitia with or without an inner endothelium.

Eighty-five percent occur in the anterior circulation, and 15% in the posterior circulation. They are evenly divided among midline, right, and left. The most common locations are the anterior or posterior communicating artery (25%–30% each, depending on the study), middle cerebral artery (20%), and basilar artery (10%). Multiple aneurysms occur in 20%, usually at mirror locations.

CLINICAL PRESENTATION

The overall risk of aneurysm rupture is 0.5% to 1% per year. This risk is dependent on size, history of prior ruptured aneurysm, and location. The risk is 0.5% to 1% per year if less than 7 mm in diameter and 1% to 2% per year if greater than 7 mm in diameter; the risk then increases with increasing size. Previous subarachnoid hemorrhage from another aneurysm is associated with 1% to 2% per year, regardless of size, and an 8- to 10-fold relative risk increase in posterior circulation and posterior communicating artery. Tobacco smoking is associated with a 3- to 10-fold increased risk of rupture and is the only environmental factor definitively linked with rupture.

TREATMENT

Treatment involves a team approach with the neurologist, neurointerventionalist, and neurosurgeon to consider potential aneurysm clipping versus endovascular coiling or observation.

REFERENCES

The International Study of Unruptured Intracranial Aneurysms Investigators. (1998). *N Engl J Med*, *339*, 1725–1733.

International Subarachnoid Aneurysm Trial (ISAT) study group. (2002). *Lancet*, *360*, 1267–1274. and *366*, 809–817, 2005.

CEREBRAL CORTEX

The cerebral cortex (from the Latin word for bark) is made up of a total of six lobes, five of which are exposed on the surface of the cerebral hemispheres, and are named according to the respective abutting skull bones. The sixth lobe (insular) is located internal to the lateral sulcus mantle of gray matter on the cerebral surface. Based on the difference in number of cell layers, the cerebral cortex can be divided into allocortex (three layers), mesocortex (three to six layers), and isocortex (six layers). The isocortex can further be divided into functionally relevant areas (Brodmann areas) based on cytoarchitectonics. Fig. 16 shows Brodmann areas in lateral and medial views.

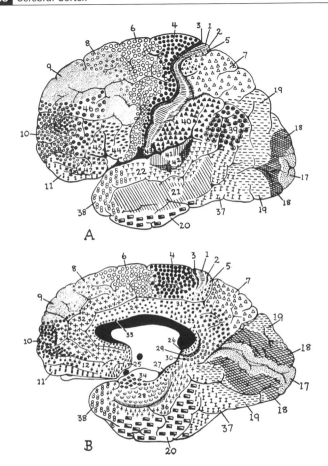

FIGURE 16

Brodmann's cytoarchitectural map of cerebral cortex, indicating major functional areas. 4, Primary motor strip; 3, 1, and 2, sensory strip; 17, primary visual cortex; 18 and 19, visual association cortex; 8, frontal eye fields; 6, premotor cortex; 41 and 42, auditory cortex; 5 and 7, somesthetic association cortex. Areas 13 to 16 (not shown) make up the insula. Labeling is from anterior to posterior. (A) Lateral view of brain. (B) Medial view of brain. (From Carpenter, M. B. (1991). *Core text of neuroanatomy*, ed 4. Baltimore: Williams & Wilkins.)

REFERENCE

Simić, G., & Hof, P. R. (2015). In search of the definitive Brodmann's map of cortical areas in human. *J Comp Neurol, 523*(1), 5–14.

CEREBRAL HEMORRHAGE, INTRACRANIAL HEMORRHAGE, SUBARACHNOID HEMORRHAGE

EPIDEMIOLOGY

Primary intracranial hemorrhage (ICH) accounts for 10% to 15% of all strokes. The annual incidence is 10 to 20 cases per 100,000 people with a prevalence of 37,000 to 52,000 cases per year in the United States. ICH is more common in persons older than 55 years of age, men, African-Americans, and Japanese. Chronic hypertension is a common cause, often due to lipohyalinosis of the small intraparenchymal arteries, resulting in arteriolar wall weakness and subsequent rupture. Locations of hemorrhage in order of frequency are as follows: putamen (35%–50%), subcortical white matter (30%), cerebellum (15%), thalamus (10%–15%), and pons (5%–12%). The active bleeding usually lasts only a short time, and later clinical deterioration is most often ascribed to surrounding edema and ischemia, rather than continued hemorrhage; however, up to 25% of patients have hematoma expansion.

INTRACRANIAL HEMORRHAGE RISK FACTORS

Risk factors are hypertension, excessive use of alcohol, low serum cholesterol (<160 mg/dL), amphetamine and cocaine use, and genetic predilection (mutation of a subunit of factor XIII, β amyloid deposition in blood vessels, and presence of e_2 and e_4 alleles of apolipoprotein E) and cerebral amyloidosis.

CLINICAL FEATURES

The clinical presentation correlates with anatomic location, size, and degree of associated mass effect (Table 22). Headache is a frequent accompanying symptom. Classic symptoms vary by location:

1. Putamenal hemorrhage is associated with dense ipsilateral hemiplegia, hemianesthesia, and homonymous hemianopsia with aphasia or neglect (depending on which hemisphere is involved). There is also decreased level of consciousness (disproportionate to the weakness), ipsilateral eye deviation, and normal pupils.
2. Thalamic hemorrhage can be highly variable and may produce dense contralateral hemisensory loss with variable hemiparesis, contralateral homonymous hemianopia, vertical or lateral-gaze palsies (including "wrong way" deviation), and occasionally, nystagmus.
3. Cerebellar hemorrhage is associated with severe occipital headache, sudden nausea and vomiting, gait changes, and truncal ataxia. It is a potential neurosurgical emergency when brainstem compression is imminent or for lesions greater than 3 cm in diameter. Emergency decompressive surgery may be indicated to relieve signs of brainstem compression or acute hydrocephalus.
4. Pontine hemorrhage causes coma, pinpoint pupils (reactive to light), bilateral extensor posturing, and impaired ocular motility.

C

CEREBRAL HEMORRHAGE

TABLE 22

CLINICAL PRESENTATION OF INTRACRANIAL HEMORRHAGE

Location	Pupils	Eye Movements	Motor and Sensory Deficits	Other
Putamenal	Normal or dilated if herniation	Ipsilateral conjugate deviation	Contralateral hemiparesis or sensory loss	Decreased consciousness
Caudate	Ipsilaterally constricted	Conjugate deviation ± ptosis	Transient hemiparesis	Headache, confusion
Thalamic	Small, poorly reactive	Upgaze palsy, lids retraction, medial and downward deviation	Mild hemiparesis, sensory loss	Aphasia, if left thalamus involved
Pontine	Constricted but reactive	Horizontal gaze palsy	Quadriplegia	Coma
Cerebellar	Ipsilateral slight constriction	Sixth nerve palsy, contralateral conjugate deviation	Ipsilateral limb ataxia, no hemiparesis	Gait ataxia

DIAGNOSIS

I. The size is estimated based on the computed tomography (CT) findings using the simple volumetric formula: ABC/2 (A = width, B = length, C = height). Angiography may be necessary to exclude underlying vascular malformation or tumor.

MANAGEMENT

Immediate attention must be directed at the ABCs: airway, breathing, and circulation. Patients with a Glasgow coma score (GCS) of 8 or less or an impaired gag reflex need rapid sequence intubation. Sedation with short-acting drugs (midazolam) prevents the intracranial pressure (ICP) spikes and allows frequent neurologic checks.

I. Blood pressure management is critical. Judicious lowering of the BP is indicated, although the BP goals and agents to use are controversial. Many authors favor the calcium channel blocker nicardipine starting at 3 to 5 mg/hour to keep systolic BP 140 to 160 mm Hg or mean arterial pressure (MAP) around 100 mm Hg to keep cerebral perfusion pressure above 60 mm Hg. Other agents that are easily titratable with limited ICP changes have been used: labetalol, enalapril, and hydralazine. Patients with chronic severe hypertension with autoregulation curve shifted to the right require higher MAP.

II. Adequate ventilation, oxygenation, and pulmonary/pharyngeal toilet must be maintained.

III. Antiedema agents (osmotic diuretics or hypertonic saline) may be used. Mass effect may be managed medically with hyperosmolar therapy, typically only for up to three days. Patients who are not clinically improving or holding stable may require surgical decompression.

IV. Intraventricular instillation of thrombolytic agents to aid dissolution of mainly intraventricular clot remains controversial.

V. Procoagulants such as factor VII (rFVIIa) have not yielded favorable clinical results that can be reproduced.

VI. Neurosurgical evaluation should be obtained for superficially located cerebral hemorrhages and all cerebellar hemorrhages, for placing ICP monitors, external ventricular drainage for obstructive hydrocephalus and intraventricular hemorrhage and possibility of intraventricular recombinant tissue plasminogen activator.

VII. Other supportive measures: Prophylactic use of anticonvulsant agents is no longer recommended in the treatment of patients with ICH. Clinical seizures should be treated, and patients for whom subclinical seizures are suspected should be evaluated with continuous electroencephalogram monitoring for at least 48 hours, if available. Maintain adequate fluid and electrolyte balance. Raise the head of the patient's bed 30 degrees, barring contraindications due to spinal injury. Correct underlying coagulopathy if present. Prophylaxis for stress ulcer involves proton pump inhibitor, and for deep vein thrombosis pneumatic sequential compression devices are needed.

C

CEREBRAL HEMORRHAGE

PROGNOSIS AND COMPLICATIONS

Death from ICH is usually due to mass effect with herniation or brainstem compression and brainstem hemorrhages. Common ICH complications are hematoma expansion (20%–40% within the first 24 hours, 25% within the first hour), intraventricular extension, and edema with shift, obstructive hydrocephalus, and increased ICP. ICH has the highest mortality rate of all strokes (23%–58% at 6 months). The main predictors of fatality are (1) GCS at presentation; (2) hematoma volume; and (3) intraventricular extension. Mortality rate varies from 17% (GCS > 9 and hematoma volume < 30 mL) to 90% (GCS < 9 and hematoma volume > 60 mL). A survivor's long-term functional prognosis may be better than for infarction because there is more reversible injury. The 2015 American Heart Association/American Stroke Association (AHA/ASA) guideline recommends not discussing new do not resuscitate (DNR) status on ICH patients until, at the earliest, hospital day 2. They specify, "Current prognostic models for individual patients early after ICH are biased by failure to account for the influence of withdrawal of support and early DNR orders."

Other causes of intraparenchymal hemorrhage (Table 23) include the following:

   I. Trauma (accounts for up to 50% of nonhypertensive cerebral hemorrhage)
   II. Ruptured arteriovenous malformation
   III. Ruptured aneurysm with parenchymal extension
   IV. Metastatic carcinoma, especially lung, choriocarcinoma, melanoma, and renal adenocarcinoma
   V. Primary neoplasms (glioblastoma multiforme, pituitary adenoma)
   VI. Embolic infarction with secondary hemorrhage (up to one third of embolic infarcts)
   VII. Hematologic disorders, including leukemia, lymphoma, thrombocytopenic purpura, aplastic anemia, sickle cell anemia, hemophilia, hypoprothrombinemia, afibrinogenemia, and Waldenström macroglobulinemia
   VIII. Anticoagulant therapy
   IX. Cerebral amyloid angiopathy. This usually presents as multiple, recurrent hemorrhages in the white matter or cortex, sparing deep gray matter (as opposed to hypertensive hemorrhages). Amyloid angiopathy may be the cause in 5% to 10% of sporadic intracerebral hemorrhages. It is associated with dementia in about 30% of cases; familial cases are associated with mutations in the amyloid precursor protein on chromosome 21 (Dutch and Icelandic forms). Attempts at surgical evacuation are usually futile because the vessels are very fragile, bleeding is very difficult to control, and there is a high incidence of recurrent hemorrhages.
   X. Vasculopathies such as lupus, polyarteritis nodosa, and granulomatous arteritis
   XI. Cortical vein thrombosis with secondary hemorrhage
   XII. Drugs, including methamphetamine, amphetamine, pseudoephedrine, phenylpropanolamine, and cocaine

TABLE 23

CHARACTERISTICS OF SPONTANEOUS INTRACRANIAL HEMORRHAGE

Cause	Clinical History	Annual Recurrence Rate
Hypertension (HTN)	Longstanding uncontrolled HTN, middle-aged patients	<2%
Amyloid angiopathy	Preexistent dementia, presents in sixth to eighth decades of life	21%–31%
Intracranial aneurysm	Peak age for rupture 50 years	50% within 6 months, 3% per year afterward
Arteriovenous malformation	Preexistent headaches, seizures, prior to 40 years of age	2%–4% without surgical correction
Cavernous angioma	Preexistent symptoms prior to 30 years of age	0.5%–1% initial, 4.5% afterward
Venous angioma	Broad range of age with a peak in the fourth decade	First rate of bleed 0.15%, recurrence rate undetermined
Brain tumors	Malignant astrocytomas, metastatic malignant melanoma, choriocarcinoma, renal cell carcinoma, thyroid cancer	1%–15% overall estimate of bleeding
Drugs of abuse (cocaine, amphetamine, ecstasy)	Peak incidence in the third through fifth decades	Unknown

C

CEREBRAL HEMORRHAGE

Other forms of ICH

Subarachnoid hemorrhage occurs with an incidence of 15:100,000 with peak incidence at 55 to 60 years of age. The majority of cases are due to rupture of cerebral aneurysm or trauma (see Aneurysm for further discussion).

Subdural hemorrhage (SDH) may be acute or chronic. Acute SDH is usually due to trauma with tearing of bridging veins in the subdural space. There may be an initial loss of consciousness with regaining of consciousness (lucid interval) followed in several hours by progressive deterioration of mental status and headache. Lateralizing signs may be present. Diagnosis is based on clinical course, emergency CT (appears as hyperdensity over cortex), and if necessary, angiography. Treatment consists of neurosurgical evacuation and correction of underlying coagulopathies (if present). Dialysis patients and alcoholics are particularly prone to develop SDH.

Chronic SDH is less clearly related to trauma and may follow minor head trauma in the elderly and in patients on anticoagulants. Symptoms and signs resemble those in acute SDH but develop gradually over several days to months. Lateralizing signs are common. Mental status changes may suggest dementia. Diagnosis is as for acute SDH, although the lesion on CT is usually hypo- or isodense. Treatment is neurosurgical evacuation. The prognosis for survival and recovery in surgically treated patients is generally good, but SDH may recur.

Acute epidural hemorrhage results from skull fracture with laceration of the middle meningeal artery and vein. The clinical course is similar to acute SDH but is more rapidly progressive. Rapid herniation, respiratory depression, and death may ensue. The diagnosis is established emergently as for acute SDH. The CT appearance is a convex hyperdensity. This hemorrhage is a neurosurgical emergency and is treated by immediate evacuation.

REFERENCES

Bradley, W. G., Daroff, R. B., Fenichel, G. M., & Jankovic, J. (2004). *Neurology in clinical practice,* ed 4. Philadelphia: Butterworth-Heinemann.

Hemphill, J. C., III, et al. (2015). Guidelines for the management of spontaneous intracerebral hemorrhage. *Stroke, 46,* 2032–2060.

CEREBRAL PALSY

Cerebral palsy (CP) refers to a heterogenous group of early-onset nonprogressive disorders of the central nervous system manifested primarily by neuromotor impairment. It is the most common cause of physical impairment in children. CP shares a significant overlap with many developmental conditions, and is thus a diagnosis of exclusion with five key elements: (1) a *group* of disorders with (2) abnormality in fetal/infant brain, which is (3) permanent, although not unchanging, (4) nonprogressive, and (5) affecting movement/ motor function. It is often accompanied by multiple comorbidities (particularly its severe forms), e.g., cognitive impairment, epilepsy (30%), hearing (20%) or vision loss (25%–30%), feeding difficulty, and behavioral disturbances.

Risk factors for development of CP include probable genetic disorders (up to one-third), prematurity, intrauterine growth restriction, maldevelopment, placental abnormalities, intrauterine infections, perinatal stroke, tight nuchal cord, multiple gestations, prolonged shoulder dystocia, and intrapartum hypoxia.

CP classification has been traditionally based on neurologic examination into different forms, including spastic, dyskinetic, ataxic, hypotonic, and atonic. The more recent Gross Motor Function Classification System is based on differences in ambulation, from level I (most able) to level V (least able).

The mainstay of treatment is physical therapy and orthoses. Surgery involves tendon release and transfer. Spasticity is treated with baclofen, diazepam, clonidine, tizanidine, or botulinum toxin injections. Dyskinesia treatment is challenging, but trihexyphenidyl and intrathecal baclofen can be tried. Seizure treatment must account for higher sensitivity to sedative and cognitive effects or antiepileptic drugs in CP patients.

Prognosis depends on the severity of the disease; however, improved medical care has extended the quality of life for even the most affected patients.

REFERENCES

Smithers-Sheedy, H., Badawi, N., Blair, E., et al. (2014). What constitutes cerebral palsy in the twenty-first century? *Dev Med Child Neurol*, 56(4), 323–328. https://doi.org/10.1111/dmcn.12262.

MacLennan, A. H., Thompson, S. C., & Gecz, J. (2015). Cerebral palsy: causes, pathways, and the role of genetic variants. *Am J Obstet Gynecol*, 213(6), 779–788. https://doi.org/10.1016/j.ajog.2015.05.034.

CEREBRAL SALT-WASTING SYNDROME

Cerebral salt-wasting syndrome (CSW) is defined as renal sodium wasting leading to hyponatremia and a decrease in extracellular fluid volume.

Not all patients with hyponatremia have syndrome of inappropriate ADH secretion (SIADH) with resultant free water retention; instead, they have inappropriate natriuresis.

CSW is associated with numerous intracranial pathologies, such as primary cerebral tumors, carcinomatous meningitis, head trauma following intracranial surgery, and pituitary surgery, but it has most commonly been studied as subarachnoid hemorrhage. The mechanism underlying this association has not yet been clearly identified. The following mechanisms have been proposed: renin–angiotensin–aldosterone system, sympathetic nervous system hypothesis, and natriuretic peptide theory, including atrial natriuretic peptide, brain natriuretic peptide, C-type natriuretic peptide, and dendroaspis natriuretic peptide.

It is important to recognize this syndrome as CSW is one of the most commonly encountered electrolyte disturbances in the neurologic intensive care unit, and the treatment is different from SIADH. It is not possible to distinguish CSW from SIADH based on serum and urine laboratory findings alone. Differentiation is done by careful assessment of volume status (Table 24).

TABLE 24

DIFFERENTIAL DIAGNOSIS OF CEREBRAL SALT-WASTING SYNDROME AND SYNDROME OF INAPPROPRIATE ADH SECRETION

Variable	CSW	SIADH
Urine osmolality	↑ (>100 mOsm/kg)	↑ (>100 mOsm/kg)
Urine sodium concentration	↑ (>40 mmol/L)	↑ (>40 mmol/L)
Extracellular fluid volume	↓	↑
Body weight	↓	No change or ↑
Fluid balance	Negative	Neutral to slightly +
Urine volume	No change or ↑	No change or ↓
Hematocrit	↑	No change
Albumin	↑	No change
Serum bicarbonate	↑	No change or ↓
Blood urea nitrogen	↑	No change or ↓
Serum uric acid	No change or ↓	↓
Sodium balance	Negative	Neutral or +
Central venous pressure	↓ (<6 cm H_2O)	No change or slightly + (6–10 cm H_2O)
Wedge pressure	↓	No change or slightly ↑

CSW, cerebral salt-wasting, *SIADH*, syndrome of inappropriate antidiuretic hormone secretion.
Manzanares, W., Aramendi, I., Langlois, P. L., & Biestro, A. (2015). Hyponatremia in the neurocritical care patient: an approach based on current evidence. *Med Intensiva*, *39*(4), 234–243.
Braun, M. M., & Mahowald, M. (2017). Electrolytes: sodium disorders. *FP Essent*, *459*, 11–20.

Classical signs and symptoms of hypovolemia include hypotension, orthostatism, lassitude, increased thirst, and muscle cramps but all lack specificity. If there is any doubt regarding the diagnosis, fluid restriction should be instituted. Then, if the natriuresis persists, cerebral salt-wasting should be suspected and treated appropriately. The syndrome responds to vigorous sodium and water replacement. Other therapies such as vasopressin antagonists have recently been suggested with promising results, although long-term studies will be needed.

REFERENCES

Cerdà-Esteve, M., Cuadrado-Godia, E., Chillaron, J. J., et al. (2008). Cerebral salt wasting syndrome: review. *Eur J Int Med*, *19*, 249–254.
Yee, A. H., Burns, J. D., & Wijdicks, E. F. M. (2010). Cerebral salt wasting: pathophysiology, diagnosis, and treatment. *Neurosurg Clin N Am*, *21*, 339–352.

CEREBROSPINAL FLUID

FORMATION

Cerebrospinal fluid (CSF) is produced mainly by the choroid plexuses (95%) but also in the interstitial space and ependyma (5%). The rate of CSF formation is about 500 mL/day, and total CSF volume is 150 mL (50% intracranial, 50% spinal). Secretion is an energy-requiring process related to ion exchange (Na/K). Production is also dependent on the cytosolic enzyme carbonic anhydrase. Therefore carbonic anhydrase inhibitors (e.g., acetazolamide,

TABLE 25

NORMAL VALUES FOR LUMBAR FLUID

Age	Protein (mg/dL)	Glucose (mg/dL)	Cell (Count/mm^3)	Lymph/PMN (Ratio)	Opening Pressure (mm CSF)
Preterm	115	50	9	40/60	
Term	90	52	8	40/60	80–100
Child	5–40	40–80	0–5		60–200
Adult	20–40	50–70	0–5	100/0	60–200
Ventricular	6–15				
Cervical	20–30				

IgG/albumin ratio (CSF IgG/Alb) upper limit: 0.27.

IgG/albumin index (CSF IgG/Alb)/(serum IgG/Alb) upper limit: 0.60.

Myelin basic protein upper limit: 4 ng/mL.

Corrections

WBC: Reduce WBC by one cell for every 700 RBC (if hematocrit is normal) or: WBC (corr) = WBC(csf)– WBC(blood) ∞ RBC(csf)/RBC(blood).

Protein: Subtract 1 mg/mL for every 1000 RBC.

CSF, Cerebrospinal fluid; *PMN*, polymorphonuclear leukocyte; *RBC*, red blood cell; *WBC*, white blood cell.

C

CEREBROSPINAL FLUID

furosemide, topiramate) substantially reduce CSF formation. CSF is absorbed primarily by arachnoid villi extending into the dural venous sinuses. Normal CSF opening pressure during lumbar puncture (LP) should be less than 20 cm H_2O (Table 25).

APPEARANCE

Normal CSF is clear and colorless (specific gravity 1.007, pH 7.33–7.35); when cell counts reach approximately 200 white blood cells (WBCs)/mm^3 or 400 red blood cells (RBCs)/mm^3, it may become cloudy. Viscous CSF can result from large numbers of cryptococci within the CSF, secondary to their polysaccharide capsules. Clot or pellicle formation occurs with elevated protein. Froin syndrome refers to clot formation in the setting of complete spinal block and very high protein. CSF is perceived as grossly bloody with cell counts greater than 6000 RBC/mm^3, and at cell counts of more than 500, xanthochromia appears, which refers to the yellow, pink, or orange coloration of the CSF corresponding to the breakdown products of RBCs. Oxyhemoglobin released from RBCs can be detected within the supernatant fluid within 2 to 4 hours after the release of blood into the subarachnoid space; it reaches a maximum at about 36 hours and disappears in about 7 to 10 days. Supernatant fluid may, however, remain clear for up to 12 hours after a subarachnoid bleed. CSF can be analyzed with spectrophotometry or by visual inspection to rule out xanthochromia. The differential diagnosis of xanthochromia includes hyperbilirubinemia, hyperproteinemia, hypercarotenemia, and drugs (e.g., rifampin), though if there is clinical suspicion of subarachnoid hemorrhage (SAH) in the setting of a possible sentinel bleed or thunderclap headache, management should be directed toward a hemorrhagic cause such as a ruptured aneurysm.

CYTOLOGY

Cytologic analysis must be done soon after LP. Prompt refrigeration is necessary. Lymphocytes are the predominant leukocyte forms in normal CSF. An occasional granulocyte is seen in normal fluid and is not necessarily pathologic if the total WBC count is normal (0–3 cells/mm^3). A few or moderate numbers of granulocytes may occur following spinal anesthesia, myelography, or other intrathecal injections, or with trauma, hemorrhage, or infarct in the absence of infection.

No RBCs should be present in normal CSF. In a traumatic spinal tap, it is important to differentiate whether the WBCs are truly elevated or whether they are present in the same WBC/RBC ratio as in the peripheral blood. In a nonanemic patient, as an approximation, subtract 1 WBC for every 700 RBCs. Fishman's formula can be used for correction of WBC counts in the presence of significant anemia or peripheral leukocytosis. It estimates the WBC count in the CSF before the LP (actual WBC$_{CSF}$ = WBC$_{CSF}$ ∞ RBC$_{CSF}$/RBC$_{blood}$). Detection of tumor cells is enhanced by collection of large volumes of CSF (20 mL), repeated CSF examination, and cisternal taps in suspected basilar meningitis.

CEREBROSPINAL FLUID PROTEIN

CSF protein is a nonspecific indicator of disease. Normally, the blood-brain barrier keeps serum proteins out of the CSF (normal adult, 15–45 mg/dL). Many central nervous system (CNS) diseases disrupt the barrier, allowing entrance of serum protein and consequently elevation of CSF protein (see Table 21). Increases greater than 500 mg/dL are rare and occur mainly in spinal block, meningitis, arachnoiditis, and SAH. Metabolic conditions such as myxedema and diabetic neuropathy and Guillain-Barre syndrome may cause an increase in protein levels.

The major immunoglobulin in normal CSF is IgG. The IgG index and synthesis rate correct for serum IgG. Elevated levels may result from production within the CNS in various immune response disorders. Oligoclonal bands are not specific to one diagnosis and may indicate the presence of an immune-mediated pathologic process such as multiple sclerosis or, very rarely, subacute sclerosing panencephalitis. Serum should be drawn in conjunction with CSF collection to confirm that the oligoclonal banding is unique to the CSF. Oligoclonal bands occur in 80% to 90% of patients with clinically definite multiple sclerosis, but oligoclonal bands are less important than the clinical history and imaging findings in making the diagnosis. Myelin basic protein, a product of oligodendroglia, may be increased by any processes that result in myelin breakdown, such as stroke or anoxia; elevated levels are not a specific marker of demyelinating disease. Low CSF protein may occur with dural leaks and in benign intracranial hypertension. Protein in cisternal CSF is 50% of the lumbar value and is even lower (25%) within the lateral ventricles.

GLUCOSE

Glucose is derived from serum and is a reflection of the previous 4 hours of systemic glucose levels. Normal CSF to blood ratio is 0.6 with a usual value of 40 to 80 mg/dL. Simultaneous serum glucose level should be done. Hypoglycorrhachia occurs in bacterial, fungal, or tuberculosis meningitis, and inflammatory processes such as sarcoidosis, carcinomatous meningitis, and SAH. The mechanism of hypoglycorrhachia in meningeal disorders is related to an increase in anaerobic glycolysis in brain and spinal cord and, to a variable degree, polymorphonuclear leukocytes (PMNs) as well as an inhibition of glucose entry from altered glucose membrane transport across the blood brain barrier.

COMPLICATIONS OF LUMBAR PUNCTURE

Headache

Headache may occur immediately after LP or with persistent dural CSF leak, and occurs in about 5% to 10% of LP procedures. Onset is 5 minutes to 4 days after LP. Pain is related to positioning and may be diminished or relieved when the head is lowered and exacerbated by sitting up. Post-LP headache usually resolves spontaneously, the majority within 1 week, but may persist up to several months. These headaches are more common in women and younger patients. Provoking factors are related to larger needle size, use of the traditional beveled spinal needles, larger amounts of CSF obtained, and failing to replace the stylet before removing the needle. Preventive measures include use of the smallest gauge needle, insertion of the needle bevel parallel to the dural fibers of the posterior longitudinal ligament, and the use of nontraumatic needles.

Treatment of an established post-LP headache involves bed rest, adequate hydration (particularly if nausea and vomiting occur), and analgesics. Caffeine 300 to 500 mg PO and theophylline may be used. Intractable cases often respond (>80%) with an epidural blood patch by injection of 10 mL of the patient's freshly drawn blood into the epidural space, where it can clot. There is no evidence that extended bedrest after an LP prevents post-LP headache, contrary to popular belief.

Brain Herniation

Brain herniation may occur immediately or up to 12 hours after an LP in patients with supratentorial mass lesions and midline shift or obstructing posterior fossa tumors.

Bleeding

Spinal subdural, epidural, and SAH may occur in patients treated with anticoagulants or those with thrombocytopenia or bleeding diatheses.

Diplopia

Rare transient unilateral or bilateral abducens palsy can cause diplopia.

C

CEREBROSPINAL FLUID

Others

Radicular irritation, meningitis, and implantation of epidermoid tumor cells are also complications of LP.

Lumbar Puncture Contraindications

Contraindications include infection over the site of entry, coagulopathy, presence of a known or suspected intracranial mass especially with midline shift, and noncommunicating hydrocephalus (always try to obtain computed tomography [CT] before procedure). For patients with elevated intracranial pressure due to pseudotumor cerebri, CSF drainage via LP can be both diagnostic and therapeutic. In patients for whom the diagnosis of bacterial meningitis is suspected, the Infectious Disease Society of America guidelines recommend performing a CT brain prior to LP in patients with focal neurologic deficits, new onset seizures, suspicion for mass lesions, papilledema, alterations in consciousness, or immunocompromised states. Obtaining a CT prior to LP in patients without the above red flags should not delay prompt antibiotic therapy and worsens outcomes if bacterial meningitis goes untreated.

REFERENCES

Chu, K., et al. (2014). Spectrophotometry or Visual Inspection to Most Reliably Detect Xanthochromia in Subarachnoid Hemorrhage: Systematic Review. Ann Emerg Med, 64(3), 256–264.e5.

Arevalo-Rodriguez, I., Ciapponi, A., Munoz, L., Roqué i Figuls, M., Bonfill Cosp, X. (2013). Posture and fluids for preventing post-dural puncture headache. Cochrane Database of Systematic Reviews, Issue 7. Art. No.: CD009199. https://doi.org/10.1002/14651858. CD009199.pub2.

CHANNELOPATHIES

DEFINITION AND PATHOPHYSIOLOGY

Ion channels consist of multiple subunits, each with very similar structure but different electrophysiologic characteristics. The differing neuronal expression and combination of these subunits into complexes gives rise to enormous diversity in the properties and distribution of ion channels, which is reflected in the variety of diseases that make up the neurologic channelopathies (Table 26). Disorders of ion channels (channelopathies) are increasingly being identified, making this a rapidly expanding area of neurology. Ion channel function may be controlled by changes in voltage (voltage gated), chemical interaction (ligand gated), or mechanical perturbation.

I. Voltage-gated channelopathies causing inherited muscle diseases include the nondystrophic myotonias and familial periodic paralyses. Paramyotonia congenita is due to mutation in the gene coding for the α_1 subunit of the sodium channel; Thomsen disease (autosomal dominant myotonia congenita) and Becker disease (autosomal recessive myotonia congenita) are allelic disorders associated with mutations in a gene coding for skeletal muscle chloride channel. Familial hyperkalemic periodic

TABLE 26

CHANNELOPATHIES: MUSCLE AND NEURONAL DISEASES

Type of Channel	Channel	Disease
	Muscle Diseases Related to Channelopathies	
VOLTAGE-GATED		
Na^+ channels	α subunit of Na_v 1.4 (skeletal muscle)	Hyper- and hypokalemic periodic paralysis
		Paramyotonia congenita and other myotonic disorders
K^+ channels	α subunit of Kir2.1 inward rectifier (skeletal and smooth muscle)	Andersen syndrome
	Accessory subunit MiRP2 (assembles with K_V 3.4)	Hypokalemic periodic paralysis
Ca^{2+} channels	α subunit of Ca_V 1.1 (skeletal muscle Dihydropyridine-sensitive channel)	Hypokalemic periodic paralysis
	Ryanodine receptor (sarcoplasmic channel)	Malignant hyperthermia
		Malignant hyperthermia
Cl^- channels	ClC1 (skeletal muscle chloride channel)	Myotonia congenita (dominant and recessive)
LIGAND-GATED		
Nicotinic ACh R	α_1 subunit (skeletal muscle)	Congenital myasthenic syndromes
	β_1 subunit (skeletal muscle)	Congenital myasthenic syndromes
	δ subunit (skeletal muscle)	Congenital myasthenic syndromes
	$\in$ subunit (skeletal muscle)	Congenital myasthenic syndromes
	Neuronal Diseases Related to Channelopathies	
VOLTAGE-GATED		
Na^+ channels	α subunit of Na_v1.1 (somatic sodium channel)	Generalized epilepsy with complex febrile seizures
	α subunit of Na_v1.2 (axonal sodium channel)	Severe myoclonic epilepsy of infancy
	β_1 subunit of sodium channels	

Continued

CHANNELOPATHIES

C

TABLE 26

CHANNELOPATHIES: MUSCLE AND NEURONAL DISEASES—CONT'D

Type of Channel	Channel	Disease
K^+ channels	α subunit of $K_V 1.1$ (axonal/presynaptic delayed rectifier)	Generalized epilepsy with complex febrile seizures
		Generalized epilepsy with febrile seizures plus
	M-type potassium channel subunit (with KCNQ3)	Episodic ataxia type 1
	M-type potassium channel subunit (with KCNQ2)	Benign familial neonatal convulsions
		Benign familial neonatal convulsions
Ca^{2+} channels	α subunit of $Ca_V 2.1$ (P/Q-type channel in cerebellar neurons and presynaptic terminals)	Familial hemiplegic migraine
		Episodic ataxia type 2
		Spinocerebellar ataxia type 6
LIGAND-GATED		
Nicotinic ACh R	β_2 subunit of nicotinic receptors (with $\alpha 4$)	Autosomal dominant nocturnal frontal lobe epilepsy
	α_4 subunit of nicotinic receptors (with $\beta 2$)	Autosomal dominant nocturnal frontal lobe epilepsy
Glycine receptors	α_1 subunit (spinal cord inhibitory synapses)	Familial hyperekplexia
$GABA_A$ receptors	γ_2 subunit (brain inhibitory synapses)	Generalized epilepsy and complex febrile seizures
GLIAL		
Gap-junction proteins	Connexin 32 (paranodal myelin)	X-linked Charcot-Marie-Tooth disease

paralysis is due to mutations in the same sodium channel gene as that affected in paramyotonia congenita, while familial hypokalemic periodic paralysis results from mutations in the gene coding for the α_1 subunit of a skeletal muscle calcium channel.

The first demonstration that channelopathies could affect nerves as well as muscles came in 1995, when researchers discovered that episodic ataxia type 1, a rare autosomal dominant disease, results from mutations in one of the potassium channel genes. The impairment of potassium channel function, which normally limits nerve excitability, results in the rippling of the muscles (myokymia) of the face and limbs seen in this disease. Episodic ataxia type 2, also autosomal dominant, is not associated with myokymia but responds dramatically to acetazolamide, an unexpected feature it shares with many channelopathies. The suspicion that it might be a channelopathy was confirmed when mutations in a gene coding for the α_1 subunit of a brain-specific calcium channel were found. Mutations in this same gene can also cause familial hemiplegic migraine and spinocerebellar degeneration type 6. It is unclear how different mutations of the same gene can give rise to such different phenotypes. In the case of myotonia congenita and familial hyperekplexia, point mutations in the same gene can result in either autosomal recessive or dominant inheritance.

II. Ligand-gated channelopathies that have recently been described include familial startle disease, which is due to mutations of the α_1 subunit of the glycine receptor, and dominant nocturnal frontal lobe epilepsy, which is due to mutations of the α_4 subunit of the nicotinic acetylcholine receptor. A gene for familial paroxysmal choreoathetosis has been mapped to a region of chromosome 1p where a cluster of potassium channel genes is located.

III. Acquired channelopathies are caused by toxins and autoimmune phenomena. The marine toxin ciguatoxin, which contaminates fish and shellfish, is a potent sodium channel blocker that causes a rapid onset of numbness, intense paresthesias and dysesthesia, and muscle weakness. Antibodies to peripheral nerve potassium channels may result in neuromyotonia (Isaac syndrome). Lambert-Eaton myasthenia, which is associated with small cell carcinoma of the lung in 60% of cases, is caused by autoantibodies directed against a presynaptic calcium channel at the neuromuscular junction and against multiple calcium channels expressed by lung cancer cells. The abnormalities seen in Guillain-Barré syndrome, chronic inflammatory demyelinating polyneuropathy, and perhaps multiple sclerosis could also be explained by sodium channel dysfunction. Neuromyelitis optica is characterized by autoantibodies to the aquaporin-4 channel.

CLINICAL PRESENTATIONS

Several of the channelopathies have surprisingly similar clinical features, illustrated in Fig. 17. Typically, there are paroxysmal attacks of paralysis,

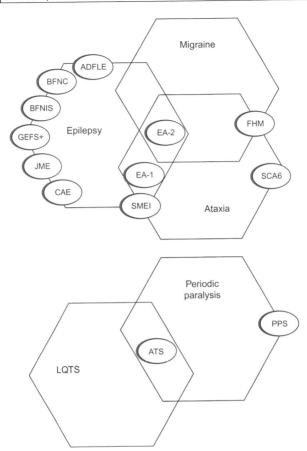

FIGURE 17

Channelopathies: overlap of signs between different diseases. *ADFLE,* Autosomal-dominant nocturnal frontal lobe epilepsy; *ATS,* Andersen/Tawil syndrome; *BFNC,* benign familial neonatal convulsions; *BFNIS,* benign familial neonatal-infantile seizures; *CAE,* childhood absence epilepsy; *EA-1,* episodic ataxia type 1; *EA-2,* episodic ataxia type 2; *FHM,* familial hemiplegic migraines; *GEFS,* generalized epilepsy with febrile seizures-plus; *JME,* juvenile myoclonic epilepsy; *LQTS,* long *QT* syndromes; *PPS,* periodic paralysis syndromes; *SCA6,* spinocerebellar ataxia type 6; *SMEI,* severe myoclonic epilepsy of infancy. (From Bernard, G., & Shevell, M. I. (2008). Channelopathies: a review. *Pediatr Neurol, 38*(2), 73–85.)

dystonia, myotonia, migraine, and ataxia precipitated by physiologic stressors. A channelopathy may cause an abnormal gain of function (such as myokymia, myotonia, and epilepsy) or an abnormal loss of function (such as weakness or numbness) depending upon whether loss of channel function leads to excessive membrane excitability or to membrane inexcitability.

TREATMENT

Many of the channelopathies respond predictably to membrane stabilizing drugs such as mexilitine and acetazolamide. Antiepileptic drugs such as carbamazepine and oxcarbazepine have been successful in treating paroxysmal kinesigenic and nonkinesigenic dyskinesias. The neuronal specificity of ion channels allows the potential for targeted drug therapy akin to the selective receptor agonists and antagonists currently available: 3,4-diaminopyridine, a potassium channel blocker, can relieve symptoms in patients with Lambert-Eaton syndrome. Dalfampridine is a similar drug, marketed in the United States and approved to improve walking by increasing walking speed in patients with multiple sclerosis. The use of this drug is contraindicated in patients with any history of seizure. Specific channel modulating drugs are currently being developed for migraine, chronic pain, and cardiac dysrhythmias and may be useful for neurologic channelopathies.

REFERENCES

Bernard, G., & Shevell, M. I. (2008). Channelopathies: a review. *Pediatr Neurol*, *38*(2), 73–85.

Erro, R., Bhatia, K. P., Epay, A. J., & Striano, P. (2017). The epileptic and nonepileptic spectrum of paroxysmal dyskinesias: Channelopathies, synaptopathies, and transportopathies. *Mov Disord*, *32*(3), 310–318.

CHEMOTHERAPY, NEUROLOGIC COMPLICATIONS

This section lists the neurotoxic signs caused by agents commonly used in patients with cancer.

I. **Acute encephalopathy:** corticosteroids, methotrexate (MTX), ara-C, cisplatin (rare), vincristine, L-asparaginase, procarbazine, 5-FU (with levamisole), nitrosoureas (high dose), cyclosporine, interleukin 2, ifosfamide/mesna, interferons, tamoxifen, VP-16 (high-dose), paclitaxel, OKT3, tipifarnib

II. **Chronic encephalopathy:** MTX, carmustine (1,3-Bis(2-chloroethyl)-1-nitrosourea [BCNU]) (intra-arterial), ara-C, carmofur, fludarabine, thiotepa (high dose)

III. **Posterior reversible leukoencephalopathy (PRES):** bevacizumab, cisplatin, carboplatin, paclitaxel, melphalan (high dose), cytarabine, filgrastim, erythropoietin, cyclosporine, tacrolimus, MTX (intrathecal [IT]), cyclophosphamide, ifosfamide, gemcitabine, immunosuppressants, sorafenib

IV. **Central nervous system demyelination:** MTX, 5-FU (with levamisole), fludarabine (can induce promyelocytic leukemia, particularly in chronic lymphocytic leukemia patients), cladribine

V. **Stroke/stroke-like/TIA:** MTX, L-asparaginase, cisplatin (with 5-FU), interleukin 2, bevacizumab, cyclosporine

VI. **Visual loss/other cranial neuropathy:** tamoxifen (retinopathy), gallium nitrate, nitrosoureas (intra-arterial), cis-platinum (cortical blindness), vincristine, irinotecan (dysarthria but rare), bevacizumab (optic neuropathy), fludarabine (cortical blindness)

VII. **Cerebellar dysfunction/ataxia:** ara-C, 5-FU, procarbazine, hexamethylmelamine, vincristine, cyclosporine A

VIII. **Aseptic meningitis:** IVIG, levamisole, monoclonal antibodies, metrizamide, OKT3, ara-C (IT), MTX (IT), bortezomib, corticosteroids (IT)

IX. **Seizures:** MTX, VP-16 (high dose), OKT3 antibody, cis-platinum, vincristine, L-asparaginase, nitrogen mustard, BCNU, dacarbazine, N-(phosphonacetyl)-L-aspartate (PALA), mAmsa, busulfan (high dose), cyclosporine, ifosfamide, chlorambucil, paclitaxel, vincristine (rare), MTX

X. **Myelopathy:** MTX (IT), ara-C (IT), thiotepa (IT), cyclosporine

XI. **Peripheral neuropathy:** ara-C (rare), carboplatin (rare), cisplatin (sensory), cyclosporine, docetaxel, hexamethyl, ifosfamide, interferon-α, melamine, methyl-G, mitotane oxaliplatin (acute dysesthesia), paclitaxel, procarbazine, suramin, thalidomide, vincristine (subacute to chronic; almost 100%), vinorelbine, VP-16, VM-26, 5-FU (rare), 5-azacytidine, bortezomib, epothilones, ifosfamide, MTX (lumbosacral polyradiculopathy via IT)

XII. **Myopathy:** vincristine (subacute), cyclosporine, corticosteroids

XIII. **Cerebral venous thrombosis:** L-Asparaginase

XIV. **Cerebral hemorrhage:** bevacizumab

XV. **Multifocal leukoencephalopathy:** ara-C, 5-FU

XVI. **Leukoencephalopathy:** fludarabine, carmustine (IA), MTX,

XVII. **Chronic neuropsychiatric syndrome:** interferon-α

XVIII. **Headaches:** corticosteroids, retinoic acid, tamoxifen

REFERENCES

Dropcho, E. J. (2010). Neurotoxicity of cancer chemotherapy. *Semin Neurol., 30*(3), 273–286.

Nolan, C. P., & DeAngelis, L. M. (2015). Neurologic complications of chemotherapy and radiation therapy. *Continuum, 21*(2), 429–451.

CHIARI MALFORMATIONS

Pathologist Hans Chiari described four types of cranial malformations. Chiari type II is also known as the Arnold-Chiari malformation.

PRESENTATION

Occipital headache (especially with straining and coughing) and lower cranial nerve palsies develop during adolescence or adulthood.

Type I: Cerebellar tonsils are herniated below foramen magnum (3 mm, mean of 13 mm vs. normal mean of 1 mm); this type is associated with syringomyelia and bony deformities.

Type II: Cerebellar vermis, fourth ventricle, and medulla are displaced inferiorly and deformed; associated with spina bifida and lumbar meningomyelocele, polymicrogyria, heterotropias, syringomyelia, hydromyelia, enlargement of the foramen magnum, elongation of the cervical arches, platybasia, basilar invagination, assimilation of the atlas, and Klippel-Feil anomaly. Symptoms begin in infancy or early childhood, most commonly presenting as hydrocephalus or respiratory distress.

Type III: This type includes cervical spina bifida, cerebellar herniation through the defect, and a dystrophic posterior fossa; it is rarely compatible with postnatal life.

Type IV: Fundamentally different from the other three, in the Chiari IV malformation there is no herniation of brain below the foramen magnum. Instead, there is hypolasia of the cerebellum, and an occipital encephalocele.

DIAGNOSIS

Magnetic resonance imaging (MRI) shows tonsils below the foramen magnum and blockage of cerebrospinal fluid flow; myelography and computed tomography may also be indicated.

TREATMENT

New onset symptoms or deteriorating symptoms may be referred for decompressive surgery, which is better if done within 2 years of symptoms onset. Asymptomatic patients with Chiari Malformation type I discovered incidentally could be managed conservatively with clinical and magnetic resonance imaging (MRI) surveillance.

REFERENCES

Langridge, B., Phillips, E., & Choi, D. (2017). Chiari Malformation Type 1: A Systematic Review of Natural History and Conservative Management. *World Neurosurg J.* https://doi.org/10.1016/j.wneu.2017.04.082.

Tubbs, R. S., Demerdash, A., Vahedi, P., et al. (2016). Chiari IV malformation: correcting an over one century long historical error. *Childs Nerv Syst*, *32*, 1175.

C

CHIARI MALFORMATIONS

CHILD NEUROLOGY: HISTORY, AND PHYSICAL EXAMINATION

I. History: Acute or insidious, focal or generalized, progressive or static process? At what age did the problem begin? These questions are all helpful in generating a differential diagnosis.

A. Birth history

1. Prenatal—infections [especially TORCH, which includes Toxoplasmosis, Other (syphilis, varicella-zoster, parvovirus B19), Rubella, Cytomegalovirus (CMV), and Herpes], maternal complications (hypertension, bleeding, preterm labor), medications or toxin exposure (drugs, alcohol, cocaine, tobacco, herbal, isotretinoin, other drugs).

2. Perinatal—gestational age, birth weight, length, head circumference, mode and presentation of delivery, maternal medications during delivery, Apgar scores, complications of delivery, resuscitation.

3. Postnatal—length of neonate's hospital stay, concomitant illnesses (jaundice, infection, seizures, IVH, respiratory problems/mechanical ventilation), newborn metabolic screen, hearing screen.

B. Developmental history: Gross motor, fine motor, speech, social skills, behavioral. These findings are very helpful in determining timing and progression of the underlying process. Remember to ask specifically about regression, to adjust for prematurity, and that girls typically achieve milestones earlier than boys (Fig. 18; Table 27 discuss developmental milestones and red flags). As the child gets older, behavioral and academic history should also be obtained.

C. Family history: Epilepsy, dysmorphisms, ataxia, early stroke, deafness, unexplained deaths or miscarriages, birth marks, intellectual disability, developmental delay, learning and behavioral disorders, genetic or chromosomal defects, psychiatric disorders, and consanguineous marriages. Be aware of racial and ethnic background as many disorders vary in frequency between populations.

D. Social history: Ask about home, school, drugs, alcohol, sex, and abuse. When speaking to teenagers, parents may be out of the room if the child chooses.

II. General physical examination: Observation of the child during the interview is critical (facial or bodily dysmorphism, developmental delays, gait abnormality, unusual motor movements). In younger children, we would recommend performing as much of the examination as possible on the parent's lap. Save painful or irritating portions of the examination until the end.

FIGURE 18

Denver II Development Screening Test. (Courtesy of W. K. Frankenburg, MD.) *See foldout for the figure.*

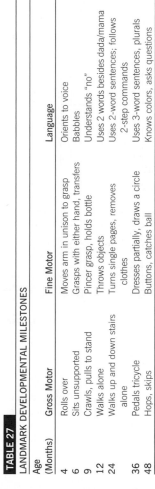

Denver II Development Screening Test. (Courtesy of W. K. Frankenburg, MD.)

TABLE 27

LANDMARK DEVELOPMENTAL MILESTONES

Age (Months)	Gross Motor	Fine Motor	Language	Social
4	Rolls over	Moves arm in unison to grasp	Orients to voice	Enjoys looking around
6	Sits unsupported	Grasps with either hand, transfers	Babbles	Recognizes strangers
9	Crawls, pulls to stand	Pincer grasp, holds bottle	Understands "no"	Explores, plays pat-a-cake
12	Walks alone	Throws objects	Uses 2 words besides dada/mama	Imitates, comes when called
24	Walks up and down stairs alone	Turns single pages, removes clothes	Uses 2-word sentences; follows 2-step commands	Parallel play
36	Pedals tricycle	Dresses partially, draws a circle	Uses 3-word sentences, plurals	Group play, shares toys
48	Hops, skips	Buttons, catches ball	Knows colors, asks questions	Tells "tall tales"

CHILD NEUROLOGY: HISTORY, AND PHYSICAL EXAMINATION

C

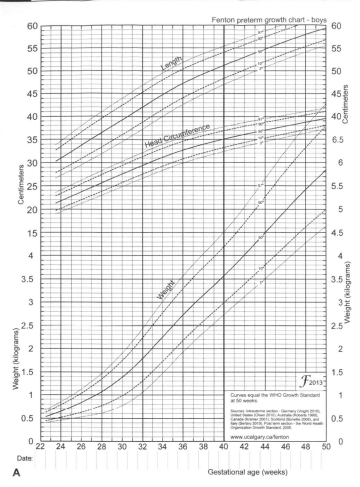

FIGURE 19

Continued

A. Measure weight, length, and head circumference and plot on the growth curves (Figs. 19–21). Average head circumference for full-term newborn at birth is 35 cm, and average growth is 1 cm per month over the first year. Height is roughly half of adult height by two years.

DIRECTIONS FOR ADMINISTRATION

1. Try to get child to smile by smiling, talking or waving. Do not touch him/her.
2. Child must stare at hand several seconds.
3. Parent may help guide toothbrush and put toothpaste on brush.
4. Child does not have to be able to tie shoes or button/zip in the back.
5. Move yarn slowly in an arc from one side to the other, about 8" above child's face.
6. Pass if child grasps rattle when it is touched to the backs or tips of fingers.
7. Pass if child tries to see where yarn went. Yarn should be dropped quickly from sight from tester's hand without arm movement.
8. Child must transfer cube from hand to hand without help of body, mouth, or table.
9. Pass if child picks up raisin with any part of thumb and finger.
10. Line can vary only 30 degrees or less from tester's line.
11. Make a fist with thumb pointing upward and wiggle only the thumb. Pass if child imitates and does not move any fingers other than the thumb.

12. Pass any enclosed form. Fail continuous round motions.

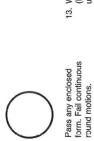

13. Which line is longer?
    (Not bigger.) Turn paper upside down and repeat.
    (pass 3 of 3 or 5 of 6)

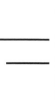
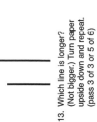

14. Pass any lines crossing near midpoint.

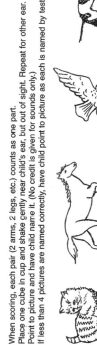

15. Have child copy first. If failed, demonstrate.

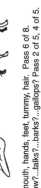

When giving items 12, 14, and 15, do not name the forms. Do not demonstrate 12 and 14.

16. When scoring, each pair (2 arms, 2 legs, etc.) counts as one part.
17. Place one cube in cup and shake gently near child's ear, but out of sight. Repeat for other ear.
18. Point to picture and have child name it. (No credit is given for sounds only.)
    If less than 4 pictures are named correctly, have child point to picture as each is named by tester.

19. Using doll, tell child: Show me the nose, eyes, ears, mouth, hands, feet, tummy, hair. Pass 6 of 8.
20. Using pictures, ask child: Which one flies?...says meow?...talks?...barks?...gallops? Pass 2 of 5, 4 of 5.
21. Ask child: What do you do when you are cold?...tired?...hungry? Pass 2 of 3, 3 of 3.
22. Ask child: What do you do with a cup? What is a chair used for? What is a pencil used for?
    Action words must be included in answers.
23. Pass if child correctly places and says how many blocks are on paper. (1,5).
24. Tell child: Put block on table; under table; in front of me, behind me. Pass 4 of 4.
    (Do not help child by pointing, moving head or eyes.)
25. Ask child: What is a ball?...lake?...desk?...house?...banana?...curtain?...fence?...ceiling? Pass if defined in terms of use, shape, what it is made of, or general category (such as banana is fruit, not just yellow). Pass 5 of 8, 7 of 8.
26. Ask child: If a horse is big, a mouse is ____? If fire is hot, ice is ____? If the sun shines during the day, the moon shines during the ____? Pass 2 of 3.
27. Child may use wall or rail only, not person. May not crawl.
28. Child must throw ball overhand 3 feet to within arm's reach of tester.
29. Child must perform standing broad jump over width of test sheet (8 1/2 inches).
30. Tell child to walk forward, ⟵⟶⟶⟶⟶ heel within 1 inch of toe. Tester may demonstrate.
    Child must walk 4 consecutive steps.
31. In the second year, half of normal children are non-compliant.

OBSERVATIONS:

Denver Developmental Materials, Inc.
P.O. Box 371075
Denver, Colorado 80237-5075
Tele. #: (303) 355-5075
(800) 419-4729

Catalog #2115   TO REORDER CALL: (800) 419-4729

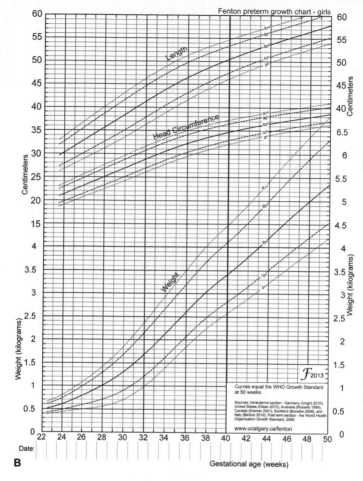

FIGURE 19—Cont'd

Fenton preterm growth charts, boys (A) and girls (B): weight, length, and head circumference. (Courtesy of Tanis Fenton, PhD.)

B. Look for any dysmorphic features (low-set ears, epicanthal folds, colobomas, midline defects, abnormal body shape or structure). Evaluate head shape, palpate the fontanels and sutures, and auscultate for bruits. In neonates, look for external trauma such as cephalohematoma, subgaleal hematoma, or caput succedaneum.

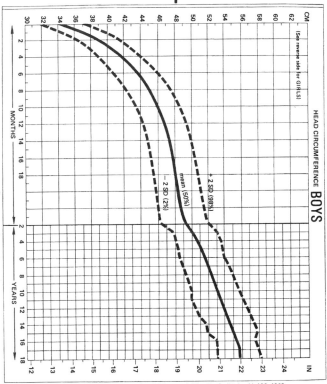

Ref: NELLHAUS, G., Composite International & Interracial Graphs, Pediatrics 41:106, 1968

BOYS

FIGURE 20

Head circumference, boys. (From Nellhouse G: Pediatrics 41:106, 1968. Used with permission.)

Name _____

Birth Date _____

Notes:

PATIENT INFORMATION:

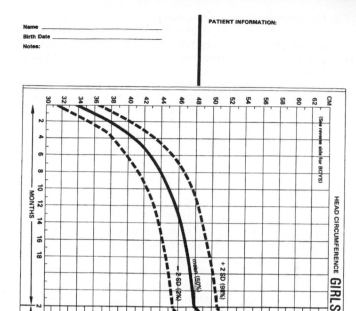

GIRLS

FIGURE 21

Head circumference, girls. (From Nellhouse G: *Pediatrics* 41:106, 1968. Used with permission.)

    C. Thorough ophthalmologic examination for cataracts, red reflex, chorioretinitis, optic nerve atrophy, papilledema, cherry red spot, retinitis pigmentosa, and retinal hemorrhages (often resulting from the birth process or trauma) should be performed. Ophthalmology consult may be necessary.

    D. Examine skin for any neurocutaneous stigmata; heart for signs of congestive heart failure or murmurs; abdomen for hepatosplenomegaly; back for scoliosis, sacral dimple, or hair tufts; and extremities for joint contractures or deformities.

III. Neurologic examination: Examination needs to be adapted to the age of the child. Older children are typically quite cooperative and their examination is similar to that for an adult.

    A. Mental status: Be aware of feeding and nap cycles, which may affect the child's mental state.

    B. Speech: Developmental milestones (both receptive and expressive); no words by 18 months is a red flag.

    C. Cranial nerves: Pupillary light reflex present at 29 to 30 weeks; optokinetic nystagmus present at 36 weeks (lack of this response may be a sign of gross visual impairment); oculovestibular reflexes present at 30 weeks; spontaneous extraocular eye movement at 32 weeks; rooting reflex (sensory V) present at 34 weeks; suck reflex reflects a combination of CN V, IX, X, and XII function and is present at 34 weeks; assess tongue for atrophy/hypertrophy and fasciculations.

    D. Motor: Observe resting posture, spontaneity and symmetry of movements. Much can be learned by just watching the child play and exploring the environment. Tone depends on level of alertness and gestational age and has a flexor progression in terms of gestational age (floppy at 28 weeks, strong flexor tone at term). Tone should be tested in both horizontal and vertical suspension as well as with traction from the supine position to assess head lag. Arching of the neck and back, scissoring of legs on vertical suspension, as well as fisting is indicative of increased tone. Hypotonic infants "slip through your fingers" at the shoulders, legs will flop apart in a frog-leg posture in supine position, and head will lag, as infant is pulled from supine to sitting by gentle arm traction. Formal manual muscle testing may be performed in older children.

    E. Deep tendon reflexes are present at 33 weeks. Look for asymmetries. Cross-adductor reflex is normal until 1 year of age. Five to 10 beats of ankle clonus is normal up to 3 months of age.

    F. Primitive reflexes (Table 28): Look for asymmetries, absence, or persistence. Occasionally these will be helpful in localization, but usually more useful for assessing general development.

TABLE 28

PRIMITIVE REFLEXES IN NEONATES AND INFANTS

Reflex	Response	Appears (Age)	Disappears (Age in Months)
Palmar grasp		28 weeks	4–5
Moro reflex (drop baby's head suddenly in relation to trunk)	Opens hands, extends and abducts upper extremities and draws them together	28–32 weeks	4–5
Gag		32 weeks	Persists
Suck		34 weeks	4
Tonic neck (rotate infant's head to the side while chest is maintained flat)	Arm and leg extend on side toward which face is rotated, flexion of limbs on opposite side; abnormal: asymmetric or obligatory and sustained pattern	34 weeks	4
Reflex stepping (baby supported in upright position)		35 weeks	5
Crossed adductor		35 weeks	7
Plantar grasp		Birth	9–12
Extensor plantar response (Babinski)		Birth	10
Placing (dorsum of foot placed against edge of table)		1 day	Covered by voluntary action
Landau reflex (lift baby with one hand under its trunk, face downward)	Reflex extension of vertebral column → baby lifts head above horizontal	3 months	24
Parachute response (suspend child horizontally about the waist, face down)	Arms extend and fingers spread	4–9 months	Covered by voluntary action

C

CHILD NEUROLOGY: HISTORY, AND PHYSICAL EXAMINATION

REFERENCES

Daroff, R. B., Jankovic, J., Mazziotta, J. C., & Pomeroy, S. L. (Eds.), (2015). *Bradley's neurology in clinical practice*, ed 7. Elsevier.

Fenton, R. T., & Kim, H. J. (2013). A systematic review and meta-analysis to revise the Fenton growth chart for preterm infants. *BMC Pediatrics*, *13*, 59.

CHOREA

Chorea is an involuntary, irregular, random, hyperkinetic movement that flows from one body part to another much like a dance (which is the meaning of its Greek origin *choreia*). Chorea is distinguished from other movement disorders by the random timing and distribution. The movements are often incorporated into deliberate movements by the patient that may camouflage the disorder. Grimacing and respiratory grunts may be manifestations. Determining the etiology of chorea is necessary as some are treatable and even reversible. A systematic method of assessing chorea is based on genetic versus nongenetic causes. Nongenetic causes may then be further divided into metabolic/endocrine, toxin and medication-related, infectious, autoimmune, vascular, and miscellaneous. While there is some overlap between these categories, having a systematic approach will minimize the risk of diagnostic inaccuracy.

GENETIC/HEREDITARY

While Huntington disease (HD) is the most common genetic/hereditary cause of chorea, clinicians should be aware of the numerous HD phenocopies including Huntington disease like (HDL) 1-3, HDL 4 (spinocerebellar ataxia type 17 or SCA17), and C9orf72-related HD phenocopy. Other genetic/hereditary causes of chorea include benign hereditary chorea (TITF-1 gene mutation), neuroacanthocytosis, McLeod syndrome, dentatorubral-pallidoluysian atrophy, neuroferritinopathy, aceruloplasminemia, SCA1, SCA2, SCA3 (Machado-Joseph disease), Wilson disease, pantothenate kinase-associated neurodegeneration (PKAN), Friedreich ataxia, pallidonigroluysian atrophy, lubag disease (TAF1) olivopontocerebellar atrophy, ataxia-telangiectasia, ataxia oculomotor apraxia types 1 and 2, and tuberous sclerosis of basal ganglia.

METABOLIC/ENDOCRINE

Metabolic and endocrine causes include adrenal insufficiency, hyper/hypocalcemia, hyper/hypoglycemia, hypomagnesemia, hypernatremia, liver failure, uremia, vitamin B_1, B_3, or B_{12} deficiency, or pregnancy (chorea gravidarum).

TOXIC/MEDICATION

The most common toxic causes include alcohol intoxication/withdrawal, anoxia, carbon monoxide, manganese, mercury, thallium, and toluene. Numerous medications have been reported to cause chorea including amantadine, amphetamine, anticonvulsants, antihistamines, central nervous system stimulants (methylphenidate, pemoline, cyproheptadine, cocaine), dopamine agonists, dopamine-receptor blockers, levodopa, levofloxacine, theophylline, tricyclic antidepressants, corticosteroids, and valproic acid.

INFECTIOUS
Infectious etiologies include AIDS-related disease such as toxoplasmosis, progressive multifocal leukoencephalopathy, and HIV encephalitis. Bacterial causes include diphtheria, Scarlet fever, Sydenham chorea, and whooping cough. Encephalitis include B19 parvovirus, herpes-6 virus encephalitis, Japanese encephalitis, measles, mumps, West Nile River encephalitis. Parasites and protozoa include neurocysticercosis, malaria, Whipple disease, and syphilis.

AUTOIMMUNE
Immune-mediated causes are vast and include acute disseminated encephalomyelopathy, anti-GABA B receptor antibody, anti-NMDA receptor encephalitis, antiphospholipid syndrome Behçet disease, celiac disease, human papilloma virus vaccine, LGI1 antibody, various paraneoplastic syndromes, sarcoidosis, Sjögren syndrome, SC and variants, contraceptive-induced chorea, and systemic lupus erythematosus.

VASCULAR
Vascular causes include brainstem/putamenal cavernous malformations, Moyamoya syndrome, polycythemia vera, pontine and other intraparenchymal hemorrhage, postpump chorea (cardiac surgery), posterior reversible encephalopathy syndrome, stroke, and subdural hematoma.

MISCELLANEOUS
Other miscellaneous causes include brainstem glioma, cerebral palsy, cerebrospinal fluid shunt-induced, extrapontine myelinolysis, intratumoral chemotherapy catheter, kernicterus, multiple sclerosis, physiological chorea of infancy (<12 months old), Buccal-oral-lingual dyskinesia, edentulous orodyskinesia, senile chorea (likely multifactorial), and post-traumatic brain injury.

TREATMENT OF CHOREA
Identifying the cause of choreic movements is of critical importance as many of the aforementioned etiologies are treatable with agents such as antibiotics, nutritional supplementation, or removal of an offending agent. Despite the absence of evidence to confirm the efficacy of neuroleptics, a trial of an atypical neuroleptic is a reasonable first line therapy. Although no disease-modifying treatments exist, symptomatic management for Huntington disease chorea may include tetrabenazine (initial: 12.5 mg/day; testing for CYP2D6 function required for doses above 50 mg/day), amantadine (300 to 400 mg/day),

C

CHOREA

clonazepam (0.5 to 6 mg/day), or riluzole (200 mg/day). Other agents with less clear benefit include Coenzyme Q10, creatine, nabilone, or clozapine. Mood stabilizers such as selective serotonin reuptake inhibitors may also be tried.

REFERENCES

Armstrong, M. J., & Miyasaki, J. M. (2012). Evidence-based guideline: pharmacologic treatment of chorea in Huntington disease: Report of the Guideline Development Subcommittee of the American Academy of Neurology. *Neurology*, *79*(6), 597–603.
Cardoso, F. (2017). Autoimmune choreas. *J Neurol Neurosurg Psychiatry*, *88*(5), 412–417.

CHROMOSOMAL DISORDERS

Chromosomal abnormalities have been reported to occur in 4% to 34% of individuals with mental retardation (MR). Diagnosis of these abnormalities is important in terms of defining prognosis, establishing risk of recurrence, avoiding further unnecessary testing, and providing families with an answer as to the cause of their child's problems. Significant advances in cytogenetics have substantially improved our diagnostic yield. Current cytogenetic testing options include routine karyotyping (high-resolution chromosomal banding analysis), individual fluorescence in situ hybridization (FISH) assays, subtelomeric FISH assay, comprehensive genomic hybridization (chromosomal microarray analysis), and whole exome sequencing. Indications for routine chromosomal analysis include intellectual disability and developmental delay (DD), microcephaly, multiple congenital anomalies or dysmorphisms, sexual ambiguity, abnormal skin pigmentation, family history of MR or miscarriages, or suspected genetic syndrome (see Table 29).

Specific guidelines regarding the type and resolution of chromosomal analysis required are still debated, but at minimum all cases of intellectual

---

TABLE 29

COMMON CLUES TO THE NEED FOR CHROMOSOMAL ANALYSIS

FAMILY HISTORY
- Recurrent miscarriage
- Infertility
- Family history of developmental delay, mental retardation, and/or multiple congenital anomalies
- Family history of balanced chromosome rearrangement

CLINICAL FACTORS
- Low birth weight, congenital microcephaly, and dysmorphic features
- Multiple congenital anomalies
- Hemihypertrophy and/or significant body asymmetry
- Pigmentary dysplasia (streaky hyper-/hypopigmentation)
- Infertility and/or delayed puberty
- Unexplained developmental impairment or autistic spectrum disorder

From Descartes, M., Korf, B. R., & Mikhail, F. M. (2017). Chromosomes and chromosomal abnormalities. In K. F. Swaiman, et al. (Eds.), *Swaiman's pediatric neurology*, ed. 6 (pp. 268–276). Elsevier.

disability and DD without known cause deserve routine karyotyping. Further testing can be guided by clinical suspicion based on phenotypic findings characteristic of known syndromes (see later descriptions) via individual FISH (microdeletions, duplications, and subtelomeric rearrangements) or DNA analysis for specific gene abnormalities. If the patient does not fit any syndromic description and routine karyotyping is normal, comprehensive genomic hybridization may be of benefit. It encompasses all abnormalities that would be detected on routine chromosomal analysis and multiple individual FISH assays (all microdeletions, duplications, and telomeres), along with some single gene disorders.

I. Single gene disorders
   A. Fragile X: second most common inherited cause of MR after Down syndrome (1/4000 to 1/9000 boys and 1/7000 to 1/15,000 girls).
      • Presentation: MR, long face with prominent chin, large ears, and macro-orchidism after puberty. Macrocephaly is frequently present. Hyperactivity and delayed speech in the young child. Autism seen in 8% to 15% of children. X-linked recessive inheritance, but some female carriers may have MR. DNA analysis shows an expanded number of CGG trinucleotide repeats in the FMR-1 gene on the X chromosome.
   B. Rett syndrome: 1 in 10,000 females
      ○ Presentation: Normal development in the first 6 to 18 months followed by regression in social, fine, and motor skills. MR, language regression, loss of purposeful hand movement (replaced by stereotypical hand wringing), acquired microcephaly (deceleration in head growth), seizures, and spastic diplegia. X-linked disorder caused by mutations (exons 1–4, 85%) or deletions (10%) in the MECP2 gene. Phenotypic expression is quite variable, and occurrence has rarely been reported in males with MR. Both mutations and deletions are detectable with DNA analysis of the MECP2 gene.

II. Trisomies
   A. Trisomy 21 (Down syndrome): 1 in 800 births; 95% of Down syndrome is secondary to trisomy 21, with the rest caused by either translocation (most commonly between chromosome 21 and chromosome 14) or mosaicism.
      • Presentation: MR, hypotonia, infantile spasms, oblique palpebral fissures, median epicanthal fold, Brushfield spots (accumulation of fibrous tissue appearing as light-colored spots encircling the periphery of the iris), low-set ears, thick protruding tongue, bilateral simian creases, short extremities and digits, heart anomalies, GI anomalies (duodenal atresia), and upper cervical spine malformation. In later life, these patients develop Alzheimer's disease with progressive cognitive decline with neuritic plaques and neurofibrillary tangles. They are also at risk for stroke in childhood

   due to congenital heart disease. Seizures are also common in later
   adult life.
B. Trisomy 13: 1 in 7000 births
   • Presentation: Severe MR, microcephaly, microphthalmos,
     holoprosencephaly, craniofacial anomalies, low-set dysplastic ears,
     polydactyly, cutis aplasia, "rocker bottom feet," and congenital heart
     disease.
C. Trisomy 18 (Edward syndrome): 1 in 4000 births
   • Presentation: Severe MR, microcephaly, brain grossly and
     microscopically normal in 50%, long narrow skull, low-set
     dysplastic ears, second finger overlies third, thumb distally
     implanted and retroflexible, heart anomalies, polycystic
     kidneys.
III. Subtelomeric rearrangements: Approximately 6% to 7% of patients with
   moderate MR have a subtelomeric chromosomal abnormality.
   Abnormalities are detected on telomeric FISH assay.
   • Presentation: Intrauterine growth retardation, postnatal failure to thrive
     or overgrowth, two or more facial dysmorphic features, one or more
     nonfacial dysmorphic features or congenital anomalies, and family
     history of MR.
IV. Microdeletion syndromes
   A. DiGeorge (DG)/velocardiofacial (VCF) syndrome
      o Presentation: Mild to moderate MR, cardiac defects (conotruncal),
        thymic aplasia/hypoplasia, and hypocalcemia. VCF syndrome has
        MR, with cleft palate, cardiac defects, hypotonia, dysmorphic facies,
        short stature, and velopharyngeal incompetence. Significant overlap
        occurs between these two syndromes, as well as extreme phenotypic
        variability. Both syndromes are associated with 22q11.2 deletion
        (95%) and are detected by FISH analysis. DG syndrome has also
        been associated with a second deletion of 10p13p14.
   B. Prader-Willi syndrome (PWS)
      o Presentation: MR, infantile hypotonia and failure to thrive, short
        stature, small hands and feet, micropenis and cryptorchidism,
        childhood onset obesity secondary to hyperphagia, blond hair, blue
        eyes, fair skin, and almond-shaped palpebral fissures. About 70% of
        cases are secondary to a paternal deletion in the 15q11-q13
        chromosome, which may be detected using FISH analysis. Other
        chromosomal abnormalities associated with PWS include maternal
        uniparental disomy of chromosome 15 (25%) and nonexpression of
        the paternal genes on the same chromosome (2%). Neither of these
        abnormalities is detected by FISH; thus it is recommended that
        when PWS is suspected, testing via DNA methylation be performed.
        This will detect all of the previously mentioned abnormalities.
   C. Angelman syndrome (AS)
      o Presentation: Severe MR, microbrachycephaly, large mouth,
        prognathia "puppet-like" ataxic gait, absent speech, seizures, and

paroxysms of laughter. About 70% of cases are due to a maternal deletion in the 15q11-q13 chromosome which may be detected using FISH analysis. Other chromosomal abnormalities associated with AS include paternal uniparental disomy of chromosome 15 (3%–5%), mutations in the UBE3A gene (5%), and nonexpression of the paternal genes on chromosome 15 (7%–9%). None of these abnormalities is detected by FISH, and thus, it is recommended that when AS is suspected, testing via DNA methylation be performed; if negative, then further DNA sequence analysis for UBE3A mutations should be performed.

D. Smith-Magenis syndrome (SM)
   o Presentation: MR, brachycephaly with midface hypoplasia, self-abusive behavior. SM is associated with deletions on 17p11.2 detectable by FISH assay.

E. Williams syndrome
   o Presentation: MR, "elfin facies," blue eyes with stellate pattern iris, congenital heart disease (particularly supravalvular aortic stenosis), intermittent hypercalcemia, loquacious personality, and hoarse voice; 90% are associated with deletions of the elastin gene on 7q11.23 detectable by FISH assay.

V. Sex chromosomal abnormalities

A. XO (Turner syndrome) (1 in 2000 females): Usually normal intelligence (but frequently problems with visuospatial skills), short stature, broad chest with widely spaced nipples, low posterior hairline, webbed neck, congenital lymphedema, cubitus valgus, ovarian dysgenesis.

B. XXY (Klinefelter syndrome) (1 in 500 males): Mild MR, learning disabilities, language disorder, behavior disorders, intention tremor, tall with long limbs, hypogonadism with hypogenitalism, gynecomastia.

C. XYY: Borderline MR, learning disabilities, behavior disorders, tall stature.

D. XXX: MR without other specific findings.

REFERENCES

Daroff, R. B., Jankovic, J., Mazziotta, J. C., & Pomeroy, S. L. (Eds.), (2015). *Bradley's neurology in clinical practice*, ed 7. Elsevier.

Dulac, O., Lassonde, M., & Sarnat, H. B. (Eds.), (2013). *Pediatric neurology, Part I/II/III, ed 1 (Handbook of Clinical Neurology, vol. 111/112/113)* Elsevier.

COMA (See also BRAIN DEATH, CARDIOPULMONARY ARREST, AND AAN GUIDELINE APPENDIX)

Consciousness is the state of awareness of self and surroundings. Loss of awareness with concomitant defects in arousal constitutes coma or, when less pronounced, a state of lethargy, stupor, and obtundation. Coma is neither a unitary state nor an etiologic diagnosis. Its presence suggests specific dysfunction of both hemispheres or dysfunction of the brainstem reticular activating system, or both. The mechanism of dysfunction may be a structural lesion (supratentorial or subtentorial), a metabolic disturbance, or psychogenic.

Coma evaluation requires a detailed medical history and a general physical examination to establish potential causes. In addition to complete chemistry tests, blood cell count, and coagulation panels, blood gas levels [observe color and request carbon monoxide (CO) level], toxicology screens (on blood, urine, and gastric contents), thyroid function tests, cortisol level, and cultures should be obtained at the time of initial evaluation of coma of unknown cause. Emergency management is outlined in Table 30.

The neurologic examination is focused toward determining the pathophysiologic features by distinguishing the location and degree of central nervous system dysfunction, including the following.

I. Level of consciousness: Response to voice, shaking, or pain. Consider status epilepticus, akinetic mutism, vegetative state (VS), locked-in (de-efferented) syndrome, and psychogenic states (see below).

II. Brainstem function
   A. Pupils: Light reflex tests for cranial nerves II and III (midbrain).
      1. Anisocoria: Horner syndrome suggests hypothalamic or lateral medullary dysfunction; without Horner syndrome, and if there are associated ocular motility deficits, consider transtentorial herniation.

TABLE 30

EMERGENCY MANAGEMENT OF COMA OF UNKNOWN CAUSE

1. Ensure oxygenation. Clear airway, suction, perform bag-valve-mask ventilation, and intubation as needed. Immobilize cervical spine prior to neck extension until C-spine injury is excluded. Atropine, 1 mg IV, may prevent vagally mediated bradyarrhythmias during intubation.
2. Maintain circulation with fluids and pressors to keep mean arterial pressure above 100 mm Hg. Continuous ECG monitoring is necessary.
3. Thiamine, 100 mg IV, followed by glucose 25 g (50 mL D_{50}) IV, immediately after blood is drawn (large volume) for diagnostics.
4. Treat intracranial hypertension if suspected.
5. Stop seizures when present (see Epilepsy).
6. Restore acid-base balance.
7. Treat drug overdose.
   a. For suspected opiate overdose: naloxone (Narcan) 0.4 mg IV, repeat as necessary if effective (short half-life) or in 5 min.
   b. For suspected anticholinergics (e.g., tricyclics), physostigmine, 1 mg IV.
   c. For suspected benzodiazepine overdose, flumazenil starting at 0.2 mg IV over 30 seconds. Failure to respond to a total dose of 5 mg makes it unlikely that coma is due to benzodiazepines.
8. Exclude intracranial masses by CT (uncontrasted). MRI may be performed when stable.
9. Normalize body temperature.
10. Treat infection if suspected (see Meningitis).
11. Specific therapy should be instituted as soon as a diagnosis is established.

2. Miosis: Common in toxic or metabolic encephalopathy (preserved light reflex is a hallmark of metabolic coma) and central herniation with supratentorial mass lesion. Pinpoint, barely reactive pupils suggest acute pontine lesion or opiate use.

3. Mydriasis: In association with absent light reflex and (sometimes) irregular pupils, suggests dorsal midbrain dysfunction. Atropine or sympathomimetics commonly given during resuscitation may cause mydriasis.

4. Fixed, midposition pupils suggest midbrain nuclear (third cranial nerve) dysfunction.

B. Eye movements: Assess conjugacy, spontaneous movements, gaze deviation or preference, nystagmus. Oculocephalic responses and vestibulo-ocular testing with ice water and head elevated 30 degrees evaluate brainstem connections of cranial nerves III, VI, and VIII. Presence of nystagmus without ocular deviation to the irrigated ear on caloric testing suggests psychogenic coma, because it indicates integrity of brainstem and hemispheric pathways. Roving eye movements suggest an intact brainstem. Ocular bobbing and its variants suggest pontine lesions.

C. Corneal or sternutatory reflexes test cranial nerves V and VII (pons).

D. Gag (pharynx) or cough (larynx-trachea) reflexes test cranial nerves IX and X (medulla).

III. Breathing patterns

A. Breathing patterns are of little localizing value but aberrant breathing patterns are common and may be a false localizing sign in cases of coexisting metabolic derangement (e.g., metabolic acidosis and hypoxia cause reactive hyperventilation, simulating neurogenic hyperventilation).

1. Cheyne-Stokes respirations consist of cyclically increasing, then decreasing respiratory depth and rate, separated by apneic phases. It results from the interaction of an increased ventilatory drive to P_{CO_2} and a decreased forebrain stimulus for respiration, when P_{CO_2} is decreased. It suggests bilateral cerebral hemispheric or diencephalic dysfunction but may be produced by an encephalopathic state, or severe congestive heart failure.

2. Central neurogenic hyperventilation is attributed to brainstem injury. Tachypnea is more common and is usually associated with hypocapnia and hypoxemia. It often resolves with correction of the metabolic abnormalities, whereas central neurogenic hyperventilation does not. Tachypnea with brainstem disease may be associated with neurogenic pulmonary edema.

3. Apneustic breathing consists of prolonged "jamming" of respiration in inspiratory and expiratory phases. Although rare, it is seen with dorsolateral pontine lesions at the level of the sensory trigeminal nucleus.

    4. Ataxic breathing consists of generally slow, irregular respirations with variable amplitude and can progress rapidly to complete apnea. It is due to bilateral lesions of the reticular formation in the caudal dorsomedial medulla, where the respiratory rhythm is generated. Medullary compression, usually caused by acute lesions, may result in respiratory arrest, leading to cardiovascular collapse.

IV. Sensorimotor function

    A. Spontaneous activity. Assess for volitional movement, choreoathetosis, posturing (arms decorticate or flexor vs. decerebrate or extensor), asterixis, myoclonus, and seizures.

    B. Response to noxious stimuli (listed in order of increasing severity of coma). Lateralizing features of response should be noted.

        1. Purposeful.

        2. Flexion withdrawal.

        3. Abnormal flexion (decorticate posturing): Usually slow, stereotyped flexion of arm, wrist, and fingers with shoulder adduction and variable leg extension.

        4. Abnormal extension (decerebrate posturing): Extension of wrist and arm with adduction and internal rotation of shoulder; extension and internal rotation of leg with plantar flexion of foot.

        5. No response.

    C. Tone: Assess for flaccidity, rigidity, spasticity, clonus, and paratonia.

    D. Tendon reflexes: Assess for asymmetry, increase, or decrease in response.

The Glasgow coma scale quantitates level of consciousness. It is easy to use and reliable, with low interobserver variability (Table 31). Because the scale does not assess brainstem reflexes, it does not communicate a

TABLE 31

GLASGOW COMA SCALE

Category	Response	Score[a]
Eye opening	Open spontaneously	4
	To verbal command	3
	To pain	2
	Do not open	1
Best motor response	Obeys to verbal command	6
	Localizes pain	5
	Flexion withdrawal	4
	Flexion-abnormal (decorticate)	3
	Extension-abnormal (decerebrate)	2
	No response	1
Best verbal response	Oriented and converses	5
	Disoriented and converses	4
	Verbalizes	3
	Vocalizes	2
	No response	1

[a]Total score ranges from 3 to 15.

complete neurologic assessment but is useful for rapid identification, reliable communication, serial quantitation, and aid in assessing prognosis, particularly when used in evaluation of posttraumatic coma.

CAUSES OF COMA
I. Supratentorial lesion
   A. Presentation
      a. Supratentorial mass with diencephalic or brainstem compression
      b. Early focal cerebral dysfunction
      c. Rostral to caudal progression with signs referable to one area at a time
      d. Asymmetrical motor signs
      e. Third-nerve palsy preceding coma (early herniation)
   B. Etiologies
      a. Hemorrhage: epidural, subdural, subarachnoid, intracerebral; hypertensive, vascular malformation
         Infarction: thrombotic or embolic arterial occlusion, venous thrombosis
      b. Tumor: primary, metastatic
      c. Abscess: intracerebral, subdural
      d. Closed head injury: edema, diffuse axonal injury
II. Infratentorial lesion
   a. Compressive: cerebellar hemorrhage, infarct, tumor, or abscess; posterior fossa subdural, extradural hemorrhages, basilar aneurysm
   b. Destructive: brainstem hemorrhage, infarction, tumor, demyelination, or abscess
III. Diffuse brain dysfunction
   A. Presentation
      a. Confusion and stupor precede motor signs
      b. Motor signs usually symmetrical
      c. Pupillary reactions usually preserved (except with certain drugs and toxins; see Pupil)
      d. Asterixis, myoclonus, tremor, and seizures are common
      e. Acid-base disturbance with hypoventilation or hyperventilation is common
   B. Etiologies
      a. Intrinsic: encephalitis, progressive multifocal leukoencephalopathy, meningitis, concussion, ictal or postictal state, herniation
      b. Hypoxic or metabolic: anoxia, ischemia, nutritional (e.g., Wernicke syndrome), hepatic encephalopathy, uremia, pulmonary disease, nonketotic hyperglycemic hyperosmolar coma, ketoacidosis, disseminated intravascular coagulation, hypoglycemia, Addison disease, myxedema, thyrotoxicosis, panhypopituitarism
      c. Toxic, drug-induced: opiates, amphetamines, cocaine, psychedelics, tricyclics, phenothiazines, lithium, benzodiazepines, methaqualone, glutethimide, barbiturates, alcohol, ibuprofen, aspirin

C

COMA

      d. Acid-base disorders: hypo-osmolarity or hyperosmolarity; hyponatremia or hypernatremia, hypocalcemia or hypercalcemia, hypophosphatemia, lactic acidosis, cerebral edema

      e. Hypothermia, hyperthermia

      f. Remote effects of cancer (paraneoplastic): limbic encephalitis, thalamic degeneration

   D. Psychogenic coma

     A. Presentation

       a. Psychogenic unresponsiveness

        1. Lids tightly closed

        2. Pupils reactive or dilated (factitious mydriatics)

        3. Oculocephalic responses highly variable; nystagmus and arousal occur with caloric stimuli

        4. Motor tone normal or inconsistent

        5. Breathing normal or rapid

        6. Reflexes nonpathologic

        7. Normal electroencephalogram (EEG)

     B. Etiologies

       a. Conversion reaction

       b. Catatonic stupor

       c. Malingering

III. Other states of consciousness related to coma

   A. **Vegetative state:** Subacute or chronic condition after severe brain injury characterized by wakefulness, sleep-wake cycles, and eye opening to auditory stimuli, without evidence of consistent cognitive function or response to stimuli. Blood pressure and respirations are maintained. VS may follow coma and persist for years (duration > 1 month is called *persistent vegetative state*). About one third of patients eventually become more responsive (more common in traumatic than in hypoxic cases). May occur with forebrain, occipital, hippocampal, or diffuse cerebral or cerebellar destruction.

   B. **Minimally conscious state (MCS):** Defined as a condition of severely altered consciousness in which minimal but definite behavioral evidence of self or environmental awareness is demonstrated. Although MCS patients can demonstrate cognitively mediated behaviors, they occur inconsistently, but are reproducible on extended assessments. Distinguishing between VS and MCS is difficult because precisely reproducing behaviors may be quite difficult. However, the difference may imply different prognosis.

     Behaviors reported in MCS include following simple commands, yes/no responses, appropriate smiling or crying in response to stimuli, reaching and touching objects purposefully, and visual pursuit or fixation.

   C. **Akinetic mutism:** Subacute or chronic condition characterized by seeming alertness, yet minimal vocalization or movement even with noxious stimuli. May occur with cingulate, limbic, corpus striatum, globus pallidus, thalamic, or reticular formation damage.

D. **Locked-in syndrome:** Intact consciousness plus quadriplegia and lower cranial nerve dysfunction. Voluntary vertical, and sometimes horizontal, eye movements are preserved. Usually occurs with ventral pontine infarcts, tumors, hemorrhages, or myelinolysis; ventral midbrain infarction; head injury; or severe neuromuscular disease. May be transient or chronic.

IV. Prognosis in coma, excluding psychogenic, traumatic, and drug-related causes, is usually poor. Prediction is less reliable in cases of intoxications and trauma but more precise after cardiopulmonary arrest (see Cardiopulmonary Arrest). In general, the longer coma lasts, the lower the chance for regaining independent function.

A. Prediction: Several standard measures, such as Glasgow coma scale, and case series may predict prognosis in coma, Outcome and mortality vary by etiology and widely varying estimates may be obtained from various case series.

Levy et al. reported on 500 patients, excluding known trauma or drug intoxication.

1. At 6 hours after onset of coma, absence of any of the following was associated with less than 5% chance of good recovery:
   a. Pupillary light reflex
   b. Corneal reflexes
   c. Oculocephalic reflexes
   d. Vestibulo-ocular reflexes (calorics)
2. One day after onset, no patients with absent corneal reflexes had satisfactory recovery.
3. Three days after onset, no patient with absence of pupillary reflexes, corneal reflexes, or motor function had satisfactory recovery.
4. Predictors of good outcome are less reliable than negative predictors.
   a. Six hours after onset, moaning or better verbal response plus pupillary, corneal, or oculovestibular responses: 41% of patients had good recovery.
   b. One day after onset, with inappropriate or better words plus any three of pupillary, corneal, oculovestibular, or motor responses: 67% had good recovery.
   c. Three days after onset, with inappropriate or better words plus corneal and motor responses: 74% had good recovery.
   d. Seven days after onset, with eye opening to pain plus localizing motor response: 75% had good recovery.

B. Overall outcome (at 1 year):
   1. 16% of patients were back to independent life.
   2. 11% were severely disabled.
   3. 12% were in a VS.
   4. 61% died without recovery.

REFERENCES

Horsting, M. W., Franken, M. D., Meulenbelt, J., van Klei, W. A., & de Lange, D. W. (2015). The etiology and outcome of non-traumatic coma in critical care: a systematic review. *BMC Anesthesiology*, *15*, 65. https://doi.org/10.1186/s12871-015-0041-9.

Posner, J. B., Saper, C. B., Schiff, N., & Plum, F. Stupor and Coma, ed 4. Oxford University Press, New York, NY.

COMPLEX REGIONAL PAIN SYNDROME (REFLEX SYMPATHETIC DYSTROPHY)

DEFINITION AND CLINICAL FEATURES

Complex regional pain syndrome (CRPS) is a disorder of the extremities which is characterized by pain, sensory, sudomotor and vasomotor disturbances, trophic changes, and impaired motor function (Table 32). Two types of CRPS have been identified. In CRPS type I, there is no definable nerve lesion. CRPS type I represents the majority (90%) of clinical cases. In CRPS type II, a definable nerve lesion is present, limiting its responsiveness to treatment.

TABLE 32

SIGNS AND SYMPTOMS OF COMPLEX REGIONAL PAIN SYNDROME

Region	Signs/Symptoms
Sensory	Spontaneous burning or stinging pain (80%) occurring with active or passive movements
	Pain spreads beyond initial site of injury
	Mechanical hyperesthesia (65%) e.g., clothes resting on skin
	Mechanical allodynia (74%)—pain with light touch or brushing
	Mechanical hyperalgesia (100%)—exaggerated response to pinprick
	Temperature allodynia—tested with cool or warm test tubes of water
	Extreme sensitivity to temperature changes
	In CRPS II, electrical sensation or shooting pain is common
	Hypoesthesia in affected nerve distribution with extreme allodynia; cold allodynia is also more common
	Foreign feeling of affected limb (30%)
Vasomotor	Asymmetry of color (66%) and temperature (56%)
	Sympathetic hypofunction—skin is red, hot, and dry
	Sympathetic hyperfunction—skin is cold, blue, pale or mottled, and sweaty
	Thermography may reveal a 1∞C difference
Sudomotor and edema	Asymmetry in sweating (53%)
	Limb edema (80%)
	Smooth-handled instrument will glide more easily over sweaty area than a dry area

Continued

TABLE 32

SIGNS AND SYMPTOMS OF COMPLEX REGIONAL PAIN SYNDROME—CONT'D

Region	Signs/Symptoms
Motor	Decreased range of motion (70%)
	Weakness (56%–77%)
	Tremor (9%–20%) and myoclonus
	Exaggerated reflexes on affected side (40%)
	Focal dystonia (14%)
	Contractures and fibrosis if chronic in late stages
Trophic	Trophic changes in skin (20%), hair (9%), nails (9%)
	Osteoporosis on x-ray

CRPS, Complex regional pain syndrome.

ETIOLOGY AND PATHOGENESIS

CRPS is often preceded by some kind of injury, including fracture (25%–47%), soft tissue injury (40%), myocardial infarction (12%), or stroke (12%). Sometimes, no precipitating event is found (5%–10%). Female–male ratio is 4:1. Proposed mechanisms include trauma-related cytokine release, exaggerated neurogenic inflammation, sympathetically maintained pain, and cortical reorganization in response to chronic pain.

DIAGNOSIS

CRPS remains a clinical diagnosis. Diagnostic criteria for CRPS by the International Association for the Study of Pain are listed here:

I. Preceding noxious event to the affected limb, with (CRPS I) or without (CRPS II) an obvious nerve lesion

II. Continuing pain, allodynia, or hyperalgesia not limited to a single nerve territory and disproportionate to the inciting event

III. Presence of edema, skin blood flow (temperature), or sudomotor (sweat) abnormality, motor symptoms, or trophic changes on the affected extremity

IV. Other diagnoses are excluded

Three stages of CRPS have been identified: Stage I (acute phase) includes pain, temperature changes, and hyperalgesia. Stage II (dystrophic phase) has worsening of stage I symptoms. Stage III (atrophic phase) usually includes irreversible tissue damage with thin skin, thickened fascia, muscle contracture, joint stiffness, diffuse osteoporosis, limb movement reduction, and allodynia.

The following tests support the diagnosis: Comparative x-ray examination may reveal spotty osteoporotic changes. Three-phase bone scan (scintigraphy) reveals tracer uptake in late images suggesting increased bone metabolism. Magnetic resonance imaging (MRI) can exclude other causes (e.g., septic or inflammatory arthritis). Measurement of cutaneous temperature by thermography or infrared thermometer shows difference of 1°C between

C

COMPLEX REGIONAL PAIN SYNDROME

affected and unaffected limb is present in 75% to 98% of patients with reflex sympathetic dystrophy. Autonomic testing of resting skin temperature (RST), resting sweating output test, and quantitative sudomotor reflex test have been reported to have high sensitivities and specificities.

TREATMENT

All treatment should be focused primarily on functional restoration. Blocks, psychotherapy, and drugs are reserved for situations of failure to progress or in significant concomitant problems such as depression. Physical, occupational, and recreational therapy and vocational rehabilitation are geared to minimize edema, normalize sensation (desensitization maneuvers), promote normal positioning, decrease muscle guarding, and increase functional use of each extremity to improve functional use of the extremity to increase independence in work, leisure, and activities of daily living.

Neuropathic pain is treated with nonsteroidal anti-inflammatory drugs, tricyclic antidepressants (amitriptyline and nortriptyline), or anticonvulsants (gabapentin, pregabalin). For severe refractory pain, opioids may be used. Nasal calcitonin (300 IU daily) and bisphosphonates (e.g., clodronate IV 300 mg qd for 10 days) can improve motor function and pain control. Palmidronate and alendronate are alternatives. A short course of corticosteroids may be tried, such as prednisone 60–80 mg daily for 2 weeks. Evidence for corticosteroids is limited, and long-term use has not been demonstrated to be effective.

Postganglionic blocks (intravenous regional blocks), ganglion blocks (lumbar sympathetic and stellate ganglion blocks), and preganglionic blocks (epidural block) may be transiently effective in a selected group. If repeated blocks are required, surgical sympathectomy is an option. Predictors of response to sympathetic blocks include abnormal QSART and RST, cold allodynia, and a positive effect from a single sympathetic block. Dorsal spinal cord stimulator and implantable peripheral nerve stimulator may be used if conventional treatment fails to improve pain control.

REFERENCES

Chevreau, M., et al. (2017). Bisphosphonates for treatment of Complex Regional Pain Syndrome type 1: a systematic literature review and meta-analysis of randomized controlled trials versus placebo. *Joint Bone Spine*, *84*(4), 393–399. https://doi.org/10.1016/j.jbspin.2017.03.009. Epub 2017 Apr 11.

Harden, R. N., Swan, M., King, A., Costa, B., & Barthel, J. (2006). Treatment of complex regional pain syndrome: functional restoration. *Clin J Pain*, *22*(5), 420–424.

COMPUTED TOMOGRAPHY

Computed tomography (CT) combines conventional x-ray with a digitized, computerized reconstruction technique that yields multiple two-dimensional images of the body. Tissues are assigned absorption coefficients (CT or

TABLE 33

COMPUTED TOMOGRAPHY DENSITY

Moiety	Hounsfield Units
Bone	600–2000
Freshly congealed blood	50–100
Gray matter	37–41
White matter	30–34
Cerebrospinal fluid (CSF)	8–18
Water	0
Adipose	−100 to −60
Air	−1000 to −600

From Blumenfeld, H. (2010). *Neuroanatomy through clinical cases.* Sunderland: Sinaur Associates Publishers.

C

COMPUTED TOMOGRAPHY

Hounsfield numbers) by the computer and are displayed along a grey scale (low radiodensity, dark; high radiodensity, bright) (Table 33). The range of CT numbers displayed can be manipulated to focus on certain structures (e.g., bony structures or intracranial contents) by "windowing." The window width (WW) determines the range of CT numbers displayed, and the window level determines the center of the WW.

Nonenhanced CT (NECT) of the brain is primarily used for the detection of hemorrhage, acute infarcts, or masses. Hemorrhage is initially hyperdense (white), gradually becomes isodense (gray and equal to brain tissue), and finally hypodense (black) over time. Findings of acute infarction include hyperdensity within an occluded vessel (especially the middle cerebral artery), loss of gray-white matter differentiation, effacement of sulci, and hypodensity involving both the gray and white matter (Table 34). Masses, unless they are hypercellular (i.e., lymphoma, meningioma), can be difficult to detect on NECT. Secondary signs of mass effect, such as midline shift, edema within the white matter, and hydrocephalus are readily seen on NECT. However, a contrast-enhanced CT or magnetic resonance image (MRI) is more sensitive in detecting masses.

Iodinated intravenous (IV) contrast material enhances (brightens) many normal vascular structures (large vessels, choroid plexus, tentorium, and falx) as well as highly vascular pathologic structures (tumors, metastases, lymphoma). "Ring" enhancement (white rim around a dark core) is seen with metastases, abscess, gliomas, subacute infarcts, contusions, demyelinating plaque, radiation necrosis, acquired immune deficiency syndrome (AIDS)-related central nervous system (CNS) disease, lymphoma, and resolving hematomas.

CT angiography allows visualization of the intra/extracranial vasculature. It is performed with a rapid bolus of IV contrast agent to enhance the vessels in order to acquire axial images, which can be further reviewed in any plane on a computer workstation. It is useful for the detection of aneurysms, evaluation of vascular dissection, and measurement of the degree of stenosis of a vessel. However, conventional angiography remains the gold standard, particularly for detecting small (<3 mm) aneurysms, revealing beading of vessels in vasculitis,

TABLE 34

COMPUTED TOMOGRAPHY FINDINGS IN STROKE

	Infarct	
Duration	Without Contrast	With Contrast
Hyperacute (<1 day)	Normal or obscuration of lentiform nuclei	Hyperdense vessel sign, blurring of gray-white junction, and/or no enhancement effacement of gyri
Acute (1–7 days)	Vaguely defined hypodensity, best seen after 3–4 days	No enhancement maximal edema and mass effect
Subacute enhancement (8–21 days)	Hypodensity less evident "brain fogging"; decreased mass effect and edema	Gyral (peaks at week 3)
Chronic (>21 days)	Hypodensity sharply defined, negative mass effect, isodense to CSF	Enhancement usually in 6–7 weeks

	Intraparenchymal Hemorrhage	
Duration	Appearance	Mass Effect
Acute (0–3 days)	Homogeneous hyperdensity	+++
Subacute		
Early (3 days to 3 weeks)	Enlarging hypodense periphery with hyperdense center	++
Late (3–5 weeks)	Hypodense periphery; isodense center	+
Chronic (>5 weeks)	Hypodense periphery; hypodense center several months[a]	±

[a]Ring enhancement is present from week 1 to week 7.

and characterizing arteriovenous malformations (AVMs). CT is preferred to MRI for evaluating patients in the acute setting (with the exception of cord compression). However, CT is less sensitive than MRI in detecting subtle areas of tumor, infarct, or demyelination, as well as brainstem/cerebellar lesions, old hemorrhage, leptomeningeal enhancement, and spinal cord abnormalities. It is the modality of choice for those unable to undergo MRI because of metal devices (aneurysm clips, cochlear implants, pacemakers), claustrophobia, or agitation.

REFERENCES

Blumenfeld, H. (2010). *Neuroanatomy through clinical cases.* Sunderland: Sinaur Associates Publishers.

Jadhav, A. P., & Jovin, T. G. (2012). Vascular imaging of the head and neck. *Semin Neurol., 32*(4), 401–410.

C

CONVERSION DISORDER

Conversion disorder or functional neurological symptom disorder (FNsD) is defined as a psychiatric illness in which symptoms and signs affecting voluntary motor or sensory function cannot be explained by a neurological or general medical condition. Generally, conversion disorder differs from FNsD in that typically a psychological stressor is deemed responsible for symptoms. The neurobiology of these disorders remains largely unknown.

PRESENTATION

Conversion disorder symptoms range widely in frequency, duration, and level of distress; however, it is important to note that *symptoms experienced are real and often debilitating.* The core symptoms are those of motor or sensory function or episodes of altered awareness. Common examples include blindness, paralysis, dystonia, psychogenic nonepileptic seizures, blackouts, anesthesia, swallowing difficulties, motor tics, difficulty walking, hallucinations, dysphonia, dysarthria, and dementia. Other symptoms also commonly occur in patients with conversion disorder; however, these are not defined by neurological deficit. These include chronic pain, fatigue, sleep disturbance, poor memory, concentration, nausea, irritable bowel syndrome, depression, and anxiety. A history of sexual abuse is very common.

DIAGNOSIS

The diagnostic criteria for conversion disorder in the Diagnostic and Statistical Manual of Mental Disorders-5 emphasize the importance of positive physical criteria in making the diagnosis.
1. One or more symptoms of altered voluntary motor or sensory function.
2. Clinical findings provide evidence of incompatibility between the symptom and recognized neurological or medical conditions.
3. The symptom or deficit is not better explained by another medical or mental disorder.

CONVERSION DISORDER

4. The symptom or deficit causes clinically significant distress or impairment in social, occupational, or other important areas of functioning or warrants medical evaluation.

The diagnosis of FNsD should be made on the basis of positive features in the history and examination, not on the absence of disease (Table 35). Key concepts to remember include:

1. FNsD is a diagnosis of inclusion not exclusion.
2. FNsD signs demonstrate the potential for reversibility.
3. FNsD signs demonstrate the functional role of attention and the benefit of distraction.

TREATMENT
Once diagnosis is confirmed, the key to successful treatment is the establishment of a strong therapeutic physician-patient alliance and the incorporation of a multidisciplinary goal-oriented treatment program including psychotherapy, physical therapy, and medication to treat underlying psychiatric issues. Follow-up evaluations and consideration of the etiology of newly emergent symptoms are also critical components of successful treatment.

REFERENCES
Ali, S., Jabeen, S., Pate, R. J., et al. (2015). Conversion disorder-mind versus body: a review. *Innov Clin Neurosci, 12*, 27–33.

Stone, J., & Carson, A. (2011). Functional neurologic symptoms: assessment and management. *Neurol Clin, 29*, 1–18. vii.

CONFUSIONAL STATE (See DELIRIUM)
Please refer to "Delirium".

CRAMPS

DEFINITION
Muscle *cramps* are sudden, temporary, involuntarily forcibly contracted or overshortening of muscle that causes mild-to-excruciating pain, attended by visible or palpable knotting of muscle, relieved by passive stretching or massage. This contrasts to muscle *spasm*, defined as a sustained involuntary muscle contraction, with or without pain, that cannot be terminated by voluntary relaxation.

ETIOLOGY
Muscle cramps are caused by ectopic discharges from nerves or nerve terminals due to hyperexcitability of the nerves, damage to the central mechanisms responsible for controlling potentiation, or damage to the nerve itself and/or associated muscle unit. When the motor system is stressed, such as with neurodegenerative disease, neuromuscular disease, or physiologic stress (dehydration, electrolyte imbalance, excessive exercise, etc.), cramps become more frequent.

TABLE 35

POSITIVE SIGNS IN FUNCTIONAL DISORDERS

FUNCTIONAL NEUROLOGICAL DISORDER

Hoover's sign	Hip extension weakness that returns to normal with contralateral hip flexion against resistance
Hip abductor sign	Hip abduction weakness that returns to normal with contralateral hip abduction against resistance
Evidence of inconsistency	For example, weakness of ankle plantar flexion on the bed but able to walk on tiptoes
Global pattern of weakness	Global weakness affecting extensors and flexors equally
Give way weakness	Patient transiently has normal power, but then the limb gives way, sometimes just before it is touched

FUNCTIONAL MOVEMENT DISORDER OR PSYCHOGENIC MOVEMENT DISORDER

Tremor entrainment test	Unilateral tremor is asked to copy a rhythmical movement with their unaffected limb: the tremor in the affected hand either "entrains" to the rhythm of the unaffected hand, stops completely, or the patient is unable to copy the simple rhythmical movement.
Tremor distractibility	Using mental tasks such as calculate serial 7s can temporarily abolish tremor or change frequency. Voluntary ballistic movements of unaffected hand often stops tremor briefly during the movement.
Attempted immobilization	Attempting to immobilize the affected limb often makes a functional tremor worse. Likewise, loading the limb with weights tends to make the tremor worse, whereas organic tremor tends to improve with this maneuver.
Cocctivation sign	Presence of voluntary coactivation of agonist and antagonist muscles
Coherence analysis	If functional tremor is present in more than one limb, it usually has the same frequency. In contrast, organic tremor usually has slightly different frequencies.
Fixed dystonic posture	A typical fixed dystonic posture, characteristically of the hand (with flexion of fingers, wrist, and/or elbow) or ankle (with plantar and dorsiflexion)
Functional hemifacial overactivity, pseudoptosis	Orbicularis oculis or orbicularis oris over-contraction appears with forehead weakness with a depressed eyebrow. A similar appearance of lower facial weakness can occur because of overactivity of the platysma. Features enhanced on examination by sustained voluntary contraction of facial or periocular muscles.

Continued

C

CRAMPS

TABLE 35

POSITIVE SIGNS IN FUNCTIONAL DISORDERS—CONT'D

Balance/gait	Dragging gait with external or internal hip rotation. Tightrope walker's gait where the arms are outstretched like a tightrope walker, often with lurches to one side and the other but good recovery of balance. Astasia-abasia with normal limb power and sensation on the bed but inability to stand. Crouching gait, which requires better strength and balance than a normal gait. Grab onto walls, chairs, or "fall" into bed, but will avoid a complete fall or injury.
Reduced postural sway with distraction	Abnormal sway that resolves during tasks such as assessing numbers written on the back or using a phone

PSYCHOGENIC NON-EPILEPTIC SEIZURES OR NON-EPILEPTIC ATTACK DISORDER

Prolonged attack of motionless unresponsiveness	Paroxysmal motionlessness and unresponsiveness lasting longer than a minute
Long duration	Attacks lasting longer than 2 minutes without any clear-cut features of focal or generalized epileptic seizures
Closed eyes	Closed eyes during an attack, especially if there is resistance to eye opening
Ictal weeping	Crying either during or immediately after the attack
Memory of being in a generalized seizure	Ability to recall the experience of being in a generalized shaking attack
Presence of an attack resembling epilepsy with a normal EEG	A normal electroencephalogram (EEG) does not exclude frontal lobe epilepsy or deep foci of epilepsy but does provide supportive evidence.

VISUAL SYMPTOMS

Fogging test	Vision in the unaffected eye is progressively "fogged" using lenses of increasing diopters while reading an acuity chart. A patient with good acuity at the end of the test must be seeing out of their affected eye.
Tubular visual field	The patient has a field defect of the same width at 1 m as at 2 m

DIAGNOSTIC APPROACH

The first diagnostic step is to determine whether the patient exhibits concordant neuromuscular signs and symptoms. These include muscular weakness/rigidity/atrophy/myotonia, loss of voluntary control including twitching/spasms, sensory abnormalities including numbness/tingling/myopathic pain or joint deformities. The second step should distinguish distribution between localized muscle cramps from generalized cramps. Frequently localized muscle cramps are related to nerve/root compression or motor neuropathy. Generalized muscle cramps are invariably associated with generalized disturbances such as electrolytes, osmolarity, etc. In the assessment of muscle cramps, electromyography (EMG) is valuable in distinguishing a true cramp (motor unit hyperactivity) from contracture (electrically silent), tetany (sensory and motor unit hyperactivity), or dystonia (agonist and antagonist recruitment) (Table 36). Typically, the EMG signature of a cramp consists of a crescendo of high-frequency, high-amplitude motor unit potentials which causes an interference pattern.

1. Physiological cramps (i.e., without neuromuscular signs)
    a. **Presentation:** Physiologic cramps can occur in both skeletal and smooth muscle. Usually they involve single muscles rather than groups, with clinical examination typically significant for visible or palpable hardening of the associated muscle. Sequelae include muscle soreness and swelling with elevated serum creatine kinase (CK).
    b. **Etiology:**
        i. Dehydration
        ii. Metabolic: hyponatremia, hypomagnesemia, hypocalcemia, glucose

C

CRAMPS

TABLE 36

ELECTROMYOGRAPHICAL DIFFERENCES

True cramp (motor unit hyperactivity):
- Idiopathic cramp
- Lower motor neuron disease
- Hemodialysis cramp
- Heat cramp
- Fluid- and electrolyte-related
- Drug-induced cramp

Contracture (electrically silent):
- Metabolic myopathy
- McArdle disease
- Thyroid disease

Tetany (sensory and motor unit hyperactivity):
- Hypocalcemia
- Respiratory alkalosis
- Hypomagnesaemia
- Hypokalemia
- Hyperkalemia

Dystonia (simultaneous contraction of agonist and antagonist muscles):
- Occupational cramp
- Drug-induced cramp

  iii. Endocrine: thyroid (hyper- or hypo-); adrenal insufficiency, uremia

  iv. Liver dysfunction

  v. Pregnancy: frequently during the last trimester of pregnancy

  vi. Familial cramp syndromes (Satoyoshi syndrome, HANAC, Becker muscular dystrophy, type II muscle fiber predominance, etc.)

  vii. Medications/drugs: nifedipine, cimetidine, beta-agonists, ethanol, clofibrate, penicillamine, and diuretics

 c. **Treatment:** Invariably reversing the systemic disorder of an acquired cramp or symptomatic management (Table 37)

2. Toxin-related cramps

 a. **Tetanus:** Tetanospasmin, a neurotoxin secreted by *Clostridium tetani*, interferes with central-mediated gamma amino butyric acid (GABA) and glycine release, producing hyperexcitability of lower motor neurons.

  i. **Presentation:** Rapidly progressive, generalized, continuous tonic contractures with superimposed painful spasms and autonomic instability. Tonic spasms of the masticatory muscles (trismus or lockjaw) is common. The spasms may be triggered by sensory stimuli or emotional stress.

  ii. **Laboratory findings:** EMG is similar to stiff-person syndrome.

  iii. **Treatment:** Supportive; ventilatory support, tetanus antitoxin, diazepam, or curare may be used. Intensive care monitoring is necessary to address autonomic dysfunction, (cardiac dysrhythmias; labile blood pressure).

  iv. **Prognosis:** Mortality 20% to 50%.

 b. **Strychnine:** Component of rat poison, inhibits glycine release in the central nervous system causing stiffness and muscle spasms and generalized tonic-clonic seizures.

  i. **Laboratory findings:** Detected in urine and gastric fluid

  ii. **Treatment:** Supportive

  iii. **Prognosis:** Good

 c. **Cholinesterase intoxication:** Cholinesterase inhibition suppresses enzyme action causing excessive buildup of acetylcholine at the synaptic cleft.

TABLE 37

TREATMENTS FOR CRAMPS

Normalize metabolic abnormalities
Quinine sulfate: 260 mg qhs or bid
Carbamazepine: 200 mg bid or tid
Phenytoin: 300 mg qd
Tocainide: 200–400 mg bid
Verapamil: 120 mg qd
Amitriptyline: 25–100 mg qhs
Vitamin E: 400 IU qd
Riboflavin: 100 mg qd
Diphenhydramine: 50 mg qd
Calcium: 0.5–1 g elemental Ca++ qd

i. **Presentation:** Excessive actions of the parasympathetic nervous system, SLUDGE (salivation, lacrimation, urination, diarrhea, gastrointestinal distress, emesis)—seen excessive therapy for myasthenia gravis, snake venoms, organophosphate poisoning (often suicide attempts), and nerve gases such as sarin and VX

ii. **Treatment:** Decontamination and supportive with mainstay medical therapy: atropine, pralidoxime (2-PAM), and benzodiazepines

iii. **Prognosis:** Mortality 20%

3. Neuromuscular disorders

a. **Motor system disorders:** Increased lower motor neuron excitability with spread of ectopic motor unit potentials to nearby nerve terminals

  i. Acquired motor neuropathies:
    1. Spinal stenosis, plexopathy, radiculopathy, polyneuropathies

  ii. Hereditary motor neuron disorders:
    1. Spinal muscular atrophy, bulbar motor neuron syndromes, hereditary motor neuropathy

  iii. Lesions of anterior horn cells
    1. Amyotrophic lateral sclerosis, poliomyelitis, West Nile virus

b. **Spontaneous activity syndromes**

  i. **Stiff-person syndrome:**
    1. **Presentation:** Adult onset of uncontrolled fluctuating proximal rigidity typically in axial muscles with progression to limbs over time present only during wakefulness. Cramping is extremely painful, often provoked by movement, noise, or other sensory stimuli. Palpable paraspinal contractions and hyperactive deep tendon reflexes, but spasticity and weakness are absent.
    2. **Diagnosis:** EMG: continuous activity in agonist and antagonist muscles with normal motor unit morphology. Antibodies to glutamic acid decarboxylase are found in serum and cerebrospinal fluid in 80% of cases.
    3. **Treatment:** First line agents: high-dose benzodiazepines. Second line agents include baclofen, valproic acid, and gabapentin. Immunosuppressive therapies with plasma exchange, immunoglobulin, prednisone, azathioprine. Refractory cases have used botulinum toxin injection, oral dantrolene.

  ii. **Neuromyotonia** (Isaac syndrome):
    1. **Presentation:** Insidious onset of generalized muscle stiffness, generalized myokymia with variable excessive sweating, dysarthria, dysphagia, and paresthesias, but pain is not usually present.
    2. **Diagnosis:** EMG shows short continuous bursts of motor unit activity at 10 to 100 Hz, often associated with autoimmune channelopathies.
    3. **Treatment:** Phenytoin, carbamazepine, dantrolene, or immunomodulation. Motor activity is not altered by spinal or proximal nerve block.

C

CRAMPS

      iii. **Cramp-fasciculation syndromes**

         1. **Presentation:** Subacute or chronic history of diffuse fasciculations and cramps. Similar to tetany but without metabolic disturbance and similar to hyperexcitable nerve syndrome with less prominent lancinating pain and paresthesias

         2. **Treatment:** Carbamazepine

4. Contractures (electrically silent cramps)

   a. **Inherited Metabolism Disease:** Glycogenoses (myophosphorylase deficiency, McArdle disease), lipidoses, and carnitine palmitoyltransferase (CPT) deficiency)

      i. **Presentation:** Abnormal muscle activity precipitated by exercise (glycogenoses and CPT deficiency) or fasting (CPT deficiency). Characterized as electrically silent contractures on EMG.

      ii. **Treatment:** High-carbohydrate diet for phosphorylase deficiency and a high-carbohydrate/low-fat diet for CPT deficiency.

   b. **Rippling muscle disease** is a rare disease that may be acquired (autoimmune) or congenital (autosomal dominant or recessive).

      i. **Presentation:** Involuntary muscle stiffness, hypertrophy of large muscles with myoedema, and visible muscle contractions. Cardiac subtype may present with heart failure and dysrhythmias.

      ii. **Treatment:** Those that lack family history or those associated with thymoma respond to immunomodulation or thymectomy, respectively.

   c. **Brody syndrome**

   d. **Myoedema**

REFERENCES

Jansen, P. H., Gabreëls, F. J., & van Engelen, B. G. (2002). Diagnosis and differential diagnosis of muscle cramps: a clinical approach. *J Clin Neuromuscul Dis*, *4*(2), 89–94.

Young, G. (2009). Leg cramps. *BMJ Clin Evid*, *26*. pii: 1113.

CRANIAL NERVES

The cranial nerves and their functions and innervations are listed in Table 38. Expanding on this list, Table 39 shows the clinical features of lesions in these nerves. The cranial nerves are anatomically in close proximity to one another, so it is useful when evaluating a patient to look for cranial nerve deficits within the same area when evaluating for a mass lesion versus other causes, such as ischemia, connective tissue disease, or demyelinating processes.

REFERENCES

Ropper, A. H., Samuels, M. A., & Klein, J. P. (2014). Diseases of the cranial nerves. In *Adams & Victor's principles of neurology*, ed (p. 10). New York: McGraw-Hill.

White, J. S. (2004). *USMLE road map neuroscience.* New York: Lange/McGraw-Hill.

TABLE 38

CRANIAL NERVES AND THEIR FUNCTIONS

Nerve	CNS Nucleus	Function/Innervation
I	Olfactory bulb	Smell
II	Lateral geniculate nucleus	Vision
III	Oculomotor nucleus	Extraocular muscles except superior oblique and lateral rectus
	Edinger-Westphal nucleus	Sphincter pupillae and ciliary muscle
IV	Trochlear nucleus	Superior oblique muscle
V	Spinal and main sensory nucleus	Sensory from face, deep tissues of head and neck, dura mater, and tympanic membrane
	Mesencephalic nucleus	Muscle spindles; mechanoreceptors of face and mouth
	Trigeminal motor nucleus	Muscles of mastication and tensor tympani
VI	Abducens nucleus	Lateral rectus muscle
VII	Facial motor nucleus	Muscles of facial expression and stapedius
	Spinal trigeminal nucleus	Sensory from external ear and tympanic membrane
	Solitary nucleus	Taste from anterior 2/3 of tongue
	Superior salivatory nucleus	Salivary and lacrimal glands
VIII	Cochlear and vestibular nuclei	Balance and hearing
IX	Nucleus ambiguous	Muscles of pharynx
	Spinal trigeminal nucleus	Sensory from external ear, tympanic membrane, and posterior 1/3 of tongue
	Solitary nucleus	Taste from posterior 1/3 of tongue
	Solitary and spinal trigeminal	Carotid body and sinus; sensation from nasal nuclei and oral pharynx
	Inferior salivatory nucleus	Parotid gland
X	Nucleus ambiguous	Muscles of larynx and pharynx
	Spinal trigeminal nucleus	Sensory from external ear
	Solitary nucleus	Taste buds of epiglottis
	Solitary and spinal trigeminai	Parasympathetics from thoracic and abdominal viscera; sensory from larynx and pharynx
	Dorsal motor nucleus	Parasympathetics to thoracic and abdominal viscera
XI	Nucleus ambiguous	Muscles of larynx and pharynx
	Accessory nucleus	Sternocleidomastoid and trapezius
XII	Hypoglossal nucleus	Intrinsic tongue muscles

CNS, Central nervous system.

CRANIAL NERVES

C

TABLE 39

CRANIAL NERVES: CLINICAL FEATURES OF LESIONS

Nerve	Name	Type	Function	Clinical Features of Lesions
I	Olfactory	Sensory	Smell	Anosmia
II	Optic	Sensory	Vision	Anopsia (visual field defects)
III	Occulomotor	Motor	All eye muscles (except lateral rectus and superior oblique)	Diplopia, external strabismus
				Loss of parallel gaze
			Adduction (medial rectus muscle)	Ptosis
			Upper eyelid elevator	Mydriasis; loss of motor limb light reflex with CN II
			Constricts pupil	Loss of accommodation
			Accommodates	Mydriasis seen first in compressive lesions
				Pupillary sparing "down and out" lesions suggestive of ischemia
IV	Trochlear	Motor	Superior oblique; depresses and abducts eyeball	Weakness looking down when eye adducted
			Intorsion	Head tilts away from lesion side
V	Trigeminal	Mixed	General sensation (touch, pain, temperature) of forehead/scalp, cornea	Sensory loss forehead/scalp
	V1-ophthalmic		General sensation of palate, nasal cavity, maxillary face, maxillary teeth	Loss of sensory limb blink reflex with CN VII
	V2-maxillary		General sensation of anterior 2/3 of tongue, mandibular face, mandibular teeth,	Loss of sensation in innervated areas
	V3-mandibular		Motor to muscles of mastication (temporalis, masseter, medial & lateral pterygoids) plus anterior belly of digastric, mylohyoid, tensor tympani; tensor palatine	Loss of sensation in innervated areas
				Weakness in chewing; jaw deviates to lesion nerve

VI	Abducens	Motor	Lateral rectus; abducts eye	Diplopia; internal strabismus; loss of parallel gaze, "pseudoptosis" False localizing sign with elevated intracranial pressure, especially with bilateral CN VI palsies
VII	Facial	Mixed	Muscles of facial expression (orbicularis oculi and oris, platysma, buccinator, stapedius)	Weakness of facial muscles Loss of motor limb of blink reflex Hyperacusis Central lesion: lower facial weakness Peripheral lesion: upper and lower facial weakness
VIII	Vestibulocochlear	Sensory	Balance and hearing	Tinnitus, impaired hearing, vertigo
IX	Glossopharyngeal	Mixed	Muscles of larynx and pharynx	Loss of taste in posterior tongue, absence of gag reflex, dysphagia
X	Vagus	Mixed	Pharynx, larynx, vocal cords, heart rate	Tachycardia, vomiting, slowed respirations, vocal cord and laryngeal paralysis
XI	Spinal Accessory	Motor	Shoulder shrug, contralateral head turn	Weakness of head turn, shoulder weakness
XII	Hypoglossal	Motor	Supplies tongue muscles, thyroid cartilage, and hyoid bone	Deviation toward lesion, lingual dysarthria, hemiatrophy

C

CRANIAL NERVES

CRANIOCERVICAL JUNCTION (See also ARNOLD-CHIARI MALFORMATION)

Dysfunction localized to the craniocervical junction (CCJ) usually results from abnormalities involving the foramen magnum, occipital bone and/or the first two cervical vertebrae. The congenital abnormalities of CCJ can be structure specific, such as Arnold-Chiari malformations, or part of widespread systemic involvement (e.g., achondroplasia, osteogenesis imperfecta). Acquired abnormalities of CCJ can result from trauma or a disease process (rheumatoid arthritis, Paget disease, malignancy, multiple sclerosis).

Clinical presentation is usually that of a chronic dysfunction because acute lesions usually become evident with respiratory arrest, and may include various combinations of the following: head and neck pain; spastic quadriparesis; dorsal column dysfunction; a syringomyelia pattern of deficits; cranial nerve palsies; Lhermitte phenomenon (electrical sensation running down the back on neck flexion); cerebellar signs; vertebrobasilar symptoms (syncope, vertigo, and drop attacks); downbeat nystagmus, and hydrocephalus with papilledema. However, some individuals with abnormalities of the CCJ may be asymptomatic.

Evaluation requires magnetic resonance imaging or computed tomography of the brain and cervical spine, and occasionally a CT myelogram. Treatment is based on the underlying cause.

CRANIOSYNOSTOSIS

Craniosynostosis describes the premature closure of suture(s) while the brain is still growing, resulting in an abnormal skull shape. Depending on the suture(s) that close prematurely, the skull takes on a characteristic shape (Table 40). The normal structure of the sutures and fontanelles is shown in Fig. 22.

Most cases are sporadic (85%) and of uncertain etiology. Craniosynostosis may be seen in association with metabolic disorders (rickets, mucopolysaccharidoses, hyperthyroidism, hypercalcemia, and

TABLE 40

CRANIOSYNOSTOSIS: SUTURE AFFECTED, HEAD SHAPE, AND DESCRIPTION

Suture Affected	Head Shape	Description
Sagittal	Scaphocephaly	60%; boys > girls; may be familial; neurologically normal
Coronal	Brachycephaly	20%; girls > boys; affected in Apert-Crouzon disease (5% of all cases of craniosynostosis)
Single coronal or lambdoidal	Plagiocephaly	Distinguish from deformational plagiocephaly
Metopic	Trigonocephaly	Varies in severity; may result in hypertelorism; may be associated with mental retardation
Multiple	Oxycephaly	Seen in Carpenter syndrome

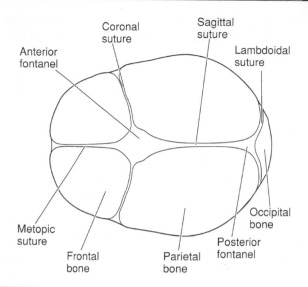

FIGURE 22

Normal appearance of newborn sutures and fontanelles (From Jarvis, D. A. (2011). Examining the head and neck. In Goldbloom R, *Pediatric clinical skills* (pp. 89–100, Figure 7.2A). Philadelphia: Saunders.

hypophosphatemia), hematologic disorders (sickle cell, thalassemia, and polycythemia vera), or intrauterine fetal skull compression. Plagiocephaly must be distinguished from the much more common (1 per 300 births) deformational plagiocephaly. Deformational plagiocephaly has increased as a result of campaigns to prevent sudden infant death syndrome and is related to the position of sleeping in infants.

Clinical presentation depends on the underlying cause, but most cases are associated with hydrocephalus. Evaluation includes palpation of the calvarial bones (palpable ridging) and skull x-rays (band of increased density at site of prematurely closed suture), ultrasonography (for screening), computed tomography (provides superior visualization of bone structure, but to minimize exposure to ionizing radiation should be reserved for complex cases), or magnetic resonance imaging (if suspected intracranial abnormality).

Treatment depends on the underlying cause; some cases may require surgery or ventriculoperitoneal shunting. Surgery can correct cosmetic appearance and increase cranial vault size. Timing involves a balance of ability to tolerate surgery versus acute and chronic issues to be addressed through surgery (e.g., hydrocephalus, cognitive, visual, cosmetic).

Prognosis depends on the underlying cause. There are no clear data indicating that surgery improves cognitive outcome.

REFERENCES

Kabbani, H., & Raghuveer, T. S. (2004). Craniosynostosis. *Am Fam Physician*, 69, 2863–2870.

Kim, H. J., Roh, H. G., & Lee, L. I. (2016). Craniosynostosis: updates in radiologic diagnosis. *J Korean Neurosurg Soc*, 59(3), 219–226.

CREUTZFELDT-JAKOB DISEASE; OTHER HUMAN PRION DISEASES

Prion disorders, also known as transmissible spongiform encephalopathies, comprise a group of diseases that cause rapid degeneration of neurons and universal fatality. They can be sporadic, inherited, or—less commonly—acquired by manner of infectious spread. Proteinaceous infectious particles, or prions, are an aberrant isoform protein (PrP^{Sc}) of a normally expressed, highly conserved mammalian membrane surface glycoprotein (PrP^{C}) encoded by a single gene on the short arm of chromosome 20. This occurs due to misfolding of the normal alpha-helical protein structure to an abnormal beta-pleated sheet. It is hypothesized that this conformational change from PrP^{C} to PrP^{Sc} occurs spontaneously, although in familial forms, the mutation occurs from a mutant prion protein *(PRNP)* gene. The PrP^{Sc} protein then binds to other normal PrP^{c} proteins inducing a conformational change and perpetuating spread. The PrP^{Sc} isoform is a protease-resistant proteinaceous infectious agent which aggregates intracellularly, affecting synaptic transmission and inducing dendritic swelling, leading to pathologic spongiosis, neuronal loss, and gliosis. In Creutzfeldt-Jakob disease (CJD), Gerstmann-Sträusseler-Scheinker syndrome (GSS), kuru, and some cases of sporadic CJD, extracellular aggregation and polymerization of PrP^{Sc} form pathognomonic amyloid kuru plaques. Identification by the protease-resistant PrP^{Sc} occurs with immunohistochemical staining or Western blot. Human diseases caused by prions include the following:

I. Creutzfeldt-Jakob disease is characterized by rapidly progressive dementia. It initially presents with fatigue, disordered sleep, cognitive decline, confusion, ataxia, aphasia, visual loss, hemiparesis, or amyotrophy. Signs of cerebellar, pyramidal, and extrapyramidal involvement develop in most patients.
   A. Sporadic CJD (85% of CJD cases) occurs worldwide with an incidence of 1 per million per year worldwide. Men and women are equally affected, and onset of disease is between 55 and 75 years of age. There is no evidence of geographic or seasonal clustering.
   B. Familial or inherited CJD (15% of CJD cases) affects younger patients and is autosomal dominant (short arm of chromosome 20).

C. Infectious or iatrogenic CJD has been reported after transplants of cadaver-derived dura mater, injection of cadaver-derived growth hormone and gonadotropic hormone, stereotactic implantation of depth electroencephalogram (EEG) electrodes, inoculation, corneal grafting, and other invasive medical procedures.

Diagnosis is suggested by rapid progression of dementia and development of myoclonic jerks, particularly startled myoclonus in response to acoustic or tactile stimulus. EEG findings may be normal or demonstrate nonspecific slow waves in the early stages. Later in the course, periodic biphasic or triphasic synchronous complexes (classically 1 Hz), often correlating with myoclonic jerks, may develop over a slow background rhythm. These periodic complexes carry a sensitivity of 67% and a specificity of 86% and are less likely to be present in familial cases. Cerebrospinal fluid (CSF) studies are usually normal or may show mildly elevated protein. Immunoassay for 14-3-3 protein in the CSF has a sensitivity and specificity of greater than 90% (false-positive in stroke, subarachnoid hemorrhage, intracranial hemorrhage (ICH), tumors, meningoencephalitis due to rapid neuronal loss). Diffusion-weighted magnetic resonance imaging is the most sensitive sequence for abnormal cortical ribbon sign (although can also be seen on fluid-attenuated inversion recovery [FLAIR]). There will also be hyperintensity of the neocortex, thalamus, and striatum. Biopsy shows pathologic findings of spongiform changes (intracellular vacuolation of neutrophils, primarily in neocortical and deep gray matter), neuronal loss, and reactive gliosis. There is no therapy, and mean survival time is 5 months, with 80% of infected persons dying within 1 year.

II. Atypical CJD has prominent amyotrophic or ataxic features with slow progression, longer duration of symptoms, and an absence of typical EEG changes, which causes diagnostic uncertainty. Differential diagnosis includes amyotrophic lateral sclerosis, multiple sclerosis, and paraneoplastic cerebellar degeneration. Rapid progressive dementia with myoclonus should be differentiated from other neurodegenerative diseases, such as Alzheimer disease, as well as infectious diseases, such as human immunodeficiency virus (HIV), tertiary syphilis, subacute sclerosing panencephalitis, and encephalopathies due to heavy metals or other toxins.

III. Variant CJD is a novel form of CJD that is believed to be acquired from cattle affected by bovine spongiform encephalopathy (BSE), also known as mad cow disease, which was first reported after an epidemic in the United Kingdom. The disease is acquired by eating meat or meat products contaminated with BSE. It affects younger adults (mean age is 29 years) and presents with prominent behavioral manifestations, persistent paresthesias and dysesthesias, and a similar periodic EEG pattern. Ataxia, dementia, and myoclonus appear during the terminal stage of the disease (Table 41 compares variant CJD with sporadic CJD).

C

CREUTZFELDT-JAKOB DISEASE

TABLE 41

COMPARISON OF VARIANT AND SPORADIC CREUTZFELDT-JAKOB DISEASE

Clinical Features	Variant CJD	Sporadic CJD
Mean age of onset	29 years	60 years
Mean survival time	14 months	4 months
Early psychiatric symptoms	Common	Unusual
Painful sensory symptoms	Common	Rare
Later cerebellar ataxia	All	Many
Dementia	Commonly delayed	Typically early
Electroencephalogram	Nonspecific slowing	Biphasic and triphasic periodic complexes
MRI (mainly in variant CJD)	Signal in pulvinar region	Signal in basal ganglion of thalamus and putamen
Cerebrospinal fluid 14-3-3 concentration	High in 50% of patients	High in most patients
Histopathology of brain	Many florid plaques	No amyloid plaques
Immunostaining of tonsils	Positive	Negative
Polymorphism at codon 129	All homozygotes (M/M)	Homozygosity and heterozygosity

CJD, Creutzfeldt-Jakob disease; *MRI*, magnetic resonance imaging.
Adapted from Johnson, R. T. (2005). Prion disease. *Lancet Neurol 4*, 635.

IV. Kuru is an endemic form of prion disease associated with cannibalism, as part of the funeral ceremony common to the Fore tribe of Papua New Guinea. It was first reported by Gajdusek in the 1950s. In Fore language, kuru means "to tremble or shake," which graphically describes a symptom of the disease. Cessation of cannibalism since the 1950s has gradually eliminated the disease.

V. GSS is familial with autosomal dominant inheritance (point mutation of PrP gene on chromosome 20) and presents with ataxia, dementia, aphasia, and extrapyramidal symptoms. The course is similar but slower than CJD, and death occurs in 4 to 10 years.

VI. Fatal familial insomnia is characterized by early intractable insomnia, followed by dysautonomia, ataxia, and dementia. The disease affects mainly the thalamic nuclei and is associated with an autosomal dominant mutation of codon 178 of the *PRNP* gene. Symptoms occur between 20 and 70 years, and death occurs within 1 to 2 years.

REFERENCES

Cutsforth-Gregory, J., & Aksamit, A. (2015). Prion disorders: Creutzfeldt-Jakob disease and related disorders. In K. Flemming & L. Jones (Eds.), *Mayo Clinic neurology board review*, ed 1 (pp. 649–654). New York: Oxford University Press.

Gaudino, S., Gangemi, E., Colantonio, R., Botto, A., Ruberto, E., Calandrelli, R., et al. (2017). Neuroradiology of human prion diseases, diagnosis and differential diagnosis. *Radiol Med, 122*(5), 369–385.

DEGENERATIVE DISEASES OF CHILDHOOD

Degenerative diseases of childhood may be classified in a number of ways, as they represent a heterogeneous set of disorders. Widespread availability of genetic testing has shed light both on multiple genes causing similar phenotypes, but also milder late-onset and adult forms of many of these disorders.

I. Diseases that predominantly affect white matter (present with long tract signs [spasticity and hyperreflexia], optic atrophy, cortical blindness, or deafness)

A. Metachromatic leukodystrophy: autosomal recessive (AR); arylsulfatase A deficiency or saposin B deficiency; diffuse demyelination and accumulation of metachromatic granules; age of onset 2 to 5 years; with peripheral neuropathy; magnetic resonance imaging (MRI) characteristically shows sparing of arcuate fibers.

B. Krabbe disease: AR; beta-galactosidase deficiency; globoid cells; age of onset 4 to 6 months; restlessness, irritability and progressive stiffness; optic atrophy; hyperacusis; peripheral neuropathy; MRI—arcuate fibers spared and parieto-occipital lobes involved early, high-density basal ganglia.

C. Adrenoleukodystrophy (ALD): X-linked recessive; acyl coenzyme A (Acyl-CoA) synthetase deficiency resulting in accumulation of very long-chain fatty acids; *ABCD1* gene mutation; single peroxisomal enzyme deficiency; childhood ALD—neurologic symptoms before adrenal insufficiency; adrenoleukomyeloneuropathy—spinal cord and nerves involved, age of onset in 20s to 30s, paraparesis and adrenal dysfunction almost at the same time; MRI—occipital lobes and splenium of the corpus callosum affected, marked contrast enhancement; pathologically, three distinct zones are identified: innermost zone with necrosis, intermediate zone of active demyelination and inflammatory changes, and peripheral zone consisting of demyelination without inflammation.

D. Pelizaeus-Merzbacher disease: X-linked recessive; deficient proteolipid protein 1 (PLP1) expression; newborn—nystagmus and opsoclonus; axial hypotonia; tongue fasciculations; ataxia. Childhood onset—dementia, tremor and choreoathetosis; MRI—hypomyelination, perivascular white matter spared producing a "tigroid pattern"; involves arcuate fibers. A similar disorder is found with *GJA12* mutations- called Pelizaeus-Merzbacher like disease.

E. Alexander disease: sporadic; *GFAP* mutations. Neuropathology shows Rosenthal fibers; macrocephaly; MRI—frontal lobe hyperintensities, basal ganglia or brainstem involvement (+) contrast enhancement.

F. Canavan disease: AR; aspartoacylase deficiency; normal for first 1 to 2 months, then by 6 months develop macrocephaly, hypotonia, seizures, and loss of early milestones; widespread vacuolation; MRI—near or total lack of myelin, involves arcuate fibers.

G. Cockayne syndrome: AR; defective DNA repair; microcephaly, large ears, sunken eyes, joint contractures, delayed psychomotor development; age of onset 2 years; retinitis pigmentosa, progeria; MRI—hypomyelination, perivascular calcification in basal ganglia and cerebellum.

H. Chédiak-Higashi syndrome: AR; mutations in *CHS1* gene; lysosomal disorder resulting in neutrophil dysfunction with impaired phagocytosis leading to defective bactericidal abilities; intracytoplasmic inclusions in neutrophils and neurons, most prominent in pons and cerebellum; albinism, pancytopenia, susceptibility to infection, nystagmus, hepatosplenomegaly; mental retardation, cerebellar and long tract signs, cranial and peripheral neuropathy.

II. Neuroaxonal dystrophy: mutations of *PLA2G6* gene, neuroaxonal spheroids along axons, especially neuromuscular junction; onset between 1 and 2 years, upper and lower motor neuron signs. Cognitive and motor regression, seizures, progressive motor sensory neuropathy, and hypotonia.

J. Phenylketonuria: AR; phenylalanine hydroxylase deficiency; developmental delay, hyperactive deep tendon reflexes, lighter pigmentation, musty odor. MRI—arcuate fibers spared, optic radiations most affected. Often detected in newborn screening surveillance monitoring; mental retardation results if not treated early. Treatment with low phenylalanine diet—must avoid aspartame, an artificial sweetener that contains phenylalanine; evidence is accumulating that a low phenylalanine diet must be maintained lifelong to avoid precipitating cognitive decline.

III. Diseases that predominantly affect gray matter (present with myoclonus, seizures, and cognitive impairment)

A. Lipidoses

1. Tay-Sachs disease (GM2 gangliosidosis): AR; hexosaminidase A deficiency; mainly found in Ashkenazi Jews; onset 3 to 6 months, excessive startle, macrocephaly, macular cherry-red spot; MRI—hyperintense signal in caudate, thalamus, and putamen on T2-weighted images. A late-onset variant presenting as an ataxic syndrome is also present.

2. Gaucher disease: AR; glucocerebrosidase deficiency; type III—early to mid-childhood, seizures, ataxia, dementia, subacute neuronopathy; hepatosplenomegaly. Enzyme therapy has been developed. Parkinson disease is also associated with glucocerebrosidase mutations.

3. Niemann-Pick disease: AR; sphingomyelinase deficiency. Type A—infantile, hypotonia, pulmonary interstitial disease, organomegaly, macular cherry-red spot. Type B—neurologically normal. Type C—mutation in gene *NPC1* and *NPC2*. Between 3 and 8 years of age, presents with spasticity, seizure, vertical gaze paresis, ataxia, and dementia.

B. Neuronal ceroid-lipofuscinosis: "fingerprint" inclusions of lipofuscin within cytosomes on electron microscopy of leukocytes; presents with dementia, vision loss, ataxia, myoclonus, seizures; infantile, late infantile (photoconvulsive response at 3 Hz on EEG, juvenile (Batten disease), adult (Kufs disease).

C. Mucopolysaccharidoses

1. Hurler syndrome: AR; α-L-iduronidase deficiency; mucopolysaccharides accumulate in neurons (meganeurites) and in histiocytes (gargoyle cells) in perivascular spaces; gargoyle-like facies, dwarfism, kyphosis, corneal clouding, mental retardation, hepatosplenomegaly, severe psychomotor deterioration, death within 5 to 10 years of onset; MRI—macrocrania, thick dura, perivascular "pits"; concave or "hooked" thoracolumbar vertebrae.

2. Hunter syndrome: X-linked recessive; iduronate 2-sulfatase deficiency; spinal cord compression, hydrocephalus, optic nerve compression, cervical myelopathy, hearing impairment, thick dura, perivascular "pits."

3. Sanfilippo syndrome: AR; heparin-N-sulfatase deficiency; normal until age 2 to 6 years, then progressive dementia; hyperactive, aggressive, insomnia; spastic and movement disorder; death in second to third decade of life.

IV. Diseases that primarily affect gray and white matter

A. Leigh disease (subacute necrotizing encephalopathy): mitochondrial disorder with no male-male transmission; spongiosis, demyelination, astrogliosis and capillary proliferation in basal ganglia, brainstem, and spinal cord; infantile—onset at age 2 years of hypotonia, vomiting, and seizures; childhood; adult—fifth to sixth decades; MRI—hyperintense foci in globus pallidus (GP), putamen, and caudate.

B. Myoclonic epilepsy with ragged-red fibers: mitochondrial; muscle biopsy—ragged red fibers; myoclonic epilepsy, myopathy, progressive external ophthalmoplegia, multiple infarcts in cortex and white matter.

C. Mitochondrial encephalomyopathy, lactic acidosis, and stroke-like episodes: mitochondrial; myopathy, encephalopathy, lactic acidosis, stroke-like episodes, migrainous headaches, large and multifocal infarcts mainly in parietal and occipital lobes.

D. Kearns-Sayre syndrome: mitochondrial; elevated pyruvate; progressive external ophthalmoplegia, cerebellar ataxia, heart block, and

D

DEGENERATIVE DISEASES OF CHILDHOOD

pigmentary retinopathy. Treatment is supportive with pacemaker and coenzyme Q10; progressive disease; death is common in third and fourth decade from central nervous system or cardiac complications.

E. Alpers disease: etiology uncertain: hypoxic injury versus AR inheritance. Onset before age 6 years; myoclonic seizures appear early, then mental retardation and spasticity or opisthotonus.

F. Menkes disease: X-linked recessive; *ATP7A* gene mutation; defective transmembrane copper transport; seizures, hypotonia develops into spastic quadriparesis; light-colored and brittle hair, hyperextensible joints, skeletal anomalies; susceptible to sepsis, heat-intolerant. Decreased serum copper and ceruloplasmin. Supportive and replacement therapy with copper histidine.

G. Zellweger syndrome: AR; multiple peroxisomal enzymes; craniofacial abnormalities, hypotonia, severe weakness, seizures, and apnea. MRI—heterotropia, pachygyria, or polymicrogyria. Supportive treatment.

V. Diseases that predominantly affect basal ganglia (present with movement disorders)

A. Huntington disease: autosomal dominant (AD); CAG repeat with age of onset inversely proportional to age of onset; chorea, dystonia, myoclonus, ataxia, dementia, and personality changes, atrophy of caudate and enlarged frontal horns of lateral ventricle. The Westphal variant may present in teenage years with an akinetic-rigid syndrome. Poor prognosis with 10 to 15 years survival from time of diagnosis. Chorea may be treated with tetrabenazine or deutetrabenazine.

B. Neurodegeneration with brain iron accumulation· AR and due to multiple genes. Iron deposits in GP and substantia nigra (SN); dystonia, mental retardation, stiff gait, equinovarus, dementia, retinitis pigmentosa, optic atrophy; low signals in GP and SN on T2-weighted images MRI, low signal surrounds region of high signal "eye of tiger" sign. Iron chelation has been studied, but clinical effects minimal or absent.

C. Fahr disease: AD; first 2 years mental retardation and movement disorder; microcephaly, hypertonia. MRI—prominent calcification in basal ganglia, dentate nuclei, centrum semiovale, and subcortical white matter. Calcifications can be seen in multiple conditions, including TORCH syndrome.

D. Wilson disease: chromosome 13, AR; P-type ATPase deficiency, *ATP7B* gene mutation. Defect in copper metabolism with decrease in ceruloplasmin and serum copper. Copper deposits in liver and basal ganglia; onset 8 to 16 years. Parkinsonism, seizures, ataxia, dementia, hemolytic anemia, liver dysfunction, and Kayser-Fleischer rings. Treatment is zinc, penicillamine, and tetrathiomolybdate.

E. Dystonia musculorum deformans: AD; most common genetic cause of childhood dystonia. Age of onset before 20 years. Focal dystonia in limb progressing to generalized. Treatment with anticholinergic medication (see Dystonia).

F. Aminoacidurias

1. Glutaric aciduria type 1: AR; glutaryl-CoA dehydrogenase deficiency (lysine to tryptophan); macrocephaly, dystonia, and dyskinesia; MRI—high-signal changes in basal ganglia and caudate; affects mitochondrial activity and preferentially involves basal ganglia leading to "bat wing" dilatation of sylvian fissures. Treatment includes protein and lysine restriction, and carnitine and riboflavin supplementation.

2. Methylmalonic acidemia: AR; secondary to blockage of conversion of methylmalonic acid (MMA) to succinyl-CoA leading to MMA accumulation; poor feeding and hypotonia, hyperammonemia, and ketoacidosis; MRI—hyperdensities in GP. Protein restriction.

REFERENCES

Daroff, R. B., Jankovic, J., Mazziotta, J. C., & Pomeroy, S. L. (Eds.), (2015). *Bradley's neurology in clinical practice*, ed 7. Elsevier.

Dulac, O., Lassonde, M., & Sarnat, H. B. (Eds.), (2013). *Handbook of Clinical Neurology: vol. 111/112/113. Pediatric neurology, Part I/II/III*, ed 1. Elsevier.

DEMENTIA (See also AAN GUIDELINE SUMMARIES APPENDIX)

Dementia is a clinical syndrome characterized by loss of multiple cognitive functions and emotional abilities in an individual with previously normal intellect and clear consciousness (i.e., in the absence of delirium). Though there is evidence of declining age-specific incidence of dementia in the Western world, the worldwide prevalence is expected to continue to increase due to increased life expectancy.

In its latest iteration, the *Diagnostic and Statistical Manual of Mental Disorders* (Fifth Edition) changed the previous diagnosis of dementia and cognitive disorder categories to neurocognitive disorders (NCDs), separating cognitive impairments into major and mild categories (see Tables 42 and 43). Major cognitive impairment (dementia) is characterized by significant cognitive decline in at least one cognitive domain that interferes with daily function (Table 44). It is classified by etiology and presentation into Alzheimer dementia, frontotemporal lobar dementia, Lewy body disease, and other conditions (Table 45). It excludes patients with isolated deficits, such as aphasia or apraxia, and symptoms that occur during delirium.

D

DEMENTIA

TABLE 42

DSM-5 DIAGNOSTIC CRITERIA FOR MAJOR NEUROCOGNITIVE DISORDER (PREVIOUSLY DEMENTIA)

A. Evidence of significant cognitive decline from a previous level of performance in one or more cognitive domains (learning and memory, language, executive function, complex attention, perceptual-motor, or social cognition)

B. The cognitive deficits interfere with independence in everyday activities. At a minimum, assistance should be required with complex instrumental activities of daily living, such as paying bills or managing medications

C. The cognitive deficits do not occur exclusively in the context of delirium

D. The cognitive deficits are not better explained by another mental disorder (e.g., major depressive disorder, schizophrenia)

TABLE 43

DSM-5 DIAGNOSTIC CRITERIA FOR MILD NEUROCOGNITIVE DISORDER (PREVIOUSLY COGNITIVE DISORDERS—NOS)

A. Evidence of modest cognitive decline from a previous level of performance in one or more cognitive domains (complex attention, executive function, learning and memory, language, perceptual motor, or social cognition) based on:

  a. Concern of the individual, a knowledgeable informant, or the clinician that there has been a mild decline in cognitive function; and

  b. A modest impairment in cognitive performance, preferably documented by standardized neuropsychological testing or, in its absence, another quantified clinical assessment.

B. The cognitive deficits do not interfere with capacity for independence in everyday activities (i.e., complex instrumental activities of daily living such as paying bills or managing medications are preserved), but greater effort, compensatory strategies, or accommodation may be required.

TABLE 44

DIAGNOSIS OF DEMENTIA

Dementia is diagnosed when there are cognitive or behavioral (neuropsychiatric) symptoms that:

1. Interfere with the ability to function at work or at usual activities; and

2. Represent a decline from previous levels of functioning and performing; and

3. Are not explained by delirium or major psychiatric disorder;

4. Cognitive impairment is detected and diagnosed through a combination of (1) history-taking from the patient and a knowledgeable informant and (2) an objective cognitive assessment, either a "bedside" mental status examination or neuropsychological testing. Neuropsychological testing should be performed when the routine history and bedside mental status examination cannot provide a confident diagnosis.

5. The cognitive or behavioral impairment involves a minimum of two of the following domains:

  a. Impaired ability to acquire and remember new information—symptoms include: repetitive questions or conversations, misplacing personal belongings, forgetting events or appointments, getting lost on a familiar route.

Continued

D

TABLE 44

DIAGNOSIS OF DEMENTIA—CONT'D

b. Impaired reasoning and handling of complex tasks, poor judgment—symptoms include: poor understanding of safety risks, inability to manage finances, poor decision-making ability, inability to plan complex or sequential activities.

c. Impaired visuospatial abilities—symptoms include: inability to recognize faces or common objects or to find objects in direct view despite good acuity, inability to operate simple implements, or orient clothing to the body.

d. Impaired language functions (speaking, reading, and writing)—symptoms include: difficulty thinking of common words while speaking, hesitations; speech, spelling, and writing errors.

e. Changes in personality, behavior, or comportment—symptoms include: uncharacteristic mood fluctuations such as agitation, impaired motivation, initiative, apathy, loss of drive, social withdrawal, decreased interest in previous activities, loss of empathy, compulsive or obsessive behaviors, and socially unacceptable behaviors.

TABLE 45

CONDITIONS CAUSING DEMENTIA

1. Potentially reversible causes of dementia
   a. Neoplasms (gliomas and meningiomas)
   b. Metabolic disorders (hypo/hyperthyroidism, renal failure, hepatic failure, Cushing disease, Addison disease, Wilson disease, and hypopituitarism)
   c. Trauma (subdural hematoma)
   d. Toxins (alcohol, heavy metals, and organic poisons)
   e. Infections (bacterial/fungal/viral/parasitic meningoencephalitis, neurosyphilis, HIV, and brain abscess)
   f. Autoimmune disorders (systemic lupus erythematosus, multiple sclerosis, and vasculitis)
   g. Drugs (antidepressants, anxiolytics, sedatives, anticonvulsants, anticholinergics, and antiarrhythmics)
   h. Nutritional deficiencies (thiamine, folate, vitamin B_{12} and vitamin B_6)
   i. Psychiatric disorders (depression, schizophrenia, and mania)
   j. Other disorders (normal pressure hydrocephalus, Whipple's diseases, sleep apnea, and sarcoidosis)
2. Irreversible causes of dementia
   a. Degenerative diseases (Alzheimer disease, frontotemporal dementia, Huntington's disease, progressive supranuclear palsy, Parkinson's disease, diffuse Lewy body disease, olivopontocerebellar atrophy, ALS-parkinsonism-dementia complex, Hallervorden-Spatz disease, Kufs disease, adrenoleukodystrophy, and metachromatic leukodystrophy)
   b. Vascular dementia (multiple small/large infarcts, Binswanger's disease, CADASIL; see later discussion)
   c. Traumatic (dementia pugilistica and TBI)
   d. Infectious (CJD, postencephalitic dementia, and progressive multifocal leukoencephalopathy)

CADASIL, Cerebral autosomal dominant arteriopathy with subcortical infarcts and leukoencephalopathy; *CJD*, Creutzfeldt-Jakob disease.

Examination for dementia should include assessment of multiple areas of cognitive performance, including memory, language, perception, praxis, attention, judgment, calculation, and visuospatial functions. The presence of psychiatric features (affective disorder, hallucinations, delusions, and anxiety) must also be sought. Questions about the patient's activities and self-care capabilities should be obtained from collateral sources of information (caregiver). Acquiring family history is essential. Short, standardized mental status tests such as the Mini-Mental State Examination are widely used. Mild cognitive deficits may require more extensive neuropsychologic testing. Depression is common and treatable. It should be screened for in all patients being evaluated for dementia.

According to the latest guidelines from the American Academy of Neurology (see Appendix), laboratory workup should include a vitamin B_{12} level and thyroid function test, as B_{12} deficiency and hypothyroidism are common in the elderly. A complete blood count (CBC) and chemistry panel are often performed. Screening for syphilis is not recommended unless the patient has a clear risk factor or history of a prior syphilitic infection, or lives in one of the few areas in the United States where syphilis is frequently seen. Computed tomography (CT) or magnetic resonance imaging (MRI) of the brain is used to rule out structural lesions. Other tests (EEG, lumbar puncture, HIV titer, serologic testing for vasculitis, heavy metal screening, angiography, brain biopsy) are indicated only if suggested by the history or examination. In younger adults, dementia may be caused by late-onset childhood metabolic diseases, and special studies may be required.

ALZHEIMER DISEASE

Alzheimer disease (AD) is the most common etiology for dementia in adults, accounting for 50% to 60% of cases. AD is characterized by progressive cognitive and functional deficits. In the United States, its prevalence is 11% by age 65, and 32% by age 85. Incidence can double every 4.4 years after age 60. The biggest risk factors are advanced age and female sex (which may be explained by the fact that women typically live longer than men), though family history, hypertension, diabetes, smoking, low socioeconomic status, stress, endocrine dysfunction, low education level, and head injury also increase risk. Lower risk has been suggested in those taking nonsteroidal anti-inflammatory drugs (NSAIDS), postmenopausal women on estrogen replacement therapy, individuals with a higher education level or socioeconomic status, individuals engaging in mentally demanding tasks, and those with apolipoprotein E (*APOE*) ε2 genotype.

Clinical Presentation

Early symptoms of AD include difficulty remembering recent conversations, names, or events, and apathy and depression. Subtle decreases in the ability to focus attention and recall remote events become more prominent with disease progression. Later, there is disorientation, confusion, poor judgment, and personality changes. Delusions and hallucinations may occur. Language decline (particularly word finding in spontaneous speech) and anomia (especially for parts of objects) impair communication. Ultimately, impairments in visuospatial dysfunction, apraxia, and complications from difficulty speaking, walking, and aspiration lead to mounting morbidities and mortality.

Pathology

AD is associated with progressive extracellular accumulation of β-amyloid peptide (Aβ) plaques in the brain, and twisted strands of intracellular tau protein tangles. While the exact mechanism is unknown, this accumulation is associated with decline in choline acetyltransferase activity, as well as neurodegeneration throughout the brain, particularly in the hippocampus and posterior cingulate, lateral parietal, and medial frontal cortices.

Genetics

AD develops at an earlier age in patients with various genetic mutations, particularly those coding for amyloid-β precursor protein *(AβPP)* on chromosome 21, presenilin 1 (PSEN1) on chromosome 14, and presenilin 2 (PSEN2) on chromosome 1. Additionally, APOE handles lipid metabolism and trafficking, and serves as the primary modulator of cholesterol in the brain. It has multiple isoforms associated with both early- and late-onset familial AD (see Table 45), with the APOE ε4 being the largest known genetic risk factor (Table 46). To date, over 20 additional genes have been associated with late-onset AD.

Diagnosis

Diagnostic criteria for dementia are outlined in Table 44. In AD, the onset of dementia is insidious and worsens over time. Patients meeting these criteria may be diagnosed with AD with reasonably high sensitivity (81%), and specificity (70%). Clinical diagnostic criteria have been revised into probable and possible AD (Table 47). While autopsy remains the only definitive

D

DEMENTIA

TABLE 46

GENETIC FACTORS LINKED TO ALZHEIMER DISEASE RISK

Genetic Factor	Chromosome Involved	Age at Onset (years)
Down syndrome	21	>35
Amyloid precursor protein mutation	21	45–66
Presenilin 1 mutation	14	28–62
Presenilin 2 mutation	1	40–85
Apolipoprotein ε4	19	>60

From Martin, J. B. (1999). Molecular basis of the neurodegenerative disorders. *N Engl J Med, 340*(25), 1970–1980.

TABLE 47

DIAGNOSIS OF ALZHEIMER DISEASE

PROBABLE AD DEMENTIA:

1. Patient meets criteria for dementia described earlier in the text, and in addition, has the following characteristics:
   a. Insidious onset. Symptoms have a gradual onset over months to years, not sudden over hours or days;
   b. Clear-cut history of worsening of cognition by report or observation; and
   c. The initial and most prominent cognitive deficits are evident on history and examination in one of the following categories.
      i. Amnestic presentation: It is the most common syndromic presentation of AD dementia. The deficits should include impairment in learning and recall of recently learned information. There should also be evidence of cognitive dysfunction in at least one other cognitive domain, as defined earlier in the text.
      ii. Nonamnestic presentations:
         1. Language presentation: The most prominent deficits are in word-finding, but deficits in other cognitive domains should be present.
         2. Visuospatial presentation: The most prominent deficits are in spatial cognition, including object agnosia, impaired face recognition, simultanagnosia, and alexia. Deficits in other cognitive domains should be present.
         3. Executive dysfunction: The most prominent deficits are impaired reasoning, judgment, and problem solving. Deficits in other cognitive domains should be present.
   d. The diagnosis of probable AD dementia should not be applied when there is evidence of (a) substantial concomitant cerebrovascular disease, defined by a history of a stroke temporally related to the onset or worsening of cognitive impairment; or the presence of multiple or extensive infarcts or severe white matter hyperintensity burden; or (b) core features of Dementia with Lewy bodies other than dementia itself; or (c) prominent features of behavioral variant frontotemporal dementia; or (d) prominent features of semantic variant primary progressive aphasia or nonfluent/agrammatic variant primary progressive aphasia; or (e) evidence for another concurrent, active neurological disease, or a non-neurological medical comorbidity or use of medication that could have a substantial effect on cognition.
2. Probable AD dementia with increased level of certainty
   a. Probable AD dementia with documented decline:
      i. In persons who meet the core clinical criteria for probable AD dementia, documented cognitive decline increases the certainty that the condition represents an active, evolving pathologic process, but it does not specifically increase the certainty that the process is that of AD pathophysiology.
      ii. Probable AD dementia with documented decline is defined as follows: evidence of progressive cognitive decline on subsequent evaluations based on information from informants and cognitive testing in the context of either formal neuropsychological evaluation or standardized mental status examinations.

Continued

TABLE 47

DIAGNOSIS OF ALZHEIMER DISEASE—CONT'D

3. Probable AD dementia in a carrier of a causative AD genetic mutation
   a. In persons who meet the core clinical criteria for probable AD dementia, evidence of a causative genetic mutation (in *Amyloid precursor protein [APP]*, *Presenellin-1 [PSEN1]*, or *Presenellin-2 [PSEN2]*), increases the certainty that the condition is caused by AD pathology. The workgroup noted that carriage of the $\varepsilon4$ allele of the apolipoprotein E gene was not sufficiently specific to be considered in this category.

POSSIBLE AD DEMENTIA:

1. Atypical course: Atypical course meets the core clinical criteria in terms of the nature of the cognitive deficits for AD dementia, but either has a sudden onset of cognitive impairment or demonstrates insufficient historical detail or objective cognitive documentation of progressive decline, OR
2. Etiologically mixed presentation: Etiologically mixed presentation meets all core clinical criteria for AD dementia but has evidence of (a) concomitant cerebrovascular disease, defined by a history of stroke temporally related to the onset or worsening of cognitive impairment; or the presence of multiple or extensive infarcts or severe white matter hyperintensity burden; or (b) features of Dementia with Lewy bodies other than the dementia itself; or (c) evidence for another neurological disease or a non-neurological medical comorbidity or medication use that could have a substantial effect on cognition

AD, Alzheimer disease.

From McKhann, G. M., Knopman, D. S., Chertkow, H., et al. (2011). The diagnosis of dementia due to Alzheimer's disease: recommendations from the National Institute on Aging-Alzheimer's Association workgroups on diagnostic guidelines for Alzheimer's disease. *Alzheimers Dement*, 7(3), 263–269.

---

diagnostic tool, biomarkers such as reduced $A\beta$ and elevated tau levels in the cerebrospinal fluid, the advent of high-resolution molecular MRI, and positron emission tomography (PET) demonstrating $A\beta$ deposits and reduced fluorodeoxyglucose (FDG)-uptake in the medial, basal, and lateral temporal lobes, and medial parietal cortex, suggest a high likelihood of AD.

Differential Diagnosis

It is important to note other features that may indicate atypical dementia. Vascular dementia, the second most common cause of dementia, can be distinguished from AD based on evidence of strokes on neuroimaging, abrupt onset, stepwise deterioration, focal neurologic signs and symptoms, and risk factors for stroke. Pick disease, or frontotemporal dementia (FTD), features early disinhibited behavior and frontal lobe dysfunction, with asymmetrical frontal or temporal lobe atrophy on neuroimaging. Lewy body dementia may present with psychosis, or with extrapyramidal signs such as tremor or rigidity. Creutzfeldt-Jakob disease is characterized by rapidly progressive dementia with myoclonus or seizures.

D

DEMENTIA

Treatment

To date, only three cholinesterase inhibitors (donepezil, rivastigmine, and galantamine) and one N-methyl-D-aspartate (NMDA) receptor antagonist (memantine) have been demonstrated to have therapeutic efficacy with acceptable side effects in multiple large randomized controlled clinical trials (see Therapeutic Appendix Dementia). Cholinesterase inhibitors potentiate the activity of acetylcholine released by surviving neurons, though unfortunately, only have a modest degree of clinical effect. Memantine is typically used in moderate to severe AD and in conjunction with cholinesterase inhibitors, or when cholinesterase inhibitors are poorly tolerated, and serves to combat glutamatergic neuronal excitotoxicity while still preserving the receptor.

While there is currently no medication that has been found to slow progression of AD, there is ongoing research into therapies that inhibit amyloid production, directly target Aβ or tau proteins, and reduce inflammation and oxidative stress in the hopes that they may decrease amyloid-β load in the brain and slow disease progression.

Symptom Management

Much of treatment is therefore focused on symptom management. Behavioral symptoms can be disruptive and require careful investigation. Treatment for any underlying medical condition (e.g., urinary tract infection) and thorough review of the medication list should be sought before starting any psychoactive drugs. Depression can be treated with tricyclic antidepressants (e.g., imipramine or amitriptyline) or selective serotonin reuptake inhibitors (e.g., fluoxetine or sertraline). If psychosis is present, neuroleptics should always be used with extreme caution in the elderly. As a class, all antipsychotics are associated with an increased risk of death when used to treat psychosis in elderly patients with dementia. These medications carry a black box warning to this effect. Counseling and social planning in the face of increasing disability are important facets of long-term management.

VASCULAR DEMENTIA

Vascular dementia refers to dementia caused by vascular disease. This is the second most common cause of dementia, accounting for approximately 20% of cases. Patients diagnosed as having vascular dementia, however, do not constitute a homogeneous group. Lacunar infarcts, cortical infarcts, intracerebral hemorrhage (ICH), intraventricular hemorrhage (IVH), subarachnoid hemorrhage (SAH), leukoaraiosis, and neuronal loss in the hippocampus, neocortex, and basal ganglia after global cerebral anoxia or ischemia can all lead to vascular dementia. Diagnostic criteria for ischemic vascular dementia therefore include the following:

I. Dementia involving memory loss, executive dysfunction, focal cortical signs, personality changes, and affective changes

II. Cerebrovascular disease demonstrated by history, clinical examination, or brain imaging

III. Evidence that the two conditions are causally related by a temporal relationship, abrupt or stepwise deterioration, or specific brain imaging findings, indicating damage to regions important for higher cerebral function

Supportive clinical features include history of cerebrovascular risk factors, early appearance of gait disturbance and urinary incontinence, and frontal lobe, extrapyramidal and pseudobulbar features. Subtypes of vascular dementia worth mentioning include the following:

I. Multi-infarct dementia (MID) is caused by multiple infarcts affecting both the cortical or subcortical areas and by multiple lacunar infarcts. The modified Hachinski ischemic scale (Table 48) may help to differentiate MID from AD.

II. Binswanger disease (subacute arteriosclerotic encephalopathy) consists of periventricular demyelination of the cerebral white matter in demented patients with a history of hypertension. Previously considered rare, it is now diagnosed more often because of brain imaging. Leukoaraiosis is a frequent finding in nondemented elderly patients and therefore the diagnosis should only be considered in patients with leukoaraiosis who are demented with no other obvious cause for the dementia.

III. Cerebral autosomal dominant arteriopathy with subcortical infarcts and leukoencephalopathy (CADASIL) is a familial nonarteriosclerotic, nonamyloid arteriopathy characterized by recurrent subcortical ischemic

D

DEMENTIA

TABLE 48

CLINICAL FEATURES OF ISCHEMIC SCORE (MODIFIED HACHINSKI SCALE)

Feature	Point Value
Abrupt onset	2
Stepwise deterioration	1
Fluctuating course	2
Nocturnal confusion	1
Relative preservation of personality	1
Depression	1
Somatic complaints	1
Emotional incontinence	1
History of presence of hypertension	1
History of strokes	2
Evidence of associated atherosclerosis	1
Focal neurologic symptoms	2
Focal neurologic signs	2

Score 4 suggests primary degenerative dementia; score 7 suggests vascular dementia.

Modified from Rosen, W. G., Terry, R. D., Fuld, P. A., et al. (1980). Pathological verification of ischemic score in differentiation of dementias. *Ann Neurol, 7*(5), 486–488.

strokes starting in the third or fourth decade leading to pseudobulbar palsy, subcortical dementia, and early MRI abnormalities, and is associated with a high frequency of migraine. The inheritance is autosomal dominant and is localized to the NOTCH3 gene on chromosome 19.

DEMENTIA WITH LEWY BODIES

Dementia with Lewy bodies (DLB) is currently the preferred term to describe diffuse Lewy body disease, Lewy body dementia, and cortical Lewy body disease. Lewy bodies are spherical eosinophilic intracytoplasmic neuronal inclusion bodies with a pale halo as seen in the substantia nigra of Parkinson disease patients. Cortical Lewy bodies contain alpha-synuclein, a presynaptic protein of unknown function, and can be found in association with AD histopathologically, especially in senile plaques. DLB is the third most common subtype of dementia. Age of onset is 50 to 70 years. The central feature required for the diagnosis of DLB is progressive cognitive decline of sufficient magnitude to interfere with normal or occupational function. Prominent or persistent memory impairment may not necessarily occur in the early stages, but is usually evident with progression. Core features include fluctuating cognition with pronounced variations in attention and alertness, recurrent visual hallucinations that are typically well formed and detailed, and spontaneous motor features of parkinsonism. Features supporting the diagnosis include repeated falls, syncope, transient loss of consciousness, neuroleptic sensitivity, systematized delusions, and hallucinations in other modalities. A diagnosis of DLB is less likely in the presence of stroke, evident as focal neurologic signs or on brain imaging, and evidence on physical examination and investigation of any physical illness or other brain disorder sufficient to account for the clinical picture. Clinical diagnosis is often suspected in patients with parkinsonism and dementia, particularly those with visual hallucinations or excess sensitivity to the extrapyramidal effects of neuroleptics. Definitive diagnosis is by autopsy.

FRONTOTEMPORAL DEMENTIA

FTD consists of a clinically and pathologically heterogeneous group of neurodegenerative disorders collectively referred to as "tauopathies," which also includes corticobasal ganglionic degeneration and progressive supranuclear palsy (PSP). These have in common degeneration of the frontal and temporal lobes. Behavioral changes, including disinhibition, impulsiveness, social inappropriateness, apathy, and withdrawal are early and prominent features. These behavioral changes provide the most important clue allowing the differentiation of this condition from AD. Language disturbances may also appear early, whereas visuospatial function remains intact until later in the disease. Neuroimaging may allow the visualization of focal atrophy, but the disease can often be recognized clinically before changes on routine imaging are apparent. SPECT demonstrates hypoperfusion in the frontal and temporal lobes before atrophy is evident on structural imaging.

FTD includes the following subtypes:

I. FTD is also known as Pick disease (which is also used to refer to the entire entity of FTD). Both sexes are affected equally and the typical age of onset is between 40 and 80 years. It is characterized by motor speech disorders and verbal stereotypy. Language impairments such as abundant unfocused speech (logorrhea), echo-like spontaneous repetition (echolalia), and compulsively uttered repetitive phrases (palilalia) are often seen in conjunction with the behavioral disturbances and represent focal involvement of the frontal lobes. There is marked personality deterioration with antisocial behaviors. Visuospatial skills are remarkably preserved until late in the disease. Pick cells (chromatolytic ballooned neurons) and Pick bodies (argyrophilic cytoplasmic inclusions) are classic pathologic findings.

II. PSP is characterized by postural instability, supranuclear gaze palsy, progressive supranuclear gaze palsy, mild dementia, and progressive axial rigidity. Typically presents in the 60s, with progression to death within 5 to 8 years. Gait instability (a "drunken sailor" or "dancing bear" walk) or frequent falls are often the earliest symptoms. Parkinsonism may be present, manifest as stiffness and bradykinesia. Tremors are often absent. There is usually a poor or absent response to levodopa. Neuronal and glial tau protein accumulation may be found in basal ganglia, diencephalon, brainstem, and cerebellum autopsy.

III. Primary progressive aphasia (PPA) is characterized by nonfluent speech production with phonologic and grammatical errors in the absence of decline of other aspects of cognition. Difficulties in reading and writing may also occur, but comprehension is relatively preserved. PPA is related to left frontal lobe involvement.

IV. Semantic dementia (SD) is characterized by progressive loss of word meanings with severe impairment of naming and word comprehension but fluent speech output. SD is primarily related to left temporal lobe involvement, but when the right temporal lobe involvement is out of proportion to other areas, patients present with prosopagnosia, an inability to recognize familiar faces.

V. Corticobasal degeneration (CBD) is FTD with extrapyramidal apractic supranuclear palsy presentation. CBD is a clinical syndrome characterized by asymmetrical rigidity, apraxia, and the alien limb phenomenon.

VI. FTD with parkinsonism (FTD-P) is a clinical syndrome linked to chromosome 17, with autosomal dominant inheritance. Initially, behavioral abnormalities appear without memory loss, but they are eventually followed by progressive dementia and parkinsonism.

VII. FTD with motor neuron disease (FTD-MND), an increasingly recognized clinical syndrome. In these patients, motor findings may precede, or coincide with, or follow the development of cognitive and behavioral changes.

REFERENCES

Hane, F., Lee, B. Y., & Leonenko, Z. (2017). Recent progress in Alzheimer disease research, part 1: pathology. *J Alz Dis*, *57*, 1–28.

Hane, F., Robinson, M., Lee, B. Y., et al. (2017). Recent progress in Alzheimer disease research, part 3: diagnosis and treatment. *J Alz Dis*, *57*, 645–665.

DELIRIUM (ACUTE CONFUSIONAL STATE)

Delirium, also known as acute confusional state, is a syndrome characterized by an acute change in mental status consisting of inattention and disturbance in cognition that develops over a short period of time and tends to fluctuate. Unlike the slow, insidious progressive onset of dementia, delirium is acute in onset (hours to days), includes interspersed lucid intervals, and is generally reversible if the causative factor is rapidly corrected. However, it can lead to prolonged hospitalization, severe impact on caregivers, and consistently associated with increased mortality. Delirium is also an independent risk factor for long-term cognitive decline and dementia. While hospitalization alone can cause delirium (prevalence ranges from 6% to 56% in hospitalized patients and up to 80% in intensive care unit [ICU] patients), predisposing factors that can facilitate onset and worsen severity include visual impairment, illness severity, underlying cognitive impairment, and dehydration (Table 49).

Many causes of delirium have been proposed, including neuroinflammation, neuronal aging, oxidative stress, neurotransmitter deficiency, neuroendocrinopathy, diurnal dysregulation, and network

TABLE 49

PREDISPOSING AND PRECIPITATING FACTORS FOR DELIRIUM

Predisposing Factors	Precipitating Factors

Dementia or preexisting cognitive impairment	Medications
	  Polypharmacy
	  Psychoactive medication use
	  Sedative hypnotic use

History of delirium	Use of physical restraints
Functional impairment	Use of bladder catheter

Sensory impairment
  Vision impairment
  Hearing impairment
	Physiologic and metabolic abnormalities
	  Elevated BUN/creatinine ratio
	  Abnormal sodium, glucose, or potassium

Comorbidity/severity of illness	Infection
Depression	Any iatrogenic event
History of transient ischemia/stroke	Major surgery
Alcohol abuse	Trauma or urgent admission
Older age	Coma

Fong, T., Davis, D. D., Growdon, M. E., et al. (2014). The interface of delirium and dementia in older persons. *Lancet Neurol*, *14*(8), 823–832.

disconnectivity. However, these theories are likely complementary. It is suggested that a final common pathway underlying the cause is associated with deficiencies in acetylcholine and melatonin availability, excess dopamine, norepinephrine, and/or glutamate release, and alterations (increases or decreases) in serotonin, histamine, and gamma-aminobutyric acid (GABA).

Delirium manifests as a reduced ability to direct, focus, and shift attention, which impairs other areas of cognition leading to confusion and disorganized thinking. Speech is often rambling, tangential, and circumlocutory with abnormal rate, dysarthria, anomia, perseveration, hesitation, and repetition. Dysgraphia, dyscalculia, and constructional deficits are common. Perceptual distortions may lead to illusions and unpleasant visual hallucinations. Associated features such as tremor, myoclonus, or asterixis may also appear, necessitating workup of other causes. Delirium can be subtyped based on psychomotor change into hypoactivity (psychomotor retardation), hyperactivity (agitation, hallucinations, and autonomic overactivity), or mixed (alternating between hypoactive and hyperactive).

Workup should include extensive evaluation for causes and contributing factors. Recent medication changes, metabolic disturbances (e.g., glucose, blood urea nitrogen [BUN]), infection (systemic and central nervous system [CNS]), head trauma, and seizures are common causes of confusional states. As such, medication review, serum electrolytes, glucose, blood count with differential, urine studies, acid-base status, thyroid and hepatic function, and toxicity should initiate evaluation. Further assessment—particularly in immunocompromised patients—with blood, urine, sputum, and cerebrospinal fluid (CSF) cultures may be warranted. Due to risk of nonconvulsive status epilepticus, EEG testing should be obtained, particularly if initial testing is unremarkable. This may demonstrate generalized slowing (reflecting encephalopathy), triphasic waves (classically indicating hepatic disturbance), β-activity (particularly from benzodiazepine usage), or a variety of other patterns. Imaging can help assess for stroke, infection, or autoimmune etiologies. Unilateral or bilateral damage to the fusiform and lingual gyri, as well as lesions of the nondominant posterior parietal and inferior prefrontal regions, may produce a confusional state.

Management should be directed at eliminating the cause of delirium, with attention to environmental interventions (avoiding sensory deprivation or overstimulation), fluid and electrolyte balance, nutritional status, medication review, and infectious workup and treatment. While avoidance of treatment with medication is ideal, haloperidol and low dose antipsychotics (quetiapine, risperidone, olanzapine) can be used for agitation and confusion. Acetylcholinesterase inhibitors—while not scrutinized in controlled trials— may be useful in dementia patients with acute worsening of mental state. Other medications such as valproate, ondansetron, and melatonin may be safe and effective in treatment and risk reduction. Dexmedetomidine and clonidine are useful in ICU setting for delirium.

D

DELIRIUM (ACUTE CONFUSIONAL STATE)

REFERENCES

Daroff, R. B., Jankovic, J., et al. (2016). Delirium. *Bradley's neurology in clinical practice,* ed 7. Philadelphia: Elsevier.

Wilber, S. T., & Ondrejka, J. E. (2016). Altered mental status and delirium. *Emerg Med Clin North Am, 34*(3), 649–665.

DEMYELINATING DISORDERS

Demyelinating diseases may be peripheral, such as Guillain-Barré syndrome (GBS), or multifocal motor neuropathy, or they may affect the central nervous system (CNS), such as multiple sclerosis (MS). Demyelinating disorders involve the destruction of normally formed myelin or oligodendroglia, in contrast to the so-called dysmyelinating diseases (e.g., leukodystrophies) in which myelin is abnormally formed. Many demyelinating disorders, such as MS and acute disseminated encephalomyelitis (ADEM), appear to be immune-mediated, although pathogenesis remains an enigma.

Demyelinating diseases are classified as:

I. Autoimmune/Immune-Mediated
   A. Primary diseases of myelin
      1. MS is the most common demyelinating disease and is discussed in greater detail elsewhere in this text.
      2. Neuromyelitis optica (NMO) spectrum disorder, also known as *Devic's disease*, most commonly manifests as optic neuritis and transverse myelitis (but not necessarily at same time), and in some cases involves brain parenchyma, often confounding the diagnosis. Sometimes overlooked core clinical features also include intractable nausea, vomiting, or hiccups (the area postrema syndrome), symptomatic narcolepsy, and symptomatic cerebral syndromes. There are proposed diagnostic criteria for patients with core clinical features for both seropositive and seronegative patients for the anti-aquaporin-4 channel antibody. A proportion of patients who are seronegative should be checked for antibodies to the myelin oligodendrocyte glycoprotein (MOG) antibody, which can cause similar symptoms in a relapsing course but is usually associated with better recovery. NMO is sometimes misdiagnosed as MS, but the treatments differ greatly. Disease modifying drugs for MS have been known to worsen NMO, so diagnostic accuracy is crucial.
      3. Schilder disease—a rapidly progressive sporadic disease—results in bilateral, massive hemispheric demyelination and is seen mainly in children and adolescents.
      4. Balo concentric sclerosis, a possible variant of MS, results in acute demyelination in a concentric pattern evident on magnetic resonance imaging (MRI).

5. Tumefactive demyelinating lesions mimic the appearance of mass lesions, and can cause extensive vasogenic edema, along with a tendency to have a hemorrhagic appearance as well. Characteristically, these lesions have an incomplete ring enhancement on MRI post-gadolinium sequences.

6. GBS, also known as acute inflammatory demyelinating polyradicular neuropathy (AIDP), is discussed elsewhere.

7. Chronic inflammatory demyelinating polyradicular neuropathy is of insidious progression and follows a more polyphasic course than AIDP. Like AIDP, it is also characterized by a demyelinating neuropathy with areflexia and albuminocytologic dissociation in the cerebrospinal fluid (CSF). Patients are often treated with long-term courses of intravenous immunoglobulin or plasma exchange.

8. Multifocal motor neuropathy is an asymmetric, demyelinating motor neuropathy characterized by weakness without sensory loss in two or more nerves. Motor conduction block is present on electrodiagnostic testing. CSF may contain anti-GM1 antibodies or elevated protein. Intravenous immunoglobulin is an effective treatment.

B. Parainfectious or postvaccination

1. ADEM, a monophasic, inflammatory demyelinating disorder, can occur shortly after measles, varicella, rubella, or other viral illnesses, after vaccination, or after immunizations.

2. Acute hemorrhagic leukoencephalitis, a hyperacute necrotizing form of ADEM, occurs usually after upper respiratory tract infections, and clinicopathologic features are more tissue destructive.

3. Site-restricted, uniphasic, acute inflammatory demyelinating disorders include transverse myelitis, optic neuritis, cerebellitis, and Bickerstaff brainstem encephalitis.

4. Chronic or recurrent parainfectious or postvaccination encephalomyelitis.

II. Infectious

A. Progressive multifocal leukoencephalopathy (most commonly seen in human immunodeficiency virus/ acquired immunodeficiency syndrome (HIV/AIDS) patients and MS patients with elevated JC virus titers after prolonged natalizumab or other disease-modifying treatments).

B. Subacute sclerosing panencephalitis is a devastating encephalitic condition following infection with measles. It generally occurs in children and adolescents. The suggested treatment includes ribavirin and interferon; however, 95% of cases are fatal.

C. Human T-lymphotropic virus causes spastic leg weakness due to spinal cord demyelination. It has a high-risk population of IV drug abusers, prostitutes, and hemodialysis patients. It is endemic to the Equator, southern Japan, and South America.

D

DEMYELINATING DISORDERS

III. Nutritional
  A. Alcohol or tobacco amblyopia
  B. Central pontine myelinolysis
  C. Marchiafava-Bignami syndrome, demyelination of the corpus callosum seen in chronic alcoholics
  D. Vitamin B12 deficiency, which usually manifests as paresthesias, weakness, gait ataxia with proprioceptive and vibratory sensory loss. There may be systemic changes such as macrocytosis.
IV. Toxic or metabolic
  A. Anoxia or hypoxia
  B. Carbon monoxide poisoning
  C. Mercury intoxication (Minamata disease)
  D. Radiation therapy
  E. Methotrexate, especially with radiation therapy
V. Hereditary demyelinating disorders
  A. Metachromatic leukodystrophy, diagnosed as arylsulfatase-A deficiency. Variable presentation depending on age of onset.
  B. Krabbe disease (globoid cell leukodystrophy) is a deficiency of galactosyl ceramidase. It presents with severe developmental delay. It is usually fatal in early childhood, though hematopoietic stem cell transplantation has shown promise in asymptomatic patients.
  C. Adrenoleukodystrophy is a mutation of the ABCD1 gene with X-linked inheritance. There are characteristic confluent white matter lesions surrounding occipital–parietal white matter. Treatment has been successful with hematopoietic stem cell transplantation (HSCT) in select patients.
    Lorenzo oil may delay disease progression in patients with early or mild disease, but neurologic deterioration should prompt consideration for HCST.
  D. Vanishing white matter disease is caused by the mutation of one of the EIF2B (1–5) genes. It presents with rapid progressive neurologic decline, including ataxia, and spasticity. It often follows an infection, stress, or injury.
  E. Alexander disease is due to a mutation of glial fibrillary acid protein (GFAP) on chromosome 17q21. Infants present with macrocephaly, seizures, failure to thrive, spasticity, and developmental delay. Rosenthal fibers are classically seen on pathology. There is no proven treatment besides supportive care.
  F. Canavan disease or aspartoacylase deficiency; infants present with lethargy, poor suck, poor cry, and hypotonia that eventually progresses to spasticity and macrocephaly. It is diagnosed by testing urine N-acetylaspartic acid. There is no effective treatment
  G. Organic and amino acid deficiencies
  H. Gaucher disease is a lysosomal storage disease caused by glucocerebrosidase deficiency. Variable presentation with three

phenotypes, GD1, GD2, and GD3. Types 2 and 3 are more likely to have neurologic manifestations such as ocular palsies, abnormal saccades, hypertonia, poor swallow, and seizures. Type 3 is of later onset than type 2, but is often difficult to distinguish.

I. Leber hereditary optic neuropathy is a maternally derived mitochondrial DNA mutation affecting mostly males with subacute onset of vision loss in their second decade of life. There is no proven treatment.

J. Niemann–Pick disease. Types A and B are due to sphingomyelinase deficiency, typically characterized by hepatosplenomegaly, developmental delay, interstitial lung disease, and a macular "cherry-red spot" on fundoscopic exam. Type C involves impaired transport and processing of low-density lipoprotein cholesterol with either NPC1 or NPC2 mutations. Type C should be suspected in patients with hepatic failure, interstitial lung disease, gelastic cataplexy, or supranuclear gaze palsies. The diagnosis can be confirmed via genetic testing or fibroblast cell culture. Miglustat is thought to slow the neuropsychiatric manifestations of Niemann–Pick Type C.

K. Tay–Sachs disease is caused by a deficiency of hexosaminidase A. It is an autosomal recessive disease that usually results in death due to neurologic decline before the age of 5. It is most common in the Ashkenazi Jewish population. It may also present with ataxia, spasticity, and cognitive decline in adults in the late-onset Tay–Sachs form.

REFERENCES

Kim, H. J., Paul, F., Lana-Peixoto, M. A., et al. (2015). MRI characteristics of neuro-myelitis optica spectrum disorder: an international update. *Neurology, 84*, 1165–1173.

Parikh, S., Bernard, G., Leventer, R. J., et al. (2015). A clinical approach to the diagnosis of patients with leukodystrophies and genetic leukoencephelopathies. *Mol Genet Metab, 114*(4), 501–515.

DERMATOMES

The following summarizes the landmarks for various dermatomes (Fig. 23):

I. Cervical
   A. C2—Occiput and tops of ears
   B. C3—The nape of the neck, the throat, and lobe of the ear
   C. C4—The clavicle
   D. C6—The thumb and lateral aspect of the forearm
   E. C8—The 5th finger and medial aspect of the hand

II. Thoracic
   A. T1—The medial aspect of the forearm
   B. T2—Below the clavicle

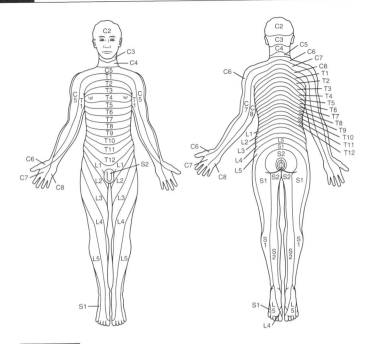

Dermatome map. (From Magee, D., Zachazewski, J., & Quillen, W. (2008). *Pathology and intervention in musculoskeletal rehabilitation*. Figure 12.3. Maryland Heights, Missouri: Saunders Elsevier, 2008.)

    C. T5—The nipple
    D. T10—The navel
    E. T12—The iliac crest
III. Lumbar
    A. L1—The groin
    B. L2—The anterior and lateral aspect of the thigh
    C. L3—The knee and inner thigh
    D. L4—The medial leg and malleolus
    E. L5—The big toe and lateral leg
IV. Sacral
    A. S1—The heel and posterior leg
    B. S2—The posterior thigh
    C. S3—The buttocks
    D. S5—The anus

REFERENCES

Downs, M. B., & Laporte, C. (2011). Conflicting dermatome maps: educational and clinical implications. *J Orthop Sports Phys Ther*, *41*(6), 427–434.

O'Brien, M. D. (2010). *Aids to the examination of the peripheral nervous system,* 5th ed. Edinburgh: Saunders Elsevier.

DIABETES INSIPIDUS

Diabetes insipidus (DI) is related to disturbances in the antidiuretic hormone (ADH, also called arginine vasopressin). ADH is a protein secreted by the magnocellular neurons of the hypothalamus. The ADH has two main sites of action: V1 vascular receptor causing vasoconstriction and V2 renal collecting ducts receptor causing water retention. The ADH secretion is regulated by intravascular volume, neural factors (pain, emesis, or stress), and medications such as chemotherapy, phenytoin, or antidepressants.

There are two forms of DI:

1. Central DI is the most common form, mainly secondary due to low ADH secretion by the posterior pituitary gland; however, in nephrogenic DI, ADH secretion is normal but tubules cannot respond to ADH. Common causes of central DI include head trauma, surgery, and destructive processes involving the hypothalamus, including tumors, sarcoidosis, tuberculosis, and eosinophilic granuloma; it can also be idiopathic.
2. Nephrogenic DI is most often associated with metabolic or toxic processes, including severe hypokalemia, hypercalcemia, lithium, and other drugs (e.g., demeclocycline, amphotericin, and foscarnet). It can also be congenital.

DI usually presents with severe polyuria and mild hypernatremia; extreme thirst and polydipsia are also common.

DIAGNOSIS

I. Low urine osmolality (50–100 mOsm/L) or specific gravity
II. Large urinary output (3–4 mL/kg/hour)
III. Increased serum sodium
IV. Water deprivation test: water deprivation followed by the administration of desmopressin (deamino-delta-D-arginine vasopressin [DDAVP]), an ADH analog, can help to differentiate central from nephrogenic DI. Central DI will be responsive to desmopressin, whereas nephrogenic DI will not.

TREATMENT

I. Both central and nephrogenic DI: hydration, replacing the free water deficit (oral or intravenous) in an amount equivalent with the urinary output.
II. Central DI: desmopressin can be given by nasal spray, orally, or by injection; chlorpropamide can increase ADH secretion and enhances the effect of ADH.

D

DIABETES INSIPIDUS

III. Nephrogenic DI: treat underlying causes; correct electrolyte abnormalities; can also use thiazide diuretics.

REFERENCES

Lu, H. A. (2017). Diabetes insipidus. *Adv Exp Med Biol, 969*, 213–225.
Robertson, G. L. (2016). Diabetes insipidus: differential diagnosis and management. *Best Pract Res Clin Endocrinol Metab, 30*(2), 205–218.

DIALYSIS (CENTRAL NERVOUS SYSTEM COMPLICATIONS)

There are three main neurologic syndromes related to dialysis:

I. *Dialysis disequilibrium syndrome* is the acute onset of neurologic manifestations during or after hemo- or peritoneal dialysis. Symptoms involve restlessness, headache, confusion, anorexia, cramps, and even coma. Generalized seizures may also occur, and electroencephalogram (EEG) changes reflect the degree of uremia before dialysis and consist of bursts of rhythmic delta waves and occasionally spike-and-wave complexes. While the exact etiology remains unknown, it is thought to occur due to substantial urea gradients following hemodialysis; namely, cerebrospinal fluid (CSF) concentrations of urea remain elevated compared to blood, following hemodialysis. This creates an osmotic gradient causing water to move into the central nervous system (CNS), generating cerebral edema and increased intracranial pressure (ICP). Pediatric populations are particularly susceptible, likely owing to smaller volume of distribution of urea. While treatment is supportive (aimed at lowering ICP), the syndrome is usually self-limited, and recovery usually occurs in a few days. However, profound symptoms may be difficult to reverse, and mortality is high. Prevention involves early initiation of dialysis (when uremia is less profound), slower rate of dialysis, and hemofiltration (convective removal) over dialysis (diffusive removal).

II. *Dialysis dementia syndrome* occurs in chronic dialysis patients. While improved practices have made it rare, it is considered a fatal encephalopathy initiating with speech hesitancy/arrest and memory changes, followed by personality changes, delusions, hallucinations, asterixis, ataxia, myoclonus, and seizures. EEG findings are characteristic of 2- to 4-second bursts of high-voltage, irregular, frontally dominated generalized delta waves, accompanied by frontal sharp waves, spikes, and triphasic waves on normal or minimally slow background. The syndrome may be related to elevated aluminum levels in the dialysate fluid, as removal of aluminum from dialysate products has markedly reduced the frequency of this syndrome. Deferoxamine (an aluminum chelator) is used to treat, though may precipitate/exacerbate encephalopathy in patients with very high serum aluminum levels.

III. *Other CNS complications of dialysis*: Dialysis encephalopathy (multisystem disease that includes vitamin D-resistant osteomalacia, myopathy, and anemia), Wernicke encephalopathy due to diffusive removal of thiamine, subdural hematomas due to hemoconcentration, confusional states from hyperosmolarity, hypercalcemia, hypophosphatemia, and drug intoxication. Patients with chronic renal failure often have multiple risk factors for cerebrovascular disease. Cognitive function, particularly in attention and concentration as well as memory function, is often abnormal with individual with lowered glomerular filtration rate (GFR) (chronic kidney disease [CKD] stage III or higher), and especially in patients with end-stage renal disease on dialysis.

REFERENCES

Daroff, R. B., Jankovic, J., Mazzotta, J. C., et al. (2016). *Bradley's neurology in clinical practice,* ed 7. Philadelphia: Elsevier.

Zepeda-Orozco, D., & Quigley, R. (2012). Dialysis disequilibrium syndrome. *J Pediatric Nephrol, 27,* 2205–2211.

DISSEMINATED INTRAVASCULAR COAGULATION

Disseminated intravascular coagulation (DIC) is a clinical and laboratory diagnosis based on findings of coagulopathy and/or fibrinolysis. DIC is a clotting disorder complicating many diseases and is most commonly associated with obstetric catastrophes, hemolysis from acute hemolytic transfusion reaction, malignancies, massive trauma, and bacterial sepsis. It is less commonly associated with immunologic disturbances, diabetic ketoacidosis, tissue damage (stroke, brain hemorrhage, meningitis, etc.), or shock. In each case, potent thrombogenic stimuli, such as tissue factor or endotoxin, trigger the coagulation cascade and activate platelets. Fibrin then deposits in the microcirculation, causing ischemia, red blood cell (RBC) damage, hemolysis, and secondary fibrinolysis.

DIC can be either an explosive and life-threatening bleeding disorder or relatively mild and subclinical. Most often, patients have hemorrhagic or thrombotic complications in venipuncture sites or distal extremities. Neurologic complications can affect any portion of the brain or spinal cord with hemorrhage or thrombosis, producing a fluctuating encephalopathy, commonly with focal findings. Confusion, delirium, stupor, and coma may occur with hemiparesis, hemianopia, ataxia, aphasia, seizures, and focal brainstem disease.

Laboratory manifestations include elevated prothrombin time and partial thromboplastin time, low platelets, decreased fibrinogen (consumptive), and elevated fibrin split products and D-dimer (due to fibrinolysis). Anemia, fragmented RBCs, and schistocytes may be found.

Treatment consists of correcting the underlying cause. Active bleeding requires fresh-frozen plasma and cryoprecipitate to replenish clotting factors and platelet transfusions to correct thrombocytopenia.

REFERENCES

Aminoff, M. J. (1989). *Neurology and general medicine* (pp. 204–205). Edinburgh: Churchill Livingstone.

Schwartzman, R. J., et al. (1982). Neurologic complications of disseminated intravascular coagulation. *Neurology, 32*(8), 791–797.

DIZZINESS

Dizziness is a nonspecific, ill-defined term commonly used by patients to describe a variety of subjective or objective experiences, such as faintness, unsteadiness, vertigo, and lightheadedness. An accurate account of what the patient is describing, a detailed medical history, and reproduction of the patient's symptoms by means of provocative maneuvers (e.g., hyperventilation, Barany maneuver, stooping over, measuring orthostatic blood pressures) help suggest the following more specific etiologic categories:

 I. Vertigo: The illusion of self-motion or environmental motion (see Vertigo).
 II. Syncope or presyncope: The sensation of impending faint or loss of consciousness. Causes include cardiac arrhythmia, carotid sinus hypersensitivity, postural hypotension (diabetic autonomic neuropathy or side effect of antihypertensive, diuretic, dopaminergic, or other drugs), anemia, and Addison disease (see Syncope).
 III. Disequilibrium: Loss of balance without various subjective movement sensations of head. Causes include cerebellar or proprioceptive disturbances and muscle weakness.
 IV. Dizziness due to causes other than those previously mentioned may be described as lightheadedness, floating, wooziness, faintness, or some other sense of altered consciousness. Causes include the following:
 A. Hyperventilation syndrome. Hyperventilation is one of the most common causes of dizziness or lightheadedness. Circumoral and digital paresthesias are frequently associated. Symptoms may be reproduced during hyperventilation. Occasionally a patient has positional vertigo with hyperventilation (see Hyperventilation, Vertigo).
 B. Multiple sensory deficits. Two or more of the following are usually present: visual impairment (often caused by cataracts), neuropathy, vestibular dysfunction (see Vertigo), cervical spondylosis, and orthopedic disorders that interfere with ambulation. Patients may complain of lightheadedness when walking and turning. Holding the examiner's finger lightly may provide enough additional sensory input to relieve the symptoms. Patients are often elderly or diabetic, or both. Proprioceptive deficits and gait apraxia should be excluded during the evaluation.
 C. Psychogenic dizziness (not associated with hyperventilation). Patients complain of vague lightheadedness, mental fuzziness, or difficulty in thinking. They may be depressed or anxious. Dizziness is usually

continuous rather than episodic. Patients may state that all or none of the maneuvers performed during physical examination produce dizziness.

D. Severe anemia or polycythemia may cause symptoms of lightheadedness or dizziness.

E. Drugs may produce symptoms of dizziness that are not necessarily related to orthostatic changes in blood pressure or presyncope. These drugs include antiarrhythmics, anticonvulsants, antidepressants, antihistamines, antihypertensives, antiparkinsonian agents, hypnotics, hypoglycemics, phenothiazines, alcohol, and tobacco.

F. Endocrinologic disorders (hypoglycemia, Addison disease, hypopituitarism, and insulinoma).

Treatment of dizziness depends on the underlying cause. For evaluation and management of vertigo, see Vertigo.

D

DYSARTHRIA

REFERENCES

Ropper, A. H., Samuels, M. A., Klein, J. P. (Eds.), 2014. *Adams & Victor's principles of neurology*, ed 10, Ch 15. New York: McGraw-Hill.

Choi, K. D., Lee, H., & Kim, J. S. (2016). Ischemic syndromes causing dizziness and vertigo. *Handb Clin Neurol, 137*, 317–340.

DYSARTHRIA

Dysarthria is an alteration in speech quality. By definition, there is no defect of the cortical language pathways in dysarthria. Language expression, reading, writing, and comprehension are preserved. This disorder of speech is produced by disturbance of the coordination of the muscles of speech, most often indicating a subcortical lesion, rather than a cortical lesion seen in different aphasias. Several patterns of dysarthria are recognized: pyramidal (spastic), extrapyramidal (rigid), ataxic (cerebellar), neuromuscular (flaccid), hypophonia, tremulous voice, and stuttering. Whether the cause is buccal, lingual, or labial is helpful as well, which can be assessed by having the patient repeat phonetic sounds such as "ca-ca-ca," "la-la-la," or "ma-ma-ma." Although each has differing sound characteristics to the trained ear, it is often necessary to assess corroborating neurologic deficits such as limb ataxia, involvement of cranial nerves, or brisk jaw jerk or gag reflex to distinguish the speech patterns (ataxic, flaccid, and spastic, respectively). Acute dysarthria is most often seen in stroke, and can produce nonspecific "slurred" speech, that is typically nonlocalizing, as dysfunction at any level from cortex to muscles can produce it, underscoring the importance of a complete neurologic examination for associated deficits to aid in localization.

Characteristic lesions and disease states that produce dysarthria include:

1. Bilateral corticobulbar lesions
2. Basal ganglia lesions
3. Cerebellar lesions (scanning or explosive speech)

4. Hypophonia and bradykinesia in Parkinson disease
5. Bilateral cranial nerve lesions
6. Muscle weakness as caused by neuromuscular junction, muscle, or mitochondrial disease
7. Upper and lower motor neuron lesions in amyotrophic lateral sclerosis
8. Lesions to lower portion of the precentral gyrus or frontal lobe lesions ("frontal dysarthria")

REFERENCES

Rampello, L., Patti, F., Zappia, M. (2016). When the word doesn't come out: a synthetic overview of dysarthria. *J Neurol Sci, 369*, 354–360.

Ropper, A. H., Samuels, M. A., Klein, J. P. (Eds.), 2014. *Adams & Victor's principles of neurology*, ed 10, Ch 23. New York: McGraw-Hill.

DYSKINESIA; TARDIVE (See also THERAPEUTIC APPENDIX)

Tardive dyskinesia (TD) is an iatrogenic movement disorder that is associated with prolonged use of certain medications, most famously antipsychotics. Patients present with abnormal involuntary movements of the mouth, face, trunk, and/or extremities. It is distinguished from other extrapyramidal side effects of antipsychotic medications in that it generally occurs after the patient has been using the medication for some time.

Diagnosis requires a history of exposure to a medication known to be associated with TD. Characteristic movements (e.g., lip smacking, tongue thrusting, or chorea) will be evident on exam. The Abnormal Involuntary Movement Scale is a tool to help diagnose and quantify TD. Several subtypes or variants of TD have been described, including tardive dystonia, tardive akathisia, tardive tremor, tardive blepharospasm, tardive myoclonus, tardive tics and tourettism, and tardive gait.

The symptoms of TD may be difficult to treat. Withdrawing the causative agent has not been shown to be an effective treatment. The American Academy of Neurology has published an evidence-based guideline regarding treatment of TD and related syndromes. After a review of the available literature, Bhidayasiri et al. found Level B evidence that clonazepam and gingko biloba each probably improve tardive syndromes, and Level C evidence that amantadine and tetrabenazine might be considered as treatment. Risperidone was not recommended as treatment, as it may cause tardive symptoms. Many other treatments were evaluated, but Bhidayasiri et al. found insufficient evidence for recommendations regarding their use.

REFERENCES

Bhidayasiri, R., et al. (2013). Evidence-based guideline: treatment of tardive syndromes: report of the Guideline Development Subcommittee of the American Academy of Neurology. *Neurology, 81*(5), 463–469.

Guy W. *ECDEU Assessment manual for psychopharmacology—revised (DHEW publ no ADM 76-338)*. Rockville, MD: US Department of Health, Education, and Welfare.

DYSPHAGIA

Dysphagia—impaired swallowing—can originate from disturbances in the mouth, pharynx, or esophagus and can involve mechanical, musculoskeletal, or neurogenic mechanisms. Dysphagia can lead to superimposed problems such as inadequate nutrition, dehydration, recurrent upper respiratory infections, and frank aspiration with consequent pneumonia and even asphyxia.

Clinically, dysphagia is divided into two types, oropharyngeal and esophageal, based on characteristics of the symptoms.

I. Oropharyngeal dysphagia is manifested by difficulty transferring food through the mouth with the following features: occurs immediately after the initiation of swallowing and is associated with repetitive swallows, drooling, food spillage, hypersalivation, coughing, choking, dysarthria, nasal regurgitation, and dysphonia. There are two important subcategories to consider in oropharyngeal dysphagia: mechanical and neurogenic/neuromuscular.

II. Esophageal dysphagia is characterized by the sensation of food lodging in the suprasternal notch or behind the sternum after swallowing and occurs several seconds after initiating a swallow. The type of esophageal dysphagia is further subdivided into categories based on whether it occurs with solid food only (mechanical obstruction) or with both solids and liquids (neurogenic/neuromuscular).

The four key historical questions are (1) What types of food cause symptoms? (2) Is the course progressive or a new onset? (3) Is there a prior history of reflux disease? (4) Is there pain with swallowing? Regurgitation of undigested food and halitosis may indicate a Zenker diverticulum.

Therapy for dysphagia is dependent on the specific mechanism responsible for the dysphagia, underlying etiologic disease process, and patient/family desires.

MECHANICAL DYSPHAGIA
I. Oral
   A. Amyloidosis
   B. Congenital abnormalities
      a. Intraoral tumors
      b. Lip injuries (burns, trauma)
      c. Macroglossia
      d. Scleroderma
      e. Temporomandibular joint dysfunction
      f. Xerostomia (Sjögren syndrome)
      g. Cleft lip and palate
   C. Infection (oral thrush)
II. Pharyngeal
   A. Cervical anterior osteophytes
   B. Infection (diphtheria, pharyngitis)
   C. Thyromegaly

    D. Retropharyngeal abscess
    E. Retropharyngeal tumor
    F. Zenker diverticulum
    G. Eagle syndrome
  III. Esophageal
    A. Aberrant origin of the right subclavian artery
    B. Caustic injury
    C. Esophageal carcinoma
    D. Esophageal diverticulum
    E. Esophageal infection (*Candida albicans*, herpes simplex virus, cytomegalovirus, varicella-zoster virus, and tuberculosis)
    F. Esophageal intramural pseudodiverticula
    G. Esophageal stricture
    H. Esophageal ulceration
    I. Esophageal webs or rings
    J. Scleroderma
    K. Radiation-induced scarring
    L. Gastroesophageal reflux disease
    M. Hiatal hernia
    N. Metastatic carcinoma
    O. Posterior mediastinal mass
    P. Thoracic aortic aneurysm
    Q. Severe congestive heart failure
    R. Cardiomegaly
    S. Severe chronic obstructive pulmonary disease
    T. Eosinophilic esophagitis

NEUROGENIC DYSPHAGIA
  I. Oropharyngeal
    A. Arnold-Chiari malformation
    B. Neurodegenerative disorders
        a. Corticobasal degeneration
        b. Dementia with Lewy bodies
        c. Huntington disease
        d. Multiple system atrophy
        e. Neuroacanthocytosis
        f. Parkinson disease
        g. Progressive supranuclear palsy
        h. Wilson disease
    C. Central pontine myelinolysis
    D. Cerebral palsy
    E. Drug-related (cyclosporine, tardive dyskinesia, and vincristine)
    F. Infectious
        a. Brainstem encephalitis (Listeria, Epstein-Barr virus)
        b. Diphtheria
        c. Poliomyelitis

    d. Progressive multifocal leukoencephalopathy
    e. Rabies
  G. Mass lesions (abscess, hemorrhage, metastatic tumor, and primary tumor)
  H. Motor neuron disease
    a. Amyotrophic lateral sclerosis
  I. Multiple sclerosis
  J. Peripheral neuropathic processes
    a. Charcot-Marie-Tooth disease
    b. Guillain-Barré syndrome (Miller-Fisher variant)
  K. Spinocerebellar ataxias
  L. Stroke
  M. Syringobulbias
II. Esophageal
  A. Achalasia
  B. Autonomic neuropathies
    a. Diabetes mellitus
    b. Familial dysautonomia
    c. Paraneoplastic syndromes
  C. Basal ganglia disorders
    a. Parkinson disease
  D. Chagas disease
  E. Esophageal motility disorders
  F. Scleroderma

NEUROMUSCULAR DYSPHAGIA

I. Oropharyngeal
  A. Inflammatory myopathies
    a. Dermatomyositis
    b. Inclusion body myositis
    c. Polymyositis
  B. Mitochondrial myopathies
    a. Kearns-Sayre syndrome
    b. Mitochondrial neurogastrointestinal encephalomyopathy
  C. Muscular dystrophies
    a. Duchenne
    b. Facioscapulohumeral
    c. Limb-girdle
    d. Myotonic
II. Oculopharyngeal
  A. Neuromuscular junction disorders
    a. Botulism
    b. Lambert-Eaton syndrome
    c. Myasthenia gravis
    d. Tetanus

B. Scleroderma
C. Stiff-man syndrome
D. Oculopharyngeal dystrophy
III. Esophageal
A. Amyloidosis
B. Inflammatory myopathies
a. Dermatomyositis
b. Polymyositis
C. Scleroderma
D. Sarcoidosis
Functional esophageal disorders

EVALUATION OF DYSPHAGIA

Oropharyngeal Dysfunction
I. Oral phase dysfunction
A. Screening tests
a. Clinical examination
b. Cervical auscultation
c. 3-ounce water swallow (i.e., bedside swallow test)
B. Primary test: modified barium swallow
II. Pharyngeal phase dysfunction
A. Screening tests
a. Clinical examination
b. 3-ounce water swallow
c. Timed swallowing
B. Primary test: modified barium swallow test
C. Complementary tests
a. Pharyngeal videoendoscopy
b. Pharyngeal manometry
c. Electromyography
d. Videomanofluorometry
e. laryngoscopy
Esophageal Dysfunction
A. Primary test
a. Videofluoroscopy
b. Upper endoscopy
B. Complementary test: esophageal manometry
Additional laboratory testing and imaging studies to confirm the underlying infectious (e.g., syphilis, Candida), metabolic (e.g., Cushing disease, and thyrotoxicosis), or neuromuscular conditions (e.g., myopathy, myasthenia gravis, and multiple sclerosis).

REFERENCES

Baijens, L. W., Clavé, P., Cras, P., et al. (2016). European Society for Swallowing Disorders—European Union Geriatric Medicine Society white paper: oropharyngeal dysphagia as a geriatric syndrome. *Clin Interv Aging*, *11*, 1403 1428.

Cabib, C., Ortega, O., Kumru, H., et al. (2016). Neurorehabilitation strategies for post-stroke oropharyngeal dysphagia: from compensation to the recovery of swallowing function. *Ann N Y Acad Sci, 1380*(1), 121–138.

DYSTONIA

DEFINITION

"A movement disorder characterized by sustained or intermittent muscle contractions causing abnormal movements, postures, or both; are typically patterned, twisting, or tremulous; and are initiated or worsened by voluntary action and associated with overflow muscle activation." (Movement Disorders Society international consensus, 2013)

KEY FEATURES

- Dystonia is a hyperkinetic movement disorder caused by involuntary muscle contractions.
- *Overflow* is the induction of dystonia by action in a separate or distal set of muscles.
- Tremor can mimic dystonia. Unlike tremor, dystonia has directionality and task-specificity (e.g., will not occur performing other tasks). Tremor tends to be more rhythmic.
- Dystonia can be alleviated by a *geste antagoniste* (sensory trick), e.g., touching the face, which is often incidentally discovered by the patient; dystonias also typically remit during sleep.
- Adult-onset dystonias more commonly affect the upper body segments (face, neck, arms), and onset is gradual over minutes; presentations with atypical features may warrant further investigations for alternative etiology.

   Classification of dystonias occurs across two axes (Table 50).

NOTABLE DYSTONIA SYNDROMES AND GENETIC CAUSES

Early-onset torsion dystonia (*DYT-TOR1A*) and adolescent-onset dystonia of mixed type (*DYT-THAP1*): most common inherited dystonias, both autosomal dominant, typically presenting in adolescence as focal dystonia (leg); *also known as DYT1: torsion dystonia found worldwide but often identified in Ashkenazi Jews.* Usually begins in childhood or adolescence with involuntary posturing of the trunk, neck, or limbs, and becomes generalized. May present into adulthood:

- Adult onset focal/segmental dystonias: cervical dystonia (torticollis), blepharospasm, spasmodic dysphonia, vocal tremor, arm dystonia, task-specific (writer's cramp, musician's dystonia, golfer's dystonia/yips)
- Dystonia-parkinsonism: dopa-responsive dystonia (DRD), Wilson disease, neurodegeneration with brain iron accumulation. DRD typically presents as childhood-onset, generalized dystonia, parkinsonism,

TABLE 50

CLASSIFICATION OF DYSTONIAS

Axis I: Clinical features		Axis II: Etiology	
Age of onset:	Infancy, childhood, adolescence, or early/ late adulthood	*Nervous system pathology:*	Degeneration, static lesion(s), or none
		Inherited or acquired:	Autosomal dominant, autosomal recessive, X-linked, mitochondrial
Body distribution:	Focal, segmental, multifocal, generalized, or hemidystonia.		Stroke, hemorrhage, traumatic brain injury, perinatal injury, infection, toxic/metabolic, neoplastic, or psychogenic
Temporal pattern:	Static or progressive. Persistent, action-specific, diurnal, or paroxysmal.	*Idiopathic:*	Familial or sporadic
Associated features:	Isolated Combined with other movement disorder		

Modified from Albanese, A., Bhatia, K., Bressman, S. B., et al. (2013). Phenomenology and classification of dystonia: a consensus update. *Mov Disord*, 28(7), 863–873.

and hallmark is dramatic therapeutic response to levodopa. GTP cyclohydrolase 1 mutations are the most common genetic cause of DRD.

Diagnostic workup: Labs (directed based on clinical suspicion) can include complete blood count (CBC), electrolytes, erythrocyte sedimentation rate/C-reactive protein, antinuclear antibodies, serum copper/ceruloplasmin, rapid plasma reagin, and genetic testing. Imaging with magnetic resonance imaging brain and/or spine to evaluate for structural lesions.

Treatment: Treating the underlying/primary disease (e.g., copper antagonism in Wilson disease). Symptomatic treatment with carbidopa/levodopa trial (diagnostic and therapeutic for DRD), tetrabenazine, trihexyphenidyl, clonazepam, baclofen, botox. Diphenhydramine for acute dystonic reactions. Some patients may benefit from deep brain stimulation.

REFERENCES

Albanese, A., Bhatia, K., Bressman, S. B., et al. (2013). Phenomenology and classification of dystonia: a consensus update. *Mov Disord*, 28(7), 863–873.

Balint, B., & Bhatia, K. P. (2015). Isolated and combined dystonia syndromes - an update on new genes and their phenotypes. *Eur J Neurol*, 22, 610–617.

E

ELECTROCARDIOGRAM AND CARDIAC EFFECTS OF NEUROLOGICAL DISORDERS

Changes in electrocardiographic rhythm and morphology and cardiac structure may occur with acute or chronic central nervous system diseases. In subarachnoid hemorrhage (SAH), large upright or deeply inverted T waves and prolonged QT intervals are characteristic. These changes may be mediated by a sympathetic surge associated with hypothalamic involvement and can cause myocardial ischemia, stunning, and infarction (with creatine kinase elevations, troponin elevations, and regional wall motion abnormalities). Electrocardiogram changes can be seen in neuromuscular disorders and muscular dystrophies (e.g., Friedreich ataxia, myotonic dystrophy, mitochondrial disorders, Pompe disease), migraine, brain tumor, head injury, and stroke (both as cause and effect). Many other conditions affect autonomic function (postural orthostatic tachycardia syndrome, Lewy body disease), and the electrocardiogram may be affected by medications that have cholinergic effects or prolong the QT interval. In epileptic patients, cortical stimulation of the left insula leads to bradycardia and depressor effects, but the opposite effect can be seen with right insular stimulation.

Abnormal cardiac rhythms, most commonly atrial fibrillation, are associated with embolic strokes along with increased stroke risk with patent foramen ovale, and cardiomyopathies. The prevalence of atrial fibrillation below age 55 years in the United States is less than 0.5%, rising to 6% for individuals older than 65 years.

ELECTROENCEPHALOGRAPHY

The electroencephalogram (EEG) is the difference in voltage between two different recording locations plotted over time. An EEG signal consists of inhibitory and excitatory postsynaptic potentials of pyramidal cells generated in the brain cortex. This activity reflects the major influence of subcortical structures, especially the brainstem reticular formation and intralaminar and reticular nuclei of the thalamus, generating the three normal states of consciousness: waking, non-rapid eye movement sleep, and rapid eye movement (REM) sleep. EEG is clinically useful in large part because it provides real-time information regarding brain physiology, rather than structure.

I. The normal, adult, waking EEG may contain the following:
   A. Alpha rhythm (8 to 13 Hz): Present occipitally in nearly all adults, it appears during relaxed wakefulness with eyes closed and attenuates with eye opening or mental effort. EEG attenuation and reactivity is a sign of better prognosis when evaluating encephalopathy. Posterior

rhythm below 8 Hz is considered abnormal after age 8, abiding by the "eight by eight" rule.

B. Beta activity (>13 Hz): This is a normal finding unless its amplitude consistently exceeds 25 mV, which may suggest the presence of benzodiazepines, barbiturates, or chloral hydrate. Beta is enhanced over skull defects (breach rhythm, sometimes appearing quite "spiky") and depressed in areas of focal brain injury and over subdural, epidural, or subgaleal fluid collections.

C. Slow wave activity: Theta and delta activity. The presence of theta activity (4 to 7 Hz) waves in an awake adult's EEG recording is generally considered abnormal—concerning for mild encephalopathy. Their appearance is one of the hallmarks of the onset of drowsiness. Normal elderly individuals may have a limited amount of intermittent temporal theta. Activity slower than 4 Hz (delta) should not be present in the waking adult record.

D. Mu rhythm: A rhythm of alpha frequency that is located centrally. It attenuates with contralateral extremity movement. It originates from the sensorimotor cortex.

E. Lambda waves: Low voltage, occipital sharps that appears only with eyes open, associated with searching eye movements.

F. Features that prompt considerations of normal variants: high frequency spiking (6 Hz and above), monomorphic rhythms (repetitive waves of similar shape and wavelength), and their disappearance during deeper sleep. Other benign patterns appearing during waking or drowsiness include posterior occipital sharp transients of sleep, small sharp spikes/benign epileptiform transients of sleep, positive occipital sharp transients of sleep, rhythmic temporal theta bursts of drowsiness (psychomotor variant), posterior slow waves of youth, subclinical rhythmic electrographic discharge of adults, 14- and 6-Hz positive bursts, 6-Hz phantom spike and wave, and wicket spikes.

G. Hyperventilation (HV) response: A physiologic increase in generalized slowing occurs with prolonged HV, particularly in children, and is accentuated with hypoglycemia. Abnormalities during HV include focal slowing or epileptiform discharges.

H. Photic stimulation response: Normal photomyoclonic responses consist of muscular contractions, typically orbicularis oculi, elicited by each flash. Abnormal photoparoxysmal responses, bursts of generalized epileptiform discharges that may outlast the flash stimuli, are indicative of generalized epilepsy or an inherited EEG trait.

II. The normal, adult, sleep EEG may contain the following:

A. Wakefulness EEG: Features include (1) posterior alpha rhythm is present when eyes are closed, disappears with eye opening; (2) anterioposterior gradient of voltage and frequency. Anteriorly, waves are of lower voltage and higher frequency. Posteriorly, waves are of higher voltage and lower frequency.

B. Drowsiness: Features include subtle slowing of the posterior rhythm and slow roving lateral eye movement of drowsiness.

C. Stage I sleep: Defined by midline sharp waves called vertex waves.

D. Stage II sleep: Marked by the appearance of sleep spindles, rhythmic 12- to 15-Hz waves with a waxing and waning morphology, and K complexes, large biphasic sharp transients maximal over the vertex, often precipitated by external stimuli.

E. Stages III and IV sleep: Defined by the presence of delta waves 2 Hz or slower, greater than 75 μV, occurring between 20% and 50% of a 30-s epoch (stage III) or over 50% (stage IV).

F. REM sleep: Defined by relatively low-voltage desynchronized EEG, muscular atonia, and bursts of REMs.

III. EEG artifacts:

A. Eyeblink artifact: Sharp, downward waveform in the frontal leads (Fp1-F3 and Fp2-F4) with rapid decrease in amplitude in the subsequent electrodes, F3-C3 and F4-C4 respectively.

B. Muscle artifact: Fast wave that "turns the channel black" and does not have an electric field, i.e., not present in adjacent electrodes.

C. Other EEG artifacts include a lateral eye movement artifact, nystagmus artifact, electrode pop, sweat artifact, pulse artifact, 60 Hz artifact, EKG artifact and special movement artifact (hiccup, chewing, and glossokinetic).

IV. EEG abnormalities (Fig. 24i–v)

A. Epilepsy: Interictal epileptiform activity, consisting of spikes, sharp waves, or spike-wave complexes, is strongly but not absolutely correlated with epilepsy. Thus, the presence of such activity does not unequivocally indicate a diagnosis of epilepsy, nor does its absence exclude it. Nevertheless, their presence, in combination with clinical information, frequently allows one to make a diagnosis in terms of recognized electroclinical syndromes (see Epilepsy). Ictal discharges, or electrographic seizures, provide irrefutable evidence of an epileptic seizure disorder. In generalized epilepsies, electrographic seizures may consist of a prolonged run of otherwise typical interictal discharges, but this is rarely the case in partial epilepsies, and the ictal patterns have their own morphology that is usually characterized by evolution in frequency and amplitude. The absence of an ictal EEG pattern during a typical, generalized convulsion provides strong evidence of a nonepileptic event (see Epilepsy), but this is less true for auras, focal motor, or sensory seizures, and complex partial seizures.

B. Focal brain lesions: The presence of continuous, focal, polymorphic delta activity, especially in combination with depression of ipsilateral background rhythms, strongly suggests a focal lesion. However, an area of focal dysfunction, as may be seen following a complicated migraine or focal seizure, should also be considered. Periodic lateralized epileptiform discharges (PLEDs) are frequently associated with irritative lesions, such as acute cerebral infarcts or encephalitis.

E

ELECTROENCEPHALOGRAPHY

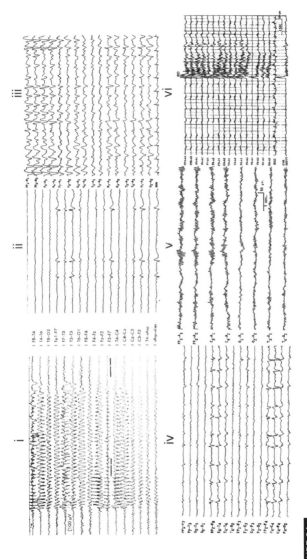

FIGURE 24

Examples of electroencephalogram abnormalities.

(i) Typical 3 seconds spike and wave seen in absence seizure. (ii) Left mesial temporal epilepsy with interictal focal discharges. (iii) Triphasic waves. (iv) Periodic lateralized epileptiform discharge. (v) Alpha coma. (vi) Burst suppression.

C. Diffuse encephalopathies: The EEG has a high sensitivity for detecting global cerebral dysfunction but is nonspecific as to etiology. Exceptions include Alzheimer disease and human immunodeficiency virus encephalopathy, in which the EEG may remain normal until late in the course of the disease. Early changes include slowing of the alpha rhythm and the appearance of generalized theta activity; more severe cases show generalized polymorphic delta, frontal intermittent rhythmic delta activity (FIRDA), and a lack of normal reactivity. Triphasic waves are seen in hepatic or other metabolic encephalopathies and may be periodic. Other conditions associated with periodic discharges include Creutzfeldt-Jakob disease (most patients have periodic sharp discharges, occurring with a period of about 1 second, within 12 weeks of diagnosis) and subacute sclerosing panencephalitis (periodic, generalized, slow waves, or sharp and slow complexes, with a period of about 5 to 10 seconds).

D. Coma: Findings include lack of normal background, reactivity, or state changes, in combination with continuous generalized polymorphic delta activity, FIRDA, low-voltage patterns, and periodic discharges. These may include PLEDs or triphasic waves or a burst-suppression pattern (bursts of electrical activity separated by periods of diffuse voltage suppression, indicative of severe diffuse cerebral dysfunction). In patients with a coma following seizures, electrographic status epilepticus should be ruled out. Alpha coma, with generalized, invariant, unreactive alpha frequency activity, is associated with toxic or metabolic insults and cerebral anoxia and must be distinguished from normal alpha rhythms present in those with a "locked-in state."

E. Brain death: Confirmatory evidence includes the demonstration of electrocerebral silence (ECS), under proper technical conditions, in the appropriate clinical context. Conditions associated with reversible ECS include overdose of central nervous system depressants, hypothermia, cardiovascular shock, metabolic and endocrine disorders, and very young age.

REFERENCES

André-Obadia, N., et al. (2015). Continuous EEG monitoring in adults in the intensive care unit (ICU). *Neurophysiol Clin*, *45*(1), 39–46.

Marcuse, L. V., et al. (2016). *Rowan's primer of EEG,* ed 2. London: Elsevier.

ELECTROLYTE DISORDERS

Symptoms are usually more severe with acute changes than chronic alterations in electrolyte levels. Occasionally, chronic disturbances may produce signs and symptoms opposite from the acute state. In general, central nervous system (CNS) dysfunction occurs with abnormalities of sodium, peripheral nervous system dysfunction with abnormal potassium levels, and combinations of both with abnormalities of calcium, magnesium, and phosphate. Management is directed at treatment of the primary disorder and correction of the electrolyte abnormality. Neurologic findings usually disappear with appropriate therapy (Table 51 lists signs and symptoms).

TABLE 51

COMPARISON OF ELECTROLYTE DISORDERS

Electrolyte Disorder	Causes	Symptoms
Hypernatremia	Water loss Sodium retention Impaired thirst or access to water Poor release of ADH	Restless Confused Poor arousability Seizures (rare)
Hyponatremia	Fluid loss (sweat, polyuria, diarrhea, third space) Fluid overload (CHF, renal failure) Medications (diuretics) Iatrogenic (excess intravenous fluids) SIADH Hypoaldosteronism	Headache, nausea Muscle cramps Seizures Reduced consciousness
Hyperkalemia	Poor elimination (renal failure, mineralocorticoid insufficiency) Iatrogenic Excess potassium release from cells (trauma, burns, status epilepticus)	Rare symptoms Nonspecific weakness Paresthesias
Hypokalemia	Excess gastrointestinal or urinary excretion Distribution away from extracellular space (insulin, β-agonists)	Myalgias Weakness Hyporeflexia
Hypercalcemia	Hyperparathyroidism (primary, secondary, or tertiary) Malignancy Thyrotoxicosis	Headache Fatigue Myalgias Psychiatric symptoms
Hypocalcemia	Renal failure Parathyroid deficiency Acute pancreatitis Hypomagnesemia Rhabdomyolysis Tumor lysis syndrome Vitamin D deficiency Critically ill patients	Paresthesias Chvostek sign Trousseau sign Tetany Altered mental status

Continued

TABLE 51

COMPARISON OF ELECTROLYTE DISORDERS—Cont'd

Electrolyte Disorder	Causes	Symptoms
Hyperphosphatemia	Renal failure Rhabdomyolysis Tumor lysis syndrome Hypoparathyroidism	Similar to effect of hypocalcemia (high serum concentration of phosphorous lowers the calcium level)
Hypophosphatemia	Impaired absorption Alkalosis Refeeding syndrome Burns Chronic alcoholism Medications (catecholamines, thiazide diuretic, antacid)	Perioral paresthesias Polyneuropathy Inability to wean from ventilator
Hypermagnesemia	Excess magnesium intake (patients with eclampsia or renal failure)	Nausea, vomiting Dry mouth Flushing Generalized weakness, hyporeflexia (severe)
Hypomagnesemia	Critically ill patients Low magnesium intake Poor absorption Excess excretion by kidneys (e.g., diuretics)	Tremor Myoclonus Ataxia Tachycardia, sweating, dilated pupils Seizures (severe)

ADH, Antidiuretic hormone; *CHF*, congestive heart failure; *SIADH*, syndrome of inappropriate secretion of antidiuretic hormone.

Adapted from Hocker, S. E. (2015). Electrolyte disturbance and acid-base imbalance. In K. D. Flemming & L. K. Jones (Eds.), (2015). *Mayo Clinic Neurology Board review: clinical neurology for initial certification and MOC* (pp. 741–745). Oxford University Press.

SODIUM

Sodium is the main determinant of serum osmolality (Osm) and extracellular fluid volume. Neurologic symptoms are dependent on the time lag necessary for the brain to compensate for rapid changes in serum Na^+ concentration, and Osm.

I. Hyponatremia: Acute decreases of Na^+ levels to 130 mEq/L may produce symptoms, whereas chronic changes to 115 mEq/L may be asymptomatic. Acute hyponatremia (<115 mEq/L) with seizures carries a high mortality rate and necessitates rapid (over a 6-hour period) correction to 120 to 125 mEq/L (with hypertonic saline or normal saline and furosemide). Rapid correction to levels greater than 120 to 125 mEq/L may result in central pontine myelinolysis, a disorder described in alcoholics but also occurring in children and adults with liver disease, severe electrolyte imbalances, malnutrition, anorexia, burns, cancer, Addison disease, and sepsis.

There is symmetrical focal myelin destruction predominantly involving the basal central pons. Asymptomatic chronic hyponatremia usually requires no immediate intervention and is managed by correction of the underlying condition.

II. Hypernatremia: Neurologic symptoms develop when the serum Na^+ level rises above 160 mEq/L or serum Osm is greater than 350 mOsm/kg. Level of consciousness correlates well with the degree of hyperosmolality. Sudden increases in serum Osm may produce decreased brain cell volume, with mechanical traction on cerebral vessels causing subcortical, subdural, or subarachnoid hemorrhage. Cerebrospinal fluid protein levels may be high without pleocytosis, and the electroencephalogram (EEG) is normal or mildly slowed. Hypernatremia resulting from diabetes insipidus may occur with tumors involving the hypothalamus or pineal region, as well as with basilar meningitis, encephalitis, ruptured aneurysms, sarcoidosis, trauma, or surgery. Treatment for hypernatremia includes isotonic solutions to reduce the serum Na^+ level by no more than 1 mEq/L every 2 hours during the first 2 days of treatment. Rapid infusion of hypotonic solutions may cause cerebral edema and seizures.

POTASSIUM

Almost 60% of total body K^+ is located within muscle; therefore, predominantly muscular symptoms occur with altered K^+ levels.

I. Hypokalemia most commonly occurs with diuretic use but also occurs with gastrointestinal losses, mineralocorticoid excess, and rarely, thyrotoxicosis. Muscle weakness usually develops with serum levels of 2.5 to 3.0 mEq/L, with structural muscle damage occurring at levels below 2.0 mEq/L. Hypokalemia and hypocalcemia frequently coexist, with cancellation of neuromuscular manifestations. Treatment of one condition in isolation may produce symptoms of the other. Electrocardiogram (ECG) and cardiac abnormalities are common and may require intensive care unit (ICU) monitoring and treatment. Treatment includes increasing dietary K^+, supplements of potassium chloride (KCl), and the use of K^+-sparing diuretics.

II. Hyperkalemia is relatively uncommon but may occur in familial hyperkalemic periodic paralysis (see Periodic Paralysis). Quadriparesis may develop with levels greater than 6.8 mEq/L, and levels greater than 7.0 mEq/L are life-threatening due to cardiac toxicity. Potassium levels greater than 6.0 mEq/L require ICU monitoring and immediate therapy with administration of glucose and insulin, cation exchange resins, or calcium gluconate.

CALCIUM

Plasma Ca^{2+} is a stabilizer of excitable membranes in the central and peripheral nervous systems and in muscle. Ca^{2+} concentrations are closely controlled through the combined effects of parathyroid hormone, calciferol, and calcitonin on intestine, kidney, and bone.

I. Hypocalcemia occurs in neonates, patients with renal failure, and after thyroid or parathyroid surgery. The "tetany syndrome" originates in the peripheral nerve axon and initially becomes evident with distal and perioral tingling. Distal tonic spasms (carpopedal spasms) may progress to laryngeal stridor and opisthotonus if severe. The EEG is diffusely slow with an exaggerated response to photic stimulation. ECG abnormalities are also common. Treatment consists of oral calcium supplements. Acute treatment of hypocalcemia with tetany or seizures may require 10% IV solutions of calcium gluconate or CaCl. Underlying disorders should be corrected, if possible. Hypocalcemia often coexists with hypomagnesemia. In such cases, total serum calcium levels may be normal, but ionized calcium levels may be low.

II. Hypercalcemia: Malignant neoplasms are the most common cause of increased serum Ca^{2+} levels. Mental status alterations occur with total serum levels greater than 14 mg/dL. Serum calcium levels need to be adjusted for serum albumin levels which are often low in chronically ill patients. Myopathy or carpal tunnel syndrome may occur in association with hyperparathyroidism.

Treatment: Saline hydration and furosemide are recommended. Occasionally, mithramycin (suppresses bone resorption) or calcitonin (suppresses bone resorption and increases urinary Ca^{2+} excretion) are required.

MAGNESIUM

Ninety-eight percent of Mg^{2+} is intracellular. Magnesium is necessary for the activation of various enzymes. Extracellular Mg^{2+} affects central and peripheral synaptic transmission. Acute changes in serum levels may not reflect total body stores.

I. Hypomagnesemia occurs most commonly as a result of excess renal loss (chronic alcoholism, diuretics), but may also be the result of decreased intake or absorption. Neurologic symptoms usually develop at levels below 0.8 mEq/L. The presence of seizures requires treatment with parenteral $MgSO_4$. Oral Mg^{2+} supplements may suffice in less severe cases. Calcium gluconate should be available when giving IV $MgSO_4$, as transient hypermagnesemia may cause respiratory muscle paralysis (see also hypocalcemia, above).

II. Hypermagnesemia, an uncommon disorder, usually occurs with increased intake and renal failure. Deep tendon reflexes may be lost at levels of 5 to 6 mEq/L, and CNS depression occurs at levels above 8 to 10 mEq/L. Muscular paralysis is due to neuromuscular blockade.

Paralysis treatment may be accomplished by small amounts of parenteral calcium gluconate and hydration. Otherwise, discontinuation of Mg^+-containing preparations is indicated. If renal function is severely impaired, dialysis may be necessary. Magnesium infusions are often given as treatment for seizures associated with eclampsia. Serum magnesium levels need to be closely monitored in this situation.

E

ELECTROLYTE DISORDERS

PHOSPHATE

Hypophosphatemia is often complicated by multiple abnormalities of electrolytes, nutrition, and acid-base balance. The syndrome commonly occurs in malnutrition and chronic alcoholism, especially after the infusion of glucose or hyperalimentation solutions.

Acute hypophosphatemia may not reflect decreased total body stores and may produce neurologic symptoms if severe (<1.5 mEq/L). Chronic hypophosphatemia is usually moderate (1.5–2.5 mEq/L) and may not be symptomatic unless acute stresses (alcohol withdrawal, burns, binding of phosphate in the gut) cause sudden decreases below the moderate level.

REFERENCES

Diringer, M. (2017). Neurologic manifestations of major electrolyte abnormalities. *Handb Clin Neurol, 141*, 705–713.

Hocker, S. E. (2015). Electrolyte disturbance and acid-base imbalance. In K. D. Flemming & L. K. Jones (Eds.), *Mayo Clinic Neurology Board review: clinical neurology for initial certification and MOC* (pp. 741–745). New York: Oxford University Press.

ELECTROMYOGRAPHY AND NERVE CONDUCTION STUDIES

Electrodiagnostic testing of nerve and muscle with nerve conduction studies (NCS) and electromyography (EMG) is used to localize lesions in the peripheral nervous system, to differentiate primary nerve and muscle disorders, to provide insight for underlying pathophysiology of peripheral nervous system disorders, and to assess its severity and temporal course.

NERVE CONDUCTION STUDIES

NCS are performed by recording action potentials with a surface electrode over the skin (Table 52). Both motor and sensory components of nerves can be studied.

Motor NCS involve stimulating a peripheral nerve and recording the action potential from a muscle innervated by that nerve—because this induced action potential conducts in the same direction as physiologic motor nerve signals, it is referred to as "orthodromic." Compound muscle action potential (CMAP) is signal recorded as results from depolarization of all muscle fibers innervated, hence it is termed compound.

Sensory NCS are usually done antidromically, by stimulating a peripheral nerve proximally and recording from a distal site innervated by that nerve; for some sensory nerves, orthodromic recording is also possible. The recorded response is called a sensory nerve action potential (SNAP).

The amplitude, duration, shape, and latency of CMAPs or SNAPs are all noted for comparison to expected normalized values or morphology. Conduction velocities are calculated for SNAPs by dividing the distance between stimulating and recording electrodes by the time required for action potential conduction. For CMAPs, because the latency recorded includes not only nerve transmission velocity but also neuromuscular junction transmission time, conduction velocity is calculated by dividing the distance between two

TABLE 52

ROUTINE NERVE CONDUCTION STUDIES IN NEUROMUSCULAR DISORDERS

Disorder	Amplitude	Distal Latency	Conduction Velocity	F and H Wave Latencies
Polyneuropathy				
Axonal	↓	NL	>70%	Mild ↑
Demyelinating	NL or ↓	NL or ↑	<50%	↑
Myopathy	NL or ↓ motor	NL	NL	NL
Radiculopathy	NL or ↓ motor	NL	>80%	NL or ↑
	NL sensory			
Neuromuscular transmission defect				
Presynaptic type	NL or ↓ motor	NL	NL	NL
	NL sensory			
Postsynaptic type	NL	NL	NL	NL
Motor neuron disease	↓ motor	NL	>70%	NL or ↑
	N1 sensory			
Upper motor neuron disease	NL	NL	NL	NL

NL, Normal.

stimulation sites (proximal and distal) by the difference in conduction time between the distal stimulus site and the recording site. Normal values of NCS vary with different physiologic factors, most importantly with temperature and age. Normal nerve conduction velocities are approximately 50 m/second in the upper limbs and 40 m/second in the lower.

Repetitive nerve stimulation is another form of electrodiagnostic testing that is helpful in the diagnosis of neuromuscular junction disorders. Repetitive stimulation focuses on the change in the CMAP amplitude, if any, that results from stimulating the motor nerve multiple times per second. With slow (3 Hz) repetitive stimulation, more than a 10% drop in CMAP amplitude is often seen in both myasthenia gravis and Lambert-Eaton myasthenic syndrome (LEMS). With fast (50 Hz) stimulation, an increase in CMAP amplitude of over 50% would be diagnostic of a presynaptic neuromuscular junction disorder such as LEMS or botulism. This increment is not seen in myasthenia gravis. The order of testing in suspected neuromuscular junction disease is therefore typically first slow then fast repetitive stimulation. These studies are challenging to perform: acetylcholinesterase medications must be withheld, tissue temperature carefully attended to, and for anatomic and technical reasons the study is usually done on facial nerve and musculature or the spinal accessory nerve and trapezius. Since 50 Hz stimulation is quite painful, a more commonly used test is to evaluate the increase in CMAP amplitude after 10 seconds of maximal muscle contraction. Single-fiber EMG is the most sensitive test of NMJ transmission (Table 53). Jitter is the variability in interpotential difference between two muscle fiber action potentials during

TABLE 53
ELECTRODIAGNOSTIC STUDIES HELP TO DIFFERENTIATE THE NEUROMUSCULAR
JUNCTION DISORDERS

	MG	LEMS
SNAPs	Normal	Normal
CMAPS	Normal	Low amplitudes
Slow RNS (2 to 3 Hz)	Decrement of CMAP amplitudes (greater than 10%)	There may be decrement of CMAP amplitudes
Rapid RNS (20 to 50 Hz) or exercise	No CMAP increment (may show further decrement)	Increment of CMAP amplitudes (atleast 50%)
EMG	Normal	Normal
Jitter (on SFEMG)	Present	Present

consecutive discharges of the same motor unit. Increased jitter is present in
patients with NMJ abnormalities, but cannot differentiate between MG and
LEMS.

F waves are low-amplitude late responses due to antidromic activation of
motor neurons (anterior horn cells) following peripheral nerve stimulation,
which then cause orthodromic impulses to pass back along the involved motor
axons, also called *backfiring* of axons. It is called the F wave because it was first
noted in intrinsic foot muscles. The latency of the *F* wave is usually 25 to 32
milliseconds in the upper limbs and 45 to 56 milliseconds in the lower. *F*
waves are useful for evaluating peripheral neuropathies with predominantly
proximal involvement, such as the acute and chronic inflammatory
demyelinating polyneuropathies, in which distal conduction velocities may be
normal early in the disease. The H reflex is the other clinically recordable late
response. It is the electrical homologue of checking ankle-jerk reflex on
physical exam. It is the result of a monosynaptic reflex arc with an afferent
component mediated by large, fast-conducting group 1a fibers, and an efferent
component mediated by alpha motor neurons. For practical and anatomic
reasons, the only routinely tested H reflex is in the S1 segment, recorded after
tibial nerve stimulation in the popliteal fossa. Typical latency is 30
milliseconds. The loss of the H reflex is nonspecific—it can be simply a function
of age (it is normally absent over age 60), or it can result from a very large
number of disorders.

ELECTROMYOGRAPHY
EMG records electrical activity in individual and collective muscle fibers,
yielding more information on the localization and pathophysiology of peripheral
nervous system disorders. NCS on the other hand record electrical activity from
entire nerves at once and cannot study individual neurons. An EMG evaluation
requires the examiner to carefully select the appropriate muscles to test on the
basis of a thorough history and physical examination, and results of NCS.

For each of the muscles being studied, the first part of the examination is to assess insertional and spontaneous activity at rest. Once the insertional and spontaneous activity has been assessed, the examiner will ask the patient to slowly contract the muscle, and the motor unit action potentials (MUAPs) are evaluated. MUAPs are assessed for duration, amplitude, and numbers of phases. Then, the number of MUAPs and their relationship to the firing frequency (recruitment and activation pattern) are evaluated.

INSERTIONAL ACTIVITY

Insertional activity occurs when a needle is quickly moved through the muscle and creates depolarization of muscle fibers which is visualized on the monitor as high-frequency, positive and negative spikes (with an associated "crisp" noise). Normal insertional activity typically lasts only a few hundred milliseconds. Decreased insertional activity is seen in muscle atrophy because fewer muscle fibers are available to respond to needle insertion. Any electrical activity lasting longer than 300 milliseconds is considered increased insertional activity which may be seen in neuropathic disorders that result in denervation and several myopathic conditions that result in necrosis of the muscle fibers, such as inflammatory myopathies.

SPONTANEOUS ACTIVITY

Recognition of abnormal spontaneous activity can provide helpful information for the diagnosis:

1. The distribution of abnormal spontaneous activity may suggest the neuroanatomic localization of the lesion (e.g., mononeuropathy, radiculopathy).
2. Certain types of spontaneous activity are associated with specific disorders, for example, myotonic discharges in myotonic dystrophy and hyperkalemic periodic paralysis (see below).
3. The amount of spontaneous activity or the presence of spontaneous activity may provide information regarding the time course and severity of the lesion (e.g., presence of fibrillation potentials begins 2 to 3 weeks after the acute nerve injury).

Spontaneous activity may originate from individual muscle fibers, or from entire motor units.

Fibrillation potentials and positive sharp waves are brief, rhythmic discharges from individual denervated muscle fibers, and indicate acute or ongoing impaired innervation. They are not seen on EMG testing until 2 weeks or more after denervation occurs. They are usually graded on a scale from zero to four, where zero means that no such potentials are present and 4 + means that these spontaneous potentials fill the entire screen. They can be seen in neurogenic disorders (neuropathies, radiculopathies, motor neuron disease, etc.), myopathic disorders (especially in inflammatory myopathy and muscular dystrophics), and in severe disorders of the neuromuscular junction (such as botulism or therapeutic chemodenervation with botulinum toxin).

E

ELECTROMYOGRAPHY AND NERVE CONDUCTION STUDIES

Complex repetitive discharges (high-frequency, regular-firing, multiserrated repetitive discharges with abrupt onset and termination, creating a characteristic "machine-like" sound) result from the depolarization of a single muscle fiber followed by ephaptic spread to adjacent denervated fibers. This occurs in a wide variety of chronic neurogenic disorders (poliomyelitis, motor neuron disease, radiculopathies, and neuropathies) and myopathic disorders (Duchenne and limb-girdle dystrophy, polymyositis, and hypothyroidism). These potentials are usually not seen on EMG testing until 6 months or more after an injury.

Myotonic discharges are characterized by waveforms with waxing and waning amplitude and frequency, creating a "dive bomber" sound on the recording. They arise from single muscle fibers, but many fibers may fire myotonic discharges simultaneously. They are typically seen in myotonic dystrophy, myotonia congenita, paramyotonia congenita, hyperkalemic periodic paralysis, acid maltase deficiency, diazocholesterol toxicity, clofibrate toxicity, and rarely in polymyositis and colchicine toxicity.

Fasciculations are random single spontaneous discharges from a whole motor unit. On EMG, fasciculations have the morphology of single MUAP. They can appear as normal MUAPs, or they can be complex and large if they represent a pathologic motor unit. Fasciculations are nonspecific, and can be seen in radiculopathies, entrapment neuropathies, motor neuron disease such as amyotrophic lateral sclerosis (ALS), metabolic disorders such as thyrotoxicosis, and anticholinesterase overdoses. Although fasciculations involving superficial muscles can be visible on clinical examination, EMG helps record fasciculations from deeper muscles that are not clinically visible.

Myokymic discharges are rhythmic, grouped, spontaneous repetitive discharges of the same motor unit. These repeating bursts of MUAPs have a characteristic sound like that of soldiers marching. They may be recorded in facial muscles (facial myokymia) associated with Bell palsy or brainstem lesions resulting from multiple sclerosis, brainstem glioma, or vascular disease. Appendicular myokymia is associated with radiation plexopathy. Rarely, it may be seen in Guillain-Barré syndrome, radiculopathy, chronic entrapment neuropathy, and gold toxicity.

Neuromyotonic discharges are high-frequency (150–250 Hz) decrementing, repetitive discharges of a single motor unit that create a characteristic "pinging" sound on EMG recording. These are rare and are seen only with chronic neuropathic diseases (e.g., poliomyelitis and adult-onset spinal muscular atrophy) and syndromes of continuous motor unit activity, such as in Isaac syndrome.

Cramps are sustained involuntary muscle contractions caused by the activation of multiple motor units that occur in normal subjects (especially in distal lower extremity muscles) and in many neurogenic and metabolic disorders, including ALS, electrolyte imbalances, hypothyroidism, pregnancy, and uremia (see Cramps). Electrically, cramps are high-frequency discharges of motor units.

VOLUNTARY MOTOR UNIT POTENTIALS

Once the muscle has been assessed for insertional and spontaneous activity, the motor units are analyzed by asking the patient to slowly contract the muscle. The pattern of MUAP abnormalities will allow determination of whether the disorder is a neuropathic or a myopathic process and often helps to ascertain the time course and severity of the lesion. Assessment of MUAPs involves evaluation of the morphology or shape of individual units, and the timing of unit firing—that is, MUAP recruitment and activation.

The morphology of MUAPs provides much information into the health of the muscle being studied. Although the normal appearance of MUAPs will vary slightly from muscle to muscle, a typical MUAP is about 5 to 15 milliseconds in duration, between 0.1 and 2 mV in amplitude, and has 2 to 4 phases.

Short-duration, small-amplitude, polyphasic MUAPs occur in disorders with atrophy or loss of muscle fibers in the motor unit. Thus, they are present in myopathic disorders and in severe cases of neuromuscular transmission disorders (e.g., botulism). In early reinnervation, after severe denervation in which the newly sprouting axons only begin to reinnervate a few muscle fibers, the MUAP will also be small, short duration, and polyphasic but with reduced recruitment ("nascent" MUAP).

Long-duration, large-amplitude, polyphasic MUAPs occur with increased number or density of muscle fibers, or a loss of synchrony of fiber firing within a motor unit such as in chronic neuropathic processes (e.g., motor neuron disease, chronic radiculopathies, chronic axonal neuropathies, and chronic entrapment neuropathy).

MUAPs are considered polyphasic if they have 5 or more phases. Polyphasia is a measure of synchrony of the firing of muscle fibers within the same motor unit. This is a nonspecific measure and may be abnormal in both myopathic and neuropathic disorders. In normal muscles, up to 5% to 10% of MUAPs may be polyphasic (up to 25% in the deltoid).

Unstable MUAPs are MUAPs that change in morphology from one instance to the next. This may occur due to blocking of individual muscle fiber action potentials within the motor unit. This may be seen in disorders of neuromuscular transmission, myositis, muscle trauma, reinnervation, and rapidly progressive neurogenic atrophy.

The temporal characteristics of MUAP recruitment and activation are also important in the analysis of an EMG. Recruitment and activation are two different processes that the nervous system uses to increase the force of a contraction.

In activation, individual motor units are driven to fire at a faster rate. Poor activation of MUAPs is recognized by motor units firing slowly. As this process is centrally mediated, reduced activation is attributable to upper motor neuron lesions or lack of effort.

Recruitment refers to the orderly addition of motor units as activation increases. Decreased recruitment presents as a small number of units firing with a high frequency. Decreased recruitment occurs when there is a decreased number of available motor units; the remaining motor units will fire at a faster frequency to increase the muscle force. This occurs in any peripheral neuropathic process, including neuropathies, radiculopathies, motor neuron disease, and trauma. The term "early recruitment" is used to describe the recruitment pattern seen in myopathies; when the force generated by each individual motor unit is decreased, more motor units must be recruited to generate the same amount of force.

The normal firing rate of most motor units, before additional units are recruited, is 10 Hz. *Recruitment ratio* is another term used to describe the firing rate of a motor unit. This ratio is the rate of firing of the most rapidly firing motor unit (in Hz) divided by the number of units firing. A recruitment ratio of over 8 is considered abnormal and suggests a neurogenic process.

REFERENCES

Preston, D. C., & Shapiro, B. E. (2013). *Electromyography and neuromuscular disorders: clinical-electrophysiologic correlations*, ed 3. New York: Elsevier.

Rubin, D. I. (2012). Needle electromyography: basic concepts and patterns of abnormalities. *Neurol Clin*, *30*(2), 429–456.

EMBRYOLOGY OF THE CONGENITAL MALFORMATIONS OF THE BRAIN AND SPINE

I. Dorsal induction

A. Primary neurulation: 3 to 4 weeks' age of gestation (AOG); notochord and chordal mesoderm induce neural plate, neural plate closes forming neural tube, and tube closes beginning at medulla and proceeds rostrally and caudally. Defects at this stage may cause *craniorachischisis; myeloschisis* (failure of closure of neural tube or vertebral arch); *anencephaly* (absent calvaria and brain, brainstem and cerebellum present); *encephalocele* (meninges and brain parenchyma protrude through skull defect); *myelomeningocele* (meninges and spinal cord protrude through defect in vertebral arch); *Chiari malformation*; and *hydromyelia* (focal dilation of central spinal cord canal).

B. Secondary neurulation: 4 to 5 weeks' AOG; notochord and mesodermal interactions form dura, pia, vertebrae, and skull. Defects at this stage may cause *myelocystocele; diastomyelia* (splitting of spinal cord by mesodermal band); *meningocele/lipomeningocele; lipoma; dermal sinus with or without cyst; tethered cord/tight filum terminale; anterior dysraphic lesions* (neurenteric cyst); and *caudal regression syndrome*.

II. Ventral induction: 5 to 10 weeks' AOG; prechordal mesoderm induces face and forebrain; cleavage of prosencephalon; formation of optic vesicles and olfactory bulbs/tracts; telencephalon gives rise to cerebral hemispheres, ventricles, caudate, and putamen; diencephalon gives rise to thalami, hypothalamus, and globus pallidus; rhombencephalon gives rise to cerebellar hemispheres and vermis; myelencephalon gives rise to medulla and pons. Defects at this stage may cause *holoprosencephaly* (failure of cleavage of embryonic forebrain into paired cerebral hemisphere with absence of the interhemispheric fissure); *septo-optic dysplasia* (rudimentary septum pellucidum, hypoplasia of optic nerve and chiasm); *arhinencephaly; olfactory bulb and tract aplasia; facial anomalies; cerebellar hypoplasias/dysplasias (Joubert syndrome, rhombencephalosynapsis, tectocerebellar dysplasia);* and *Dandy-Walker malformation* (enlarged posterior fossa, hyogenesis or agenesis of the cerebellar vermis, and cystic dilatation of the fourth ventricle).

III. Neuronal proliferation, differentiation, and histogenesis: 2 to 4 months' AOG; germinal matrix forms at 7 weeks; cellular proliferation forms neuroblasts, fibroblasts, astrocytes, and endothelial cells; choroid plexus is formed; *cerebrospinal fluid (CSF)* production begins. Defects at this stage may cause *microcephaly; megalencephaly; aqueductal stenosis; arachnoid cysts;* and *congenital vascular malformations.*

IV. Cellular migration: 2 to 5 months' AOG; neuroblasts migrate from germinal matrix along radial glial fibers; cortical layers form from deep to superficial; gyri and sulci form; commissural plates form corpus callosum and hippocampal commissure. Defects at this stage may cause *schizencephaly* (lateral clefts through cerebral hemispheres extending from cortex to ventricles); *lissencephaly* (absence of gyri); *pachygyria* (abnormally wide and thick gyri); *micro/polymicrogyria* (small gyri with increased number and abnormal lamination); *heterotropias* (ectopic collections of gray matter); *Lhermitte-Duclos syndrome* (diffuse enlargement of the cerebellar cortex); and *agenesis of the corpus callosum.*

V. Neuronal organization: 6 months postnatal; neuronal alignment, orientation, and layering; dendrites proliferate; synapses form.

VI. Normal myelination begins during the fifth fetal month. It proceeds in a highly predictable and orderly manner: caudal to cephalad, dorsal to ventral, and central to peripheral. Sensory tracts myelinate first.

A. Birth (full term): medulla, dorsal midbrain, inferior and superior cerebellar peduncles, posterior limb of internal capsule, and ventrolateral thalamus.

B. One month: deep cerebellar white matter, corticospinal tracts, pre/postcentral gyrus, optic nerves, and tracts.

C. Three months: brachium pontis, cerebellar folia, ventral brainstem, optic radiations, anterior limb of internal capsule, occipital subcortical U fibers, and corpus callosum splenium.

D. Six months: corpus callosum genu, paracentral subcortical U fibers, and centrum semiovale (partial).

E. Eight months: centrum semiovale (complete except some frontotemporal areas) and subcortical U fibers (complete except for most rostral frontal areas).

F. Eighteen months: essentially like adults.

G. Twenty years: peritrigonal region. Defects at this stage may be due to metabolic, demyelinating, and dysmyelinating disorders.

VII. Acquired degenerative, toxic, or inflammatory lesions may occur at any stage, causing injury to otherwise normally formed structures. These may result in defects such as *hydranencephaly* (remnant cerebral hemisphere is a paper-thin membrane sac composed of glial tissue filled with CSF covered with leptomeninges); *hemiatrophy; multicystic encephalomalacia;* or *periventricular leukomalacia*.

REFERENCES

Daroff, R. B., Jankovic, J., Mazziotta, J. C., & Pomeroy, S. L. (Eds.), (2016). *Bradley's neurology in clinical practice*, ed 7. Philadelphia: Elsevier.

Lerman-Sagie, T., & Leibovitz, Z. (2016). Malformations of cortical development: from postnatal to fetal imaging. *Can J Neurol Sci, 43*(5), 611–618.

ENCEPHALITIS

Encephalitis is an inflammation of the brain related to infectious, postinfectious, or demyelinating states. It can occur as an *acute febrile illness* associated with headache, seizures, lethargy, confusion, coma, ocular motor palsies, ataxia, abnormal movements, and myoclonus. Alternatively, it may present as a *slowly progressive afebrile disease*. With viral infections, the meninges (meningoencephalitis) or the spinal cord (encephalomyelitis) are often involved. Compared with the high frequency of systemic viral infection, encephalitis is an uncommon complication. Prognosis of viral encephalitis depends on the causative agent and the use of antiviral agents. Variable degrees of residual effects include impaired cognition and memory, behavioral changes, hemiparesis, or seizures. Transmission of viruses can be from humans (e.g., HIV), animals (e.g., rabies), mosquitoes (e.g., St. Louis and Japanese encephalitis), ticks (e.g., Central European encephalitis), or other arthropods. Endemic causes in the United States are herpes simplex, West Nile virus (WNV), and rabies. Japanese B encephalitis is the most common epidemic infection outside North America. Arthropod-borne viruses (arboviruses) can be sporadic or epidemic. Viruses enter the CNS by one of two routes—hematogenous (most common) or neuronal. Risk factors are summarized in Table 54.

Diagnosis can be made from patient history alone (Table 55 discusses the diagnostic work-up). The season may help determine the pathogen. CSF usually shows a pleocytosis (mostly mononuclear cells) and mildly elevated protein. Glucose tends to be normal. RBCs can be found in certain types of encephalitis (e.g., herpes simplex). Acute and convalescent antibody levels from serum and CSF are typically only useful retrospectively. Polymerase chain reaction (PCR) testing facilitates the identification of causative agents.

VIRAL ENCEPHALITIS

I. *Herpes simplex encephalitis* (HSV type 1) is the most common cause of fatal viral encephalitis in the Western world. Most cases represent reactivation of latent trigeminal ganglion infection. HSV-2 causes most

TABLE 54

RISK FACTORS FOR ENCEPHALITIS

Risk Factor	Suspected Pathogen
Mosquito bites	Alphavirus Western equine, Eastern equine, Venezuelan equine
	Flavivirus: St. Louis, West Nile
	Bunyavirus: La Crosse, California
Tick bite (Apr to Jun and Oct to Nov)	Colorado tick fever, Powassan virus, Anaplasma (aka *Ehrlichia*), Rocky Mountain spotted fever, tick-borne encephalitis, Lyme disease (borreliosis, spirochete)
Raccoon feces	*Baylisascaris procyonis*
Wild/domestic animals	Leptospirosis
Bats	Rabies
Pigs	Nipah virus
Cats	*Bartonella* henselae
Rodents	Lymphochoriomeningitis virus
Sheep/goats	Q fever
Travel	
Asia	Japanese encephalitis, Nipah virus
Europe	Tick-borne encephalitis
Africa	Lassa fever
Illness-exposures	Chickenpox
	Measles
	Influenza
	Mycoplasma pneumonia
Freshwater	*Naegleria fowleri*, leptospirosis
Soil	*Balamuthia mandrillaris*
Vaccination	Measles-mumps-rubella, vaccinia
Season	Mosquito-borne, tick-borne
Spring/summer	
Drug use, other HIV risk factor	AIDS encephalitis
Other systemic illness	Evaluate as needed for neoplastic and rheumatologic disease

Modified from Lewis, P., & Glaser, C. A. (2005). Encephalitis. *Pediatr Rev, 26*, 353–363.

E

ENCEPHALITIS

cases of encephalitis in newborns. The risk of intrapartum transmission is 30% to 50% in primary maternal infection and less than 3% with recurrent infection.

Clinical presentation consists of subacute onset with fever, headache, behavioral changes, seizures, focal signs, and later stupor and coma.

Diagnosis and evaluation: EEG usually shows periodic lateralizing epileptiform discharges (PLEDs) between the 2nd and 15th days of the illness. Spikes and slow waves are common and are often localized to the temporal lobe. A CT scan, although less sensitive than EEG, may show temporal or insular low densities and focal hemorrhages or enhancement. MRI is the neuroimaging procedure of choice and may show increased signal intensity on T_2-weighted image in the medial and inferior temporal lobe extending to the insula. CSF usually shows 5 to 500 cells; elevated

TABLE 55
SUGGESTED LABORATORY TESTING FOR ENCEPHALITIS AND ITS MIMICS

CEREBROSPINAL FLUID

Glucose, protein, cell count, differential count
Routine bacterial culture
Viral culture
Herpes simplex virus polymerase chain reaction (PCR)
Cryptococcal antigen
Enteroviral PCR
Mycoplasma PCR
Tuberculosis culture and PCR
Epstein-Barr virus (EBV) PCR
West Nile virus IgM

BLOOD

Bartonella henselae IgG
Epstein-Barr virus serology panel
Lyme IgG (in endemic areas if cranial neuropathy present)
Mycoplasma IgM
West Nile virus IgM (during mosquito season)
La Crosse virus IgM (in endemic areas, during mosquito season)
Complete blood count, differential count
Serum to be saved for comparison with convalescent specimen

NEUROIMAGING

Head CT
MRI with seizure protocol

NEUROPHYSIOLOGY

EEG
Evoked potentials
EMG (suspected Lyme disease or demyelinating disease)

OTHER

Viral cultures of nasopharynx and stool
Purified protein derivative skin test
Brain biopsy rarely necessary as a last resort (usually low yield)

Modified from Lewis, P., & Glaser, C. A. (2005). Encephalitis. *Pediatr Rev, 26*, 353–363.

protein; normal or mildly decreased glucose; and elevated opening pressure. RBCs may be seen. Antibodies to HSV are detected in the CSF 8 to 12 days after onset of the disease and increase during the first 2 to 4 weeks. Viral cultures are not useful. PCR is greater than 95% sensitive and 100% specific. *False-negative PCR results* may occur if there are RBCs in the CSF to inhibit PCR or if CSF is collected in the first 24 to 48 hours of symptoms or after 10 days of onset. A brain biopsy should be considered in those patients who do not respond to therapy or in whom other diagnoses are possible.

   Treatment with acyclovir, 10 mg/kg q 8 hr for 2 to 3 weeks, significantly reduces the risks of morbidity and death, especially if started early. Acyclovir-resistant HSV infection has been identified in immunodeficient patients.

Prognosis: If untreated, the mortality rate is about 70%, with severe neurologic sequelae in most of the survivors.

II. *Rabies* carriers include skunks, foxes, dogs, bats, and raccoons. The virus is present in saliva and transmitted by bite. *Incubation* ranges from days to months. Not everyone bitten by rabid animals contracts the disease. However, once the infection is established, death almost invariably occurs (usually within 18 days). The prodrome usually consists of headache, malaise, agitation, mental changes, seizures, dysphagia (causing hydrophobia), dysarthria, facial numbness, and spasm. The medulla and pons are most frequently and extensively involved, and paralysis may be secondary to spinal cord involvement.

Treatment consists of mechanically scrubbing wound sites with soap and benzalkonium solution and administering a human rabies immunoglobulin or human diploid cell line rabies vaccine. Death is invariable once CNS manifestations occur.

III. *Epidemic encephalitis* is mostly arthropod transmitted. Peak incidence occurs in late summer and fall. In the United States, St. Louis encephalitis and La Crosse virus (California encephalitis) are the most common. St. Louis encephalitis is found in the Ohio-Mississippi River basin, with 10% to 20% fatality rate. The La Crosse virus is the most common cause of pediatric arboviral encephalitis. Venezuelan equine encephalitis is found in the southeastern United States and has a low mortality rate; most infections result in flu-like illnesses. Eastern equine encephalitis occurs along the Gulf of Mexico and Atlantic seaboard, usually affecting horses and birds, and is rare among humans. It has a 25% to 70% mortality rate, attacking the young and very old with fulminant course. Western equine encephalitis occurs in west, southwest, and central North America. *Treatment* is aimed at brain edema and seizures. *West Nile virus* is a flavivirus that uses birds as a reservoir and is transmitted by mosquitoes. It is endemic in the Middle East, Africa, and southwest Asia. *Clinically*, it is characterized by an abrupt onset of flu-like illness. A *maculopapular rash* occurs in half of the patients. Meningitis or encephalitis is most common in older individuals and happens in less than 15% of patients. *Diagnosis* is done by a PCR or CSF culture, or identification of an antibody in the serum and CSF. WNV was first identified in the United States in New York in 1999 and an increase in the death of birds, particularly crows, can be observed during an outbreak. There is no specific treatment, and death may occur in older individuals.

IV. *Nonepidemic viral encephalitis:* Enterovirus, echovirus, coxsackievirus, poliovirus, measles, mumps, Epstein-Barr virus (EBV), rubella, varicella-zoster virus (VZV), and lymphocytic choriomeningitis virus can all cause sporadic encephalitis.

A. Slow, latent, viral infections cause slowly progressive disease with insidious onset and lack of fever. These include subacute sclerosing panencephalitis (SSPE), a form of chronic measles virus infection, progressive multifocal leukoencephalopathy (see PML below), and progressive rubella panencephalitis. SSPE has had dramatically

E

ENCEPHALITIS

decreased prevalence in countries with widespread use of the measles vaccine, but prevalence has increased with the occurrence of AIDS.

Usually occurring in children or young adults, onset is insidious with changes in cognition, vision, and behavior. Malaise and lethargy are common. Myoclonus can occur. Deterioration progresses over weeks to months with patients becoming markedly demented. CSF shows mild pleocytosis, increased protein, and occasionally decreased glucose. Neuroimaging shows generalized cortical atrophy. The EEG pattern of periodic discharges is characteristic. Pathologic studies show changes suggestive of viral invasion of gray and white matter without involvement of the hypothalamus and brainstem.

B. AIDS and immune deficiency-related encephalitis: *PML*, caused by a *polyomavirus designated JC virus* (not associated with Creutzfeldt-Jakob disease), usually occurs in patients with lymphoproliferative (leukemia, lymphoma) or granulomatous disease, or during immunosuppression. It is characterized by multifocal white matter signs, such as impaired speech, vision, and cognition, progressing to death in 1 to 18 months. PCR for JC virus in CSF has a sensitivity of 72% to 92% and specificity of 92% to 96%. MRI shows multifocal white matter lesions. Encephalitis in immunosuppressed patients may also be caused by VZV, HSV-1, EBV, human herpesvirus (HHV 6), cytomegalovirus (CMV), measles virus, or enterovirus. In VZV encephalitis, patients may have a history of shingles for days or months previously. Encephalitis CMV is rare in immunocompetent individuals, and a combination of ganciclovir and *foscarnet* has been used in treatment.

NONVIRAL ENCEPHALITIS OR ENCEPHALOMYELITIS

I. *Prion infections:* Prion (proteinaceous infectious particle) diseases are sometimes confused with encephalitides, but they are slowly progressive with insidious onset and absence of fever. They include Creutzfeldt-Jakob disease, Gerstmann-Sträussler-Scheinker syndrome, and kuru (see Creutzfeldt-Jakob disease).

II. *Rickettsia:* Epidemic, murine and scrub typhus, Rocky Mountain spotted fever, and Q fever infections.

III. *Bacteria:* Listeria infection, brucellosis, pertussis, Legionnaires disease, tuberculosis, tularemia, typhoid fever, bubonic plague, dysentery, cholera, melioidosis, psittacosis, leprosy, scarlet fever, and rheumatic fever.

IV. *Spirochetes:* Relapsing fever, syphilis (meningovascular), rat-bite fever, leptospirosis, and Lyme disease.

V. *Protozoa/metazoa:* Entamoeba, Naegleria fowleri (amoebic and treated with miltefosine), trypanosomiases, leishmaniasis, malaria, and toxoplasmosis.

VI. *Helminthic:* Ancylostomiasis, angiostrongyliasis, ascariasis, cysticercosis, echinococcosis, filariasis, schistosomiasis, and toxocariasis, trichinosis.

VII. *Miscellaneous:* Behçet disease, CNS Whipple disease, vasculitis, and Rasmussen syndrome (chronic focal encephalitis).

POSTINFECTIOUS ENCEPHALOMYELITIS

Postinfectious encephalomyelitis may follow a CNS or systemic viral infection, nonviral infection, or immunization. In the United States, varicella and upper respiratory infections (especially influenza) are most commonly associated, whereas worldwide it most commonly follows measles. A disturbance of the immune system is the presumed cause with an irreversible monophasic, demyelinating syndrome. Limited CNS forms may include acute, transverse myelitis, acute cerebellitis, and postinfectious optic neuritis. Acute hemorrhagic encephalitis *(Hurst disease)* is a severe and usually fatal form. The clinical symptoms and CSF profile are similar to that seen during direct viral infections. Treatment is with high doses of intravenous methylprednisolone. Acyclovir and ganciclovir are used if encephalitis by VZV and HHV-6 are in the differential diagnosis.

REFERENCES

Doughty, C. T., Yaetz, S., & Lyons, J. (2017). Emerging causes of arbovirus encephalitis in North America: Powassan, Chikungunya, and Zika viruses. *Curr Neurol Neurosci Rep*, *17*(2), 12.

Halperin, J. J. (2017). Diagnosis and management of acute encephalitis. *Handb Clin Neurol*, *140*, 337–347.

Mailles, A., Stahl, J. P., & Bloch, K. C. (2017). Update and new insights in encephalitis. *Clin Microbiol Infect*, *23*(9), 607–613.

ENCEPHALOPATHY

Encephalopathy is a nonspecific term for diffuse brain dysfunction, usually the result of a systemic condition. Initially, there is impaired attention, confusion, and disorientation. Later, there may be progression to stupor and coma, or it may present as coma of unknown cause. Associated features may include agitation, hallucination, myoclonus, asterixis, generalized seizures, or electroencephalogram (EEG) slowing or triphasic waves. Initial evaluation includes establishing time course and baseline function. Basic approach starts with history, vital signs, physical examination, and glucose. Additional evaluation should include review of recent medications, toxin exposure, metabolic screening, consideration of systemic or central nervous system infection, electrocardiogram, EEG, and neuroimaging.

REFERENCE

Douglas, V. C., & Josephson, S. A. (2011). Altered mental status. *Continuum (Minneap Minn)*, *17*(5), 967–983.

ENCEPHALOPATHY, PERINATAL HYPOXIC-ISCHEMIC

Hypoxic-ischemic encephalopathy (HIE) is caused by either diminished oxygen delivery or diminished brain perfusion. Timing of insult may be antepartum (20%; maternal cardiac arrest or hemorrhage), intrapartum (35%; abruptio placentae, uterine rupture, or traumatic delivery), both (35%; maternal diabetes mellitus or infection, intrauterine growth retardation), or postnatal (10%; cardiovascular compromise, persistent fetal circulation, recurrent apnea; more common in premature infants).

CLINICAL FEATURES

The signs of HIE correlate with the severity of the insults. Mild encephalopathy lasts less than 24 hours. It is characterized by hyperalertness or by mild depression of the level of consciousness, which may be accompanied by uninhibited Moro and deep tendon reflexes, signs of sympathetic overdrive, or only slightly abnormal electroencephalogram (EEG). Infants with moderate to severe encephalopathy show variation in level of alertness in the first 12 to 24 hours. Seizures occur in 70% of these infants during this period. Coma may supervene and progress to brain death by 72 hours. If the infant survives, marked hypotonia and bulbar and autonomic dysfunction persist. Term infants may demonstrate quadriparesis with predominant proximal and arm weakness. This pattern represents involvement of border zones of circulation between the cerebral arteries (anterior cerebral artery-middle cerebral artery and middle cerebral artery-posterior cerebral artery). Premature infants manifest spastic diplegia primarily due to injury of motor fibers to the leg that lie dorsal and lateral to the external angles of the lateral ventricles.

NEUROPATHOLOGY

Patterns of injury are influenced by the nature of the insult and the gestational age of the infant at the time of injury. Patterns that occur in term infants include selective neuronal necrosis (CA1 region of hippocampus, deep layers of cerebral cortex, and cerebellar Purkinje fibers), status marmoratus of basal ganglia and thalamus, parasagittal cerebral injury, and focal and multifocal ischemic brain injury. Periventricular leukomalacia represents the primary ischemic lesion of the premature infant.

DIAGNOSTIC TESTS

In preterm infants, head ultrasound (HUS) demonstrates periventricular echoes in the first day or two. After 1 to 3 weeks, lateral ventricles enlarge as these areas become cystic and gliosis supervenes. HUS in the term infant is especially accurate when used consecutively in the first weeks of life. Compared to HUS, magnetic resonance imaging (MRI) visualizes HIE injuries of basal ganglia better. Diffusion-weighted sequence on MRI detects focal cerebral ischemic injury very early in its course.

MANAGEMENT

Supportive care includes ensuring adequate oxygenation and perfusion, and seizure control.

PROGNOSIS

Predictors of poor neurologic outcome include (1) acidosis at birth, (2) persistent moderate or severe HIE, (3) neonatal seizures, (4) interictal background abnormalities such as burst-suppression, persistently low-voltage

EEG, or electrocerebral inactivity, (5) HUS findings of periventricular intraparenchymal echodensities, and (6) extensive brain edema with effacement of cerebral cortex on MRI.

REFERENCE

Rivkin, M. J. (1997). Hypoxic-ischemic brain injury in the term newborn. Neuropathology, clinical aspects, and neuroimaging. *Clin Perinatol*, 24(3), 607–625.

ENDOVASCULAR TREATMENT OF ANEURYSMS

Electrolytically detachable platinum coils (Guglielmi detachable coils [GDCs]) have been US Food and Drug Administration approved for the treatment of intracranial aneurysms since 1995. The coil is composed of a tight spiral of platinum wire that forms a circle with a predetermined diameter and length when deployed. The coils are available in a variety of sizes, lengths, and shapes. Bioactive coatings on the coils may promote endothelialization across the base of the coil mass, further excluding the aneurysm from the blood flow.

Embolization requires a number of discrete steps: (1) placement of a microcatheter within the aneurysm itself; (2) the coils are then passed through the catheter; (3) the coil fills the aneurysm lumen, excluding the aneurysm from the arterial blood flow; and (4) the coil is detached in place.

Aneurysm recurrence, either by true enlargement or by coil compaction, depends on the aneurysm size, neck width, and location. Complete embolization of small aneurysms with necks less than 4 mm wide approaches 80% to 90%, with only a neck remnant in most of the remaining aneurysms. In contrast, only 20% to 40% of giant aneurysms are completely embolized during the initial treatment. However, longitudinal assessment with repeat coiling may result in up to 80% of large or giant aneurysms embolized with good outcomes.

Temporary balloon or permanent stent placement across the aneurysm neck allows the treatment of wide-necked aneurysms by preventing coil herniation into the parent artery. These techniques also may allow tighter packing of the aneurysm, reducing their recurrence rate. Higher recurrence rates occur in aneurysms directly in line with the blood stream, such as basilar apex and middle cerebral artery (MCA) bifurcation aneurysms, due to a constant "water hammer" effect on the coil mass. Rerupture of aneurysms in patients presenting with subarachnoid hemorrhage following embolization is about 1% to 3%.

The risk of a major complication during embolization is 6% or less. Intraprocedural rupture occurs in 1% to 2% of embolizations and is treated by further coiling or parent artery sacrifice; 50% of these patients have no significant change in their status, but marked deterioration or death occurs in the other 50%. Intra-arterial thrombus/stroke and parent artery occlusion have an approximate 2% rate each. Intravascular thrombus can be treated with abciximab (GP IIb/IIIa inhibitor). Significant coil herniation may require balloon remodeling or intra-arterial stent placement to either reposition the coils within the aneurysm, or trap the coils against the vessel wall. Nevertheless, 6 to

12 weeks of antiplatelet therapy, such as Plavix and aspirin, should be given in this situation.

REFERENCES

Molyneux, A. J., et al., (2005). International subarachnoid aneurysm trial (ISAT) of neurosurgical clipping versus endovascular coiling in 2143 patients with ruptured intracranial aneurysms: a randomised comparison of effects on survival, dependency, seizures, rebleeding, subgroups, and aneurysm occlusion. *Lancet, 366*, 809–817.

Sluzewski, M., et al. (2003). Coiling of very large or giant cerebral aneurysms: long-term clinical and serial angiographic results. *AJNR, 24*, 257–262.

EPILEPSY AND WOMEN (See also CATAMENIAL EPILEPSY, EPILEPSY, AND AAN GUIDELINE SUMMARIES APPENDIX)

Epilepsy raises special concerns for women. Hormones alter expression of seizures and can alter a woman's response to antiepileptic drugs (AEDs). For example, pregnant women who have epilepsy have considerations in terms of drug metabolism and teratogenicity. Menopausal women with epilepsy have specific needs such as bone health and changes in weight. Women with epilepsy require tailored care throughout their reproductive cycle.

Women with epilepsy are at increased risk for the following:

I. Increased frequency of anovulatory menstrual cycles
II. Abnormal menstrual length
III. Greater prevalence of polycystic ovarian disease
IV. Sexual dysfunction
V. Higher incidence of miscarriages and pregnancy-related complications
VI. Seizures disrupting cortical regulation of the hypothalamic hormone release, changing the secretory pattern of the pituitary gland, and altering the peripheral release of hormones

CHECKLIST FOR WOMEN WITH EPILEPSY

I. Be alert to possibility of catamenial epilepsy.
II. Take menstrual history, and ask to keep menstrual diary.
III. Ensure adequate daily intake of calcium and vitamin D.
IV. Provide contraceptive counseling.
V. Advise prophylactic intake of folic acid at least 0.4 mg/day for women on AEDs of child-bearing age.

CONTRACEPTION

I. Women with epilepsy have a higher risk for failure of hormonal contraception due to the action of some AEDs. Failure rate in women with epilepsy may exceed 6% per year (vs. nonepilepsy failure rate of <3%) related to AED enzyme induction reducing efficacy of oral contraceptive pills (OCPs).

II. Recommendations for contraception and epilepsy:
   A. The 1998 recommendation by the American Academy of Neurology (AAN) advises estradiol dose of 50 μg for 21 days of each cycle.

B. If breakthrough bleeding occurs, patient should use a barrier method in addition to estradiol.

C. Barrier method is recommended, regardless of bleeding.

D. Norplant and transdermal patch have a higher failure rate.

E. Intramuscular (IM) medroxyprogesterone needs to be given at 8- to 10-week intervals.

PREGNANCY AND EPILEPSY

A. Prenatal care

   I. Adequate prenatal screening for patients on AEDs

   II. Neural tube defect (NTD) screening with serum α-fetoprotein at 15 to 22 weeks

   III. Structural ultrasound at 16 to 20 weeks

   IV. Amniocentesis or chorionic villus biopsy if indicated

   V. Ultrasound of fetal heart at 18 to 20 weeks

   VI. Folic acid at least 0.4 mg/day for all women of childbearing age

B. During pregnancy

   I. Measure free AED concentrations, and adjust AED dose to maintain stable free AED concentrations as pregnancy progresses (Table 56).

   II. If high doses of AED required, administer in divided doses to minimize high peak drug levels.

   III. Ensure vitamin K 10 mg/day in final 4 weeks of pregnancy to reduce the risk of neonatal hemorrhage.

C. Postpartum care

   I. Breastfeeding infants are monitored for signs of sedation and poor feeding.

   II. Vigilance is needed regarding changes in AED levels with volume shifts and sleep deprivation.

   III. Precautions to ensure mother and child safety (AEDs and breastfeeding):

TABLE 56

CHANGE IN PHARMACOKINETICS OF SELECTED ANTIEPILEPTIC DRUG DURING PREGNANCY

AED	Reported inc. clearance (%)[a]	Reported dec. in conc. (%)	Dec. free conc. (%)
Lamotrigine	65–230	—	—
Phenytoin	20–100	55–61	18–31
Carbamazepine	0–20	0–42	0–28
Phenobarbital	—	55	50
Primidone	—	55	—
Valproic acid	35–183	50	25–30[b]

AED, Antiepileptic drug.

[a]Clearance of almost all AEDs increases during pregnancy. Most AED levels normalize during the first 2 to 3 mo postpartum.

[b]Decreases only during first two trimesters; levels increase or normalize by delivery.

A. The concentrations of AEDs in breast milk are lower than those in maternal serum.

B. Infant's serum concentration, based on this factor and the AED elimination half-life in neonates, is longer than in adults.

C. Benefits of AEDs outweigh adverse effects.

D. Parents should look for lethargy and delayed milestones in children. Women with epilepsy have a higher rate of children with congenital anomalies.

MENOPAUSAL

I. Bone health

II. Measure calcium, vitamin D, PTH

III. Bone density scan at first visit and every 2 years thereafter

EPILEPSY (See also AAN GUIDELINE SUMMARIES, NEUROLOGIC EMERGENCY, AND THERAPEUTIC APPENDICES)

1 DEFINITIONS AND CLASSIFICATIONS

The epilepsies are a group of conditions marked by recurrent seizures, which are the clinical manifestations of abnormal synchronous brain electrical discharges. Based on the new 2017 ILAE classification system, epileptic seizures are classified by their onset semiology. Onset may be motor or nonmotor, and may be focal with or without awareness, generalized, or unknown (Fig. 25).

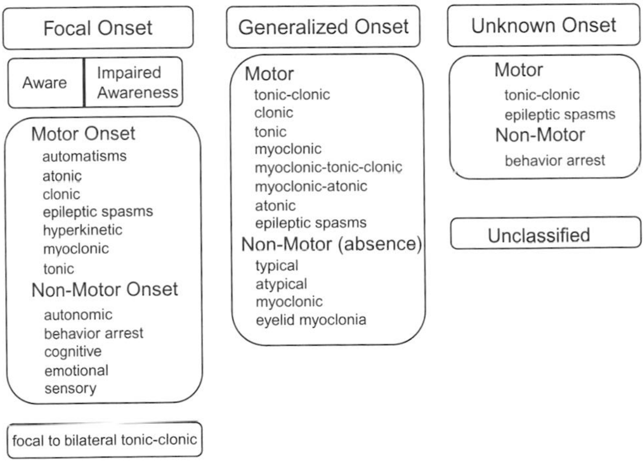

Focal Onset		Generalized Onset	Unknown Onset
Aware	Impaired Awareness	Motor tonic-clonic clonic	Motor tonic-clonic epileptic spasms
Motor Onset automatisms atonic clonic epileptic spasms hyperkinetic myoclonic tonic		tonic myoclonic myoclonic-tonic-clonic myoclonic-atonic atonic epileptic spasms	Non-Motor behavior arrest
Non-Motor Onset autonomic behavior arrest cognitive emotional sensory		Non-Motor (absence) typical atypical myoclonic eyelid myoclonia	Unclassified

focal to bilateral tonic-clonic

FIGURE 25

International classification of epileptic seizures.

DIFFERENTIAL DIAGNOSIS OF EPILEPSY

Conditions producing symptoms or signs that may be mistaken for epileptic seizures include the following: (1) syncope, (2) transient ischemic attacks, (3) migraine, (4) metabolic derangements (e.g., hypoglycemia), (5) parasomnias, (6) transient global amnesia, (7) paroxysmal movement disorders (e.g., paroxysmal dyskinesias), and (8) psychogenic nonepileptic seizures.

Psychogenic nonepileptic seizures are common and may coexist in patients with epileptic seizures. They are associated with a variety of psychiatric syndromes, including somatoform disorders, panic disorders, dissociative disorders, psychotic disorders, factitious disorders, and malingering. They may be difficult to distinguish from epileptic seizures, especially of mesial temporal, basal frontal, and supplementary motor area origin, since seizures originating from these areas may not be associated with surface EEG changes (see Electroencephalography).

SELECTED EPILEPSY SYNDROMES
Idiopathic Syndromes

I. Benign childhood epilepsy with centrotemporal spikes (BCECTS or benign rolandic epilepsy) is a common autosomal dominant syndrome producing nocturnal generalized convulsions in otherwise normal children. Focal motor or sensory seizures, often involving the face, may occur. The EEG shows characteristic interictal centrotemporal spikes. Treatment is not always required. If treated, seizures are usually easily controlled with a single antiepileptic drug. Seizures spontaneously disappear before adulthood.

II. Childhood absence epilepsy (pyknoepilepsy) occurs in genetically predisposed but otherwise normal children and is marked by typical absence seizures with a corresponding 3-Hz generalized spike-and-wave EEG discharge. Typical absences are not preceded by an aura nor followed by postictal confusion. Generalized tonic-clonic seizures may also occur. Treatment consists of ethosuximide, effective for absence seizures only, and valproic acid, effective for both isolated absence seizures and absence seizures complicated by or with generalized tonic-clonic seizures. Absence seizures rarely persist into adulthood.

III. Juvenile myoclonic epilepsy (of Janz) is a genetic epilepsy syndrome whose gene has been mapped to chromosome 6. It presents in normal teenagers with early morning myoclonic jerks and generalized tonic-clonic seizures. Sleep deprivation and photic stimulation are often activating influences. The interictal EEG typically shows 4- to 6-Hz generalized irregular spike-wave or polyspike-wave discharges with normal background. Valproate is highly effective, but relapses are the rule following drug discontinuation.

CRYPTOGENIC SYNDROMES

I. West syndrome consists of the triad of infantile spasms, developmental arrest, and the interictal EEG pattern hypsarrhythmia, consisting of very high voltage multifocal spikes, sharp waves, and slow waves in a chaotic distribution. The syndrome may be cryptogenic or symptomatic of a variety of brain insults and is generally treated with adrenocorticotropic hormone (ACTH) (either 150 units/m^2 for 14 days, followed by taper) or other corticosteroids or vigabatrine. Prognosis is unfavorable and is worse in the cryptogenic than in the symptomatic group.

II. Lennox-Gastaut syndrome is characterized by multiple, difficult to control seizure types, especially atonic seizures and atypical absences, in addition to generalized convulsions, mental retardation, and an abnormal interictal EEG with generalized 2- to 2.5-Hz slow spike-and-wave discharges. The syndrome often follows West syndrome in an affected child and is associated with a poor prognosis. Valproate is the drug of choice because of its efficacy against the multiple seizure types, and felbamate is also beneficial. Polytherapy may be necessary. Surgical section of the corpus callosum is sometimes effective in controlling drop attacks.

SYMPTOMATIC SYNDROMES

Temporal lobe epilepsy (TLE), the most common symptomatic, localization-related epilepsy, causes simple partial, complex partial, and secondarily generalized seizures as a result of ictal discharges typically arising from mesial temporal structures such as the hippocampus or amygdala. The interictal EEG often shows unilateral or bilateral, usually anterior temporal spikes. The most common associated lesion is hippocampal (mesial temporal) sclerosis; others include hamartomas, neoplasms (especially low-grade gliomas), cortical dysplasia, and vascular malformations. Magnetic resonance imaging (MRI) with thin coronal sections through temporal structures is the imaging modality of choice and may show unilateral hippocampal atrophy with enlargement of the ipsilateral temporal horn and increased hippocampal signal on T_2-weighted images, suggestive of hippocampal sclerosis. Phenytoin and carbamazepine are equally effective in treating symptomatic partial epilepsies such as TLE. Valproate is as effective in treating secondarily generalized seizures but not as effective for partial seizures. Surgical resection, typically anterior temporal lobectomy, eliminates seizures in about 70% of medically refractory patients in whom the epileptogenic lesion can be accurately localized. Vagal nerve stimulation is also effective in treating this syndrome.

Posttraumatic epilepsy typically begins 6 months to 2 years following head trauma. Risk factors include intracranial hemorrhage, depressed skull fracture, early seizures, or duration of posttraumatic amnesia greater than 24 hours. Phenytoin reduces the incidence of seizures within the first week following head trauma but is not effective as prophylaxis against the development of posttraumatic epilepsy.

OTHER SYNDROMES

I. Febrile seizures are typically generalized convulsions, occurring in children between 3 months and 5 years of age, associated with fever but without evidence of intracranial infection or defined cause. They are common, occurring in 2% to 5% of children, and tend to run in families. They usually occur during the early, rising temperature phase of an infectious illness. Most febrile seizures are simple, lasting less than 15 minutes and without focality; if the seizure is prolonged or focal, it is complex and associated with a higher risk of subsequent afebrile epilepsy. Other risk factors for seizure recurrence include more than one seizure in 24 hours, abnormal neurologic examination, and afebrile seizures in a parent or sibling. Overall, 6% to 13% of patients with two or more risk factors will develop afebrile epilepsy, compared with 0.9% without risk factors. There is no evidence that prophylactic treatment with anticonvulsants prevents future epilepsy. Phenobarbital, diazepam, and valproate (but not phenytoin or carbamazepine) reduce the rate of recurrent febrile seizures, but in most cases they are not recommended, because two-thirds of children will never have another febrile seizure and there is no evidence of mental or neurologic impairment due to febrile seizures. Rectal benzodiazepines may be useful for prevention of recurrent complicated febrile seizures.

II. Neonatal seizures are nearly always symptomatic, occurring as a result of a large number of brain insults; idiopathic syndromes are rare. The most common causes include hypoxic-ischemic encephalopathy, hypoglycemia, hypocalcemia, hyponatremia and hypernatremia, intraventricular or periventricular hemorrhage, CNS infections, cerebral malformations, inborn errors of metabolism, and drug withdrawal or intoxication. Neonatal seizures are classified clinically as subtle, tonic, clonic, and myoclonic; generalized tonic-clonic convulsions are rare in the neonatal period. Neonatal seizures commonly occur electrographically without clear clinical change and may occur clinically without a clear EEG ictal pattern. Jitteriness is a benign nonepileptic phenomenon consisting of rapid, stimulus-sensitive movements of all four extremities, abolished by passive restraint of the limbs. Treatment of neonatal seizures most commonly involves phenobarbital, phenytoin, and others (see Table 57). Hypocalcemia is treated with 5% calcium gluconate, 4 mL/kg IV, and

TABLE 57

FREQUENTLY USED MEDICATIONS FOR MANAGEMENT OF NEONATAL SEIZURES

Drug	Loading dose	Maintenance dose
Phenobarbital	20–40mg/kg in 20 minutes i.v	5mg/kg/day (target level: 40–60 mcg/ml)
Midazolam	0.05mg/kg in 10 minutes i.v	0.15 mg/kg/h (maximum dose: 0.5mg/kg/hr)
Lorazepam	0.05–0.1 mg/kg i.v	
Clonazepam	0.01 mg/kg	0.1–0.5 mg/kg per 24 h
Phenytoin/ phosphenytoin	20mg/kg in 30 minutes i.v	5 mg/kg/day (target level: 1–20 mcg/ml)

i.v, Intravenous.

From van Rooij LG, Hellström-Westas L, de Vries LS. Treatment of neonatal seizures. Seminars in Fetal and Neonatal Medicine; 2013: Elsevier; 2013. p. 209-15.

hypomagnesemia with 50% magnesium sulfate, 0.2 mL/kg IV. Pyridoxine 50 to 100 mg IV should be given if seizures continue and the cause is uncertain. Duration of treatment once seizures are controlled is controversial.

STATUS EPILEPTICUS

Generalized tonic-clonic status epilepticus (GTCSE; see Emergency appendix) is a medical emergency diagnosed either when two or more discrete seizures occur without complete recovery of consciousness or when a continuous seizure lasts at least 5 minutes. The likelihood of brain damage or death is directly related to the duration of GTCSE. GTCSE is more easily controlled when no new structural brain insult has occurred, as in withdrawal from anticonvulsants, drugs, or alcohol. More refractory cases may be seen in anoxic encephalopathy, stroke, hemorrhage, neoplasm, trauma, infection, or metabolic derangement. In general, the longer the duration of GTCSE, the more difficult it is to treat. A characteristic progression of EEG patterns in GTCSE has been described: (1) discrete seizures, (2) waxing and waning ictal discharges, (3) continuous ictal discharges, (4) continuous ictal discharges punctuated by flat periods, and (5) bilateral periodic epileptiform discharges on a flat background. In the latter stages, the patient may exhibit only subtle or no motor activity. Management of GTCSE must be carried out quickly. Treatment protocols are based on the pharmacologic properties of commonly used drugs (see Tables 58 to 63).

Absence status epilepticus (spike-wave stupor) constitutes continuous generalized spike-wave discharges with alteration of consciousness. It occurs more commonly in children with secondarily generalized epilepsy such as Lennox-Gastaut syndrome rather than with pyknoepilepsy. It may also occur sporadically in adults with no prior history of epilepsy. Treatment of the childhood condition consists of IV diazepam (0.1–0.3 mg/kg, over 2 minutes. Maximum dose 10 mg) followed by valproic acid. The adult form responds to the protocol listed for GTCSE. Because this condition is not life-threatening and residual brain damage is unproved, the use of general anesthesia is not generally recommended.

Simple partial status epilepticus (epilepsia partialis continua) most commonly involves continuous clonic focal motor seizures, but other

---

TABLE 58

COMPARISON OF MEDICATIONS COMMONLY USED TO TREAT
STATUS EPILEPTICUS

Time	Diazepam	Lorazepam	Phenytoin	Phenobarbital
To reach brain	10 sec	2–3 min	1 min	20 min
To peak brain concentration	<5 min	30 min	15–30 min	30 min
To stop status	1 min	<5 min	15–30 min	20 min
Effective half-life	15 min	6 hr	>22 hr	50–120 hr

TABLE 59

AN APPROACH TO THE TREATMENT OF GENERALIZED TONIC-CLONIC STATUS EPILEPTICUS

Action	Cumulative Time Frame
1. Stabilization and diagnosis: Secure an airway, administer oxygen, and be prepared to intubate quickly; assess vital signs, including rectal temperature, and treat hyperpyrexia appropriately; insert 2 large-bore IVs; obtain ECG, blood glucose, anticonvulsant levels, complete blood count (CBC), blood urea nitrogen (BUN), electrolytes, calcium, magnesium, phosphorus, serum and urine toxicology screens, and arterial blood gases; administer 100 mg thiamine IV and 50 mL of 50% glucose IV if necessary; obtain history and perform neurologic examination; consider possibility of nonconvulsive seizures.	0–15 min
2. Stop seizures: Lorazepam (the preferred agent due to its longer half-life) no faster than 2 mg/min, to maximum 0.1 mg/kg, no more than 8 mg. Through another IV, administer phenytoin 20 mg/kg no faster than 50 mg/min. Contraindications to phenytoin include documented allergy, significant heart block, or severe bradycardia. (If phenytoin is contraindicated, administer levetiracetam at 40–60mg/Kg or valproic acid at 20–25 mg/kg IV). ECG should be monitored continuously, and blood pressure taken frequently. If significant rhythm disturbances or hypotension occur during phenytoin infusion, reduce the rate to 25 mg/min. Fosphenytoin, a prodrug, can be used IM or IV, dosed at 20 mg/kg phenytoin equivalents, with a maximum rate of 150 mg/min. Benzodiazepines may cause respiratory depression.	15–60 min
3. If seizures persist: Following infusion of phenytoin, administer an additional 10 mg/kg phenytoin/fosphenytoin IV, no faster than 50 mg/min or try valproic acid at 20–25 mg/kg IV, at a maximum rate of 50–100 mg/min.	
4. If seizures persist: Intubate the patient, if not already done. Obtain emergency EEG monitoring; administer phenobarbital IV 2.0 mg/kg at a rate of 50–75 mg/min, until seizures stop. Carefully monitor blood pressure and ECG.	60–120 min
5. If seizures persist: Induce general anesthesia with short (thiopental) or intermediate (pentobarbital) half-life barbiturates. Pentobarbital is given IV as a 20 mg/kg loading dose (no faster than 50 mg/min), followed by initial maintenance dose of 1–3 mg/kg/hr. Midazolam (loading dose 0.2–0.3 mg/kg, with maintenance of 0.1–0.2 mg/kg/hr) or propofol (loading dose 1–2 mg/kg with a maintenance of 2–10 mg/kg/hr) anesthesia can also be employed in refractory cases. Adjust doses to achieve burst-suppression pattern on EEG with minimal blood pressure reduction. Pressor support may be required. Infusions should be utilized for at least 12 hr and used in conjunction with other antiepileptic agents.	120 min
6. Other maneuvers: Concurrently with above, treat metabolic or toxic conditions; ensure adequate hydration, keep blood glucose between 100 and 150 mg/dL and core body temperature <37.5°C. If there is clinical suspicion for new brain insult, obtain neuroimaging once GTCSE is aborted. Perform LP following neuroimaging and treat appropriately in cases suggestive of CNS infection.	

GTCSE, Generalized tonic-clonic status epilepticus.

TABLE 60

COMMON ANTIEPILEPTIC DRUGS: PRESCRIBING INFORMATION

Drug	Preparations	Average Target Plasma Concentrations (mg/L)[a]	Monotherapy Dose	Approximate Half-life	Protein Binding
Phenytoin (Dilantin)	30 mg, 100 mg caps, 50 mg tabs, 30 or 125 mg/5 mL elixirs	10–20 (6–14 in neonates to 12 weeks)	Neonates: 15–20 mg/kg, then 3–5 mg/kg/day in divided doses Infants: 15 mg/kg, then 3–5 mg/kg/day in 3–4 doses Children: 15 mg/kg, then 5–15 mg/kg/day in 2 doses Adults: 15 mg/kg, then 5 mg/kg/day, once daily	Variable	90%
Phenobarbital (Luminal)	15, 30, 60, 130 mg tabs 20 mg/5 mL elixir	15–40	Infants, children: 6–16 mg/kg, then 3–8 mg/kg/day Adults: 4–8 mg/kg, then 2–4 mg/kg/day, single dose	40–70 hr 50–120 hr	50%
Primidone (Mysoline)	50, 250 mg tabs 250 mg/5 mL elixir	5–12 (metabolized also to phenobarbital)	Children: 50 mg/day, increasing 50 mg q 3 days to 15–25 mg/kg in 2–4 doses Adults: 250 mg/day in 2 doses; start with 100 mg at bedtime and increase by 100 mg q 3 days to 10–20 mg/kg/day in 2–4 doses	10–12 hr	<5%
Carbamazepine (Tegretol)	100, 200 mg tabs 100 mg/5 mL suspension	4–12	Children: 100 mg bid, increasing 100 mg qod to 15–20 mg/kg/day in 3–4 doses Adults: 200 mg bid, increasing 100 mg qod to 7–15 mg/kg/day in 3–4 doses	5–27 hr	75%

Drug	Preparation	Level	Dosage	Half-life	Protein binding
Ethosuximide (Zarontin)	250 mg caps 250 mg/5 mL elixir	40–100	Children: 250 mg/day, increasing 250 mg q 4–7 days to 15–40 mg/kg/day in 3–4 doses Adults: 250 mg bid, increasing 250 mg q 4–7 days to 15–30 mg/kg/day in 3–4 doses	30 hr 50–60 hr	0%
Valproic acid (Depakene)	250 mg tabs 250 mg/5 mL elixir	50–100	Children: 10–15 mg/kg/day, increasing 5–10 mg/kg/day q 1 week to 15–100 mg/kg/day in 3–4 doses Adults: 10–15 mg/kg/day, increasing 5–10 mg/kg/day q 1 week to 15–45 mg/kg/day in 3–4 doses	4–14 hr 6–16 hr	75–90% (inverse to concentration)
Divalproex Sodium (Depakote)	125, 250, 500 mg tabs	50–100	Same as valproic acid except given in 2–3 doses	Same	75–90% (inverse to concentration)
Clonazepam (Klonopin)	0.5, 1, 2 mg tabs	Not usually monitored	Children: 0.01–0.03 mg/kg/day, increasing 0.25–0.5 mg q 3 days to 0.1–0.2 mg/kg/day in 3 doses Adults: 0.5 mg/day, increasing 0.5–1.0 mg/day q 3 days	18–50 hr 18–50 hr	85%
Felbamate (Felbatol)	400, 600 mg tabs 600 mg/5 mL elixir	Not usually monitored	Children (adjunctive): 15 mg/kg/day 3 or 4 times daily Adult: 1200 mg/day, increasing 600 mg q 2 weeks up to 3600 mg/day	14–20	25%

Continued

TABLE 60

COMMON ANTIEPILEPTIC DRUGS: PRESCRIBING INFORMATION—Cont'd

Drug	Preparations	Average Target Plasma Concentrations (mg/L)[a]	Monotherapy Dose	Approximate Half-life	Protein Binding
Lamotrigine (Lamictal)	25, 50, 100, 200 mg tabs	0.5–3.0 mg/mL	50 mg q hs increasing 50 mg q 2 weeks, as tolerated, divided into 2 doses	12–50 hr	55%
Levitoracetam (Keppra)	250, 500, 750 mg tabs	Not usually monitored	Children: 20–40 mg/kg Adults: 500 mg bid increasing up to 1500 mg bid	6–8 hr	<10%
Tiagabine (Gabitril) 95%	2, 4, 12, 16, 20 mg tabs	Not usually monitored	4 mg q days, increasing at weekly intervals by 4–8 mg up to 56 mg/day	4–9 hr (shorter if on hepatic)	inducing AEDs)
Topiramate (Topamax)	25, 100, 200 mg tabs 15, 25 mg sprinkle	Not usually monitored	Initial 25–50 mg/day increasing by 25–50 mg increments to 20 mg bid capsules as tolerated	20 hr	
Oxcarbazine (Trileptal)	150, 300, 600 mg tabs	4–12 (10-monohydroxy metabolite)	Children: 8–10 mg/kg/day increasing up to 20–40 mg/kg/day Adults: 150–300 mg bid up to 1200 mg bid	2 hr	40%
Zonisamide (Zonegran)	100 mg capsules	Not usually monitored	Children: 2–4 mg/kg/day Adults: 100–200 mg/day increasing up to 400–600 mg/day	60 hr	<10%
Gabapentin (Neurontin)	100, 300, 400 mg tabs 600, 800 mg tabs	Not usually monitored	300 mg/day, increasing up to 900–1800 mg/day over 2–3 days divided into 3–4 doses	5–7 hr	0%

[a]Many patients will respond at different plasma concentrations, below or above the average plasma concentrations.

TABLE 61

DOSE-RELATED ADVERSE EFFECTS OF ANTIEPILEPTIC DRUGS

Drug	Side Effects
Phenytoin	Acute: Drowsiness, ataxia, diplopia, GI complaints, choreoathetosis, nausea, hypotension (after parenteral use), heart block
	Chronic: Gingival hyperplasia, hirsutism, folate deficiency, megaloblastic anemia, osteomalacia with vitamin D deficiency, peripheral neuropathy, encephalopathy, cerebellar dysfunction, pseudolymphoma, hemorrhage in the newborn
Phenobarbital	Acute: Sedation, behavior disturbance, ataxia
	Chronic: Attentional difficulty, hemorrhage in the newborn rheumatic syndrome
Primidone	Acute: Sedation, nausea, vertigo, ataxia
	Chronic: Behavior disturbances (in children), loss of libido, attentional difficulties, hemorrhage in the newborn
Carbamazepine	Acute: Diplopia, vertigo, blurred vision, sedation, dry mouth stomatitis, hyponatremia (SIADH), headache, diarrhea, constipation, paresthesias
	Chronic: Liver enzyme induction, leukopenia, nervousness, hemorrhage in the newborn
Ethosuximide	Acute: Nausea, vertigo, vomiting, hiccups, headache
	Chronic: Insomnia, nervousness
Valproate	Acute: Sedation, GI disturbances
	Chronic: Weight gain, hepatic enzyme elevation, hyperammonemia, granulopenia, thrombocytopenia, alopecia, tremor
Clonazepam	Acute: Sedation, ataxia, irritability, hypersalivation
	Chronic: Behavior disturbances, tolerance, and withdrawal syndrome
Felbamate	Acute: GI disturbances, insomnia, headache, fatigue, nausea, vomiting
	Chronic: Weight loss
Lamotrigine	Rash, diplopia, sedation, dizziness, ataxia, headache, nausea, vomiting
Topiramate	Somnolence with confusion, psychomotor slowing, weight loss, speech disorders, ataxia, paresthesias, renal calculi
Oxcarbazine	Hyponatremia, headache, somnolence, nausea, vomiting, diplopia
Tiagabine	Somnolence, dizziness, attentional difficulties
Levetiracetam	Dizziness, somnolence, fatigue
Zonisamide	Renal calculi, kidney dysfunction, somnolence, fatigue, confusion, anorexia, ataxia, dizziness
Gabapentin	Sedation, fatigue, dizziness, nausea, weight gain, ataxia, headache and diplopia

TABLE 62

FACTORS AFFECTING SERUM CONCENTRATIONS OF ANTICONVULSANTS AND OTHER DRUG INTERACTIONS

Drug	Increased by AEDs	Increased by Other Drugs	Increased in Clinical State	Decreased by AEDs	Decreased by Other Drugs	Decreased by Clinical State	Interacts with Other Drugs
Phenytoin	Diazepam	Alcohol (acute)	Hepatic disease	Phenobarbital	Alcohol (chronic)	Acute hepatitis	Corticosteroids
	Ethosuximide	Amiodarone		Carbamazepine	Antineoplastics	Mononucleosis	Cyclosporine
	Felbamate	Amphetamines		Clonazepam	Loxepine	Pregnancy	Ketoconazole
	Oxcarbazine	Aspirin			Nicotine	Renal disease	Methadone
	Phenobarbital	Chloramphenicol			Nitrofurantoin		Oral contraceptives
	Primidone	Chlordiazepoxide			Sucralfate		Protease inhibitors
	Topiramate	Chlorpheniramine			Theophylline		Rifampin
	Valproic acid	Cimetidine			Tube feedings		Tacrolimus
		Diazepam					Trazodone
		Disulfiram					Warfarin
		Dicumarol					
		Estrogens					
		H² antagonists					
		Isoniazid					
		Methylphenidate					
		Omeprazole					
		Phenylbutazone					
		Phenothiazines					
		Propoxyphene					
		Sulfonamides					
		Tolbutamide					
		Trazodone					

Phenobarbital	Valproic acid, Phenytoin, Felbamate	Alcohol, Monoamine oxidase (MAO) inhibitors	Acidic urine, Hepatic disease, Renal disease	Clonazepam	Chloramphenicol, Dicumarol, Phenylbutazone	Alkaline urine	Chloramphenicol, Cimetidine, Folic acid, Haloperidol, Oral contraceptives, Phenylbutazone
Primidone	Valproic acid, Clonazepam	—	—	Carbamazepine, Phenytoin	—	—	Same list as Phenytoin
Carbamazepine	Felbamate (↑10, 11 Epoxide)	Cimetidine, Diltiazem, Erythromycin, Fluoxetine, Fluvoxamine, Grapefruit juice, Isoniazid, Propoxyphene, Sertraline, Verapamil	Hepatic disease	Ethosuximide, Felbamate, Phenobarbital, Phenytoin, Primidone, Valproic acid		Pregnancy	Corticosteroids, Doxycycline, Ketoconazole, Lithium, Oral contraceptives, Protease inhibitors, Quinidine, Rifampin, Tacrolimus, Thyroid hormone, Warfarin
Valproic acid	Felbamate	Salicylates	Hepatic disease	Carbamazepine, Phenytoin, Phenobarbital, Primidone, Valproic acid	Rifampin		Amitriptyline, Nortriptyline, Tolbutamide, Warfarin, Zidovudine

Continued

E

EPILEPSY

TABLE 62

FACTORS AFFECTING SERUM CONCENTRATIONS OF ANTICONVULSANTS AND OTHER DRUG INTERACTIONS—Cont'd

Drug	Increased by AEDs	Increased by Other Drugs	Increased in Clinical State	Decreased by AEDs	Decreased by Other Drugs	Decreased by Clinical State	Interacts with Other Drugs
Ethosuximide	—	—	—	Carbamazepine Phenytoin Phenobarbital Primidone	—	—	—
Clonazepam	—	—	—	Carbamazepine Phenobarbital	Antifungal agents Phenytoin	— (possibly)	—
Felbamate	—	—	—	Phenytoin Carbamazepine All hepatic inducing AEDs	—	—	—
Lamotrigine	Valproic acid	—	Hepatic disease Renal failure	Phenytoin Carbamazepine	—	—	Methotrexate
Topiramate	—	—	Renal disease	Phenytoin Carbamazepine	—	—	Carbonic anhydrase inhibitors
Tiagabine	—	—	Hepatic disease (possibly)	Carbamazepine	—	—	—
Zonisamide	—	—	Hepatic disease	Phenytoin Phenobarbital Carbamazepine	—	—	—
				Phenytoin Carbamazepine Lamotrigine	—	—	—

Levetiracetam	—	—	Renal failure	—	—	—
Oxcarbazine	—	—	Renal failure	Phenytoin Carbamazepine Lamotrigine Phenobarbital Valproic acid	—	Oral contraceptives See list for Carbamazepine
Gabapentin	—	—	Renal failure	Antacids	—	—

E

EPILEPSY

TABLE 63

IDIOSYNCRATIC ADVERSE EFFECTS OF ANTIEPILEPTIC DRUGS

Effect	Drug Type
Skin rash	All antiepileptic drugs
Erythema multiforme	All; more likely with ethosuximide
Stevens-Johnson syndrome	All
Exfoliative dermatitis	All
Systemic lupus erythematosus	Phenytoin, ethosuximide
Bone marrow depression	Most, including phenytoin, primidone, carbamazepine, ethosuximide, valproic acid, felbamate
Thrombocytopenia	Valproic acid; rare with phenytoin, phenobarbital, clonazepam
Lymphadenopathy	Phenytoin, ethosuximide
Hepatic toxicity	Valproic acid (usually in first 6 months of therapy), phenytoin, carbamazepine
Pancreatic toxicity	Valproic acid

Modified from Dreifuss, F. E. (1983). In A. A. Ward, J. K. Penry, D. Purpura (Eds.), (1983), *Epilepsy*, ed 1. New York: Raven.

manifestations such as aphasia, head and eye deviation, somatosensory changes, visual disturbances, and autonomic symptoms may occur. Ictal EEG may be normal. Focal motor status is often seen in the setting of metabolic derangements—particularly nonketotic hyperglycemia. Treatment in this case consists of correcting metabolic abnormalities. Slow loading with IV diazepam or lorazepam to avoid respiratory depression, followed by phenytoin, may also be used.

Complex partial status epilepticus may consist of repeated discrete complex partial seizures without full clearing of consciousness or as a more continuous clouding of consciousness, mimicking a confusional state. EEG is diagnostic. Treatment initially is identical to the protocol listed for GTCSE, although the use of general anesthesia (e.g., thiopental, midazolam, propofol) if initial maneuvers fail may be indicated.

Generalized convulsive status epilepticus in children is treated as in adults with the following modifications: use diazepam 0.25 mg/kg IV, no faster than 1 to 2 mg/min. If there is a delay in obtaining an IV line in a small child, this dose may be administered rectally via a feeding tube flushed with saline. Phenytoin 18 to 20 mg/kg is given IV over 20 minutes. If seizures persist, be prepared to intubate, and give phenobarbital 15 to 20 mg/kg IV no faster than 60 mg/min, with additional doses of 10 mg/kg as needed to control seizures. Recent studies have shown the benefit of valproic acid at 20 to 25 mg/kg IV in patients allergic to phenytoin or phenobarbital, or as an adjunct to these agents in convulsive status epilepticus.

Neonatal status epilepticus must be diagnosed using EEG monitoring because of the frequent dissociation between electrographic and clinical seizure activity. Treatment is as previously outlined for neonatal seizures. Diazepam 0.3 to 0.5 mg/kg IV or lorazepam 0.1 mg/kg IV may be given in refractory cases, but these drugs are contraindicated in jaundiced neonates.

ANTIEPILEPTIC DRUGS (See also AAN GUIDELINE SUMMARIES APPENDIX)

Selection of an antiepileptic drug (AED) is based on clinical and electrographic identification of seizure type. The dose is increased until seizures are controlled or clinical toxicity develops. If the drug is ineffective when taken in toxic doses, it is generally recommended to switch to another monotherapy with another agent before using drug combinations. Drug levels may be useful to answer specific questions regarding compliance, toxicity, or individual pharmacokinetics. Free levels of highly protein-bound drugs such as phenytoin, carbamazepine, and valproic acid may be helpful during hypoalbuminemic states, renal or hepatic disease, pregnancy, malignancy, sepsis, burns, or in the presence of other drugs that displace protein binding. The use of serial laboratory monitoring to prevent serious idiosyncratic reaction is of little value. It may be implemented in high-risk patients (children under age 2, especially those treated with polytherapy, patients with urea cycle defects, organic acidurias, mitochondrial disorders, GMI gangliosidosis, and neurodegenerative diseases) and in those with a history of adverse drug reactions. Abnormalities such as mild leukopenia or elevated hepatic enzymes are not predictive of severe complications. Current recommendations include the following: (1) obtain initial baseline blood work prior to initiation of therapy, including CBC with differential count, liver and kidney function tests, lipid profile, PT, PTT; (2) refrain from subsequent routine monitoring in asymptomatic patients; (3) counsel patients and family to notify you immediately should any of the following develop: bruising, bleeding, rash, abdominal pain, vomiting, jaundice, lethargy, coma, or marked increase in seizure frequency; (4) for multiply handicapped, institutionalized patients who may not be able to communicate the preceding information, annual routine blood monitoring may be of value.

REFERENCES

Fisher, R. S. (2017). The new classification of seizures by the International League Against Epilepsy. *Curr Neurol Neurosci Rep, 17*(6), 48.

Trescher, W. H., & Lesser, R. P. (2004). The epilepsies. In W. G. Bradley, R. B. Daroff, G. M. Fenichel, & J. Jankovic (Eds.), *Neurology in Clinical Practice,* ed 4 (pp. 1953–1992). Philadelphia: Butterworth Heinemann.

ERECTILE DYSFUNCTION; IMPOTENCE

PATHOPHYSIOLOGY

Penile erection is mediated by the cavernous nerves from S2 to S4 roots and is dependent on the integrity of both the paired deep arteries, which supply the corpora cavernosa, and the plexus of veins that drain it. Nitric oxide release from cavernous nerves and vascular endothelium promotes formation of cyclic guanosine monophosphate (cGMP), which stimulates smooth muscle relaxation, allowing increased arterial flow into the corpora cavernosa and resultant compression of outflow veins, facilitating rigidity. Sympathetic input from T11 to L2 constricts arterioles, reducing inflow and permitting venous drainage; this promotes detumescence and explains how sympathetic overactivity produces psychogenic impotence.

EPIDEMIOLOGY

Erectile dysfunction may affect up to 30 million men in the United States. The prevalence and severity increase with age, tripling in incidence from the 20s to the 50s. It is significantly more prevalent among neurologically disabled men, particularly those with lesions below S2 to S4, than men without neurological disability.

ETIOLOGY

1. Neurologic: multiple sclerosis (MS), spinal cord injury, pelvic nerve trauma (prostatectomy, pelvic injury, radiation).
2. Arterial: atherosclerosis, aortoiliac disease (Leriche syndrome), trauma.
3. Venous: diabetes, Peyronie disease, normal aging.
4. Endocrine: low testosterone (primary or secondary), high prolactin.
5. Pharmacologic: drugs affecting any of these systems can exacerbate the problem; neurological medications may also induce ED.
6. Vascular risk factors (diabetes, hypertension, hyperlipidemia, and smoking) increase the risk of ED.

DIAGNOSIS

Diagnosis is greatly eased if the patient reports achieving even very occasional firm, persistent erections (nocturnal, morning, with masturbation)—this removes concern for a vascular basis and suggests a psychogenic etiology. Sphincter or sensory dysfunction suggests a neurologic basis, difficulty maintaining erection suggests venous insufficiency, delay in achieving erection suggests arterial insufficiency, and painful erection suggests Peyronie disease or priapism. Examiners should look for evidence of feminization (hormonal basis) or peripheral vascular disease, abnormalities of the external genitalia, and adequacy of anal sphincter tone and the bulbocavernosus reflex.

EVALUATION

In addition to a history and physical examination, serum prolactin, testosterone, fasting glucose, and lipid panel should be evaluated. Additional work-up may include pudendal nerve sensory somatosensory-evoked potential (pSEP), penile-brachial index, penile ultrasonography, cavernosometry, and pelvic arteriogram.

TREATMENT

Medications such as sildenafil, tadalafil, and vardenafil have an overall efficacy of around 50%. These drugs inhibit the phosphodiesterase specific to the corpora cavernosa, thereby increasing cGMP. They are particularly effective in psychogenic cases and less severe organic dysfunction (including diabetes), and are also effective to a lesser extent in cases of severe organic dysfunction including spinal cord injury. They are absolutely contraindicated in patients taking nitrates, as the associated hypotension has been associated with myocardial infarction and stroke. Many case reports exist of onset of nonarteritic anterior ischemic optic neuropathy (NAION) within 36 hours of taking sildenafil. Other therapies include alprostadil penile injection (estimated efficacy for organic disorders is 80%), alprostadil intraurethral pellet (much less efficacious), and penile prosthesis (requiring surgery but effective and reliable). Testosterone supplements may help, particularly in cases of decreased libido. Yohimbine is a mixed α_1- and α_2-adrenergic receptor antagonist that works by a dual mechanism; it facilitates sexual arousal by acting on α_2-adrenergic receptors in the central nervous system (CNS) and blocks adrenergic influences at the peripheral level.

REFERENCES

Calabrò, R. S., et al. (2016). Erectile dysfunction in individuals with neurologic disability: a hospital-based cross-sectional study. *Innov Clin Neurosci*, *13*(1–2), 10–14.

Calabrò, R. S., et al. (2018). Sexual function in young individuals with multiple sclerosis: does disability matter? *J Neurosci Nurs*, *50*(3), 161–166.

EVOKED POTENTIALS

Evoked potentials (EPs) are a powerful, noninvasive and cost-effective tool for evaluating the integrity of the central nervous system. They function as adjuncts to the history and physical examination in certain settings. The advent of magnetic resonance imaging (MRI) has replaced EPs for anatomic accuracy, but they continue to be used to check the functional integrity of the nervous system, and may detect subclinical lesions, but are of little value in providing clues to the type of pathology.

The clinically useful EPs are derived from stimulation of one of the modalities of the sensory system—visual evoked potentials (VEP), brainstem auditory evoked potentials (BAEP), and somatosensory evoked potentials (SEP)—and are recorded from electrodes on the scalp. Because of the low voltage of EPs (100 times smaller than the scalp EEG), multiple stimulations with averaging and filtering are necessary to separate the signal from background noise. The actual signal recorded may be either "*near-field*" (the electrode is placed near the generator of the signal in the cortex; for example, the P100 wave of the VEP generated by the occipital cortex) or "*far-field*" (the electrode is placed far from the generator of the signal, which is volume conducted through the tissues of the body to the recording electrodes on the scalp; for example, the P11 wave of the SEP generated by the dorsal root entry zone). In general, the latency from stimulus to recorded potential is more important than signal amplitude.

EPs are usually designated by the letter "P" or "N" followed by a number. For example, "P100" is a wave of positive deflection occurring at a latency of 100 msec. By convention, "positive" is a downward and "negative" an upward needle deflection. It should be remembered that absolute latencies and standard deviations are quite laboratory specific (Fig. 26).

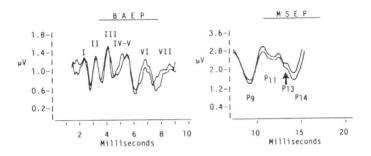

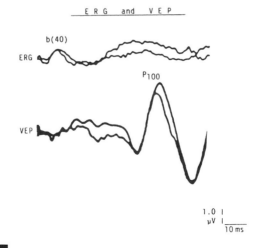

FIGURE 26

Normal evoked potentials (EPs).

Motor evoked potentials (MEP) are derived from stimulating the CNS motor system with magnetically induced or directly applied electrical current. Recordings are made from electrodes placed over muscles. MEPs have yet to gain significant clinical use and will not be discussed further.

VISUAL EVOKED POTENTIALS

VEPs are primarily used to detect anterochiasmatic lesions of the visual system; usefulness in retrochiasmatic lesions is minimal. VEPs are usually generated by checkerboard pattern-reversal stimuli that evoke large, reproducible potentials. Check sizes subtending greater than 40 degrees of arc preferentially stimulate retinal luminance channels. Those less than 30 degrees stimulate contrast and spatial frequency detectors, and those less than 15 degrees mainly stimulate the fovea. P100 is the most useful and reproducible wave. It is generated by the striate cortex as a near-field potential and recorded from electrodes placed over the occipital cortex. A significant prolongation of latency between eyes with alternate full-field monocular stimulation is evidence for anterochiasmatic disease on the side with prolonged latency. P100 may be bilaterally absent or prolonged with chiasmatic lesions. Refractive errors and macular disease can affect both the latency and amplitude of VEPs.

Electroretinograms (ERGs) are derived from stimulation of the retina with light while recording electrical activity directly from the cornea. When combined with VEPs, ERGs can be useful in prognosis for recovery of visual function and differentiation of retinal from optic nerve disease.

Flash ERGs are useful for detecting retinal lesions. Pattern ERGs (P-ERGs) utilize a checkerboard pattern-reversal stimulus. When a small enough check size is used (<2.4 degrees of arc), the major positive wave recorded from the cornea (b-wave) represents retinal ganglion cell function. The latency of "b" is about 40 msec and is prolonged or abolished by disease processes in or distal to the ganglia. When "b" is subtracted from the simultaneously recorded P100 of the VEP, retinocortical time (RCT) can be determined (RCT = P100 − b). RCT is an accurate reflection of optic nerve integrity proximal to the retinal ganglia and is independent of macular disease.

Three abnormal patterns of P-ERG/VEP have been identified:

I. Normal P-ERG, delayed VEP, and RCT: Demyelination of the optic nerve
II. Normal P-ERG, absent VEP: Acute total block of optic nerve fibers
III. Absent P-ERG, absent VEP: Severe macular disease or long-standing severe optic nerve disease with retrograde degeneration of retinal ganglion cells

There is also evidence that decreased amplitude of P-ERGs in recent optic neuritis has a poor prognosis for visual recovery, and progressive loss of P-ERG amplitude correlates with the development of optic nerve atrophy.

BRAINSTEM AUDITORY EVOKED POTENTIALS

BAEPs detect lesions of the auditory system and mid-upper brainstem. Click stimuli of 50 to 100 μs square-wave pulses to headphones or ear-inserted transducers are used to elicit seven recordable potentials at the scalp. Waves I through VII occur within 10 msec after stimulation and are generated by propagating action potentials within the eighth cranial nerve (CN VIII) and central auditory pathways. They are volume conducted to the scalp and recorded as far-field potentials. The specific generators of the waves are controversial, but most authorities follow the following schema: I—distal CN VIII; II—proximal CN VIII; III—bilateral superior olivary complex; IV—ascending auditory fibers in the rostral pons; V—inferior colliculus; VI—medial geniculate nucleus; VII—distal auditory radiations. Waves VI and VII are often unobtainable or inconsistent and are clinically useless. Waves II and IV may be buried in or fused to other waves and are not as important as waves I, III, and V. Absolute latencies are not as important as the I-III-V interpeak latencies (IPLs).

Commonly recognized abnormal BAEP patterns include the following:

I. Absence of all waves: Peripheral hearing loss, excessive background noise, technical error, brain death, and rarely in Friedreich ataxia, distal CN VIII lesions, or system atrophies.

II. Wave I only (or increased I–III IPL): Lesions of the proximal acoustic nerve or pontomedullary junction near the root entry zone such as peripheral demyelination or inflammation, cerebellopontine [CP] angle tumors, pontine glioma, multiple sclerosis (MS), leukodystrophies, neonatal anoxia, or brainstem infarct.

III. Waves I–III only (or increased III–V IPL): Lesions sparing the pontomedullary junction but affecting the pons to low midbrain. This pattern is most commonly seen with MS, lesions of pontine tegmentum, or large extra-axial masses compressing the brainstem—especially CP angle tumors opposite the stimulated ear.

IV. Increased I–III, III–V, and I–V IPL: Diffuse or multifocal disease such as demyelination, brainstem glioma, and especially hypothermia. BAEPs are usually extremely stable over wide ranges of metabolic derangement. Diffuse prolongation of IPLs should not be explained by metabolic abnormality.

SOMATOSENSORY EVOKED POTENTIALS

Somatosensory EPs (SEPs) are obtained from electrical stimulation of the median nerve at the wrist (MSEP) or the posterior tibial nerve at the ankle (PTSEP). Analysis of SEPs can give information about the integrity of the sensory component of peripheral nerves, spinal cord, brainstem, and to a lesser extent, the cortex. Recordings of far-field potentials are made over the scalp, and both near- and far-field potentials may be obtained at other points along the proximally propagating action potential.

I. MSEP: Four clinically useful "early" components of MSEPs and their presumed generators have been consistently and reproducibly identified: P9 from the distal brachial plexus; P11 from the dorsal root entry zone; P13 from the cervical cord dorsal columns; and P14 from the medial lemniscus of the brainstem. Other "late" components (such as N19, P23, N32, P40, and N60) have been identified and probably correspond to thalamic or suprathalamic generators. They are prolonged with decreasing levels of arousal and are not reproducible from person to person, or from the same person at different times or with changes of state. They also vary with different recording montages. Their usefulness is seen only when simultaneous bilateral stimulation produces asymmetries.

II. PTSEP: This is the most "laboratory specific" EP, with widely differing waveform designations and terminology. PV (propagated volley) is the designation given to the near-field potential recorded over the lower spine, which roughly corresponds to the cauda equina and lower gracile tract. N22 is probably generated by axon collaterals in the dorsal columns near the thoracolumbar junction. Later components from scalp recordings probably represent more rostral brainstem, thalamic, and cortical generators. Their usefulness is proportional to the technique and reliability of the given laboratory. As with MSEPs, PTSEPs can give localizing information pertaining to lesions along the course of propagation.

EVOKED POTENTIALS AND MULTIPLE SCLEROSIS

EPs are most useful in the evaluation of MS (1) to demonstrate sensory abnormalities when the history or physical examination is equivocal and (2) to detect subclinical lesions when demyelination is suspected in other areas of the nervous system. Less important uses are (3) to define the distribution of the disease process and (4) to monitor changes in a patient's status. When the diagnosis of MS is clinically definite, EPs will add little additional information.

Abnormal VEPs are present in about 95% of cases of optic neuritis, regardless of how remote or whether vision has returned. About 50% of MS patients have abnormal VEPs, even without clinical evidence of optic nerve involvement. About 35% of patients with progressive myelopathy have abnormal VEPs; only about 10% show abnormality after a single episode of transverse myelitis. Almost half of MS patients have abnormal BAEPs, regardless of clinical classification, and many patients without clinical findings of brainstem involvement show abnormalities. The most common abnormalities are decreased or absent wave V or increased III-V IPL. In a large study, 58% had abnormal MSEPs and 76% had abnormal PTSEPs.

The differential sensitivity of EPs in detecting white matter lesions in MS is related to the length of fiber tract being tested. As the degree of clinical certainty of the diagnosis increases from possible to probable to definite, the detection rate of lesions will be greater but the clinical usefulness may be questionable.

EVOKED POTENTIALS AND OTHER NEUROLOGIC DISEASES

Many attempts have been made to use EPs as prognostic indicators of disease and trauma. In general, results comparing the quality, size, or shape of the potentials are conflicting, and no better than following clinical examination.

E

EVOKED POTENTIALS

One study demonstrated that the complete absence of SEPs bilaterally greater than 3 days after brain injury is very highly predictive of poor outcome or death. However, there is currently no definite role for EPs in the evaluation of brain death or recovery from coma.

Intraoperatively, real-time SEPs (during spinal cord surgery or endovascular embolization) and BAEPs (during posterior fossa surgery or endovascular embolization) may provide an early indication of compromise of neural tissue. In cervical spondylosis, PTSEPs may eventually help predict which patients are more likely to develop a significant cord deficit so that early surgical intervention can be considered. Flash VEPs have been used by some centers to monitor changes in intracranial pressure, but this is controversial.

REFERENCES

Gilmore, R. (Ed.), (1988). *Neurologic clinics*. Philadelphia: WB Saunders.
Lascano, A. M., Lalive, P. H., Hardmeier, M., et al. (2017). Clinical evoked potentials in neurology: a review of techniques and indications. *J Neurol Neurosurg Psychiatry*, 88(8), 688–696.

EXTRACRANIAL ULTRASONOGRAPHY

The carotid and vertebral arteries and their branches can be evaluated with ultrasound; that is, sound with a frequency higher than 20,000 Hz. B-mode (brightness modulation) is based on the transmission of ultrasound through tissues and the reflection from tissue interfaces. Ultrasound produces a real-time two-dimensional picture of extracranial vessels in longitudinal or transverse views. It allows the measurement of vessel diameter and reveals the presence of stenosis or occlusion. High-resolution scans can determine plaque morphology, such as ulceration, calcification, or hemorrhage.

In Doppler ultrasonography, the ultrasound is reflected off moving targets (erythrocytes). Increased blood flow velocity in a stenotic arterial segment is associated with higher frequency shift, correlating with flow velocities.

Carotid duplex ultrasonography combines both techniques described above. It has excellent accuracy for the detection of stenotic processes compared with conventional angiography or magnetic resonance angiography. For arteries with more than 50% stenosis, sensitivity is approximately 94% to 100%; for occlusions, sensitivity is 80% to 96%, and specificity is 95%. However, these results vary considerably with ultrasonographic technique and machine capability. Examination of vertebral arteries allows the determination of flow direction (e.g., subclavian steal syndrome), but morphologic evaluation is not always possible.

REFERENCES

de Waard, D. D., et al. (2017). Asymptomatic carotid artery stenosis: who should be screened, who should be treated and how should we treat them? *J Cardiovasc Surg*, 58, 3–12. https://doi.org/10.23736/S0021-9509.16.09770-6.

Qu, B., & Qu, T. (2015). Causes of changes in carotid intima-media thickness: a literature review. *Cardiovasc Ultrasound*, *13*(46). https://doi.org/10.1186/s12947-015-0041-4.

EYE MUSCLES

Because of their insertional properties, the six extraocular muscles affect eye movements in the three planes relative to primary position (Table 64). In testing muscle strength, the optical axis is aligned with a muscle's main vector. The superior and inferior rectus muscles insert on the anterior globe at 23 degrees temporal to the primary position. Therefore these muscles function solely in the vertical plane only when the eye is abducted 23 degrees. The oblique muscles insert on the posterior globe at 51 degrees nasal to the primary position. Thus adduction maximizes the depressor effect of the superior oblique, whereas abduction maximizes intorsion (Fig. 27).

Diplopia testing in paralytic strabismus begins with measurement of visual acuity, confrontation visual fields, and observation of any abnormal head posture. Head tilt occurs in the direction of action of the weak muscle. Range of motion in each eye is tested in the nine cardinal positions of gaze with the opposite eye covered (ductions) and with both eyes viewing (versions). Misalignment can be seen in the corneal reflection of a penlight and can be tested in all directions of gaze (Hirschberg test).

Subjective diplopia testing relies on the principles that the disparate images are maximally separated in the main field of action of the paretic muscle and that the more peripheral image belongs to the paretic eye (Fig. 28). The Maddox rod tests primarily for phoria because it disrupts fusion; therefore, only the noncomitant deviations (unequal in different fields of gaze) should be considered abnormal. The paretic eye and the position of gaze producing the maximum separation of the images can be determined; the paretic muscle can be identified.

Objective tests include the cover-uncover test for tropia and the alternate cover test for phoria, which are performed in the primary position and in each cardinal position. Deviation of the nonparetic eye when covered (secondary

E

EYE MUSCLES

TABLE 64

ACTIONS OF EYE MUSCLES IN PRIMARY POSITION

Muscle	Primary Action	Secondary Action	Tertiary Action
Lateral rectus	Abduction		
Medial rectus	Adduction		
Superior rectus	Elevation	Intorsion	Adduction
Inferior rectus	Depression	Extorsion	Adduction
Superior oblique	Intorsion	Depression	Abduction
Inferior oblique	Extorsion	Elevation	Abduction

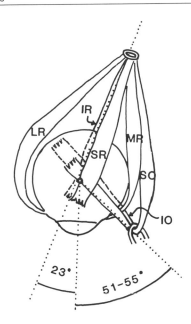

FIGURE 27

Insertion of ocular muscles of the globe. *IO*, inferior oblique; *IR*, inferior rectus; *LR*, lateral rectus; *MR*, medial rectus; *SO*, superior oblique; *SR*, superior rectus.

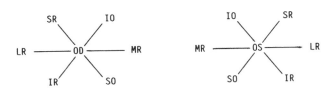

FIGURE 28

Main field of action of individual eye muscles.

deviation) is always greater than the deviation of the paretic eye when covered (primary deviation).

REFERENCE

Leigh, R. J., & Zee, D. S. (2015). *The neurology of eye movements,* ed 5. New York: Oxford University Press.

F

FACIAL NERVE, HEMIFACIAL SPASM

NEUROANATOMY

The course of the facial nerve (CN VII) is depicted in Fig. 29. The numbers in the figure refer to the following locations of the lesions:

1. Peripheral to chorda tympani in facial canal or outside stylomastoid foramen. Peripheral upper and lower facial weakness (motor aspects of CN VII) only. Usually related to trauma.
2. Facial canal (mastoid), involving chorda tympani. In addition to upper and lower facial weakness, patients have loss of taste over the anterior two-thirds of tongue and decreased salivation.
3. Facial canal, involving the stapedius nerve. Upper and lower facial weakness as in 1 and 2, plus hyperacusis.
4. Geniculate ganglion. Usually associated with pain in the ear. May have decreased lacrimation.
5. Internal auditory meatus. Complete CN VII (facial weakness; decreased taste, salivation, and lacrimation) plus CN VIII dysfunction (deafness or vestibular symptoms).
6. Extrapontine, subarachnoid. May have other cranial nerve involvement. Hemifacial spasm is more commonly associated with more proximal lesions of CN VII.
7. Pontine (nuclear or infranuclear). Millard-Gubler, Foville, and Brissaud syndromes (see Ischemia).
8. Supranuclear. Lesions may occur anywhere from mid-pons to motor cortex and are usually associated with other findings such as hemiparesis, hemisensory deficit, language disturbance, or homonymous hemianopia, depending on location. Taste, salivation, and lacrimation are not involved. Lower facial weakness is much more prominent than upper because of bilateral input to the portions of the facial nucleus controlling the upper face; input for the lower face is from contralateral cortex. Mild weakness may appear only as slight drooping of the angle of the mouth, slight widening of the palpebral fissure, or flattening of the nasolabial fold. (Table 65 compares clinical findings in the upper and lower motor neuron facial nerve weakness.)

DIFFERENTIAL DIAGNOSIS OF PERIPHERAL FACIAL PARALYSIS

Idiopathic Facial Paralysis (*Bell palsy*): the most common form (60% of cases) and is often a result of HSV-1 infection. Typified by a sudden, unilateral onset often preceded by a viral prodrome, the paralysis often regresses spontaneously in 8 to 10 weeks, with complete recovery in 85% to 90% of patients. Acyclovir and prednisone are often prescribed to treat the condition, but their use is controversial. Exposure keratitis may be ameliorated by

FACIAL NERVE, HEMIFACIAL SPASM

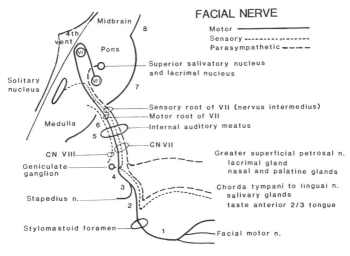

Facial nerve.

TABLE 65

CLINICAL FEATURES OF UPPER MOTOR NEURON AND LOWER MOTOR NEURON FACIAL WEAKNESS

Upper Motor Neuron Lesions	Lower Motor Neuron Lesions
Unilateral paresis of voluntary muscles of lower face with sparing of frontalis muscle	Unilateral paresis of all mimetic movements including the frontalis muscle
Facial muscle weakness less apparent with emotional than with voluntary movements	Degree of facial weakness similar with emotional and voluntary action
Preservation or accentuation of facial reflexes	Suppression of facial reflexes
Preserved taste, anterior two-thirds of tongue	Possible impairment of taste
Normal lacrimation	Possible abnormality of lacrimation

lubricating ointment but rarely requires tarsorrhaphy. *Melkersson syndrome* represents episodes of recurrent facial palsy with a deeply furrowed tongue (lingua plicata) and recurrent facial edema. Overall prognosis for this condition is good, but permanent paralysis may result after many recurrences. Aberrant regeneration of the facial nerve with resolution of the paralysis has several variations. The most common of these is involuntary tearing of the eye on the involved side when eating ("crocodile tears") or synkinesis of the facial musculature when chewing. This often takes the form of a jaw-winking phenomenon, wherein the lid closes on the involved side when the jaw opens (Marin-Amat syndrome).

Posttraumatic Facial Paralysis: Trauma is the second most common cause of peripheral facial paralysis in adults. Most often injury occurs in the intrapetrous portion. Nevertheless, traumatic lesions along the brainstem, the cerebellopontine angle (CPA), or in the parotid gland also occur.

Infectious Disorders

I. Ramsay Hunt syndrome is the third most frequent cause of peripheral facial paralysis. It is caused by herpes zoster oticus, and the symptoms are more severe than in idiopathic facial paralysis, often including dizziness, perception deafness (due to involvement of the vestibulocochlear nerve), and intense otalgia. A vesicular eruption in the external auditory canal, pinna, tragus, or soft palate confirms the diagnosis.

II. Inflammatory lesions of the middle ear include otitis media. Acute otitis media can cause a peripheral facial paralysis that resolves after antibiotic treatment or myringotomy. In chronic otitis media, facial paralysis indicates compression of the nerve by a cholesteatoma or osteitis and necessitates surgery.

III. Necrotic otitis externa (malignant otitis externa) is due to *Pseudomonas aeruginosa* infection, mostly in diabetics. The nerve is invaded through the stylomastoid foramen.

IV. Other infectious causes: Lyme disease is complicated by facial paralysis in 10% of cases; paralysis is bilateral in 25% of cases and may be the initial symptom of the disease. CN VII involvement in AIDS is nonspecific.

Tumors

Tumors may cause sudden or relapsing facial paralysis, but progressive facial paralysis with a slow onset of more than 3 weeks strongly indicates the presence of a tumor.

I. Brainstem primary or secondary tumors produce impairment in multiple cranial nerve pairs.

II. CPA and the internal acoustic meatus (IAM) can be sites of tumors. Most frequently, lesions are neurinomas of CN VIII and meningiomas (consider neurofibromatosis-2). Epidermoid tumors have cerebrospinal fluid (CSF) signal on T_1 and T_2 sequences of MRI (Table 66). Arachnoid cysts are isointense to the CSF, have sharp contours, and remain confined to the subtentorial space. Fluid-attenuated inversion recovery (FLAIR) can help detect epidermoid tumors; diffusion sequences show reduced diffusion within an epidermoid cyst compared with an arachnoid cyst.

III. Internal auditory meatus and the region of the ganglion geniculi may be sites for hemangiomas, which are small lesions associated with

TABLE 66

TOPOGRAPHIC DIAGNOSIS OF LESIONS TO THE FACIAL NERVE: CHOICE OF IMAGING PROCEDURE

Segment	Clinical Aspect/Test	Imaging Modality	Lesions
Nuclear: Pons	CN VII + CN VIII	MRI	Infarction, hematoma, multiple sclerosis, tumor, arteriovenous malformation, cavernous angioma, abscess
Cerebell-opontine angle + internal acoustic meatus	CN VII + CN VIII; audiometry: perception deafness, vestibular examination	MRI	Neurinoma of CN VIII, meningioma, epidermoid cyst, vascular compression, neurinoma of CN VII, hemangioma, glomus tumor, inflammation, fracture
Ganglion geniculi	Schirmer test	CT or MRI	Neurinoma and hemangioma of CN VII, primary or secondary cholesteatoma, cholesterol granuloma, metastasis, infection, fracture
Tympanic membrane or mastoid	Audiometry: transmission deafness, otoscopic examination, stapes reflex, gustometry	CT	Acute otitis, mastoiditis, cholesteatoma, fracture, neurinoma of CN VII, necrotic otitis externa, metastasis, glomus tumor
Parotid and endings	Often partial involvement	MRI	Often malignant parotid tumor, infection, sarcoidosis, trauma (forceps, penetrating lesion, surgery)

CT, computed tomography; *MRI*, magnetic resonance imaging.

notable clinical manifestations: perception deafness, rigidity, or facial paresis.

IV. Tympanic cavity and mastoid: Otoscopic examination can suggest tumor in the tympanic cavity and the mastoid by showing a whitish (primary cholesteatoma), grayish, or bluish (glomus) retrotympanic mass. Primary or secondary bone tumors can be seen in the petrosal bone. Metastatic tumors are the most common type.

V. Parotid gland: Every parotid mass associated with facial paralysis should suggest a malignancy.

BILATERAL PERIPHERAL FACIAL PARALYSIS

I. Sarcoidosis: facial diplegia and uveitis

II. Guillain-Barré syndrome: facial diplegia, velopharyngeal involvement, and impairment in the sensory and motor nerves of the extremities

III. Lyme disease: facial diplegia in the presence of aseptic meningitis or with a slightly erythematous indurated face resembling painless cellulitis (also referred to as *Bannwarth syndrome*)

IV. Leukosis/lymphomas: search for associated parenchymal or meningeal lesions

V. *Melkersson-Rosenthal syndrome*: see section on Idiopathic Facial Paralysis

VI. Ethylene glycol (antifreeze) toxicity: facial diplegia (temporary or permanent)

Neonatal Facial Paralysis

I. Obstetric facial paralysis is most often related to the use of forceps, but injury can be seen after spontaneous delivery or as a result of compression due to intrauterine position. The facial paralysis usually resolves in a couple of weeks. CT scanning is indicated when there is no regression after 2 months to exclude a dishpan fracture that requires early surgical decompression (before age 3 months) to be efficacious.

II. Facial paralysis due to malformations
   A. Isolated hypoplasia of CN VII
   B. Möbius syndrome is typically associated with facial diplegia and paralysis of the abducens nerves, but there are unilateral forms associated with impairment in other ipsilateral cranial nerves. It is probably caused by antenatal ischemia of the nuclei of the nerves in the brainstem.
   C. Hypoplasia of the ear often has coexistent malposition of CN VII.

HEMIFACIAL SPASM

This movement disorder is characterized by sudden, painless, involuntary clonic contractions of the muscles innervated by CN VII, usually starting with the orbicularis oculi. It is most often due to compression by vascular structures of the facial nerve at the root exit zone, which is an approximately 3-mm area beginning at the emergence of CN VII from the brainstem, at the junction of the central-type and peripheral-type myelin fibers. The vascular structures involved are, by decreasing order of frequency, the posteroinferior cerebellar artery, the vertebral artery, the anteroinferior cerebellar artery, and a vein (respectively 70%, 40%, 30%, and 20% in). Treatment usually consists of botulinum toxin injection or surgical decompression.

REFERENCES

Bradley, W. G., Daroff, R. B., et al. (2004). *Neurology in clinical practice, ed 4*. Boston: Butterworth-Heinemann.

Defazio, G., Abbruzzese, G., Girlanda, P., et al. (2002). Botulinum toxin A treatment for primary hemifacial spasm: a 10-year multicenter study. *Arch Neurol, 59*, 418–420.

F

FACIAL NERVE, HEMIFACIAL SPASM

FEMORAL NERVE

The femoral nerve arises from the combination of the posterior divisions of the ventral rami of L2, L3, and L4 spinal roots. The course of the femoral nerve runs through the psoas muscle. The femoral nerve innervates the psoas muscle, which additionally receives other branches directly from the L3 and L4 nerve roots. The nerve emerges from the psoas muscle and passes between it and the iliacus muscle. The femoral nerve is tightly covered by the iliacus fascia and is within the iliacus compartment. The femoral nerve innervates the iliacus approximately 4 to 5 cm proximal to the inguinal ligament, passes beneath the inguinal ligament just lateral to the femoral artery, and then emerges from the iliacus compartment. Just distal to the inguinal ligament, the femoral nerve ends by dividing into terminal motor and sensory branches. Motor branches supply the four heads of the quadriceps (rectus femoris, vastus lateralis, vastus medialis, and vastus intermedius) and the sartorius muscles. The sensory branches are the medial and intermediate cutaneous nerves of the thigh and the saphenous nerve. The medial and intermediate cutaneous nerves of the thigh almost immediately enter the subcutaneous space and supply sensation to the anterior and medial thigh. The saphenous nerve travels through the thigh in the adductor canal deep to the sartorius muscle, gives off the infrapatellar branch to supply cutaneous sensation to the anterior patella, emerges from the canal approximately 10 cm proximal and medial to the patella, and then runs subcutaneously along the medial leg until reaching the medial arch of the foot.

NERVE INJURY

Because the femoral nerve is actually quite short, injuries usually occur either in the retroperitoneal pelvic space or at the inguinal ligament. Most femoral neuropathies are iatrogenic. Pelvic surgical procedures are the most common cause. Injury to the nerve within the pelvis may occur when a retractor is held tightly against the pelvic wall for a prolonged period of time. Injury to the nerve at the inguinal ligament may occur with prolonged use of the lithotomy position. Femoral artery catheterization with subsequent hematoma formation may compress the femoral nerve at the inguinal ligament. Spontaneous hematomas in the iliacus compartment of the psoas muscle may compress the femoral nerve or the lumbar plexus and usually occur with excessive anticoagulation. Noniatrogenic femoral nerve neuropathies may occur in diabetes mellitus, usually as part of a more widespread polyradiculoplexopathy (i.e., diabetic amyotrophy).

NEUROPATHY

Femoral neuropathy must be distinguished from L2 to L4 polyradiculopathy and lumbar plexopathy. A lesion in any of these areas may cause weakness of knee extension, loss of quadriceps reflex, and sensory loss in the

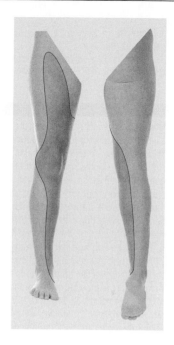

FIGURE 30

The approximate area of sensory deficits associated with lesions of the femoral nerve. *(From O'Brien, M. (2010). Aids to the examination of the peripheral nervous system, ed 5. Edinburgh: Saunders.)*

anterior and medial thigh and medial calf (see Fig. 30). In both L2 to L4 polyradiculopathy and lumbar plexopathy, weakness of hip adduction, weakness of ankle dorsiflexion, and sensory loss in the very proximal medial thigh (obturator nerve) and lateral thigh (lateral femoral cutaneous nerve) may be present, but these findings will not occur in an isolated femoral neuropathy. If the site of femoral nerve injury is intrapelvic, weakness of hip flexion is expected, while if the site is at the inguinal ligament, hip flexion will be spared. Electromyography is useful both to confirm the lesion localization and to give information about prognosis for recovery. If more than 5 or 6 days have passed since the injury (allowing Wallerian degeneration to occur) and the quadriceps compound motor action potential (CMAP) amplitude is preserved, this suggests a predominantly demyelinating process with potential for recovery within several weeks. A low CMAP amplitude suggests an axonal process and a slower recovery.

REFERENCES

Katirji, B., Kaminski, H. J., & Ruff, R. L., eds. (2014). *Neuromuscular disorders in clinical practice*, ed 2. New York: Springer.

Preston, D. C., & Shapiro, B. E. (2013). *Electromyography and neuromuscular disorders: clinical-electrophysiologic correlations, ed 3*. St. Louis: Elsevier.

FONTANEL

The anterior fontanel is an interosseous space located at the juncture of the sagittal and coronal sutures; the posterior fontanel is located at the juncture of the sagittal and lambdoidal sutures. Anterior fontanel is open at birth and usually closes between 7 and 18 months of age, with an average closing time around 17 months. Posterior fontanel is usually closed at birth. The anterior fontanel may be quite large at birth, but this has little clinical significance unless associated with palpable split sutures. If the infant has been delivered vaginally, the cranial bones may override each other and the fontanel may be difficult to palpate. When the infant cries, the fontanel may be tense and bulging. At other times, it may be soft and flat and may pulsate. A "full" or "tense" fontanel when the infant is quiet is a sign of increased intracranial pressure. Causes of delayed closure of the anterior fontanel (persistently large) include prematurity, malnutrition, increased intracranial pressure, chromosomal abnormalities (trisomies 13, 18, and 21), metabolic disorders (hypothyroidism, rickets, and hypophosphatasia), delayed ossification of cranium, and primary bone disorders (achondroplasia, cleidocranial dysostosis, and osteogenesis imperfecta). Causes of an absent or small anterior fontanel include microcephaly, craniosynostosis, and accelerated bone maturation.

REFERENCES

Daroff, R. B., Jankovic, J., Mazziotta, J. C., et al. (2015). *Bradley's neurology in clinical practice*, ed 7. Elsevier.

Idriz, S., Patel, J. H., Ameli Renani, S., et al. (2015). CT of normal developmental and variant anatomy of the pediatric skull: distinguishing trauma from normality. *Radiographics*, 35(5), 1585–1601.

FRAGILE X SYNDROME

Fragile X syndrome (FXS) is the second most common cause of mental retardation, affecting 1 in 3000 boys and 1 in 7000 girls. FXS is caused by the inactivation of the fragile X mental retardation 1 (FMR1) gene on the X chromosome resulting from the amplification of trinucleotide sequence CGG to greater than 200 copies and methylation. Of the children with FXS, 8% to 15% are affected with autism.

Physical examination may show a narrow and elongated face, a high and large forehead, a "tired" appearance (rings under eyes), a high-arched palate, large protruding ears, macro-orchidia, and joint laxity. There is developmental delay, and most FXS patients have an intelligence quotient (IQ) ranging from 35 to 50. Other neurological abnormalities include echolalic speech and pragmatic language problems. There are often difficulties with visuospatial reasoning abilities and attention, and short-term memory is affected. Behavioral difficulties include social anxiety, motor excitation, and hyperactivity. Girls with FXS may have attention deficit, learning difficulties, planning and reasoning difficulties (arithmetic tasks), anxiety, obsessive–compulsive tendencies, depression, and social withdrawal. Cognitive problems are milder in girls.

Epilepsy is seen in approximately 15% to 25%, with the electroencephalogram showing biphasic centrotemporal spikes. Sleep obstructive apnea affects 10% of patients. Male carriers with premutation (55–200 repeats) may develop a progressive neurological disorder called fragile X-associated tremor/ataxia syndrome, which is characterized by cerebellar ataxia, intention tremor, parkinsonism, peripheral neuropathy, and cognitive decline in middle age.

Supportive treatment and special education are indicated for FXS; there are no specific medications. Valproate or carbamazepine monotherapy can be used for seizures; psychotropic medications for aggressiveness; and stimulants for hyperactivity.

REFERENCES

Daroff, R. B., Jankovic, J., Mazziotta, J. C., & Pomeroy, S. L. (Eds.). (2015). *Bradley's neurology in clinical practice*, ed 7. *Elsevier*.

Dulac, O., Lassonde, M., & Sarnat, H. B. (2013). *Pediatric neurology, Part I/II/III*, ed 1. Elsevier. Handbook of Clinical Neurology, vol. 111/112/113.

FRONTAL LOBE

The frontal lobe consists of the precentral gyrus and superior, middle, and inferior frontal gyri, and contains several different functional areas: the motor, premotor, supplementary motor, and prefrontal areas. The motor cortex (Brodmann area 4) with somatotopic representation of the contralateral body (so-called homunculus) controls the voluntary movement. The giant pyramidal cells (Betz cells) in the motor cortex contribute 3% of the corticospinal tract and corticobulbar tract. The premotor and supplementary areas (Brodmann area 6) participate in programming, preparation of movement, and control of posture. The premotor cortex also includes the frontal eye field (Brodmann area 8) and the Broca area (Brodmann areas 44 and 45). The prefrontal areas lie anterior to the premotor area with extensive connections to parietal, temporal, and occipital cortices. These areas help coordinate intellect, judgment, and planning of behavior.

REFERENCES

Vanderah, T., & Gould, D. (2016). *Nolte's the human brain: an introduction to its functional anatomy,* ed 7. Philadelphia: Elsevier.

FRONTAL LOBE LESIONS AND SYNDROMES

Partial seizures, contralateral hemiplegia, and neurobehavioral syndromes may arise from different lesions of the frontal lobe. Expressive aphasia is associated with dominant frontal lobe lesion. Three behavioral (pure or mixed) syndromes have been described with prefrontal lesions:

I. *Orbitofrontal syndrome:* Judgment Center: disinhibition, impulsiveness, emotional lability, euphoria, poor judgment, and distractibility

II. *Frontal convexity syndrome:* Executive Center: apathy, psychomotor retardation, poor word-list generation, motor perseveration and impersistence, and inability to execute multistep behaviors

III. *Medial frontal and opercular syndrome:* Expression Center: paucity of spontaneous movement (abulia), sparse verbal output (Broca aphasia), lower extremity weakness, and incontinence

FRONTAL LOBE SEIZURE

Of all patients with refractory focal epilepsies (inadequate seizure control despite use of potentially effective antiepileptic drugs (AEDs) at tolerable levels for 1–2 years) referred to epilepsy surgery, 25% have frontal lobe epilepsy (FLE). Unilateral clonic, tonic asymmetric with preserved consciousness, and hyper motor seizures are specific to FLE. Abdominal auras may occur but do not evolve into an automotor seizure, thus differentiating FLE from temporal lobe seizures, and a visual aura argues against a frontal origin.

Identification of ictal semiology is key in diagnosing frontal lobe seizures, since ictal electroencephalography (EEG) is frequently falsely negative or has muscle artifacts. Interictal EEG usually reveals interictal epileptiform discharges and rhythmical midline theta, which has localizing value. High density EEG may be superior to conventional EEG in FLE, especially with midline and parasagittal regions.

REFERENCES

Beleza, P., & Pinho, J. (2011). Frontal lobe epilepsy. *J Clin Neurosci, 18,* 593–600.

Feyissa, A. M., et al. (2017). High density scalp EEG in frontal lobe epilepsy. *Epilepsy Res, 129,* 157–161.

FUNCTIONAL MAGNETIC RESONANCE IMAGING

Positron emission tomography (PET) and single photon emission computed tomography (SPECT) imaging, under the rubric of nuclear medicine, had been the only types of functional imaging available until the relatively recent advent of functional magnetic resonance imaging (fMRI). Unlike traditional MRI, which allows visualization of brain anatomy with exquisite detail, fMRI provides an avenue into imaging brain physiology and activity. Compared with PET and SPECT, fMRI has better spatial resolution with less total scan time. In addition, fMRI does not require the injection of any material, let alone a radioactive isotope.

A detailed explanation of the technical parameters of fMRI is beyond the scope of this work. In brief, among the various factors affecting signal intensity on MRI is local magnetic inhomogeneity with greater inhomogeneity, leading to more rapid loss of signal. Deoxyhemoglobin, unlike oxyhemoglobin, is paramagnetic. Paramagnetic substances increase inhomogeneity and, as expected, result in accelerated loss of signal. Autoregulation of cerebral blood flow causes increased blood flow to active regions of the brain. The increase in blood flow far exceeds the increase in oxygen extraction, resulting in a net decrease in deoxyhemoglobin in the capillary bed and venules. With the net decrease in deoxyhemoglobin comes an improvement in the local magnetic homogeneity and thus a net increase, approximately 2%, in signal intensity from the active region of the brain. That 2% can be used to map brain function.

The effective genesis of fMRI occurred in 1990, when Ogawa noted the blood oxygen level dependent (BOLD) effect on signal intensity just described. By 1992, Ogawa and associates and Kwong and associates had published the first functional images using the BOLD technique.

A cursory search of the literature reveals that fMRI has a potential role to play in seizure localization, pain management, understanding the neural connections between structures in the brain, the physiologic basis of cognition and perception, identifying psychiatric disorders, and differentiating the various forms of dementia, as well as assessing myriad other functional abnormalities of the brain.

fMRI has already improved our understanding of the organization of the brain in addition to providing a powerful tool in evaluating neurologic status. fMRI continues to make inroads into assessing neurosurgical risk; neurosurgery, in particular, depends on defining both brain structure and function.

fMRI may well become the optimal method for studying brain function in the normal, diseased, and injured states, in addition to being the least intrusive and most accurate way for assessing the potential risks of neurosurgery or radiation therapy.

REFERENCES

Buxton, R. B. (2002). *Introduction to functional magnetic resonance imaging: principles and techniques.* Cambridge: Cambridge University Press.

Huettel, S. A., Song, A. W., & McCarthy, G. (2004). *Functional magnetic resonance imaging.* Sunderland: Sinauer Associates.

G

GAIT DISORDERS

Gait depends on both maintenance of equilibrium and mechanisms of locomotion. Abnormal gait, especially in the elderly, is due to a combination of factors. A useful approach to assessing contributors to gait disorder is by localizing the level of the sensorimotor deficits and differentiating them into three groups: low, middle, and high sensorimotor level gait disorders, as shown in Table 67.

Low sensorimotor level gait disorders can be divided into peripheral sensory or peripheral motor dysfunction. In peripheral sensory impairment, an unsteady and tentative gait is commonly caused by vestibular disorders, peripheral neuropathy, proprioceptive deficits, or visual ataxia. Peripheral motor impairment results from arthritic, myopathic, and neuropathic conditions that cause deformity of the extremities, painful weight bearing (e.g., antalgic gait), and focal weakness (e.g., Trendelenburg gait in hip adductor weakness and "steppage" gait in foot drop). The resulting gait disorders are primarily compensatory, allowing patients to adapt well to the deficit.

Middle sensorimotor level gait disorders encompass hemiplegic, paraparetic, cerebellar ataxic, parkinsonian, choreic, hemiballistic, and dystonic gaits. Pyramidal, cerebellar, and basal ganglia motor systems dysfunction results in faulty execution of centrally selected postural and locomotor responses, resulting in the disruption of the sensory and motor modulation of gait. Despite the abnormal stepping pattern, gait initiation and postural reflexes are usually intact. Gait freezing is often seen in Parkinson disease, particularly when making a turn or going through a doorway. Other clinically significant aspects of the parkinsonian gait include decreased stride length, postural instability, and festination (slow, shuffling steps that slowly increase in speed, predisposing a forward fall).

High sensorimotor level gait disorders have more nonspecific gait characteristics. They are due to difficulties in frontal planning and execution, including cautious gait, frontal and subcortical disequilibrium, gait ignition failure (gait apraxia), frontal gait disorders, primary progressive freezing gait disorder, and psychogenic gait disorder. Simply holding a patient lightly by the finger during the neurologic exam can help to diagnose disorders of gait initiation. Cognitive dysfunction and behavioral aspects, such as fear of falling, play a role, particularly in cautious gait. The severity of frontal-related disorders runs a spectrum from gait ignition failure to frontal gait disorder to frontal disequilibrium, in which gait initiation difficulty and small shuffling steps progress to the point at which an unsupported stance is not possible. They are difficult to differentiate clinically and are usually the result of a lesion that affects the corticobasal ganglionic-thalamocortical loop, caused by bilateral infarction, hemorrhage, neoplasm, hydrocephalus, or a degenerative process.

TABLE 67

GAIT DISORDERS AND THEIR CLINICAL FEATURES

Type	Cause	Findings
Peripheral Sensory	Sensory Ataxia Vestibulopathy	Cautious gait, Romberg sign, associated objective sensory deficits
		Side-to-side "drifting" as if on a boat
Peripheral Motor	Pain or Joint Deformity (Antalgic)	Favors one side versus affected side, visible deformities, stooped posture, pain with weight-bearing
		Foot drop, overcompensated hip flexion
Spasticity	Hemiparesis Paraparesis	Leg swings outward (circumduction), visible limp
		Bilateral circumduction
Parkinsonism		Short, shuffling steps with festination, decreased arm swing, exaggerated tremor on affected side, decreased gait velocity. En bloc turn, postural instability
Cerebellar Ataxia		Wide based, irregular rhythm of steps
Cautious		Patient seems afraid of falling, postural stability normal
Frontal	Stroke Hydrocephalus	Impaired gait initiation, "magnetic" gait with or without cognitive or urinary symptoms
		May look like parkinsonism

G

GAIT DISORDERS

Gait disorder in the elderly frequently results from an overlap of deficits in the three sensorimotor levels. Two mechanisms appear to precipitate gait disorders, particularly in the elderly. First, "benign disequilibrium of the elderly" is a multiple sensory deficit syndrome (a combination of impairments in position and tactile sense, vision, hearing, and vestibular or baroreceptor function) causing vague dizziness or disequilibrium ("dizziness of feet") while standing, walking, or turning, but not while sitting or lying. Equilibrium improves by holding or leaning onto a wall. These patients benefit from gait training and use of an assistive device (cane or walker) and should not be medicated (meclizine, benzodiazepines) for presumed vestibular disease. A second common problem is acute deterioration in gait, balance, and postural adjustments in acutely ill, elderly patients. The ensuing "toxic-metabolic encephalopathy," caused by medications, organ failure, dehydration, electrolyte imbalance, or systemic infection, may result in varying gait difficulty and altered postural reflexes, gegenhalten (paratonia involving an involuntary resistance to passive movement) of limb and neck, diffuse myoclonus, and bilateral asterixis. Acute gait disorder may in turn be the presenting feature of acute systemic decompensation in the elderly and warrants further evaluation (i.e., stroke, myocardial infarction, or infection).

Diagnosis of gait disorders is based on history and associated neurologic findings. Isolated gait disorders in the elderly are frequently due to treatable disorders such as Parkinson disease, cervical myelopathy, or normal-pressure hydrocephalus. Gait evaluation and training by physical therapy should be initiated early. Discontinuing unnecessary medication use and home safety evaluations are pertinent in preventing future falls.

REFERENCES

Fung, V. S. (2016). Functional gait disorder. *Handb Clin Neurol*, *139*, 263–270.
Pirker, W., & Katzenschlager, R. (2017). Gait disorders in adults and the elderly: a clinical guide. *Wien Klin Wochenschr*, *129*(3-4), 81–95.

GAZE PALSY

HORIZONTAL GAZE PALSIES

A unilateral gaze palsy (for both saccadic and pursuit movements) may indicate a contralateral cerebral hemispheric (frontoparietal), contralateral thalamus, midbrain, or ipsilateral pontine lesion. Except when the pontine lesion is at the level of the abducens nucleus, either involving the nucleus itself or the paramedian pontine reticular formation, the eyes can be driven toward the side of the palsy with cold caloric stimulation of the ipsilateral ear or oculocephalic maneuvers. Hemispheric lesions characteristically produce transient defects; brainstem lesions may be associated with enduring defects. An acute cerebellar hemispheric lesion can result in an ipsilateral gaze palsy that can be overcome with caloric testing. Unilateral saccadic palsy with intact pursuit is unusual and indicates an acute frontal lesion. Unilateral impaired pursuit with normal saccades is usually due to an ipsilateral deep posterior hemispheric lesion with a contralateral hemianopia.

VERTICAL GAZE PALSIES

Vertical gaze palsies are harder to localize since there are more muscles innervated by cranial nerves II and IV. The rostral interstitial nucleus of the medial longitudinal fasciculus in the upper midbrain contains the cells that generate vertical eye movements. A medially placed lesion will result in both an up-gaze and down-gaze palsy. An isolated down-gaze palsy is often due to a bilateral or lateral midbrain lesion. Isolated up-gaze palsies occur with lesions of the posterior commissure, bilateral pretectal regions, and large unilateral midbrain tegmental lesions. In the dorsal midbrain syndrome *(Parinaud syndrome)* the paralysis of upward gaze is usually associated with convergence-retraction nystagmus, lid retraction, and light-near dissociation of the pupils. An acute bilateral pontine lesion at the level of the abducens nucleus may result in a transient up-gaze paralysis in addition to bilateral horizontal gaze palsy.

CONJUGATE EYE DEVIATIONS

Horizontal deviations are associated with acute gaze palsies as described above and with irritative cerebral foci (seizure or intracerebral hemorrhage), which usually drive the eyes to the side opposite the lesion. Ipsiversive eye and head movements, however, are reported with focal seizures. Tonic upward deviations occur in the oculogyric crisis of postencephalitic parkinsonism and, more commonly, as an idiosyncratic reaction to phenothiazines and other neuroleptics. They may also occur in coma, often anoxic encephalopathy. Downward deviations may occur transiently in normal neonates but also in infantile hydrocephalus and in adults with metabolic encephalopathy, bilateral thalamic infarction, or hemorrhage.

GERSTMANN SYNDROME

The clinical tetrad of agraphia, acalculia, agnosia to fingers, and agnosia to right-left (disorientation) defines Gerstmann syndrome. Finger agnosia may manifest as bilateral difficulties in finger naming, moving fingers to command, matching of fingers to demonstration, or recognizing stimuli ("wiggle the finger that I touch"). When all features are present, a dominant inferior parietal or posterior perisylvian lesion is highly likely. People with Gerstmann syndrome usually have other deficits as well, such as aphasia. Alexia and constructional apraxia may also accompany Gerstmann syndrome.

Gerstmann syndrome can also manifest in the context of global disease such as SLE, AIDS, or multiple sclerosis.

In children, developmental Gerstmann syndrome may occur, and the cause is often not known. It may occur with or without dyslexia. Verbal IQ among such children is often significantly higher than performance IQ.

REFERENCES
Devinsky, O. (1992). *Behavioral neurology: 100 maxims.* St. Louis: Mosby.
Mesulam, M. M. (2000). *Principles of behavioral and cognitive neurology,* ed 2. New York: Oxford University Press.

GLOSSOPHARYNGEAL NEURALGIA

Glossopharyngeal neuralgia is a rare disorder defined as severe transient stabbing pain perceived in the distribution of the glossopharyngeal nerve, including the ear, base of the tongue, tonsillar fossa, and lower jaw angle.

CLINICAL FEATURES
Attacks come in clusters of sharp, stabbing pain. The pain may be variable with a long duration and is associated with autonomic dysfunction (salivation, lacrimation, bradycardia, and syncope). Trigger points are variable and most commonly associated with swallowing, chewing, speaking, laughing, coughing, or touching particular areas of the glossopharyngeal nerve and upper sensory fibers of the vagus nerve. Onset occurs after age 40, with males and females affected equally.

DIFFERENTIAL DIAGNOSIS
The differential diagnosis of glossopharyngeal neuralgia includes underlying causes, such as oropharyngeal carcinoma, peritonsillar abscess, enlarged

styloid process (Eagle syndrome), enlarged tortuous vertebral or posterior inferior cerebellar arteries, and SUNCT syndrome (short-lasting, unilateral, neuralgiform headache attacks with conjunctival injection and tearing). The following symptoms differentiate glossopharyngeal neuropathy from glossopharyngeal neuralgia: sensory deficits in the ipsilateral posterior part of the tongue and tonsillar fossa, and a weak or missing gag reflex. In that case, an underlying cause should be identified.

DIAGNOSTIC CONSIDERATIONS
Evaluation of glossopharyngeal neuralgia should include a thorough ear, nose, and throat examination. Magnetic resonance imaging may show neurovascular compression of the glossopharyngeal nerve.

TREATMENT
Treatment is aimed at underlying causes of "symptomatic" neuralgias. Carbamazepine, phenytoin, gabapentin, or pregabalin may be used for pain management, although the response rates may vary. When pharmacological treatment fails, microvascular decompression may be considered. Other modalities include percutaneous radiofrequency (thermal) rhizotomy of the 9th and 10th nerves, surgical rhizotomy, or stereotactic radiosurgery, especially for patients who have pain caused by malignancy.

REFERENCES
Khan, M., Nishi, S. E., Hassan, S. N., Islam, M. A., & Gan, S. H. (2017). Trigeminal neuralgia, glossopharyngeal neuralgia, and myofascial pain dysfunction syndrome: an update. *Pain Res Manag*, 2017:7438326. https://doi.org/10.1155/2017/7438326. Epub 2017 Jul 30.

O'Neill, F., Nurmikko, T., & Sommer, C. (2017). Other facial neuralgias. *Cephalalgia*, *37*(7), 658–669. https://doi.org/10.1177/0333102417689995. Epub 2017 Jan 29.

GLUCOSE IMBALANCE

In contrast to other tissues, the brain normally derives its energy from carbohydrates only. Typical constellations of signs and symptoms resulting from hypo or hyperglycemia are described here.

I. Hypoglycemia
Symptoms arise from neuroglycopenia and endogenous release of catecholamines. Mild hypoglycemia produces hunger, weakness, dizziness, blurred vision, anxiety, tremor, tachycardia, pallor, diaphoresis, headache, and mild confusion. With more severe hypoglycemia, the preceding symptoms are followed by seizures (glucose <30 mg/dL) with progression to coma, pupillary dilation, hypotonia, and extensor posturing (glucose <10 mg/dL). The presence of hyperventilation may lead to paresthesias. Focal findings may mimic cerebrovascular disease. Symptoms, signs, and residual neurologic deficit depend on the rate of onset, duration, and severity of hypoglycemia. Patients with chronic hypoglycemia may have no

sympathetic symptoms but present with cognitive or behavioral disturbances. Repeated severe attacks of hypoglycemia may result in dementia because of damage to hippocampal neurons. The degree of slowing on electroencephalogram (EEG) may correlate with the severity of hypoglycemia. Glucose repletion should be accompanied by thiamine repletion in severe cases.

II. Hyperglycemia

A. Hyperglycemia is most commonly due to diabetes mellitus caused by either inadequate insulin production or insulin resistance. In patients with neurological conditions, hyperglycemia is often precipitated by stress, infection, or the therapeutic use of glucocorticoids.

Diabetic ketoacidosis evolves rapidly over a 24-hour period and is frequently accompanied by stupor or coma. Muscle cramps, dysesthesias, and diffuse abdominal pain may occur. The neurologic changes correlate best with serum osmolarity, although dehydration, acidosis, and associated electrolyte disorders contribute. For unknown reasons, hyperosmolality alone, particularly when due to hyperglycemia, may lead to continuous partial seizures, even when careful studies fail to uncover any underlying lesion. Neurologic deterioration primarily occurs in patients with an effective plasma osmolality above 320 to 330 mOsmol/kg.

The treatment of diabetic ketoacidosis may lead to fatal cerebral edema if blood osmolarity is rapidly lowered relative to brain osmolarity. Treatment may also cause hypophosphatemia, hypokalemia, and hypoglycemia.

B. Hyperglycemic hyperosmolar nonketotic state usually has more severe hyperglycemia but without ketoacidosis, resulting in central nervous system (CNS) complications due to extracellular hyperosmolarity. Neurologic manifestations are variable and include hallucinations, depression, apathy, irritability, seizures (typically transient focal or epilepsia partialis continua), flaccidity, diminished deep tendon reflexes, tonic spasms, myoclonus, meningeal signs, nystagmus, tonic eye deviations, and reversible loss of vestibular caloric responses. As the blood glucose rises above 600 mg/dL, coma may develop.

Studies indicate that hyperglycemia can lead to poor outcome in stroke patients during the acute phase, and tight control of blood sugar is recommended, though controversially, there are also studies advocating moderate hyperglycemia for favorable outcome in acute lacunar strokes. Seizures generally improve within 24 hours of rehydration and correction of hyperglycemia. EEG may show corresponding focal abnormalities, including periodic lateralized epileptiform discharges.

The initial evaluation of patients with hyperglycemic crises should include assessment of cardiorespiratory status, volume status, and mental status. In both ketotic and nonketotic hyperglycemia, care should be placed on recognizing and treating the underlying stressor, which may include stroke, myocardial infarction, infection, or other acute medical illnesses.

III. Hypoglycorrhachia, abnormally low cerebrospinal fluid (CSF) glucose concentration, is usually associated with infection, either bacterial or chronic meningitis. It may also be seen in meningeal carcinomatosis. Persistent low CSF glucose with normal serum glucose levels in a patient with seizures and developmental delay may be result of a genetic defect in glucose transport across the blood-brain barrier. These long-term neurologic sequelae may be prevented by a ketogenic diet.

REFERENCES

Kitabchi, A. E., Umpierrez, G. E., Miles, J. M., & Fisher, J. N. (2009). Hyperglycemic crises in adult patients with diabetes. *Diabetes Care*, *32*(7), 1335–1343.

Seifter, J., & Samuels, M. A. (2005). Electrolyte disorders. *Continuum Lifelong Learning Neurol*, *11*(1), 85–90.

GRAVES OPHTHALMOPATHY

INTRODUCTION AND PATHOGENESIS

Graves ophthalmopathy refers to any thyroid-associated ophthalmopathy. Approximately 50% of patients with Graves disease are found to have clinical ophthalmopathy. This condition most often affects middle-aged patients. It is more common in women, although more severe ophthalmopathy occurs in older men. Cigarette smoking is a well-established risk factor for more severe ophthalmopathy. The pathogenesis of Graves disease is complex. Genetic susceptibilities as well as environmental factors (e.g., iodine, tobacco smoke, infections, and stress) are associated with Graves disease. The autoimmunity is thought to involve both the B and T cells. Most importantly, activating autoantibodies against the thyrotropin receptor and the insulin-like growth factor 1 receptor (IGF-1R) are thought to play a key role.

CLINICAL FEATURES AND DIAGNOSIS

Main clinical features include eyelid retraction, proptosis of varying severity, diplopia, dryness, "gritty" sensation, lacrimation, photophobia, blurring of vision, and deep orbital pressure. Diplopia is due to fibrosis of ocular muscles that do not extend fully when their antagonist contracts. Fibrosis of the inferior rectus, the most frequently affected muscle, causes diplopia on vertical gaze. Other findings on examination are conjunctival chemosis and injection, and corneal exposure, which may lead to corneal perforation. Some patients have compressive optic neuropathy with decreased visual acuity, optic disk changes, visual loss, dulling of color perception, and visual field defects.

Diagnostic evaluation of thyroid eye disease begins with confirmation of Graves diagnosis with thyroid function tests, serum thyrotropin receptor antibody, and radioiodine uptake or radionuclide scan. Enlarged extraocular muscles can be assessed by CT, ultrasonography, MRI, scintigraphy with radiolabeled octreotide, gallium scanning, and thermal imaging.

TREATMENT

Most cases of thyroid ophthalmopathy resolve spontaneously, or need conservative measures. In mild cases, conservative measures such as elevation of head during sleep; lubrication; avoidance of wind, light, dust, and smoke; taping of the lids; or use of a moisture chamber while sleeping are often sufficient. Systemic glucocorticoids are used in both mild and severe disease. Rituximab has been tried in two randomized prospective trials for patients with severe disease; however, it was efficacious in only one. In a very recently published randomized, placebo-controlled trial, teprotumumab, a human monoclonal antibody inhibitor of IGF-1R, was shown to have efficacy in reducing proptosis in patients with active ophthalmopathy. Decompression surgery is indicated for present or imminent compressive optic neuropathy or ocular surface compromise. Strabismus surgery and cosmetic procedures are performed as well.

REFERENCES

Smith, T. J., & Hegedüs, L. (2016). Graves disease. *N Engl J Med*, *375*(16), 1552–1565. https://doi.org/10.1056/NEJMra1510030.

Smith, T. J., Kahaly, G. J., Ezra, D. G., et al. (2017). Teprotumumab for thyroid-associated ophthalmopathy. *N Engl J Med*, *376*(18), 1748–1761. https://doi.org/10.1056/NEJMoa1614949.

GUILLAIN-BARRÉ SYNDROME (See also NEUROPATHY)

Guillain-Barré syndrome (GBS) is an acute, autoimmune polyneuropathy, encompassing a heterogeneous group of pathologic and clinical entities with several variant forms. The annual incidence of GBS is around 1 to 3 per 100,000 population. Although it can affect both sexes and any age group, there is a bimodal distribution with peaks in young adults and the elderly and a predilection for males.

PATHOGENESIS

GBS is thought to be a postinfectious autoimmune response (molecular mimicry). The response is directed toward myelin or axon of peripheral nerves, resulting in demyelination. *Campylobacter jejuni infection* is most commonly associated with GBS. Others include cytomegalovirus, Epstein–Barr virus, human immunodeficiency virus, and Zika virus. Rare triggering events include immunization, surgery, trauma, and bone marrow transplantation.

CLINICAL FEATURES

Symptoms worsen within 4 weeks after the initial symptoms (Table 68).
- Cardinal features include progressive limb weakness, areflexia, and *albuminocytologic dissociation* on cerebrospinal fluid (CSF) analysis.
- Progressive ascending weakness typically starts at the legs but can appear in the arms or facial muscles.
- Respiratory weakness can occur, necessitating monitoring of respiratory function.

TABLE 68

CLINICAL FEATURES OF GUILLAIN-BARRÉ SYNDROME

MOTOR DYSFUNCTION

Symmetrical limb weakness (proximal, distal, global)

Neck muscle weakness

Respiratory muscle weakness

Cranial nerve paralysis: III–VII, IX–XII

Areflexia

Wasting of limb muscles

SENSORY DYSFUNCTION

Pain, numbness, paresthesia

Loss of position sense, vibration, touch, and pain

Ataxia

AUTONOMIC DYSFUNCTION

Sinus tachycardia and bradycardia

Other cardiac arrhythmias

Hypertension and orthostatic hypotension

Wide fluctuation of pulse and blood pressure

Tonic pupils, hypersalivation, anhidrosis or excessive sweating, urinary sphincter
disturbances, constipation, gastric dysmotility, abnormal vasomotor tone with
venous pooling and facial flushing

- Facial nerve palsies
- Oropharyngeal weakness
- Oculomotor weakness
- Decreased or absent reflexes
- Paresthesias in the hands and feet
- Pain due to nerve root inflammation
- Autonomic dysfunction
- Unusual features: papilledema, facial myokymia, hearing loss, meningeal signs, vocal cord paralysis, mental status changes, and syndrome of inappropriate ADH secretion.

LAB FINDINGS AND STUDIES

- CSF: elevated proteins, normal white blood cells (WBC), albuminocytologic dissociation
- Electromyography and nerve conduction study (EMG-NCS) acute polyneuropathy with demyelinating features
  - Decreased nerve conduction velocity
  - Prolonged distal motor latency
  - Increased F wave latency
  - Conduction blocks
  - Temporal dispersion
- GQ1b antibody—associated with Miller-Fisher variant of GBS
- Magnetic resonance imaging (MRI)—thickening and enhancement of intrathecal spinal nerve roots and cauda equina

VARIANTS

- Acute inflammatory demyelinating polyneuropathy
- Acute motor axonal neuropathy—*gangliosides GM1 antibodies, GD1a, GalNac-GD1a, and GD1b*
- Acute motor and sensory axonal neuropathy
- Miller-Fisher syndrome—ophthalmoplegia, ataxia, areflexia, *GQ1b antibodies*
- Bickerstaff encephalitis—encephalopathy and hyperreflexia with features of Miller-Fisher syndrome
- Pharyngeal-cervical-brachial weakness
- Paraparesis
- Acute pandysautonomia
- Pure sensory GBS
- Facial diplegia
- Acute bulbar palsy with areflexia, ophthalmoplegia, ataxia, and facial palsy
- Sixth nerve palsy and distal paresthesia

TREATMENT

Immunotherapy with plasma exchange (PLEX) or intravenous immunoglobulin (IVIG) hastens recovery from GBS. PLEX is recommended for a non-ambulatory patient with GBS within 4 weeks of onset, or for ambulant patients within 2 weeks of onset. IVIG is recommended for non-ambulant patients with GBS within 2 to 4 weeks of onset. The effects of PLEX and IVIG are equivalent, and combination of the two immunotherapies or sequential treatment is not recommended. Dosing is 0.4 g/kg bodyweight/day for 5 days. Corticosteroids have no role in GBS treatment. Supportive care, including pain control, hemodynamic monitoring, deep-vein thrombosis prophylaxis, and physical therapy, is warranted. See Table 69.

TABLE 69

CLINICOPATHOLOGIC FORMS OF GUILLAIN-BARRÉ SYNDROME

Forms of GBS	Pathology	Electrophysiologic Features	Comments
AIDP (acute inflammatory demyelinating polyneuropathy)	Lymphocytic infiltration of the peripheral nerves, segmental demyelination macrophages mediated	Segmental slowing, absent or prolonged F reflexes, increased distal latency, conduction block or abnormal temporal dispersion	Good strength recovery, permanent areflexia

Continued

TABLE 69

CLINICOPATHOLOGIC FORMS OF GUILLAIN-BARRÉ SYNDROME—CONT'D

Forms of GBS	Pathology	Electrophysiologic Features	Comments
AMAN (acute motor axonal neuropathy)	Lengthening of the Ranvier nodes, distortion of paranodal myelin, axonal dissection	Distal latencies, motor conduction velocities, F waves and sensory nerve action potentials are normal, but CMAP is reduced.	Anti-GM1, GD1a, and GD1B antibodies can be present, normo- or hyperreflexia are possible, common association with *Campylobacter* infection; usually good recovery
AMSAN (acute motor sensory axonal neuropathy)	Wallerian-like degeneration of sensory and motor fibers, little demyelination or lymphocytic infiltration	Very low M responses amplitude, inexcitable motor nerves, sensory and motor axonal dysfunction	Fulminant course, associated with *Campylobacter* infection; poor prognosis—slow and incomplete recovery
Miller-Fisher syndrome	Positive immunostain for antibodies in the paranodal region of CN III, IV, and VI, inflammation and demyelination	Reduced or absent sensory and motor nerve action potentials, absent H reflex; motor and sensory conduction velocities are normal or minimally reduced.	Although the ophthalmoplegia, areflexia, and ataxia constitute the typical picture, weakness can be occasionally seen; anti-GQ1b antibodies are usually present.

CMAP, Compound muscle action potential; *GBS*, Guillain-Barré syndrome.

REFERENCES

Jasti, A. K., Selmi, C., Sarmiento-Monroy, J. C., et al. (2016). Guillain-Barré syndrome: causes, immunopathogenic mechanisms and treatment. *Expert Rev Clin Immunol*, *12*(11), 1175–1189.

Wijdicks, E. F., & Klein, C. J. (2017). Guillain-Barré syndrome. *Mayo Clin Proc*, *92*(3), 467–479.

H

HALLUCINATIONS

Hallucinations can be defined as a "sensory precept without external stimulation of the relevant sensory organ." Hallucinations may occur in any sensory modality. It is important to distinguish hallucinations from delusions, which are false, fixed beliefs that do not directly involve a sensation. Phenomena include Lilliputian (small animals or people), Brobdingnagian (giants), and autoscopic (seeing oneself from outside) characteristics, as well as palinopsia, voices, palinacusis, crawling sensations, shooting pains, smells, and other features.

I. Differential diagnosis of visual hallucinations
   A. Ocular disorders: Hallucinations may be associated with reduced vision. These are usually formed, bright, colored images. Charles Bonnet syndrome is isolated visual hallucinations, usually of ocular causes including enucleation, cataracts, macular, choroidal, and retinal disease and vitreous traction.
   B. Central nervous system (CNS) disorders: Hallucinations may be due to lesions anywhere along the optic pathways and visual association cortices. They are also seen with midbrain disease ("peduncular hallucinosis"; complex forms, usually with other brainstem signs), dementias, epilepsy, and migraine. In narcoleptics, brightly colored hypnagogic hallucinations occur just before sleep, and hypnopompic hallucinations occur on awakening.
   C. Medical disorders: Hallucination may be seen in 40% to 75% of delirious patients; usually they are brief, nocturnal, and emotionally charged. Causes include alcohol and drug withdrawal, hallucinogens, sympathomimetics, and metabolic encephalopathies.
   D. Psychiatric disorders: Schizophrenia, mania or depression, and hysteria can produce hallucinations.
   E. Normal individuals may experience hallucinations during dreams, falling asleep, hypnosis, childhood (imaginary companion), sensory deprivation, sleep deprivation, or intense emotional experiences.
II. Differential diagnosis of auditory hallucinations
   A. Diseases of the ears or peripheral auditory nerves
   B. CNS diseases: epilepsy, neoplasms, and occasionally, vascular lesions
   C. Toxic or metabolic: alcoholic hallucinosis, encephalopathies
   D. Psychiatric: schizophrenia (60% to 90% of patients), affective disorders, conversion reactions, multiple personality disorder
III. Differential diagnosis of tactile, somatic, and phantom limb hallucinations
   A. Phantom limb is the sensation of persistent presence of an amputated extremity and is found in almost all amputees; patients usually describe the phantom limb as being numb or tingling, of normal size, correctly

aligned, with peripheral areas more prominent; the sensation may recede gradually and may be painful.

B. Tactile hallucinations occur commonly in patients with schizophrenia (15% to 50%) and affective disorder (25%). *Formication* (the sensation of insects crawling) is found in alcohol and drug withdrawal (especially sympathomimetics) and dementias.

IV. Differential diagnosis of olfactory and gustatory hallucinations

A. Medial temporal lobe lesions and complex partial seizures ("uncinate fits") may produce olfactory hallucinations. They may also occur in migraine, dementias, toxic and metabolic conditions, depression, and Briquet syndrome (20% to 25% of patients).

B. Gustatory hallucinations may be seen in manic-depressive illness, schizophrenia, Briquet syndrome, and partial seizures.

REFERENCE

Trimble, M. R., & Cummings, J. L. (Eds.), (1997). *Contemporary behavioral neurology*. Boston: Butterworth-Heinemann.

HEAD TRAUMA

EPIDEMIOLOGY

Traumatic brain injury (TBI) is a leading cause of disability and death, affecting more than 2 million people in the United States annually. Severe TBI is defined by a Glasgow Coma Score less than 9. TBI involves an initial injury and is followed by further neurologic damage that occurs over days following the initial trauma. All geographic areas should have an organized trauma system and follow published guidelines for managing TBI.

TREATMENT

Initial management of the trauma patient includes ABCI: airway, breathing, circulation, and spine immobilization. Patients with severe TBI (Glasgow Coma Scale [GCS] < 9) or who are hypoxic (arterial oxygen saturation <90%) should be intubated for airway protection and ventilatory support. The immediate goals of the initial neurologic assessment are to do a screening neurological exam; determine the severity of head injury as low, moderate, or high risk; stabilize and rule out a fracture of the cervical spine; initiate empiric treatment for increased intracranial pressure (ICP) if it is suspected; and perform an emergent CT brain and neck to rule out fractures. The goals of TBI management are to prevent secondary insults (hypoxia, hypotension) that lead to secondary neuronal injury. To date, we have no therapies that can reverse the primary neurologic injury. Maintenance of normal hemodynamic and respiratory parameters prevents secondary injury from hypotension and hypoxemia. Even a single episode of hypotension (systolic blood pressure [SBP] < 90 mm Hg) worsens outcomes in TBI, as does hypoxia (Pao_2 < 60 mm Hg). Cerebral perfusion pressure (CPP = MAP - ICP, where MAP is mean arterial pressure) should be kept greater than 60 mm Hg. Hypertension associated with wide pulse pressure and bradycardia (Cushing triad) may reflect increased ICP or focal brain stem injury. Patients who "talked and deteriorated" should be assumed to have an expanding intracranial hematoma until proven otherwise.

Intracranial pressure should be monitored in comatose patients with TBI (GCS <8). The incidence of elevated ICP increases with the depth of coma and greater neuroimaging abnormalities. There is no predictable relationship between blood pressure and ICP. Treat ICP greater than 20 mm Hg for more than 10 minutes. Hyperventilation can be used to acutely decrease elevated ICP (target arterial PCO_2 of 30 mm Hg) but has no role in chronic management. Osmotic therapy with mannitol or hypertonic saline can be used to control ICP, along with ventricular CSF drainage. Hemicraniectomy should be considered in patients with life-threatening unilateral cerebral edema. Prophylactic antiepileptic drugs should be used for the first 7 days following injury. Steroids are contraindicated for use in patients with head injury. Early enteral feeding on day 1 after injury has been shown to generally improve outcomes compared with delayed feeding.

Fever should be aggressively treated over the first few days with the goal being normothermia. There is currently no proven benefit to hypothermia. Glycemic and fever control are also a priority in acute TBI. Brain tissue oxygenation ($PbtO_2$) and jugular venous oxygen saturation ($SjvO_2$) can be monitored to ensure adequate brain oxygenation. Low-dose anticoagulation to prevent thromboembolic disease can safely be started within 48 hours after injury. Following the initial injury, physical and cognitive rehabilitative services will likely be needed on an ongoing basis. The incidence of chronic cognitive-behavioral impairment is high.

REFERENCES

Badjatia, N., Parikh, G. Y., & Mayer, S. A. (2016). Traumatic brain injury. In E. D. Louis, S. A. Mayer, & L. P. Rowland (Eds.), *Merritt's neurology*, ed 13 (pp. 364–379). Philadelphia: Wolters Kluwer.

Dutton, R. P., & McCunn, M. (2003). Traumatic brain injury. *Curr Opin Crit Care*, *9*, 503–509.

HEADACHE: MIGRAINE AND OTHER TYPES (See also AAN GUIDELINE SUMMARIES APPENDIX)

Given the range of disorders that present with headache, a systematic approach to headache classification and diagnosis is essential. Since 1988, the International Headache Society's classification has been the accepted standard for headache diagnosis. The 2017 International Classification of Headache Disorders, third edition (ICHD-3, beta, Table 70), groups headache disorders into primary and secondary headaches. The four categories of primary headache include migraine, tension-type headache (TTH), trigeminal autonomic cephalalgias, and other primary headaches. There are also eight categories of secondary headache, and a third group that includes central and primary causes of facial pain and other headaches.

TABLE 70

THE INTERNATIONAL CLASSIFICATION OF HEADACHE DISORDERS, THIRD
EDITION (ICHD-3)

I. The primary headaches
- A. Migraine
- B. Tension-type headache (TTH)
- C. Trigeminal autonomic cephalgias
- D. Other primary headaches

II. The secondary headaches
- A. Headache attributed to trauma or injury to the head and/or neck
- B. Headache attributed to cranial or cervical vascular disorder
- C. Headache attributed to non-vascular intracranial disorder
- D. Headache attributed to a substance or its withdrawal
- E. Headache attributed to infection
- F. Headache attributed to disorder of homeostasis
- G. Headache or facial pain attributed to disorder or cranium, neck, eyes, ears, nose, sinuses, teeth, mouth, or other facial or cranial structures
- H. Headache attributed to psychiatric disorder
- I. Painful cranial neuropathies and other facial pain

III. Other headache disorders (not else classified or unspecified)

From the International Headache Society 2013.

PRIMARY HEADACHE TYPES
Migraine

Migraine affects approximately 18% and 6% of US women and men, respectively. Peak prevalence occurs in middle life with lower incidence in adolescents and those older than 60 years. Nearly one-third of migraineurs experience three or more attacks per month and over half report severe impairments or the need for bedrest. Chronic migraine refers to more than 3 months of 15 or more headache days, at least eight of which are migrainous. It is important to differentiate from *medication-overuse headache* (analgesic rebound headache), which pertains to the regular intake of ergotamines, triptans, or combination analgesics on >10 days per month for >3 months. Status migrainosus refers to more than 72 hours of debilitating migraine. The term *probable migraine* may be used in patients with migrainous features not meeting diagnostic criteria for migraine.

Migraine is classified into five major categories:

I. Migraine without aura
- A. ≥5 attacks fulfilling criteria B through D
- B. Headache attacks lasting 4 to 72 hours (untreated or unsuccessfully treated)
- C. ≥2 of the following four characteristics:
  1. Unilateral location
  2. Pulsating quality
  3. Moderate or severe pain intensity
  4. Aggravation by or causing avoidance of routine physical activity (e.g., walking or climbing stairs)

D. During headache ≥1 of the following:
1. Nausea and/or vomiting
2. Photophobia and phonophobia
E. Not better accounted for by another ICHD-3 diagnosis

II. Migraine with aura

Aura refers to the complex of symptoms usually occurring prior to the onset of headache; however, symptoms may follow the initial pain phase and even continue into the headache itself. Auras may occur in the absence of headache. A diagnosis of *persistent aura without infarction* may be made when aura symptoms last ≥1 week if neuroimaging is negative for infarction. Conversely, *migrainous infarction* may be diagnosed when aura symptoms are attributed to a demonstrated ischemic brain lesion. There is a two-fold increased risk in patients suffering from migraine with aura; however, these are not migrainous infarctions. Seizures may be triggered by migraine with aura (*migraine aura-triggered seizure*).

A. ≥2 attacks fulfilling criteria B and C
B. ≥1 of the following fully reversible aura symptoms:
1. Visual (most common aura, e.g., zigzag, flashing lights, spots, or lines)
2. Sensory (second most common aura, e.g., paresthesias, numbness)
3. Speech and/or language
4. Motor (Dx: hemiplegic migraine)
5. Brainstem (e.g., dysarthria, vertigo, tinnitus, hypacusis, diplopia, ataxia, decreased level of consciousness)
6. Retinal (monocular positive and/or negative visual phenomenon, e.g., scintillations, scotomata, or blindness)
    • Other causes of monocular visual loss, including transient ischemic attack (TIA), optic neuropathy, and retinal detachment, must be ruled out
C. ≥2 of the following:
1. At least one aura symptom spreads gradually over 5 or more minutes, and/or two or more symptoms occur in succession
2. Each individual aura symptom lasts 5 to 60 minutes
3. At least one aura symptom is unilateral
4. The aura is accompanied, or followed within 60 minutes, by headache
D. Not better accounted for by another ICHD-3 diagnosis, and transient ischemic attack has been excluded

III. Familial hemiplegic migraine (FHM)
A. Mutations identified in CACNA1A, ATP1A2, and SCN1A genes
B. Aura includes motor weakness
C. First- or second-degree relative has hemiplegic migraines
D. Mistaken for epilepsy
E. May be triggered by head trauma
F. Approximately half of FHM families have chronic progressive cerebellar ataxia.
G. If no family history, then diagnosis is sporadic hemiplegic migraine.

IV. Episodic syndromes ± aura
  A. Formerly known as childhood periodic syndromes, but may be seen in adults
  B. All are characterized by normalcy between episodes
  C. Diagnoses include:
    1. Recurrent gastrointestinal disturbance
       • Attacks of abdominal pain/discomfort and/or nausea/vomiting
    2. Cyclic vomiting syndrome
       • Stereotyped episodic nausea/vomiting ± pallor and lethargy
       • Mainly seen in children
    3. Abdominal migraine (longer lasting and more severe than recurrent gastrointestinal disturbance)
       • Recurrent moderate/severe midline abdominal pain with vasomotor symptoms, nausea/vomiting
       • Lasts 2 to 72 hours
       • Normal between episodes
       • No headache during episode
    4. Benign paroxysmal vertigo
       • Sudden and resolving vertigo, no loss of consciousness
       • At least one of the following: nystagmus, ataxia, vomiting, pallor, fearfulness
    5. Benign paroxysmal torticollis
       • Recurrent head tilt to one side ± slight rotation
       • Usual onset in the first year of life
       • At least one of the following: nystagmus, ataxia, vomiting, pallor, fearfulness
       • Remits spontaneous after minutes-days

Tension-type Headache (TTH)

TTH is the most common type of primary headache, with a lifetime prevalence ranging from 30% to 78%. The ICHD-3 (beta) criteria distinguishes three subtypes: infrequent episodic TTH with headache episodes ≤1 day per month, frequent TTH with headache episodes on 1 to 14 days per month, and chronic TTH with headache ≥15 days per month, perhaps without recognizable episodes. A diagnosis of *probable tension-type headache* can be made when headache fulfills all but one of the criteria for TTH and does not fulfill criteria for migraine without aura.

  I. Infrequent episodic TTH
    A. ≥10 episodes of headache on <1 day per month on average (<12 days per year) and fulfilling criteria B-D
    B. Lasting 30 minutes to 7 days
    C. ≥2 of the following:
      1. Bilateral
      2. Pressing/tightening (non-pulsating) quality
      3. Mild/moderate intensity
      4. Not aggravated by routine physical activity (e.g., walking or climbing)

D. Both of the following:
1. No nausea or vomiting
2. No coincidence of photophobia and phonophobia (may have one or the other)
E. Not better accounted for by another ICHD-3 diagnosis
II. Frequent episodic TTH is ≥10 episodes of headache occurring on 1 to 14 days per month for >3 months on average (≥12 and <180 days per year) and fulfilling criteria B-D shared by infrequent episodic TTH
III. Chronic TTH is headache occurring ≥15 per month for >3 months on average (≥180 days per year) and fulfilling criteria B-D shared by infrequent episodic TTH

Trigeminal Autonomic Cephalalgias

This group of primary headache disorders is characterized by trigeminal activation coupled with parasympathetic activation.
I. Cluster Headache
The prevalence is ~1 in 500 individuals, and it is approximately three times more prevalent in men than women with no significant differences in clinical presentation. Onset typically occurs after age 30. Patients usually experience *cluster periods* (on average, one or two 6- to 12-week periods per year) alternating between longer periods of remission. During a cluster period, there is usually 1 to 3 attacks in a 24-hour period. It commonly wakes people from sleep. Approximately 90% of patients have this episodic form. The remainder suffer from the chronic form, during which cluster periods last for more than 1 year without remission or with remission periods lasting <1 month.
A. ≥5 attacks fulfilling B-D
B. Severe or very severe unilateral orbital, supraorbital, and/or temporal pain lasting 15 to 180 minutes (untreated)
C. ≥1 of the following:
1. ≥1 of the following ipsilateral to the headache:
   • Conjunctival injection and/or lacrimation, nasal congestion and/or rhinorrhea, eyelid edema, forehead and facial sweating/flushing, sensation of fullness in the ear, miosis and/or ptosis
2. Sense of restlessness or agitation
D. Attacks frequency Q48 hours to 8× per day for more than half of the time when the disorder is active
II. Paroxysmal hemicrania
May differentiate between episodic (attack periods of 7 days to 1 year, separated by pain-free periods ≥1 month) and chronic where paroxysms occur for ≥1 year without remission or with remission period of <1 month.
A. ≥20 attacks fulfilling B-E
B. Severe unilateral orbital, supraorbital, and/or temporal pain lasting 2 to 30 minutes

    C. ≥ 1 of the following:
- Conjunctival injection and/or lacrimation, nasal congestion and/or rhinorrhea, eyelid edema, forehead and facial sweating/flushing, sensation of fullness in the ear, miosis and/or ptosis

    D. Attack frequency ≥ 5 per day for more than half of the time

    E. Attacks are prevented absolutely by therapeutic doses of indomethacin

III. Short-lasting unilateral neuralgiform headache attacks

    A. ≥ 20 attacks fulfilling B-D

    B. Moderate/severe unilateral head pain, with orbital, supraorbital, temporal, and/or other trigeminal distribution, lasting 1 to 600 seconds and occurring as a stabbing pain (single/series) or in a saw-tooth pattern

    C. ≥ 1 of the following ipsilateral to the pain:
- Conjunctival injection and/or lacrimation, nasal congestion and/or rhinorrhea, eyelid edema, forehead and facial sweating/flushing, sensation of fullness in the ear, miosis and/or ptosis

    D. Attack frequency ≥ 1 per day for more than half of the time when the disorder is active

Within this headache type, there are *short-lasting unilateral neuralgiform headache attacks with conjunctival injection and tearing* (SUNCT) and *short-lasting unilateral neuralgiform headache attacks with cranial autonomic symptoms* (SUNA), both of which may be episodic (attacks periods lasting 7 days to 1 year, separated by pain-free periods lasting ≥ 1 month) or chronic (attack periods >1 year without remission or with remission lasting <1 month). SUNCT headaches are accompanied by both conjunctival injection and lacrimation, while SUNA headaches may be accompanied by one or neither of these. A diagnosis of *hemicrania continua* can be made when present for >3 months with exacerbations of moderate or greater intensity. This condition is also absolutely responsive to indomethacin.

Other Primary Headache Disorders

This group of miscellaneous primary headache disorders includes some mimics of potentially serious secondary headaches, which need to be carefully evaluated by imaging or other appropriate tests. Diagnosis of these headaches may only be made in the absence of any intracranial disorder.

    I. Primary cough headache

        Precipitated by coughing or other Valsalva maneuver, but not by prolonged physical exercise. Neuroimaging, with special attention to the posterior fossa and base of the skull, is mandatory to rule out secondary forms of cough headache. Normally occurs over the age of 50.

    II. Primary exercise headache

        Precipitated by any form of exercise. Normally alleviates when exertion is finished. Typically occurs under the age of 50.

    III. Primary headache associated with sexual activity

    A. Usually starts as dull bilateral ache and lasts 1 minute to 24 hours with severe intensity and/or up to 72 hours with mild intensity.

    B. ≥ 1 of the following

      1. Increasing headache intensity with increasing sexual excitement

      2. Abrupt explosive intensity just before or with orgasm

  C. With the first episode it is mandatory to rule out secondary causes such as subarachnoid hemorrhage and reversible cerebrovascular vasoconstriction syndrome.

IV. Primary thunderclap headache

  A. High-intensity headache of abrupt onset (<1 minute to max intensity).

  B. Lasts ≥ 5 minutes

  C. Important alternate diagnoses to rule out include:

- Subarachnoid hemorrhage, unruptured vascular malformation (mostly aneurysm), cerebral venous sinus thrombosis, cervicocephalic arterial dissection, pituitary apoplexy, acute hypertensive crisis, spontaneous intracranial hypotension, meningitis, embolic cerebellar infarcts, colloid cyst of the third ventricle, and reversible cerebral vasoconstriction syndromes.

V. Cold-stimulus headache

- Generalized headache following exposure of unprotected head to a very low environmental temperature. Resolves within 30 minutes after removal of cold stimulus.

VI. External-pressure headache

- Results from sustained compression of or traction on pericranial soft tissues. Common catalysts include headbands, hats, helmets, goggles, and wearing hair in a ponytail. Resolves within 1 hour of compression/traction cessation.

VII. Primary stabbing headache

- Spontaneous transient and localized stabs of pain in the head that last up to a few seconds and occur with irregular frequency from one to many times per day.

VIII. Nummular headache

- Highly variable duration of pain that is often chronic in a small circumscribed scalp area, which is sharply contoured, fixed in size and shape, round/elliptical, and 1 to 6 cm in diameter.

IX. Hypnic headache

- Recurrent headaches occurring only during sleep, resulting in wakening on ≥ 10 days per month for >3 months and lasting 15 minutes to 4 hours after wakening without autonomic symptoms or restlessness, which differentiates these headaches from cluster headaches.

X. New daily persistent headache

- Patients typically remember the day their headache began from which point it has not ceased. Characteristics may be similar to migraine, TTH, or both. Must be present for >3 months to diagnose. Two isoforms include a self-limiting (resolves within months without therapy) and refractory form that is resistant to therapy.

HEADACHE THERAPY

Three components of a systematic approach to treating headache are psychological, physical, and pharmacologic. Psychological therapy involves reassurance and counseling, as well as stress management, relaxation therapy, and biofeedback as appropriate. Physical therapy involves identifying headache triggers, such as diet, hormone variations, and stress, and whether alteration may be helpful in treating selected cases. The patient should record a headache calendar documenting the occurrence, severity, and duration of headaches; the type and efficacy of medication taken; and any triggering factors. Pharmacotherapy can be divided into two approaches: abortive and prophylactic.

Abortive (Acute) Therapy of Migraine

Migraine-specific agents (e.g., triptans, dihydroergotamine [DHE], ergotamine) are used in patients with more severe migraine and in those whose headaches respond poorly to nonsteroidal anti-inflammatory drugs (NSAIDs) or combination of analgesics. Select a non-oral route of administration for patients whose migraines present early with significant nausea or vomiting.

I. Routine analgesics (aspirin, acetaminophen, and NSAIDs, including ibuprofen, naproxen, indomethacin, etc.) are given for less severe headaches. Ketorolac may be used for more severe headaches.

II. Triptans (oral, intranasal, subcutaneous injection)
   A. Good first-line therapy for severe migraine
   B. Contraindicated in pregnancy, patients with hemiplegic migraine, or migraine with brainstem aura, or those with uncontrolled hypertension, prior stroke, or MI.
   C. Examples: almotriptan, eletriptan, frovatriptan, naratriptan, rizatriptan, sumatriptan, zolmitriptan.
   D. If symptoms persist after first dose, a second dose 2 hours later may/ may not be beneficial.

III. Narcotic analgesics should be avoided (especially as first-line treatment) but useful for occasional, severe headaches.

IV. Ergotamine (oral form less effective than rectal or parenteral administrations)
   A. Less commonly used
   B. Contraindicated in pregnancy
   C. Dosing strategy
      1. Oral
         • Symptom recognition: Ergotamine tartrate 2 mg by mouth
         • 1 hour later: Repeat first dose with an oral analgesic-caffeine combination
      2. Rectal
         • Aura onset: 1 to 2 mg rectal suppository of ergotamine tartrate
         • 1 hour later: Repeat first dose

TABLE 71

TYPICAL EMERGENCY DEPARTMENT TREATMENT PROTOCOL FOR SEVERE HEADACHE

Steps to be followed in succession separated by 15–20 min

1. IV fluids (normal saline 2–3 L bolus or 80–100 cc/hr while patient is in emergency department)
2. IV diphenhydramine 12.5–25 mg
3. IV metoclopramide or prochlorperazine 10 mg
4. IV magnesium sulfate 500–1000 mg
5. IV ketorolac 30 mg
6. If no improvement:
   - IV sodium valproate (500 mg), IV levetiracetam (500 mg), or IV methylprednisolone (200 mg)
7. IV dihydroergotamine 0.5–1.0 mg if patient has not used a triptan within 24 hr and no contraindications exist

From Rozen, T. D. (2009). Trigeminal autonomic cephalgias. *Neurol Clin, 27*, 537–556.

H

3. Dihydroergotamine (intravenous, intramuscular, subcutaneous, nasal spray) (Table 71)
   - 0.5 mg or 1 mg dose at onset that may be repeated 1 hour later not to exceed 3 mg in a 24-hour period.

V. For nausea/vomiting
   A. Metaclopramide is a good option if nausea/vomiting are a significant symptom (10 mg IM, IV, or PO 15 minutes before other analgesic agents)
   B. Prochlorperazine 25 mg IM, IV, supp
   C. Chlorpromazine 12.5 to 50 mg IM, IV, supp (obtain ECG prior for baseline QTc interval)

VI. Single-pulse transcranial magnetic stimulation (currently used only for migraine with aura)

VII. Status migrainosus
   A. Neuroleptic agents ± dihydroergotamine
   B. Magnesium sulfate 1 g IV infusion (administered in hospital setting; more helpful in migraine with aura)
   C. IV fluids for dehydrated patients
   D. Prednisolone 20 mg IV Q6 hours followed by 2- to 3-day tapering

Prophylactic Treatment of Migraine

I. Avoid inciting dietary factors such as red wine, aged cheese, chicken liver, pickled herring, tuna, sour cream/yogurt, ripe avocado, banana, smoked meats, and foods with monosodium glutamate or nitrates.
II. Eat regular balanced meals avoiding periods of hunger
III. Good sleep hygiene and regular exercise
IV. Pharmacologic therapy should be considered for those with frequent or disabling attacks.

A. Beta blockers
1. Propranolol, 20 mg PO BID and gradually increasing PRN to 80 mg TID
2. Others
   - Nadolol 80 to 240 mg/day
   - Atenolol 50 to 100 mg/day
B. Antidepressants
1. Tricyclics
   - Amitriptyline, nortriptyline, imipramine, desipramine (10–150 mg nightly at bedtime)
2. Venlafaxine (37.5 mg daily for 3 days with target 75–150 mg daily based on tolerability)
C. Antiepileptics
1. Valproic acid (250 mg BID titrated up PRN to 1 g/day). Avoid in women of reproductive age.
2. Gabapentin (100 mg TID or 300 mg QHS and titrate PRN to 2400 mg/day)
3. Topiramate (Initial: 25 mg BID; gradual titration 15–25 mg/week to 75–200 mg/day)
D. Calcium channel blockers
1. Verapamil (80–160 mg TID)
2. Others such as nifedipine, diltiazem, and nimodipine may be considered but evidence supporting efficacy is lacking.
E. Methysergide
1. This serotonin antagonist no longer available in USA or Canada
F. Others
1. Riboflavin (400 mg/day)
2. Magnesium (600 mg/day PO)
3. Aspirin (325 mg/day PO)
4. Onabotolinumtoxin A injection (only Food and Drug Administration [FDA] treatment approved for chronic migraine)
   - Doses of ≥150 mg are injected into forehead, temporalis, occipitalis, splenius, capitis, and trapezius.
5. Candesartan (up to 16 mg/day)
6. Lisinopril (10–20 mg/day)
7. Transcutaneous supraorbital nerve stimulator
8. PFO closure is NOT recommended with three negative randomized clinical trials (MIST, PIMA, and PREMIUM).

Treatment of Tension-Type Headache
I. Simple analgesics, such as acetaminophen, aspirin, and other NSAIDs are the drugs of choice for abortive therapy.
II. Prophylactic therapy is indicated for patients with chronic headaches requiring daily analgesics.
III. Stress reduction, proper neck posture, and proper sleep hygiene may be helpful.

Treatment of Cluster Headache

I. Abortive therapies
- A. Sumatriptan injection or nasal spray
- B. 100% O_2 by non-rebreather mask at 8 to 15 L/min for 15 to 20 minutes.
- C. Dihydroergotamine: intramuscular, subcutaneous, or intravenous
- D. Ergotamine: oral or suppository
- E. Zolmitriptan: nasal spray or orally (5–10 mg)
- F. 4% Intranasal lidocaine (one spray in nostril ipsilateral to pain; may repeat 10 to 15 minutes later; max: $4 \times$ per day)
- G. Greater occipital nerve blockade
- H. Olanzapine (2.5–10 mg PO per headache; useful if patient cannot use triptans and failed O_2 therapy but sedating)
- I. Chlorpromazine suppository (may use 1–2 25 mg dose)
- J. Indomethacin suppository (50 mg suppository: Q26 minutes up to 150 mg total)
- K. Subcutaneous octreotide (100 μg)

II. Preventative therapies
- A. Verapamil (initial: 80 mg PO TID; 80–960 mg/day; serial electrocardiograms necessary with doses >480 mg)
- B. Lithium carbonate (300–900 mg)
- C. Divalproex sodium extended release (500–3000 mg)
- D. Topiramate (50–400 mg although typical doses are ≤75 mg)
- E. Melatonin (9 mg QHS)

Treatment for Indomethacin-Responsive Headaches

Indomethacin 25 to 500 mg daily as for primary exercise, cough, and stabbing headaches. For hemicranias continua and paroxysmal hemicranias dosing is 25 to 50 mg TID as preventative.

Treatment of Chronic Daily and Medication Overuse Headache

I. Discontinue the offending medications, especially analgesics used to excess (tapering may be necessary).
II. Lifestyle modifications: exercise, eliminate caffeine consumption, and maintain consistent mealtime/sleep schedules
III. Treat potential coexisting mood disorders and sleep disturbances
IV. Relaxation techniques and biofeedback
V. Inpatient programs for chronic refractory patients

REFERENCES

Probyn, K., Bowers, H., Caldwell, F., et al. (2017). Prognostic factors for chronic headache: a systematic review. *Neurology, 89*(3), 291–301.

Scher, A. I., Rizzoli, P. B., & Loder, E. W. (2017). Medication overuse headache: an entrenched idea in need of scrutiny. *Neurology, 89*(12), 1296–1304.

H

HEADACHE: MIGRAINE AND OTHER TYPES

HEARING

I. Office testing of hearing should include examination of the external ear and the tympanic membranes. Auditory acuity can be grossly assessed by whispering into each ear while closing the other and by comparing the distance from the ear at which the patient and the examiner can hear a ticking watch or fingers rubbing together. Tuning fork tests are commonly used. In the *Weber test*, a 256-Hz tuning fork is placed at the midline vertex of the skull; sound referred to an ear with decreased acuity indicates conductive hearing loss. In the *Rinne test*, a tuning fork placed on the mastoid and one held in front of the ear are compared; if bone conduction is greater, conductive loss is implied. Note that tuning forks are uncalibrated and are inadequate for general screening for hearing loss.

II. Audiologic tests are used to quantitate and localize (conductive vs. sensorineural) hearing loss. Pure-tone audiogram determines auditory threshold for tones over various frequencies and intensities for both air and bone conduction. Impairment of both air and bone conduction, especially at high frequencies, indicates sensorineural hearing loss. When bone conduction is greater than air conduction, conductive hearing loss is present. Hearing is considered normal between 0 dB and 25 dB, mild hearing loss between 21 dB and 40 dB, moderate loss between 41 dB and 55 dB, moderately severe between 56 dB and 70 dB, severe between 71 dB and 90 dB, and profound above 90 dB. Other tests of loudness function are the alternate binaural loudness balance and the short-increment sensitivity index. Bekesy audiometry, tone decay tests, speech discrimination tests, the stapedius reflex (pathway from cochlea to eighth cranial nerve to facial nerve to stapedius muscle), and brainstem auditory evoked potentials (BAEPs) help distinguish conductive from sensorineural hearing loss. Rarely, cortical deafness or auditory agnosia occur with bitemporal lesions, and BAEPs are normal.

III. Causes of conductive hearing loss

    A. External ear: Congenital atresia, acquired auditory canal stenosis, trauma, chronic external otitis, osteoma or exostosis, otitis externa, external canal neoplasm

    B. Tympanic membrane: Tympanosclerosis, perforation, thickened tympanic membrane

    C. Middle ear: Otitis media, congenital ossicular abnormality, cholesteatoma, middle ear effusion, trauma, tumors, osteosclerosis, superior semicircular canal dehiscence

    D. Combined external and/or middle ear abnormalities: Treacher Collins syndrome, Pierre Robin syndrome, Crouzon disease, Apert syndrome, Goldenhar syndrome, Turner syndrome

IV. Causes of sensorineural hearing loss

    A. Chronic loud noise exposure

    B. Infections: viral (measles, mumps, cytomegalovirus), bacterial (syphilis, Lyme disease), meningitis

C. Vascular: vertebrobasilar ischemia and inferior lateral pontine infarction or basilar occlusion
D. Demyelinating disease
E. Congenital malformations: Arnold-Chiari, Klippel-Feil syndromes
F. Degenerative diseases: Hereditary ataxias, hereditary neuropathies; Refsum disease, xeroderma pigmentosum, Cockayne syndrome, Usher syndrome (retinitis pigmentosa and deafness), and other rare hereditary degenerative disorders
G. Ototoxicity: Aminoglycosides, quinine, salicylates, cisplatinum
H. Inflammatory: Vogt-Koyanagi-Harada syndrome, Behçet syndrome; sarcoidosis
I. Mitochondrial diseases: Kearns-Sayre syndrome

REFERENCE

Douglas, E. M. (2006). Assessment and management of tinnitus and hearing loss. *Continuum*, *12*(4), 135–150.

HEMIFACIAL SPASM

Hemifacial spasm is a syndrome of involuntary unilateral irregular tonic or clonic movements of the muscles innervated by the ipsilateral facial nerve. The estimated incidence is 0.78/100,000, and it is more common in women than men. Onset is usually between 40 and 50 years of age. Typically, it is a unilateral occurrence, but there are rare cases of bilateral hemifacial spasm.

CLINICAL PRESENTATION

Patients usually present with a complaint of one eye closing involuntarily. In 90% of patients, the orbicularis oculi is the first muscle affected, but eventually, other muscles innervated by the ipsilateral facial nerve also become affected. The resulting spasms occur in all ipsilateral affected muscles synchronously. In about 5% of cases, bilateral facial nerves will be affected; in these cases, the spasms of the right facial muscles are asynchronous with those of the left.

ETIOLOGY

It is presumed to be related to vascular compression of the ipsilateral facial nerve as it emerges from the pons. It is thought that this compression results in demyelination, and that adjacent demyelinated fibers of the facial nerve trigger each other to fire through ephaptic coupling. Several families of hemifacial spasms have been reported to suggest a genetic etiology or predisposition with an autosomal dominant pattern.

CLASSIFICATION

I. Primary or idiopathic hemifacial spasm—No identifiable etiology or hereditary evidence
II. Secondary hemifacial spasm
   • Bell palsy
   • Facial nerve injury—hyperactive facial motor neurons

- Demyelinating lesions
- Brain or vascular insults—brainstem tumors

III. Hemifacial spasm mimickers
- Psychogenic—one of the most common presentations of psychogenic movement disorders
- Facial tics
- Facial myoclonus
- Hemimasticatory spasms

EVALUATION

If the diagnosis is not clear from the history and physical examination, magnetic resonance imaging and magnetic resonance angiography may be helpful, but these studies are neither sensitive nor specific. Vascular abnormalities are seen in 88% of hemifacial spasm patients versus 25% of control subjects. The differential diagnosis includes tic disorders, blepharospasm, tardive dyskinesia, and facial myokymia.

TREATMENT

Neurosurgical treatment involves microvascular decompression of the offending artery. This procedure is still done, and has a high success rate. However, some patients do suffer recurrence of symptoms, and ipsilateral hearing loss is a known complication of the surgery.

Recently, the use of botulinum toxin injections has emerged as a nonsurgical treatment. It is widely used, and has a high rate of patient satisfaction. It is not a permanent solution, and injections must be repeated every 3 months. Less than 10% of cases resolve without treatment.

REFERENCES

Tan, N. C., Chan, L. L., & Tan, E. K. (2002). Hemifacial spasm and involuntary facial movements. *Q J Med*, 95(8), 493–500.

Yaltho, T. C., & Jankovic, J. (2011). The many faces of hemifacial spasm: differential diagnosis of unilateral facial spasms. *Mov Disord*, 26(9), 1582–1592.

HERNIATION

The Monro-Kellie doctrine states that intracranial volume consists of brain, blood, and cerebrospinal fluid contained within a fixed space in the skull. Subsequently, when one of these three intracranial components increases in size, or an additional component (i.e., tumor) is added, then changes in intracranial pressure (ICP) occur and may result in herniation, which is the displacement of the cerebral or cerebellar structures from their normal compartments. Most commonly, increased pressure is due to a focal lesion (i.e., tumor with cerebral edema, extra/intra-axial hemorrhage, infarct, or abscess). Some diffuse elevations of ICP, such as pseudotumor cerebri, rarely produce herniation. Other conditions produce diffuse cerebral edema, elevated

ICP, and frequent herniation (i.e., hepatic coma, meningoencephalitis, hypoxic brain injury, diffuse traumatic brain injury).

HERNIATION SYNDROMES

I. Transtentorial herniation
   a. Descending, Unilateral (Uncal): Usually occurring rapidly and from a temporal lobe mass, it pushes the uncus and hippocampal gyrus over the edge of tentorium, entrapping the oculomotor nerve and later directly compressing the midbrain. The posterior cerebral arteries may be pinched on the tentorium and cause occipital infarction (as with central herniation).
      - Kernohan notch phenomenon: Defined as ipsilateral/contralateral hemiparesis due to compression of the cerebral peduncle by the uncus, which may impinge the adjacent cerebral peduncle or push the midbrain, causing impingement of the opposite cerebral peduncle. Therefore, laterality of hemiparesis may be false-localizing.
   b. Descending, Bilateral (Central): Most often seen in the setting of a diffuse cerebral edema, a downward displacement of cerebral hemispheres and basal nuclei compresses/displaces the diencephalon and midbrain through a tentorial notch.
   c. Ascending: It is occasionally seen with posterior fossa masses and may be exacerbated by ventriculostomy. It can cause hydrocephalus and occlusion of the superior cerebellar arteries with sylvian aqueduct compression, leading to cerebellar infarctions.
II. Subfalcine (Cingulate): It is often asymptomatic and precedes central/transtentorial herniation. Protrusion of the cingulate gyrus under the falx cerebri can lead to bifrontal infarctions when anterior cerebral arteries become compromised.
III. Tonsillar: Cerebellar tonsils descend through the foramen magnum and compress the medulla and upper cervical cord. May be precipitated by a lumbar puncture in the presence of intracranial mass lesions.

These syndromes are accompanied by characteristic clinical signs that correspond to the anatomic structures involved (Table 72). Decreased level of consciousness or coma is usually the first clinical finding. There is a rostral-caudal progression of clinical signs seen with descending transtentorial herniation, indicating worsening herniation (Table 73). This begins with diencephalic involvement, followed by mesencephalic, pontine, and finally medullary involvement. Two infrequent exceptions to this orderly progression, in which signs skip from the hemispheres or diencephalon to the medulla, bypassing the rostral brainstem, are as follows: (1) acute cerebral hemorrhage, with extravasation into the ventricles, compresses the medullary respiratory center in the floor of the fourth ventricle and (2) a lumbar puncture is performed on patients with incipient transtentorial herniation, possibly inducing enough of a pressure gradient change to produce tonsillar herniation.

For treatment of herniation, see ICP.

H

HERNIATION

TABLE 72

HERNIATION SYNDROMES

Syndrome	Signs/Symptoms
Transentorial	
Descending, Unilateral (Uncal)	Ipsilateral pupil dilation, external ophthalmoplegia, contralateral hemiparesis, decerebrate posturing, variable impairment in consciousness
Descending, Bilateral (Central)	Medium sized and fixed pupils, early coma, decorticating posturing, Cheyenne-Stokes respiration, diabetes insipidus
Ascending	Nausea/vomiting, progressive stupor
Subfalcine (Cingulate)	Miotic reactive pupils, headache, contralateral leg paralysis
Tonsillar	Hypertension/bradycardia/bradypnea, coma, respiratory arrest, bilateral arm dysesthesia

REFERENCES

Berger, J. R. (2016). Stupor and coma. In R. B. Daroff, J. Jankovic, J. C. Mazziotta, & S. L. Pomeroy (Eds.), *Bradley's neurology in clinical practice,* ed 7 (pp. 34–50). Philadelphia: Elsevier.

Posner, J. B., Saper, C. B., Schiff, N., & Plum, F. (2007). *Diagnosis of stupor and coma,* ed 3. New York: Oxford Press.

HICCUPS (SINGULTUS, HICCOUGHS)

Hiccups, as they are generally called, are involuntary repetitive myoclonic contractions of the diaphragm with forceful inspiration. They are associated with laryngeal spasm and closure of the glottis, which produces the characteristic sound. Singultus is mediated by the phrenic (afferent), vagus and the thoracic nerves (efferent).

Neurologic causes include lesions around the area postrema, which include immune-mediated conditions (e.g., multiple sclerosis), infection (brainstem encephalitis), hypothalamic disease (also associated with yawning), tumors of the fourth ventricle, and cerebrovascular disease. Nonneurologic causes include gastrointestinal (reflux, achalasia, abscess, abdominal tumors, hiatal hernia), metabolic (electrolyte disturbances, uremia, diabetes), drugs (ethanol, glucocorticoids, dopamine agonists, chemotherapy, opioids, benzodiazepines, barbiturates, sulfonamides, macrolides), pulmonary or pleural irritation or malignancy, pericarditis, mediastinitis and mediastinal mass, intrathoracic abscess or tumor, and aortic aneurysms. Chronic idiopathic and psychogenic hiccups also occur. Those with persistent or refractory singultus should undergo diagnostic evaluation.

Treatment: There are no high-quality data to guide treatment, but options include treatment of the underlying condition, and various medications including valproic acid, baclofen, gabapentin, pregabalin, metoclopramide, dopamine blockers, phenytoin, carbamazepine, and benzodiazepines.

TABLE 73

ROSTRAL-CAUDAL PROGRESSION OF TRANSTENTORIAL HERNIATION

	Early Diencephalic	Late Diencephalic	Midbrain-Upper Pons	Low Pons-Upper Medulla	Medulla
Consciousness, systemic	Decreased alertness, confusion	Drowsiness, stupor, coma	Comatose	Comatose	Comatose; fluctuating pulse and blood pressure
Breathing, respirations	Eupneic with deep signs or yawns; Cheyne-Stokes	Cheyne-Stokes	Sustained regular hyperventilation; rarely, Cheyne-Stokes	Eupneic but more rapid/shallow or ataxia	Irregular/slow, gasping quality
Pupils	Small but reactive pupils	Small but reactive pupils	Midposition, often irregular, fixed	Midposition, fixed	Dilated, fixed
Eye movements	Conjugate or divergent if patient not awake. ± roving. VOR and CCT normal	Conjugate or divergent if patient not awake. ± roving. VOR and CCT normal	VOR and CCT: impaired, may be dysconjugate	VOR and CCT: no response	VOR and CCT: no response
Motor	Appropriate response to noxious stimuli; diffuse paratonia/gegenhalten; ± extensor plantar responses	Pain response may disappear or decorticate response. Initial decorticate posture is contralateral to lesion progress to bilateral.	Motionless at rest. Decerebrate posturing (contra > ipsilateral to lesion)	Motionless/flaccid, no response to noxious stimuli; bilateral lower triple flexion	Motionless/flaccid, no response to noxious stimuli; bilateral lower triple flexion

CCT, Cold caloric testing; VOR, vestibulo-ocular reflex.

HICCUPS (SINGULTUS, HICCOUGHS)

H

REFERENCES

Moretto, E. N., Wee, B., Wiffen, P. J., & Murchison, A. G. (2013). Interventions for treating persistent and intractable hiccups in adults. *Cochrane Database Syst Rev*,(1). CD008768.

Steger, M., Schneemann, M., & Fox, M. (2015). Systemic review: the pathogenesis and pharmacological treatment of hiccups. *Aliment Pharmacol Ther*, *42*, 1037–1050.

HORNER SYNDROME, COCAINE TEST

I. Pathophysiology: Horner syndrome (oculosympathetic paresis) is due to disruption at any point along the course of the sympathetic pathway from the hypothalamus to the orbit (Fig. 31). Signs are ipsilateral pupillary miosis (resulting from iris dilator weakness) most evident in dim illumination, blepharoptosis (minor, <2 mm, weakness of Müller muscle), and facial anhidrosis. Slight elevation of the lower lid (so-called "upside-down ptosis") is sometimes present, and is best appreciated when the upper eyelid is in the resting position. Other symptoms sometimes seen include pseudoenophthalmos (the impression that the eye is sunken, caused by a narrow palpebral aperture), loss of the ciliospinal reflex (dilation of the ipsilateral pupil in response to pain applied to the neck, face, and upper trunk), pupillary dilation lag (an asymmetry in pupillary redilation between the two eyes when the light source is moved away from the eye), and conjunctival hyperemia (a transient early sign of acute Horner syndrome due to sympathetic denervation and vasodilatation that is rarely present after the first few weeks). Heterochromia of the iris occurs in congenital Horner syndrome.

II. Etiology: The cause of Horner syndrome can be determined in about 60% of cases. Lesions of the first-order neuron (central) are myriad and may be due to stroke, tumor, syringomyelia, and demyelinating disease. Second-order neuron (preganglionic) causes include apical lung tumor, thyroid lesions, tuberculosis, radical neck dissection, trauma, and neck masses. Third-order neuron (postganglionic) lesions include internal carotid aneurysms, carotid dissection, cavernous sinus lesion, cluster headaches, and migraine, and do not have anhidrosis. The sympathetic fibers responsible for facial sweating and vasodilation branch off at the superior cervical ganglion from the remainder of the oculosympathetic pathway; thus, anhidrosis is not a feature of postganglionic or third-order lesions.

III. Evaluation: Cocaine (4% or 10%) eye drops are used to differentiate subtle Horner syndrome from simple anisocoria on a pharmacologic basis. Cocaine works by preventing norepinephrine reuptake at sympathetic nerve endings; the eyedrops cause normal pupils to dilate. Lesions of any part of the sympathetic pathway cause failure of pupillary dilation because of lack of norepinephrine at the nerve terminal. The day after confirming with topical cocaine, hydroxyamphetamine (no longer commercially available) or pholedrine can be used to distinguish central and preganglionic from postganglionic sympathetic lesions. This causes

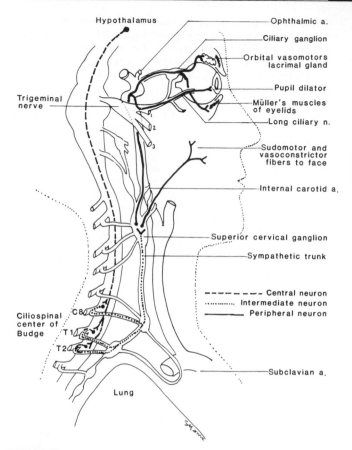

Hypothalamus

Ophthalmic a.

Ciliary ganglion

Orbital vasomotors
lacrimal gland

Pupil dilator

Müller's muscles
of eyelids

Long ciliary n.

Trigeminal
nerve

Sudomotor and
vasoconstrictor
fibers to face

Internal carotid a.

Superior cervical ganglion

Sympathetic trunk

– – – – – – Central neuron
.... Intermediate neuron
––––––––– Peripheral neuron

Ciliospinal
center of
Budge

C8

T1

T2

Subclavian a.

Lung

FIGURE 31

Oculosympathetic pathways.

mydriasis by releasing norepinephrine from the synaptic terminal, but only if the third-order neuron is intact.

Apraclonidine, a direct alpha-adrenergic receptor agonist, has been proposed as an alternative to cocaine in confirming the diagnosis of Horner syndrome. Apraclonidine has weak alpha-1 and strong alpha-2 activity; the former mediates pupillary dilation, while the latter downregulates norepinephrine release at the neuromuscular junction. In a Horner pupil, denervation supersensitivity to the alpha-1 receptor will cause that pupil to dilate (usually by about 2 mm), while alpha-2 stimulation in the normal eye will cause that pupil to constrict slightly (usually by <1 mm). Thus, one to two drops of 0.5% apraclonidine instilled in both eyes causes a reversal of anisocoria in patients with Horner syndrome. Comparison testing in small series of patients suggests that this test compares favorably with cocaine in the diagnosis of Horner syndrome.

Evaluation for central and preganglionic lesions should include careful neck palpation, apical lordotic chest x-ray views, and possibly computed tomography (CT) of the neck and chest. New-onset postganglionic Horner syndrome suggests carotid artery disease; an axial magnetic resonance imaging (MRI) of the neck with T1-weighted, fat-suppressed sequences and magnetic resonance angiography (MRA) will detect most internal carotid artery dissections. However, conventional angiography remains the gold standard. A Horner syndrome with accompanying ophthalmoparesis, particularly involving the sixth cranial nerve with no other brainstem signs, should focus the neuroimaging study (usually MRI) on the cavernous sinus. Isolated postganglionic Horner syndrome is generally benign. A new Horner syndrome in a child without obvious birth or other traumatic association should initiate an evaluation for tumor, particularly neuroblastoma. Because localization through pharmacologic testing can be incorrect and misleading, imaging of the entire sympathetic pathway is warranted if the accuracy of localization cannot be ensured. Imaging studies to consider include MRI brain, CT chest, and for carotids, an ultrasound, CT angiogram, or MRA.

IV. Treatment: Treatment should be directed at underlying disease. Blepharoptosis may be corrected surgically or with topical phenylephrine drops.

REFERENCES

Koc, F., Kavuncu, S., Kansu, T., et al. (2005). The sensitivity and specificity of 0.5% apraclonidine in the diagnosis of oculosympathetic paresis. *Br J Ophthalmol*, *89*, 1442.

Reede, D. L., Garcon, E., Smoker, W. R., et al. (2008). Horner syndrome: clinical and radiographic evaluation. *Neuroimaging Clin N Am*, *18*(2), 369–385.

HUNTINGTON DISEASE

PATHOLOGY OF HUNTINGTON DISEASE

Huntington disease (HD) is an autosomal dominant, neurodegenerative disease that belongs to the family of polyglutamine diseases (e.g., Kennedy disease, dentatorubropallidoluysian atrophy, and several spinocerebellar ataxias). It is a trinucleotide repeat disease and occurs when the CAG nucleotide (glutamine) sequence in the *huntingtin (HTT)* gene is repeated greater than 35 times, leading to a mutant genotype. While research is ongoing, the HTT protein is thought to participate in myriad cell processes, including cell trafficking, mitosis, and neurotoxicity prevention. The mHTT phenotype disrupts these processes, causing neurodegeneration to medium, spiny neurons in the caudate and putamen, as well as neurotransmitter disruption, particularly to dopamine, glutamate, and GABA. This leads to symptoms of motor, cognitive, and psychiatric disturbance.

CLINICAL HUNTINGTON DISEASE
While motor symptoms are perhaps best associated with HD, they typically trail behavioral and cognitive symptoms by up to a decade. The earliest symptoms are typically psychiatric; there is frontal lobe inhibition (impulsivity, emotional lability, and severe irritability) that progresses to abulia, loss of apathy, and emotional blandness. Cognitively, patients experience difficulties in executive tasks early on, progressing to a subcortical dementia (patients can recall memory items if cued, unlike in cortical dementia). Motor symptoms begin with choreiform/hyperkinetic movements with later development of hypokinesis, dystonia, and dysphagia, leading to aspiration pneumonia, and death.

EPIDEMIOLOGY
There is a prevalence of 5 to 10 per 100,000 individuals, with typical age of onset ranging from 30 to 50 years old, and an average duration from onset to death of 15 years. Men and women are equally affected. Anticipation is observed; there is earlier presentation and increased phenotypic severity with a greater number of CAG repeats: greater than 40 repeats causes full penetrance in adults, greater than 50 repeats presents between 20 and 30 years old, and greater than 60 repeats is associated with onset between 10 and 20 years old (juvenile HD), which is typically paternally transmitted. These patients often present with a more rapid course, which has the characteristics of rigidity, myoclonus, dystonia, and seizures more evident than chorea.

DIAGNOSIS AND TREATMENT
Diagnosis is primarily based on clinical symptomatology and a family history of disease. DNA testing can confirm the diagnosis, and computed tomography (CT) and magnetic resonance imaging (MRI) can reveal cortical and caudate nucleus atrophy. There is no treatment to delay onset or to forestall progression, but genetic counseling can play a role in family planning. Advances in gene therapy hold promise for future treatment and prevention by silencing mutant genes, thereby preventing the death of neuronal circuits and protecting against disease progression. For now, symptom management is key, and the degree of motor, psychiatric, and cognitive impairment should direct the individualization of therapy. Tetrabenazine is indicated for the treatment of chorea, although it can exacerbate concomitant depression and should be closely monitored. Alternatively, haloperidol (1–40 mg/day) and atypical antipsychotics (e.g., quetiapine, olanzapine, risperidone, aripiprazole) have shown effective management of chorea and psychosis, although prolonged use may cause dyskinesia and chorea. Amantadine, riluzole, and high-dose

benzodiazepines are also effective in treating chorea and anxiety. Some trials with antioxidants, antidepressants, and mitochondrial enhancers may be neuroprotective and favorably influence the disease course, although more studies are needed.

REFERENCES

Muller, T. (2017). Investigational agents for the management of Huntington's disease. *Expert Opin Investig Drugs*, *26*(2), 175–185.

Wyant, K. J., Ridder, A. J., & Dayalu, P. (2017). Huntington's disease-update on treatments. *Curr Neurol Neurosci Rep*, *17*(4), 33.

HYDROCEPHALUS

Hydrocephalus, literally "water on the brain," may be divided into obstructive and nonobstructive types, although all types are associated with ventricular enlargement.

Obstructive hydrocephalus is characterized by ventricular enlargement due to an accumulation of cerebrospinal fluid (CSF) under pressure. When present in a young child or infant, head circumference may cross percentile lines as expanding cerebral hemispheres separate sutures.

PATHOGENESIS

Obstruction: the following are common sites of obstruction.

- Foramen of Monroe obstruction results in expansion of the ipsilateral lateral ventricle
- Third ventricle obstruction, commonly due to tumor (e.g., colloid cyst) will cause dilation of both lateral ventricles
- Aqueduct of Sylvius obstruction will result in enlargement of third and both lateral ventricles

An increase of CSF volume within ventricles or a decrease in the rate of absorption may lead to hydrocephalus. Common clinical scenarios include subarachnoid hemorrhage, intraparenchymal hemorrhage, or brain abscess with rupture. Less common are papillomas of choroid plexus with direct overproduction of CSF, but these are usually accompanied by obstruction as well.

CLINICAL CORRELATION

In general, maximal expansion is typically seen in the frontal horns, such that frontal lobe function is affected first. Other than showing an enlarged ventricle, magnetic resonance imaging may be notable for **transependymal flow**, which represents an increase in interstitial fluid in the tissue adjacent to the lateral ventricles best seen on fluid-attenuated inversion recovery (FLAIR) and T2-weighted sequences.

Congenital or infantile hydrocephalus: the cranial bones fuse by the end of the third year. If hydrocephalus develops prior to fusion, head enlargement and diastasis (separation of sutures) may be seen. The skull carries on a typical appearance, in which the inner table may be unevenly thinned and frontal skull prominence with brachiocephaly may be seen. Clinically, the child may present with a tense anterior and posterior fontanelle, is fretful, and often has poor feeding. As hydrocephalus develops, the child may become stuporous and languid with setting-sun eye—the latter of which is due to pressure on the mesencephalic tegmentum and improves with shunting of the lateral and third ventricles. Even with an arrest in hydrocephalus, motor development may be delayed. Occult childhood hydrocephalus occurs after suture closure and may have a delayed presentation with a variable course. It may also appear after minor head trauma.

Acute hydrocephalus may develop with subarachnoid hemorrhage, intraparenchymal hemorrhage with intraventricular extension, and less commonly arteriovenous malformation and tumor. Clinically, patients may present with headache, visual abnormalities, emesis, and depression in mental status. With ongoing hydrocephalus, there may be bilateral Babinski signs, increased tone in lower limbs, and extensor posturing and coma. Papilledema may or may not be present depending on how acutely the hydrocephalus develops. Pupils may progress from normal to roving horizontally to miotic with aligned or bilateral abducens palsy and limited upward gaze. Ultimately, the pupils become dilated, oculocephalic reflex is lost, and limbs become flaccid. Treatment is via ventricular drainage or shunt placement.

H

HYDROCEPHALUS

NORMAL PRESSURE HYDROCEPHALUS

Presentation: a slowly progressive change in gait is usually the earliest clinical manifestation, which is often accompanied by urinary incontinence followed by impairment in mental functioning. Headaches are rarely present, and no papilledema will be seen.

- Gait: characterized by unsteadiness, impaired balance and **shortening of step length** resulting in difficulty with stairs and curbs, and loss of balance when turning. Patients may present with unexplained falls and report subjective weakness and fatigue in legs, though no paresis nor ataxia are found on exam.
- Cognition: frontal lobe dysfunction including apathy, and dullness in thinking and actions.
- Urination: usually the last symptom to develop. This may start as increased urinary urgency and frequency progressing to incontinence and eventually "frontal lobe incontinence" in which the patient may be apathetic to the incontinence.

Diagnosis: disproportionate enlargement of the ventricular system compared to cortical atrophy is the classic finding on imaging. Standardized gait testing, such as the "Get up and Go" test, can quantitate gait impairment. Studies have shown improvement in several neuropsychological tests post shunt, including the Mini Mental State Examination, Rey Auditory Verbal Learning Test (RAVLT), total verbal recall, RAVLT delayed verbal recall, phonemic verbal fluency, and TMT-A (trail-making test A, which looks at psychomotor speed). These tests can be done pre- and postoperatively or after lumbar puncture, which functions as a temporary shunt. The Evans' index, also called a frontal horn ratio, which is defined as the maximal frontal horn ventricular width divided by the transverse inner diameter of the skull, signifies ventriculomegaly if it is 0.3 or greater. Normal pressure hydrocephalus is more likely if the Evans' index exceeds 0.35.

Treatment: ventriculoperitoneal (occasionally ventriculoatrial, ventriculopleural, or lumboperitoneal) shunting using a one-way pressure valve is often employed. Improvement on cognitive and gait testing post-LP are important predictors of shunt success. Shunt valve pressure may need to be lowered below CSF pressure so that shunting will actually occur. In general, shunt failure is common if dementia and long-standing incontinence have developed. An x-ray shunt series can determine if the shunt tubing is in continuity. Over-shunting may result in subdural hematoma formation.

REFERENCES

Peterson, K. A., Savulich, G., Jackson, D., et al. (2016). The effect of shunt surgery on neuropsychological performance in normal pressure hydrocephalus: a systematic review and meta-analysis. *J Neurol, 263*, 1669–1677.

Ropper, A. H., Samuels, M. A., & Klein, J. P. (2014). Disturbances of cerebrospinal fluid, including hydrocephalus, pseudotumor cerebri, and low pressure syndromes. In *Adam and Victor's principles of neurology,* ed 10 (pp. 617–638). China: McGraw-Hill Education.

HYPERVENTILATION

Inspiratory patterns reflect many factors and may provide localizing information.

 I. Involuntary hyperventilation resulting from autonomic hyperactivity of brainstem respiratory centers is rare; hypoxemia, acid-base disorders, cerebrospinal fluid acidosis, increased intracranial pressure, pulmonary disease, drug effects, and voluntary hyperventilation are more common causes.

 II. Voluntary hyperventilation is usually related to anxiety. Symptoms include chest pain, palpitations, dyspnea, lightheadedness, perioral and fingertip numbness or paresthesias, cramps, gastrointestinal distress, insomnia, a feeling of fright, and occasionally syncope. Arterial blood gas levels should show a respiratory alkalosis during an attack. Reproduction of symptoms by hyperventilation is diagnostic.

 III. Posthyperventilation changes: apnea is characterized by an exaggerated apneic response to lowered $Paco_2$ seen with bilateral hemispheric dysfunction. The diagnosis is made when more than 12 seconds of apnea follows 20 to 30 seconds of voluntary hyperventilation (normal response, <10 seconds of apnea). The induction of absence seizures may occur (see Epilepsy for further discussion).

Cheyne-Stokes breathing, central neurogenic hyperventilation, and apneustic and ataxic respirations may occur during coma (see Coma for a discussion of these entities).

REFERENCE

Colice, G. L. (1989). Neurologic disorders and respiration. *Clin Chest Med*, *10*(4), 521–543.

HYPOTONIC INFANT/HYPOTONIA IN INFANCY/FLOPPY INFANT

Hypotonia in infancy is the reduced resistance to passive movement of joints; it can be caused by lesions at any level of the nervous system, including the brain, brain stem, spinal cord, peripheral nerves, neuromuscular junction, and muscle. Patient history and physical examination may help determine the site of dysfunction and identify the cause of the hypotonia (see Figs. 32 and 33).

HISTORY AND PHYSICAL EXAMINATION

History: Specific emphasis should be placed on the following: prenatal toxin/teratogen exposure, maternal diabetes, parental age, decreased fetal movement, polyhydramnios, spontaneous abortion, fetal demise, and family history of neuromuscular disease. Perinatal history of trauma, breech presentation (possibly indicative of poor fetal mobility), maternal fever, difficult delivery, and low Apgar scores are very important in terms of determining onset of hypotonia.

Physical examination: In a classic case, the hypotonic ("floppy") infant assumes a frog-leg posture (hips abducted and externally rotated and the entire length of the limbs in contact with the flat surface). There is decreased resistance to passive movement and marked head lag with traction from the supine position. In horizontal suspension, neck extension is absent, and elbow and knee flexion are minimal. In vertical suspension at the shoulders, hypotonic infants will often slip through your hands.

DETERMINING THE CAUSE (See Table 74)

Cerebral hypotonia: Decreased alertness, poor response to external stimuli, seizures, apnea, dysmorphic features, poor suck or grasp reflex, suppressed brainstem reflexes, and increased or normal deep tendon reflexes in the hypotonic infant suggest central nervous system (CNS) disease.

Anterior horn cell and peripheral hypotonia: Concomitant weakness, hypo/areflexia, and appropriate level of consciousness are more indicative of lesions of the lower motor unit. Muscle fasciculations occur with neuropathy and anterior horn cell disease.

Beyond the neonatal period, hypotonic infants frequently come to medical attention with delay in achieving motor milestones. Assessment of nonmotor-dependent activity, such as social response, smiling, and vocalization, is important in determining associated intellectual delay. Mental retardation in association with hypotonia suggests a CNS origin.

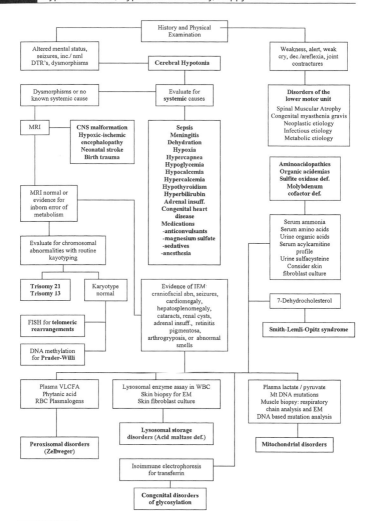

FIGURE 32

Evaluation of the hypotonic infant. *abn*, Abnormal; *DTRs*, deep tendon reflexes; *IEM*, inborn errors of mechanism; *VLCFA*, very long chain fatty acids.

Benign congenital hypotonia is a diagnosis of exclusion, with a generally good prognosis, although some affected children remain clumsy throughout development.

Laboratory studies: Lower motor neuron disease: serum enzyme, EMG, nerve conduction studies (NCS), nerve/muscle biopsy, and genetic analysis.

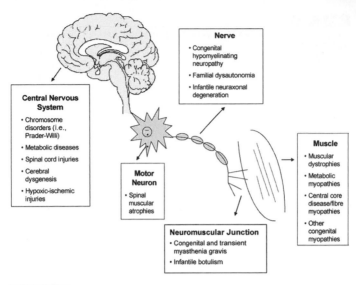

FIGURE 33

Anatomical-clinical correlation illustrating differential diagnosis of hypotonia in infancy. (From Leyenaar, J., Camfield, P., Camfield, C. (2005). A schematic approach to hypotonia in infancy. *Paediatr Child Health*, *10*(7), 397–400, Figure 1).

Upper motor neuron: EEG, evoked potential, brain imaging, specific enzymes, and endocrine evaluations.

CAUSES FOR HYPOTONIA (See Table 75 and Fig. 33).

REFERENCES

Brislin, R. P., & Theroux, M. C. (2013). Core myopathies and malignant hyperthermia susceptibility: a review. *Paediatr Anaesth*, *23*(9), 834–841.

Daroff, R. B., Jankovic, J., & Mazziotta, J. C.et al. (Eds.), (2015). *Bradley's neurology in clinical practice*, ed 7. Elsevier.

TABLE 74

DIFFERENTIATION OF CENTRAL VERSUS PERIPHERAL CAUSES OF CONGENITAL HYPOTONIA

Characteristic	Central	Peripheral
Weakness	Mild to moderate	Significant ("paralytic")
Deep tendon reflexes	Decreased or increased	Absent
Placing reaction	Sluggish	Absent
Motor delays	Yes	Yes
Antigravity movements in prone and supine	Some (less than normal)	Often absent
Pull to sit	Head lag (more than normal)	Marked head lag
Cognition/affect	Delayed	Typical
Ability to "build up" tone, e.g., tapping under knees with infant in supine to assist him/her in holding hips in adduction	Yes	No

From Harris, S. (2008). Congenital hypotonia. *Dev Med Child Neurol, 50*, 889.

TABLE 75

SELECTED CONDITIONS ASSOCIATED WITH HYPOTONIA

- Adrenoleukodystrophy (neonatal)
- Cerebellothalamospinal degeneration
- Fukuyama muscular dystrophy and encephalopathy
- Infantile neuroaxonal dystrophy
- Krabbe disease (globoid cell leukodystrophy)
- Metachromatic leukodystrophy
- Zellweger syndrome

UPPER MOTOR UNIT DISEASE (CENTRAL NERVOUS SYSTEM DISEASES)

- Acute cerebral insult
- Cerebrovascular accident (e.g., hemorrhage, thrombosis, embolism)
- Hypoxic-ischemic encephalopathy
- Infection (e.g., viral, bacterial, fungal, parasitic)
- Chromosomal abnormality
  - Angelman syndrome
  - Down syndrome
  - Prader-Willi syndrome
- Congenital motor disease (cerebral palsy)
  - Ataxia
  - Atonic diplegia or paraplegia (periventricular leukomalacia)
- Incontinentia pigmenti
- Metabolic disease
  - Carnitine deficiency
  - Cytochrome c oxidase deficiency
  - Fucosidosis
  - Gangliosidosis (GM1)

Continued

TABLE 75

SELECTED CONDITIONS ASSOCIATED WITH HYPOTONIA—CONT'D

- Hyperammonemia
- Hypercalcemia
- Hyperglycinemia
- Hyperlysinemia
- Mannosidosis
- Niemann-Pick disease
- Oculocerebrorenal syndrome (Lowe syndrome)
- Organic acidemias
- Renal tubular acidosis
- Tay-Sachs disease (and other GM2 gangliosidoses)
- Toxicity
  - Bilirubin
  - Magnesium
  - Phenobarbital
  - Phenytoin
  - Sedative drugs
- Trauma
  - Brain
  - Cord

LOWER MOTOR UNIT (PERIPHERAL NERVOUS SYSTEM DISEASES)

- Arthrogryposis multiplex congenita
- Carnitine deficiency
- Connective tissue disease, such as Ehlers-Danlos syndrome
- Anterior horn cell
  - Infantile spinal muscular atrophy
  - Kugelberg-Welander disease
  - Poliomyelitis
- Peripheral nerve
  - Familial dysautonomia
  - Guillain-Barré syndrome
  - Hereditary motor-sensory neuropathies
  - Polyneuropathy
- Neuromuscular junction
  - Botulism
  - Myasthenia gravis
  - Myasthenic syndrome
  - Neonatal myasthenia gravis (immune- and nonimmune-mediated forms)
  - Neonatal transient myasthenia gravis
- Muscle
  - Congenital myopathies (e.g., central core disease, congenital fiber type disproportion, myotubular myopathy, nemaline myopathy)
  - Glycogen storage disease (e.g., acid maltase deficiency, phosphofructokinase deficiency, phosphorylase deficiency)
  - Hypothyroidism
  - Myotonic dystrophy
  - Polymyositis

H

Swaiman, K., Phillips, J. (2017). *Swaiman's pediatric neurology*, ed 6. (p. e68, Table 5.1). Philadelphia: Elsevier.

I

IDIOPATHIC INTRACRANIAL HYPERTENSION

Idiopathic intracranial hypertension (IIH) is a disorder of unknown etiology, which is characterized by increased intracranial pressure (ICP). Other names have included benign intracranial hypertension and pseudotumor cerebri. The syndrome of IIH is characterized by clinical signs and symptoms of increased ICP but no evidence of intracranial mass, infection, hydrocephalus, or other apparent structural central nervous system pathology on neuroimaging studies and cerebrospinal fluid (CSF) examination.

EPIDEMIOLOGY

It is most common in obese women of childbearing age, and is more common in hypertensives and during pregnancy. The annual incidence has been estimated to be 3/100,000.

CLINICAL PRESENTATION

Symptoms include headache (84%), transient visual obscurations (69%), pulsatile tinnitus (52%), dizziness (51%), nausea/vomiting, photophobia (48%), neck pain (42%), or diplopia (24%).

Signs include papilledema, cranial nerve (CN) VI palsy, and visual disturbances: contrast sensitivity deficits, color vision loss, constricted visual fields, abnormal automated perimetry, contrast sensitivity defects, and abnormal visual acuity. Blind spot enlargement is characteristic.

ETIOLOGY
Idiopathic by definition

Other causes of generalized intracranial hypertension that are *not idiopathic* include venous sinus thrombosis, endocrinopathies, hyper/hypovitaminosis A, anemia, recent use of certain medications (tetracycline, indomethacin, nalidixic acid, nitrofurantoin, oral contraceptives, lithium), and prolonged use of corticosteroids. Other systemic conditions that mimic aspects of IIH include sleep apnea, pre-eclampsia, chronic obstructive pulmonary disease, right-sided heart failure, uremia, renal failure, systemic lupus erythematosus (SLE), coagulation disorders and hyperthyroidism.

DIAGNOSIS

I. If symptoms (of increased ICP) present, they may only reflect those of *generalized* intracranial hypertension or papilledema.

II. If signs (of increased ICP) present, they may only reflect those of *generalized* intracranial hypertension or papilledema.

III. Documented elevated ICP (>250 mm H_2O) measured in the lateral decubitus position (for adults).

IV. Normal CSF composition.

V. No evidence of hydrocephalus, mass, structural, or vascular lesion on magnetic resonance imaging (MRI) or contrast-enhanced computed tomography for typical patients, and MRI and magnetic resonance venography for all others.

VI. No other cause of intracranial hypertension is identified. Other radiologic findings, which are not part of the formal criteria, include flattening of the posterior aspect of the globe, empty sella, distention of the perioptic nerve sheath, and transverse venous sinus stenosis.

MANAGEMENT

I. Baseline and follow-up neuro-ophthalmologic evaluation includes visual field perimetry, optic disk stereophotographs, visual acuity, and contrast sensitivity testing.

II. In patients with IIH and mild visual loss, the use of acetazolamide (up to a maximum of 4 g/day) with a low-sodium weight-reduction diet compared with diet alone resulted in modest improvement in visual field function. Although usually well tolerated, side effects include metabolic alkalosis, paresthesias of the extremities, liver dysfunction, and allergic reactions. Other medications, such as topiramate or furosemide, may be used.

III. Weight loss is an essential component of management.

IV. Repeated high-volume lumbar punctures may provide relief, and in some cases remission, though this remains controversial.

V. Optic nerve sheath fenestration, venous sinus stenting, ventriculoperitoneal shunting in cases with rapidly progressing visual loss or intractable headaches.

VI. Steroids provide symptomatic relief, but the myriad side effects make these drugs undesirable for chronic treatment.

REFERENCES

Chan, J. W. (2017). Current concepts and strategies in the diagnosis and management of idiopathic intracranial hypertension in adults. *J Neurol*, *264*(8), 1622–1633.

Friedman, D., & Jacobson, D. (2014). Diagnostic criteria for idiopathic intracranial hypertension. *Neurology*, *59*, 1492–1495.

IMMUNIZATION, VACCINATION

Many neurologic symptoms are blamed on antecedent immunizations, but it is difficult to evaluate true causality. A common concern is when patients hear about small studies suggesting causal relationships between a vaccination and a particular disease. Studies and vaccine modification (such as the acellular pertussis vaccine) are ongoing to minimize risk to patients.

Vaccines against the following diseases and infections are currently available:

I. Anthrax: Recent studies among immunized military personnel have shown no increase in disability among those receiving the vaccine.

II. Japanese encephalitis: Acute disseminated encephalomyelitis (ADEM) has been reported to occur after vaccination. Actual incidence is unclear, as several studies show wildly different rates, ranging from 0 cases in 813,000 vaccinations to 1 in 600. Two studies showed incidence rates between 0.2 and 2 in 100,000.

III. *Haemophilus influenzae* type B: no complications have been reported.

IV. Hepatitis B: There has been public concern about increased risk of MS, but this was disproved in a large study.

V. Influenza: There may an increased frequency of Guillain-Barré syndrome (GBS) following influenza vaccination. Incidence of giant cell arteritis may also be increased.

VI. Measles: This vaccine is ordinarily combined with mumps and rubella (MMR) vaccines. Except for febrile seizures in children who are genetically predisposed, neurologic complications are uncommon but controversial. There are case reports of ADEM after measles vaccine, but that risk is very minor compared to the substantially higher risk of ADEM and subacute sclerosing panencephalitis from natural measles. In a very large study, MMR vaccine was shown to have no increase in risk of neurologic complications. A 1998 paper by Wakefield that gave rise to the belief that the MMR vaccine might be associated with increased rates of autism has been discredited and has been retracted by the Lancet.

VII. Meningococcus: There was concern for increased incidence of GBS after receiving the Menactra formulation, but two large safety trials were unable to reproduce this risk.

VIII. Pertussis: The new, acellular pertussis vaccine (diphtheria and tetanus toxoids and pertussis—DTaP) has replaced the diphtheria, tetanus toxoid, and pertussis (DTP) vaccine after many concerns about increased neurologic complications. These complications appear to be much less frequent with the new vaccine. Simple febrile seizures, with no long-term effects, can occur within 24 hours of administration. Autism, epilepsy, and hypotonic/hyporesponsive episodes, all previously related to the DTP vaccine, are much less common now.

IX. *Pneumococcus* conjugate: There is a small increase in the frequency of seizures, usually febrile, in children.

X. Poliomyelitis: Paralytic poliomyelitis is the only known complication of oral polio vaccine (OPV). It is especially a concern for immunodeficient contacts. The inactivated polio vaccine (IPV) is now replacing it in most countries to reduce this risk.

XI. Rabies: Whole-virus vaccines that contain myelin basic protein are associated with ADEM and polyneuritis within 2 weeks after immunization.

XII. Rubella: Transient arthralgias may develop in up to 40% of patients. No causal evidence exists for association with polyneuritis or other neuropathies.

XIII. Toxoids: These vaccines contain antigens from toxins, not from the microbes themselves. Tetanus and diphtheria are the most common and are often given together. Allergic hypersensitivity is the most common (though rare) complication. Demyelinating neuropathy with complete recovery has also been reported.

XIV. Smallpox: Severe, usually transient headaches are common after vaccination.

XV. Varicella: There have not been any serious neurologic complications. The theoretic concern of a shift to more serious adult zoster infections as childhood immunization wanes will be tested in the years to come.

XVI. Human papilloma virus: most common events include headache, nausea, dizziness, and syncope. Rare case reports implicate GBS and ADEM.

XVII. Other agents: Chemical vehicles, preservatives, and contamination have caused complications. Aluminum, commonly in diphtheria, tetanus, and hepatitis A and B vaccines, rarely causes a myofascitis. Mercury was used until 1999 in several preparations. Bovine products carry the risk of prion diseases but have been well monitored in the United States.

REFERENCES

Markovitz, L. E., et al. (2014). Human papillomavirus vaccination: recommendations of the Advisory Committee on Immunization Practices (ACIP). *MMWR Recomm Rep*, *63*, 1–30.

Yih, W. K., et al. (2012). No risk of Guillain-Barré syndrome found after meningococcal conjugate vaccination in two large cohort studies. *Pharmacoepidemiol Drug Saf*, *21*, 1359–1360.

INTRACRANIAL PRESSURE

BASIC CONCEPTS

Normal values of intracranial pressure (ICP) range from 5 to 15 mm Hg (torr), which equals 65 to 200 mm cerebrospinal fluid (CSF) or H_2O (conversion: 1 torr = 13.6 mm H_2O). Factors that determine the level of ICP are the volume of intracranial contents and arterial and venous pressures. After the cranial sutures fuse, the skull becomes an inelastic, closed container with a fixed total intracranial volume consisting of 3 components: brain, CSF, and blood. The *Monroe-Kellie doctrine* states that the sum of intracranial brain tissue, CSF, and blood volumes is constant; therefore, an increase in the volume of one must be compensated by an equal decrease in another compartment. Slow increases in the volume of one compartment can be compensated by decreases in the others, but a rapid rise in ICP is not well tolerated and increases the risk of herniation or the occurrence of global ischemia and is a neurologic emergency. Cerebral perfusion pressure (CPP) is critical to maintain adequate cerebral blood flow (CBF) and is calculated as a difference between mean arterial pressure (MAP) and ICP (CPP = MAP-ICP). CPP less than 50 mm Hg is detrimental to brain function and survival. Following any major cerebral injury, ICP should be maintained as close to normal as possible, to provide a margin of safety. Continuous ICP monitoring provides useful information about "pressure waves" and may be used to guide treatment. Plateau waves, consisting of episodic surges in ICP (sometimes exceeding 450 mm H_2O) can occur several times an hour, especially with pain and iatrogenic maneuvers, such as suctioning, and are associated with increased risk of herniation.

Clinical presentation of increased ICP depends on the underlying process, compartmentalized or diffuse, and whether it is acute or chronic. Manifestations of headache, papilledema, diplopia, or focal signs may occur. *Cushing's triad of bradycardia, hypertension, and slowing of respiration* may occur in patients with significant increased ICP and as such these patients will additionally have a depressed level of consciousness. If there is an element of brainstem compression or involvement of the right insula, patients may develop cardiac arrhythmias, such as atrial fibrillation, nodal and ventricular bradycardia, large T waves, prolonged QT intervals, and changes in ST segments.

CAUSES OF INCREASED INTRACRANIAL PRESSURE

Space-occupying lesions, cerebral edema (cytotoxic edema secondary to brain infarction or vasogenic edema commonly caused by tumor), trauma, intra/extra-axial hemorrhages (hemorrhagic stroke, subarachnoid hemorrhage, subdural hematoma, epidural hematoma), infections, venous sinus thrombosis, and pseudotumor cerebri may increase ICP. An acute rise in blood pressure beyond the autoregulatory curve causes an elevated ICP, as seen in hypertensive encephalopathy; chronic hypertension does not cause a change in ICP. Processes that increase venous pressures cause increases in ICP and include jugular compression (as reflected by *Queckenstedt's test* during LP), superior vena cava obstruction, congestive heart failure (CHF), or Valsalva maneuvers. Postural effects alter the pressures in the intracranial venous sinuses, which in turn alter the CSF pressure.

TREATMENT

I. *General measures:* Patients with clinical evidence of increased ICP can benefit from a few simple interventions. The most critical first step is ensuring adequate cardiopulmonary support, starting with assessment of the patient's airway, breathing, and circulation. Patients with a depressed mental status, indicated by a Glasgow Coma Scale score of less than 8, should be intubated and supported with mechanical ventilation. Elevate the head to 30 to 45 degrees above horizontal with the neck in a straight position to optimize the jugular venous drainage; equalize fluid balance, control fever (hyperthermia markedly increases CBF as a reflection of increased cerebral energy metabolism), and avoid hypotonic IV solutions. Avoid hypotension (SBP < 90 mm Hg); aim for a CPP above 60 mm Hg. If BP control is necessary, use beta blockers and calcium channel blockers, avoiding antihypertensives with known effect of increasing

ICP: nitroprusside or nitropaste. Avoid hypoxia ($Po_2 < 60$ mm Hg) and ventilate to normocarbia (Pco_2 35–40 mm Hg). All patients with clinical concern for increased ICP require emergent neuroimaging once their airway is protected and they are hemodynamically stable. A non-contrasted CT scan is a reasonable initial approach to identify the underlying pathological process to quickly determine if there is a role for neurosurgical intervention. Depending on the results of the CT brain scan, it may be appropriate for the neurosurgeon or neurointensivist to introduce an external ventricular drain (EVD) for treatment of obstructive hydrocephalus. Furthermore, an EVD provides the ability for continuous ICP monitoring as well as therapeutically draining the CSF.

II. Active measures:

A. Hyperventilation can be used as a temporary and rapid intervention for lowering ICP. Hypocarbia results in cerebral vasoconstriction and rapidly decreases ICP. The Pco_2 should be maintained between 30 and 35 mm Hg while additional therapies are considered. Prolonged hyperventilation is not effective.

B. Mannitol is given as a 20% IV solution, 0.5 to 1 g/kg over 15 minutes, and repeated at 3- to 6-hour intervals, and can be infused through a peripheral IV line. Mannitol is best used when ICP can be directly monitored; otherwise, it should be titrated to produce a serum osmolality of 320 to 340 osmol/L. Urine output should be monitored. While using mannitol, clinicians must look out for electrolyte depletion such as hypokalemia, pseudohyponatremia, volume depletion causing hypotension, and causing volume overload in CHF or end-stage renal patients. Volume depletion can be addressed by 1/1 cc urine output/ normal saline replacement. Mannitol may be used in end-stage renal patients who can be dialyzed.

C. Many centers have moved toward using hypertonic saline infusions as the hyperosmolar therapy of choice. Hypertonic saline can be temporarily infused through a peripheral line at 2% while central access is obtained. A bolus dose of 23.4% saline can be given through a central line, followed by continuous 3% infusion with frequent draws of serum sodium levels every 4 to 6 hours while the rate of infusion is being determined. Goal sodium is 155 to 160. Patients will typically benefit from hyperosmolar therapy for 3 days, after which point the therapy should be *weaned* to permit the levels to drift back to normonatremia. Do not rapidly correct the hypernatremia as this may precipitate central pontine myelinolysis.

D. Glucocorticoids are used in controlling brain edema associated with brain tumors and meningitis. Dexamethasone 0.15 mg/kg every 6 hours for 2 to 4 days should be started 10 to 20 minutes prior to or along with the first dose of antibiotics when treating bacterial meningitis in an adult. Vasogenic edema in the setting of a brain tumor should be treated acutely with 8 mg of dexamethasone q 8 hours for a total of 24 mg per 24 hours. Pending neurosurgical or radiation options, this

high dose should be maintained on a short-term basis, with weaning of the dose over days to a more typical 4 to 6 mg BID.
 E. Hypothermia (32 to 34°C) can lower ICP. However, several randomized control trials have failed to demonstrate clinical benefit.
 F. Neuromuscular blockade may be necessary, using short-acting agents such as cisatracurium.
 G. Barbiturate coma with burst suppression can decrease ICP and is a last resort medical therapy; complications include further sedation of comatose patients, hypotension often requiring vasopressors to maintain blood pressure, and sepsis. Pentobarbital may be given at 10 mg/kg IV bolus and then 5 mg IV/kg/hr titrate to 2 to 5 bursts per minute.
III. Surgical evacuation when possible offers rapid and definitive relief of intracranial hypertension. Although intraparenchymal, epidural, subdural, and subarachnoid ICP monitors can be used, the intraventricular catheter is the most accurate and allows therapeutic CSF EVD. EVD results in immediate ICP reduction, especially in cases with hydrocephalus. Indications for EVD include severe brain insult with Glasgow Coma Scale score less than 8 and an abnormal head CT. EVD is indicated, even with a normal CT, when additional factors are present, such as age over 40 years, SBP below 90 mm Hg, and decerebrate or decorticate posturing. Hemicraniectomy has been used after massive middle cerebral stroke and appears to be promising.

INTRACRANIAL HYPOTENSION

Decreased ICP may occur in the setting of CSF leakage, either spontaneously through openings in the dura to sinuses or mastoid, after lumbar puncture or neurosurgery, or through overshunting. Postural headache, similar to that observed after lumbar puncture, is a frequent symptom. Diagnosis is confirmed by demonstration of CSF leak on cisternogram or other evidence of CSF leak (positive glucose test in pharyngeal secretions). MRI may show meningeal enhancement. Spontaneous remission may occur, and treatment depends on the cause; occasionally dural graft may be necessary.

REFERENCE

Freeman, W. D. (2015). Management of intracranial pressure. *Continuum*, *21*(5), 1299–1323.

INTRACRANIAL STENOSIS

 I. *Epidemiology.* Intracranial artery stenosis (ICS) secondary to atherosclerosis is a significant cause of ischemic stroke, accounting for 5% to 10% of all ischemic strokes. The annual risk of stroke in patients with ICS is estimated at 3% to 15%, although the warfarin versus aspirin for intracranial disease (WASID) trial showed a risk of recurrent vascular events at 15% to 17%. Patients with severe stenosis of the vertebral artery, the basilar artery, or both are at particularly high risk of recurrent stroke despite antithrombotic therapy.

II. *Clinical presentation.* Stroke type can vary and depends on the artery involved and if it is related to hypoperfusion and the extent of collateral, perforator involvement, or progression to complete occlusion. The majority presents with deep infarct or watershed infarcts.

III. *Diagnosis.* In order of sensitivity and specificity, the gold standard conventional angiogram, computed tomography angiography (CTA), magnetic resonance angiogram (MRA), and transcranial Doppler ultrasound are used for diagnosis.

IV. *Treatment.* A recent study showed no difference between aspirin (ASA) (325–1300 mg daily) and warfarin, although subsequent subgroup analysis showed minor benefit of warfarin over aspirin in basilar artery and intracranial vertebral artery stenosis. Intracranial balloon angioplasty and stenting can be an option in refractory cases that continue to have symptoms despite medical therapy but come with significant risk of stroke and mortality.

REFERENCE

Chimowitz, M. I., Lynn, M. J., Howlett-Smith, H., & Stern, B. J. (2005). Comparison of warfarin and aspirin for symptomatic intracranial arterial stenosis. *N Engl J Med, 352,* 1305–1316.

ISCHEMIA (STROKE AND TRANSIENT ISCHEMIC ATTACK) (See also THE NEUROLOGIC EMERGENCY APPENDIX, ACUTE ISCHEMIC STROKE)

In the United States, stroke of all types ranked as the fifth leading cause of death in 2015, down from the third leading cause of death in 2007. A thorough medical evaluation is required for the diagnosis and management of cerebrovascular injury. The history should include age, race, family history, handedness, comorbidities, medications, time of onset, and prior pattern of neurologic deficits. History, physical examination, and imaging studies determine risk factors, localize lesions, delineate underlying pathophysiologic conditions, and guide treatment.

STROKE CLASSIFICATION

Cerebral ischemic events are classified by anatomic location, size of blood vessels (small and large vessel disease), duration of deficit, and mechanism (cardioembolic, atherosclerotic, and lacunar).

Transient ischemic attacks (TIAs) are defined by the American Heart Association/American Stroke Association as "a transient episode of neurological dysfunction caused by focal brain, spinal cord, or retinal ischemia, without acute infarction." Typically, TIAs last less than 30 minutes and commonly resolve within an hour. However, even if symptoms resolve, an acute neurovascular syndrome is considered a stroke if there is evidence of tissue damage on pathologic examination or imaging.

Completed stroke indicates that the patient has a stable neurologic deficit without evidence of progression or resolution. Completed stroke refers to the acute onset and persistence of neurologic dysfunction resulting from cerebrovascular disease (hemorrhagic or ischemic infarction).

Progressing stroke is defined as waxing and waning neurologic deficit with ultimate worsening.

Central nervous system ischemia or infarction may be described in terms of vascular anatomy (Table 76). The cerebral vasculature is divided into *anterior* (carotids) and *posterior* (vertebrobasilar) distributions. There are many variants in cerebrovascular anatomy. A congenitally incomplete circle of Willis is not uncommon; estimates of incidence range from 0.6% to 17%. Brainstem cross-sectional anatomy that correlates with many of the syndromes described in Table 77 is shown in Figs. 34 to 36. Infarctions may be concentrated along border zones ("watershed") between large vascular territories, such as the zone between the middle cerebral artery (MCA) and posterior cerebral artery or MCA and anterior cerebral artery. These *watershed infarcts* may be seen secondary to clinically significant decrease in blood pressure.

TABLE 76

SIGNS AND SYMPTOMS OF ISCHEMIC VASCULAR OCCLUSION

Artery	Signs and Symptoms
Common carotid artery (CCA)	Ipsilateral eye; distal vessels; may be asymptomatic or internal carotid artery (ICA)
Middle cerebral artery (MCA)	Contralateral hemiparesis (face and arm greater than leg); horizontal gaze palsy; hemisensory deficits; homonymous hemianopia; language and cognitive deficits (aphasia, apraxia, agnosia, neglect)
Anterior cerebral artery (ACA)	Contralateral hemiparesis (leg greater than arm and face); contralateral grasp reflex and gegenhalten; abulia; gait disorders; perseveration; urinary incontinence; may produce bilateral signs caused by involvement of a single vessel of common origin
Posterior cerebral artery (PCA)	Contralateral homonymous hemianopia (or quadrantanopia); may produce memory loss, dyslexia without dysgraphia, color anomia, hemisensory deficits, and mild hemiparesis; may be supplied by the anterior circulation
Cerebellar infarction	Dizziness, nausea, vomiting, nystagmus, ataxia
Recognition is important to detect brainstem	Compression caused by swelling; neurosurgical decompression may be lifesaving

TABLE 77

BRAINSTEM SYNDROMES

Syndrome	Localization	Clinical Features	
		Ipsilateral	Contralateral
Benedikt	Midbrain tegmentum, red nucleus, cranial nerve CN III, cerebral peduncle	CN III palsy	Hemiataxia, tremor, hemiparesis, hyperkinesia
Claude	Paramedian midbrain tegmentum, red nucleus, ND III, superior cerebellar peduncle	CN III palsy	Hemiataxia, tremor, hemiparesis
Weber	Ventral midbrain, CN III, cerebral peduncle	CN III palsy	Hemiparesis
Parinaud	Dorso rostral midbrain, posterior commissure and its interstitial nucleus	Paralysis of upward gaze and accommodation, light-near dissociation of pupil lid retraction, convergence-retraction nystagmus	
Nothnagel	Dorsal midbrain, brachium conjunctivum, CN III nucleus, medial longitudinal fasciculus	Ataxia, CN III palsy, vertical gaze palsy	
Raymond-Cestan	Medial mid-pons (paramedian branch, mid-basilar artery), middle cerebellar peduncle, corticobulbar tract, corticospinal tract, variable medial lemniscus	Ataxia	Hemiparesis (face, arm, and leg), variable sensory, variable oculomotor
One and a half	Lateral mid-pons (short circumferential artery, middle cerebellar peduncle, CN V	Ataxia, paralysis of muscles of mastication, facial hemihypesthesia	
	Paramedian pontine reticular formation or CN VI nucleus, medial longitudinal fasciculus	Horizontal gaze palsy	Internuclear ophthalmoplegia
Foville	Paramedian pontine reticular formation, CN VI and VII, corticospinal tract	Horizontal gaze palsy, CN VII palsy	Hemiparesis, hemisensory loss, internuclear ophthalmoplegia

Continued

I

ISCHEMIA (STROKE AND TRANSIENT ISCHEMIC ATTACK)

TABLE 77

BRAINSTEM SYNDROMES—CONT'D

Syndrome	Localization	Clinical Features	
		Ipsilateral	Contralateral
Millard-Gubler	Ventral paramedian pons, CN VI and VII fascicles, corticospinal tract	CN VI palsy, facial palsy	Hemiparesis
Raymond Babinski-Nageotte	Ventral pons, CN VI fascicles and corticospinal tract Dorsolateral pontomedullary junction	CN VI palsy Ataxia, hemihypesthesia in face, Horner syndrome	Hemiparesis Hemiparesis, hemihypesthesia in body, vertigo, vomiting, nystagmus
Wallenberg's	Dorsolateral medulla, vestibular nucleus, restiform body, CN V nucleus and spinal tract, CN IX and X, lateral spinothalamics, descending sympathetics	Lateropulsion; ataxia; loss of pain and temperature in face; paralysis of soft palate, posterior pharynx, and vocal cord; Horner syndrome.	Loss of pain and temperature in body
Cestan-Chenais	Lateral medulla	Ataxia; paralysis of soft palate, posterior pharynx, and vocal cord; Horner syndrome, hemihypesthesia in face	Hemiparesis, hemihypesthesia in body
Avellis	Lateral medulla, CN IX and X, lateral spinothalamics	Paralysis of soft palate, posterior pharynx, and vocal cord	Hemiparesis, hemihypesthesia
Vernet	Lateral medulla, CN IX, X, and XI	Paralysis of soft palate; paralysis of vocal cord, posterior pharynx, and sternocleido-mastoid; decreased taste over posterior third of tongue; hemihypesthesia of pharynx	Hemiparesis

Jackson	Lateral medulla, CN IX, X, XI, and XII	Paralysis of soft palate, posterior pharynx, vocal cords, sternocleidomastoid, upper trapezius, and tongue	Hemiparesis, hemihypesthesia
Tapia	Lateral medulla, CN IX, X, XII (more commonly, there is extracranial involvement)	As in Jackson syndrome, except that sternocleidomastoid and trapezius are not involved	
Preolivary	Anterior medulla, CN XII, pyramid	Tongue atrophy or weakness	Hemiparesis

Vertebrobasilar artery (VBA) brainstem syndromes are best described in terms of neuroanatomic localization. Eponymic descriptions in the literature vary.

ISCHEMIA (STROKE AND TRANSIENT ISCHEMIC ATTACK)

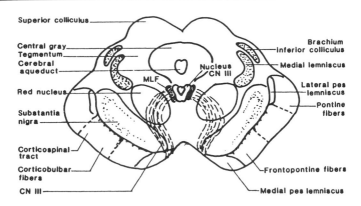

Midbrain cross-section. *MLF*, Medial longitudinal fasciculus.

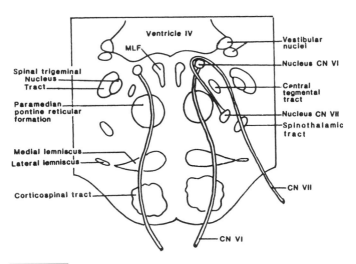

Pons cross-section. *MLF*, Medial longitudinal fasciculus.

STROKE MECHANISM AND DIFFERENTIAL DIAGNOSIS

The etiology of a stroke is associated with prognosis, and identification of the ischemic mechanism can help guide treatment, especially secondary prevention. For example, carotid endarterectomy (CEA) may be of value in strokes caused by large-artery atherosclerosis, whereas anticoagulation (AC) is

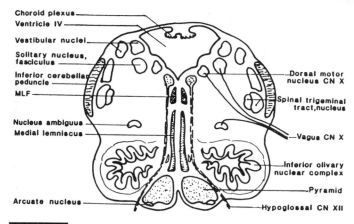

FIGURE 36
Medulla cross-section.

more likely to be of value in cardioembolic strokes in patients with atrial fibrillation (AF).

The TOAST classification defines five categories of strokes based on etiology: large-artery atherosclerosis, cardioembolism, small-vessel occlusion (i.e., lacunar stroke), stroke of other determined etiology, and stroke of undetermined etiology.

Table 78 delineates how these categories are distinguished based on clinical features and supporting tests. Testing should include brain imaging with computed tomography (CT) or magnetic resonance imaging (MRI), echocardiography or other cardiac imaging, imaging of extracranial arteries, arteriography, and laboratory tests to assess for a prothrombotic state.

Differential diagnosis of transient neurologic deficits includes syncope, hyper/hypoventilation syndromes, Meniere disease, transient global amnesia, migraine, metabolic disease (hypercalcemia and hypoglycemia), psychogenic disorders, and seizures. Patients with a history of migraine may have transient neurologic deficits with or without headache. Late-life migraine may cause fleeting visual or sensory loss in the elderly. However, in this age group, careful workup is necessary to exclude vascular causes. For instance, isolated transient vertigo or the feeling of lightheadedness in the absence of brainstem signs may indicate labyrinthine disease or orthostatic hypotension. However, particularly in patients older than 55 years, cerebrovascular disease of the posterior circulation must be seriously considered. Transient deficits may be a manifestation of seizure; when there is involuntary motor activity or a Jacksonian-like march of symptoms, TIA is a less likely diagnosis, although stroke may be heralded by a seizure.

TABLE 78

FEATURES OF TOAST CLASSIFICATION OF SUBTYPES OF ISCHEMIC STROKE

Features	Large-artery Atherosclerosis	Cardioembolism	Small-artery Occlusion (lacune)	Other Cause
CLINICAL				
Cortical or cerebellar dysfunction	+	+	−	+
Lacunar syndrome	−	−	+	+
Imaging				
Cortical, cerebellar, brain stem, or subcortical infarct > 1.5 cm	+	+	−	+
Subcortical or brain stem infarct < 1.5 cm	−	−	+	+
TESTS				
Stenosis of extracranial internal carotid artery	+	−	−	−
Cardiac source of emboli	−	+	−	−
Other abnormality on tests	−	−	−	+

TOAST, Trial of Org 10172 in Acute Stroke Treatment.
From Adams, H. P., Jr., Bendixen, B. H., Kappelle, L. J., et al. (1993). Classification of subtype of acute ischemic stroke. Definitions for use in a multicenter clinical trial. TOAST. Trial of Org 10172 in Acute Stroke Treatment. *Stroke 24*(1), 35–41.

NATURAL HISTORY AND RISK FACTORS

Identification and reduction of risk factors should be encouraged, to prevent future strokes. Risk factors may be modifiable or nonmodifiable and vary with age and race. The INTERSTROKE study identified 10 modifiable risk factors that account for about 90% of stroke risk worldwide. These include hypertension, regular physical activity, apolipoprotein (Apo)B/ApoA1 ratio, diet, waist-to-hip ratio, psychosocial factors, current smoking, cardiac causes including AF, alcohol consumption, and diabetes mellitus. These risk factors apply to all age groups, ethnic groups, and both males and females, although there are region-specific differences in the relative importance of the different risk factors.

Other risk factors that have been recognized include trauma, drug use, oral contraceptives, migraine, and spontaneous arterial dissection, prior stroke or TIAs, hypercoagulable state, vasculitis, and family history of premature death from stroke.

The prognosis in individuals with TIAs varies considerably. There is unquestionably an increased risk of stroke after a TIA. Estimates of that risk have declined since 2000, when 10.5% of patients with a TIA were noted to have had a stroke after 90 days. More recent estimates put the risk of stroke after TIA at 3.7% at 90 days, and 5.1% after 1 year.

CLINICAL AND LABORATORY EVALUATION

The National Institutes of Health Stroke Scale (NIHSS) is a commonly used means of estimating the total neurologic deficit. Attention should be given to supine blood pressure in both upper extremities, orthostatic blood pressure, cardiac examination, presence of carotid or cranial bruits and facial pulses, funduscopic examination, and evidence of peripheral emboli. Patients with carotid bruits have a higher incidence of TIA, stroke, and death from stroke compared to those without a bruit.

Radiographic evaluation: Imaging should be performed on all patients to exclude the presence of hemorrhage. In the acute setting, if the patient is a candidate for tissue plasminogen activator (tPA), CT is preferred because it is faster. If possible, MRI should not be allowed to delay the administration of tPA. MRI is more sensitive for the detection of small strokes, particularly in the brainstem and posterior fossa. Diffusion-weighted MRI is now standard, and is very sensitive and specific for detecting acute stroke. Additional techniques include MRI with perfusion-weighted images, as well as MR angiography. Cerebral angiography is still considered to be the gold standard for studying the intracranial and extracranial vasculature when there is either an unclear or potentially treatable condition. As a general guideline, patients with TIA in the carotid distribution should have angiography if they are considered candidates for surgery.

Transcranial Doppler is useful for noninvasive evaluation of the large cerebral arteries. It can demonstrate large vessel occlusion and help assess collateral flow in ischemic territories. Duplex carotid ultrasonography is also useful as an initial screening examination, especially for patients with carotid distribution ischemic events. Operator dependency is ultrasonography's main disadvantage.

Laboratory evaluation: Complete evaluation includes complete blood counts, erythrocyte sedimentation rate, blood chemistries, prothrombin time (PT), and partial thromboplastin time (PTT). One may also include syphilis screening (test CSF for neurosyphilis if syphilis is highly suspected), lipid profile, urinalysis, chest x-ray, and hemoglobin electrophoresis in patients at risk for sickle cell disease. Because AC is contraindicated in established endocarditis, serial blood cultures should be obtained if there is suspicion of endocarditis (especially in patients with artificial valves or a history of intravenous drug abuse and those with congenital heart disease).

Cardiac evaluation of stroke patients: History and examination consistent with an embolic event or history of heart disease necessitates an evaluation of possible source for artery-to-artery embolus as well as cardioembolic sources. Cerebral and cardiac atherosclerosis share many pathogenic mechanisms and risk factors. Atherosclerotic stroke survivors are more likely to die from coronary artery disease than recurrent stroke. Evaluations identify possible cardiogenic sources of embolism and detect occult coronary artery disease. Besides intracardiac sources, proximal aortic atheroma, especially mobile aortic plaques larger than 4 mm, is a strong risk factor for stroke. Transesophageal echocardiogram is most useful in identifying the cardioembolic source. Holter monitoring or cardiac event monitoring should be used if there is unconfirmed suspicion for AF.

Stroke in the Young

Additional evaluation for patients under the age of 55 and those with no clear risk factors includes cardiac evaluation as just discussed. Cardiac sources in young adults may include patent foramen ovale and atrial septal aneurysm. Mitral valve prolapse is not clearly correlated with increased stroke in the young. A search for causes of increased coagulability should be initiated before starting AC (antiphospholipid antibodies, anticardiolipin antibodies, heparin cofactor II deficiency, antithrombin III, protein C and S, activated protein C, factor V Leiden), antinuclear antibodies, serum viscosity, protein electrophoresis, ANA/rheumatologic profile, and serum homocysteine and amino acid levels. Mitochondrial studies may be indicated in selected cases such as suspected MELAS (mitochondrial encephalopathy with lactic acidosis and stroke). Peripheral blood sample may be diagnostic, searching for mutation, but muscle biopsy may be needed. Skin biopsy or genetic testing for NOTCH3 mutation in cases of suspected CADASIL (cerebral autosomal dominant arteriopathy with subcortical infarct and leukoencephalopathy) may prove to be helpful.

TREATMENT
Acute Treatment

Please see the neurologic emergency index on acute ischemic stroke.

General Measures

Prevention of secondary complications: Secondary complications in stroke patients, primarily deep vein thrombosis (DVT), urinary tract infection, and

pneumonia, may be minimized by prophylactic measures. Venous stasis may be prevented by the use of compression stockings, sequential compression devices, and subcutaneous heparin (when not medically contraindicated). The use of all three together is more effective than the use of any one alone. Both decubiti and stasis may be prevented by patient mobilization. Depressed gag reflexes or dysphagia should be carefully evaluated to avoid the risk of aspiration pneumonia. Alterations in bladder function are common after stroke and are treated as needed. Intermittent catheterization reduces the risk of infection compared to an indwelling urinary catheter.

General measures to minimize ischemia: Once prolonged ischemia occurs, little can be done to reverse neuronal death. However, the area surrounding an ischemic injury, the so-called "ischemic penumbra," is at continued risk secondary to impaired autoregulation and perfusion. Damage to this area may be reversed and is critically influenced by management choices in the first 72 hours of stroke onset. Body temperature should be aggressively controlled and kept below 37.5°C. Blood glucose should be monitored closely and maintained in the normal range, avoiding hyperglycemia and hypoglycemia.

Hypertension is common in acute stroke, but there is currently insufficient evidence to suggest how hypertension should be managed in the period immediately after a stroke. Patients who are eligible for tPA and have severe hypertension should be treated with antihypertensive agents to lower their systolic blood pressure below 185 mm Hg and their diastolic blood pressure below 110 mm Hg. Further, their blood pressure should be maintained below 180/105 mm Hg for the first 24 hours after intravenous recombinant tissue plasminogen activator (rtPA) treatment. For patients who will not receive tPA, the current AHA/ASA guidelines recommend that antihypertensive medications be withheld unless systolic blood pressure exceeds 220 mm Hg or diastolic blood pressure exceeds 120 mm Hg. Above that level, a reduction in blood pressure of 15% is suggested.

Anticoagulation Therapy

I. *Acute stroke and TIAs.* As noted above, low-dose heparin is recommended for the prevention of DVTs in the setting of acute stroke. Apart from that, there is currently insufficient evidence to recommend the use of heparinoids in the setting of acute ischemic stroke. The AAN does not currently recommend the use of heparinoids for treatment of any subset of stroke. Because recurrent stroke is relatively uncommon, particularly in the first 7 days, physicians still have no clinical basis for early initiation and use of heparin beyond anecdotal success. Complications of heparin AC include symptomatic intracranial hemorrhage, asymptomatic hemorrhagic transformation of infarction, major and minor extracranial bleeding, thrombocytopenia, and thrombophlebitis.

II. *Cardioembolic stroke.* There is good evidence that AC therapy reduces the risk of future embolization. Because the risk of stroke in patients with AF and sinus node disease is six times greater than in those without AF, patients with AF should receive AC therapy. Long-term AC therapy with warfarin requires monitoring (PT) and international normalized ratio (INR) to ensure values of 1.2 to 1.5 times the control value of PT, which translates to INR between 2 and 3. Even without a history of TIA or stroke, candidates for AC include patients with asymptomatic/symptomatic AF, AF with coexisting cardiomyopathy, mechanical prosthetic cardiac valves, symptomatic mitral valve prolapse, and intracardiac mural thrombus. When not medically contraindicated cardioversion should be considered. Short-term AC therapy is recommended in the setting of cardioversion for AF.

Many large embolic strokes (i.e., greater than two-thirds of an arterial territory) occur in association with a known cardiac source (e.g., mural thrombus). A completely satisfactory course of action is difficult to select because AC therapy may worsen the neurologic deficit and morbidity/ mortality outcome through hemorrhagic transformation. Unfortunately, withholding AC therapy may lead to repeated embolization. Management of such cases must be highly individualized. AC therapy provides no benefit in patients with embolism resulting from marantic endocarditis, calcific valves, or atrial myxoma. When embolic stroke is associated with prosthetic valve, AC therapy should be withheld while arteriography and contrasted CT scans are performed to exclude ruptured mycotic aneurysm.

III. *Use of anticoagulants.* Warfarin is commonly used. The novel anticoagulants, which include dabigatran, rivaroxaban, apixaban, and edoxaban, are also indicated for nonvalvular AF. If heparin must be used, bolus administration is avoided with cerebral embolism because of the risk of hemorrhagic complications. The heparin infusion rate is adjusted every 4 to 6 hours until obtaining a maintenance level with activated PTT of 1.5 times the control value. Patients should be monitored for evidence of excessive AC (petechiae, microscopic hematuria, occult blood in stool, signs and symptoms of retroperitoneal bleeding). Heparin can be reversed with protamine sulfate (use 10 to 15 mg IV protamine sulfate; 1 mg neutralizes 100 USP units of heparin).

The necessity of warfarin loading is controversial. Loading may result in supratherapeutic levels. Warfarin dose is typically 2 to 10 mg/day. PT is determined daily, and the dosage is adjusted to maintain an INR of 2 to 3. Valve replacement patients require an INR of 3 to 4. Higher levels of AC are associated with a greater incidence of hemorrhagic complications. Numerous factors, including many drugs and liver disease, influence the response to warfarin. After satisfactory AC is attained with warfarin, the PT should be determined at least every 2 weeks. Excessive prolongation of PT can be corrected with vitamin K; however, vitamin K reversal significantly prolongs the time required to re-attain therapeutic AC levels with warfarin. Immediate reversal is accomplished by the use of fresh-frozen plasma.

Antiplatelet Agents

Platelets play a central role in the development of thrombi and subsequent ischemic events. In one study, the rate of infarction and death with TIAs and stroke was reduced by treatment with 1200 mg/day of aspirin. Other trials show no clear evidence that aspirin doses higher than 80 mg/day show improved benefit. In addition, lower doses are associated with decreased risk of bleeding complications. Antiplatelet agents are frequently used in small vessel, noncardioembolic infarcts; however, there is no prospective data to prove efficacy of this management. Ticlopidine (Ticlid) is an antiplatelet agent that is slightly more efficacious (at 250 mg bid) than aspirin, however it is associated with serious adverse effects. The use of ticlopidine necessitates initial monitoring of complete blood cell counts every other week for the first 3 months of therapy because of the risk of neutropenia. Clopidogrel (Plavix), another antiplatelet agent, is reportedly slightly more efficacious (at 75 mg qd) than aspirin and has relatively few gastrointestinal side effects. Clopidogrel-associated thrombotic thrombocytopenic purpura has been reported. Dipyridamole is another antiplatelet agent. The slow release form in combination with 25 mg aspirin bid (Aggrenox) is more efficacious than either aspirin or dipyridamole monotherapy alone.

Ancrod is an intravenous antiplatelet agent that has been shown to be slightly more effective than placebo in treating acute stroke patients.

Thrombolytic Therapy in Acute Stroke

Since 1996, IV tPA has been approved in the United States for use in ischemic stroke patients within 3 hours of onset in a dose of 0.9 mg/kg (maximum 90 mg), with 10% administered as a bolus and the remainder infused over 1 hour. The main risk with tPA administration is brain hemorrhage. Although reports reveal a 10-fold increased risk of symptomatic brain hemorrhage within the first 36 hours after tPA, patients receiving tPA were at least 30% more likely to have only minimal or no disability at 3 months.

Current recommendations include the following: (1) emergency medical support recognition of stroke as an emergency to be able to identify more patients within the critical 3-hour window; and (2) minimal standards for stroke care facilities should include access to physician evaluation within 10 minutes, stroke expertise within 15 minutes, cranial CT scan within 25 minutes, interpretation of CT scan within 45 minutes, and intravenous tPA administration within 60 minutes of presentation. Unfortunately, only 5% of stroke victims receive tPA. Increased effort is needed to offer and administer thrombolytic therapy to qualified patients.

Contraindications to thrombolysis with tPA include: age < 18 years, SBP > 185 mm Hg or DBP > 110 mm Hg, BG < 50, INR > 1.7, platelets < 100,000/mm^3, LMWH within 24 hours, NOAC use within 48 hours, active internal bleeding, previous/recent ICH, severe head trauma within 3 months, recent intracranial or intraspinal surgery (within 3 months), CT showing hypodensity >1/3 of the cerebral hemisphere.

For patients who are within the 3- to 4.5-hour window for tPA, contraindications are: age > 80 years, NIHSS > 25, taking an oral anticoagulant regardless of INR, history of both diabetes and prior ischemic stroke.

Endovascular Therapy in Acute Stroke

Endovascular clot retrieval has been demonstrated to be an effective treatment. Patients should still receive tPA (if eligible) if they are being considered for endovascular treatment. Patients are considered eligible for endovascular therapy if all of the following criteria are met: Prestroke mRS score 0 to 1, acute ischemic stroke receiving intravenous tPA within 4.5 hours of onset in accordance with the current guidelines, occlusion of the ICA or proximal MCA (M1) causing the stroke, age $\geq$ 18 years, NIHSS score $\geq$ 6, ASPECTS score $\geq$ 6, and if treatment can be initiated (i.e., groin puncture) within 6 hours of symptom onset.

Additionally, some "carefully selected" patients with anterior circulation occlusion who cannot receive IV tPA, or who are under 18, or who have more distal occlusions, or who have a prestroke mRS score > 1, ASPECTS < 6, or NIHSS score < 6 may receive endovascular therapy, completed within 6 hours of stroke onset.

Intra-arterial (IA) tPA can be beneficial for select patients with severe stroke, if administered within 6 hours of onset. However, endovascular therapy with stent retrievers is preferred over IA tPA.

Surgical Treatment of Stroke

Carotid endarterectomy: CEA is indicated in patients with retinal or hemispheric stroke coupled with ipsilateral high-grade stenosis (70%–90%). The rate of fatal and nonfatal stroke was reduced significantly when compared to medical therapy according to the North American Symptomatic Carotid Endarterectomy Trial. Timing for surgery following acute stroke is most commonly 4 to 6 weeks; occasionally this may be shorter in unstable patients.

The Asymptomatic Carotid Atherosclerosis Study found that patients with asymptomatic carotid artery stenosis of 60% or greater reduction in diameter and whose general health makes them good candidates for elective surgery will have a reduced 5-year risk of ipsilateral stroke if CEA performed with less than 3% risk of perioperative morbidity and death is added to aggressive management of modifiable risk factors.

Hemicraniectomy: Decompressive craniectomy may involve removal of a portion of the calvaria with durotomy or a more aggressive approach with removal of the infarcted tissue as a lifesaving procedure. This procedure can reduce the compartmentalization in the intracranial pressure and prevent brainstem herniation and death. This procedure is currently experimental. Prior to such an intervention, close monitoring is required. Placement of either intracranial pressure monitors or an intraventricular catheter is used in planning for possible surgical intervention.

Bypass surgery: Previous trials of bypass surgery have been discouraging. Recent interest in bypass surgery has emerged in selected cases; those may include moyamoya disease and hemodynamic-dependent occlusion and/or stenosis in the carotid arteries with pressure-dependent neurologic deficits in patients without an alternative procedure to augment cerebral blood flow.

Endovascular therapy: stenting and angioplasty: The role of these interventions is still unclear, but they may be used in patients who are at high risk to undergo CEA or if the site of the stenosis is not amenable for surgical intervention.

REHABILITATION

Rehabilitation decreases the long-term economic cost of stroke. Rehabilitation should be initiated 24 to 48 hours after the onset of stroke. The goals of stroke rehabilitation include restoration of lost abilities (motor and psychological), prevention of stroke-related complications, quality of life improvement, and education regarding secondary stroke prevention. New techniques in rehabilitation are on the horizon, including functional electrical stimulation and constraint-induced therapy.

RECOVERY AND PROGNOSIS

Approximately 10% of stroke survivors are without disability. Another 10% of patients are institutionalized because of markedly severe disability and inability to achieve functional independence. Factors that favor a poor prognosis include hemorrhagic stroke, impaired consciousness, heavy alcohol use, older age, male sex, hypertension, heart disease, and leg weakness. Negative predictors for functional outcome include incontinence, severe inattention, severe cognitive deficits, previous stroke, global aphasia, and complex comorbidities. The mortality rates at 1 month are 17% for patients with carotid distribution and 18% for patients with vertebrobasilar territory infarction.

Most rapid neurologic and functional recovery occurs by 3 months after a stroke. Recovery is categorized in stages, and a particular stage may be prolonged or recovery may stop at any stage. Stages include the following: (1) flaccidity, (2) spasticity, (3) synergistic movements (flexor and extensor), (4) isolated movements, (5) increased muscle strength, endurance, and coordination, and (6) return of muscle tone to prestroke state. Recovery from stroke may be prolonged and late functional improvements are possible.

DIFFERENTIAL DIAGNOSIS OF CEREBRAL INFARCTION

I. Cerebrovascular thrombosis associated with vascular disease
   A. Atherosclerosis
   B. Lipohyalinosis
   C. Dissection
   D. Chronic progressive subcortical encephalopathy (Binswanger disease)

ISCHEMIA (STROKE AND TRANSIENT ISCHEMIC ATTACK)

II. Cerebral embolism
   A. Cardiac source
      1. Valvular (mitral stenosis, prosthetic valve, infective endocarditis, marantic endocarditis, Libman-Sacks endocarditis, mitral annulus calcification, mitral valve prolapse, calcific aortic stenosis)
      2. AF, sick sinus syndrome
      3. Acute myocardial infarction, left ventricular aneurysm, or both
      4. Left atrial myxoma
      5. Cardiomyopathy
      6. Acute and subacute bacterial endocarditis
      7. Prosthetic valve dysfunction
      8. Chagas disease, trichinosis
   B. Paradoxical embolism and pulmonary source
      1. Pulmonary arteriovenous malformations (including Osler-Weber-Rendu syndrome)
      2. Atrial and ventricular septal defects with right-to-left shunts
      3. Patent foramen ovale with right-to-left shunt
      4. Pulmonary vein thrombosis
      5. Pulmonary and mediastinal tumors
   C. Artery-to-artery embolism
      1. Cholesterol emboli
      2. Atheroma thrombus
      3. Complications of vascular and neck surgery
      4. Idiopathic carotid mural thrombus, emboligenic aortitis
      5. Emboli distal to unruptured aneurysm
      6. Arterial dissection
   D. Other
      1. Fat embolism syndrome
      2. Air embolism
      3. Foreign body embolism (e.g., bullets, catheter tips, etc.)
III. Arteriopathies, inflammatory
   A. Takayasu disease
   B. Allergic granulomatosis (Churg-Strauss syndrome)
   C. Granulomatosis, polyarteritis nodosa, rheumatoid arthritis, Sjögren syndrome, scleroderma, Behçet syndromes, acute rheumatic fever, inflammatory bowel disease

LACUNAR SYNDROMES

Lacunar infarcts are described as small, deep lesions on CT or MRI usually 10 mm or less in diameter with density or signal consistent with infarct. Between 10% and 24% of all strokes are lacunar. There is a greater incidence of lacunes in Asians, Blacks, and Hispanics than in Whites. Lacunar infarcts are characteristically located in the subcortical cerebrum or brainstem. Pathophysiology of lacunes can be categorized by four different mechanisms: (1) small vessel lipohyalinosis and fibrinoid degeneration, (2) decreased perfusion of penetrating arteries from proximal narrowing of larger vessels, (3) branch artery atheromatous occlusion, and (4) embolism.

Patients with lacunes frequently have a history of hypertension, diabetes, hypercholesterolemia, smoking, and atherosclerosis of large and mid-sized intracranial arteries, but there is no increased incidence of these risk factors in patients with lacunar infarcts versus other ischemic strokes. Lacunes are infrequently associated with embolism and extracranial carotid occlusive disease. Lacunes occur in the lenticular nuclei (37%), caudate nucleus (10%), thalamus (14%), internal capsule (10%), and pons (16%). Lacunes are also seen in the corona radiata, external capsule, pyramids, and other brainstem structures.

Clinical presentations of lacunar infarction (Table 79) are related to size and site of the lesion and range from asymptomatic to classic lacunar syndromes. Onset is often gradual or stepwise. Approximately 30% are preceded by transient ischemic attacks. Defined lacunar syndromes include pure motor hemiparesis, pure sensory syndrome, sensorimotor syndrome, ataxic hemiparesis, dysarthria-clumsy hand, and hemichorea/ballism.

Head CT demonstrates up to 70% of lesions within 7 days. Multiple lacunes are present in 30% of patients. MRI is more sensitive than CT. Thirty percent of lesions on imaging studies are asymptomatic. Treatment consists of antiplatelet agents, control of hypertension, and management of other vascular risk factors. Cerebral angiography is not recommended in pure lacunar syndromes. However, the absence of history or signs of hypertension (such as retinopathy and left ventricular hypertrophy) requires an aggressive workup for sources of embolus, large vessel disease, or unusual causes of stroke. Prognosis is usually favorable, but the probability of recurrence is high.

TABLE 79

MOST COMMON LACUNAR SYNDROMES

Syndrome	Localization	Clinical Features
Pure sensory stroke	Ventricular posterior thalamus	Sensory loss face, arm, leg—same side; no weakness; no visual field deficits; no "cortical" signs
Pure motor hemiparesis	Posterior limb interior capsule, basis points, cerebral peduncle	Weakness face, arm, leg—same side; no sensory loss; no visual field deficits; no "cortical" signs
Ataxic hemiparesis	Basis pontis, ventricular anterior thalamus and adjacent interior capsule	Cerebellar ataxia and weakness—same side; often leg > face
Dysarthria—clumsy hand syndrome	Basis pontis, genu interior capsule	Facial weakness, dysarthria, dysphagia, slight weakness and clumsiness of hand—same side

ISCHEMIA (STROKE AND TRANSIENT ISCHEMIC ATTACK)

THALAMIC SYNDROMES

Cerebrovascular disease is the most common cause of discrete thalamic lesions. The thalamic arteries arise from the posterior communicating arteries and from the perimesencephalic segment of the posterior cerebral arteries. The following thalamic syndromes result from infarctions and each corresponds to a different arterial territory:

Inferolateral artery (thalamogeniculate artery) infarcts with posterolateral thalamic lesions involve mainly the ventral posterior, ventral lateral, and subthalamic nuclear groups. These most commonly include hemisensory loss and pain, hemiataxia, disequilibrium, athetoid posture, and paroxysmal pain.

Tuberothalamic artery supplies the anterior regions. Neuropsychologic dysfunction occurs most commonly. Other symptoms include facial paresis for emotional movement, occasional hemiparesis, dysphasia with left-sided lesions, and hemineglect and visuospatial dysfunction with right-sided lesions. Bilateral lesions lead to lethargy, apathy, abulia, and impaired memory.

Posterior choroidal arteries supply the lateral geniculate body. With infarction, visual field deficits occur, most commonly quadrantanopia.

Paramedian arteries supply the paramedian midbrain and thalamus, including the intralaminar group and most of the dorsomedial nucleus. The triad of common changes is somnolent apathy, memory loss, and abnormalities in vertical gaze. Also, this triad is occasionally associated with akinetic mutism.

The syndrome of *Dejerine and Roussy (inferolateral thalamic syndrome)* is due to a vascular lesion in the territory of the thalamogeniculate artery. It is characterized by a mild hemiparesis, persistent hemianesthesia for touch, slight hemiataxia and astereognosis, choreoathetotic movements, and pain. *Thalamic pain syndrome* occurs contralateral to the lesion and is described as burning, aching, or boring. It is constant, but often there are paroxysmal increases, spontaneous or observed in patients with lesions in brainstem, internal capsule, basal ganglia, and subcortical parietal lobe. Treatment with tricyclic antidepressants (amitriptyline 10 to 100 mg qhs) or anticonvulsants (carbamazepine or dilantin) is sometimes effective. Conventional analgesics are ineffective.

REFERENCES

Amarenco, P., Lavallée, P. C., Labreuche, J., et al. (2016). One-year risk of stroke after transient ischemic attack or minor stroke. *N Engl J Med*, *374*, 1533–1542.

O'Donnell, M. J., et al. (2016). Global and regional effects of potentially modifiable risk factors associated with acute stroke in 32 countries (INTERSTROKE): a case-control study. *Lancet*, *388*(10046), 761–775.

L

LAMBERT-EATON MYASTHENIC SYNDROME

Lambert-Eaton myasthenic syndrome (LEMS) is an autoimmune disorder of neuromuscular transmission. *Antibodies directed at the voltage-gated calcium channels (VGCCs)* on presynaptic cholinergic nerve terminals are responsible for the disease. Calcium entry via VGCCs is required to facilitate vesicle docking and release of presynaptic acetylcholine (ACh). Antibodies to P/Q type VGCCs lead to a reduction in the release of presynaptic ACh vesicles. Presynaptic ACh stores and the postsynaptic response to individual quanta are normal.

LEMS is a rare disease that typically occurs after age 40 in males and females with near equal incidence. LEMS is often the result of a paraneoplastic phenomenon, the symptoms of which may or may not precede detection of an underlying malignancy, of which more than 80% is small-cell lung cancer. Other neoplasms associated with LEMS include leukemia and carcinomas of the rectum, kidney, stomach, and breast. LEMS may occur in the absence of cancer and is not uncommonly associated with other autoimmune diseases such as systemic lupus erythematosus, rheumatoid arthritis, and Sjögren syndrome.

CLINICAL FEATURES

Clinical features include *proximal* leg or arm weakness; muscle aching and stiffness *worsened by prolonged exercise*; and difficulty with certain movements, such as combing hair or rising from a chair. Unlike myasthenia gravis (MG), ocular and bulbar symptoms are rare but may occur. However, transient diplopia, ptosis, dysphagia, dysarthria, and neck flexion weakness can develop in later stages. Autonomic involvement is common and characterized by xerostomia, xerophthalmia, erectile dysfunction, postural hypotension, and constipation. Sensory complaints are rare.

On examination, proximal weakness of the lower limbs greater than the upper limbs is the most consistent finding. A progressive increase in strength after a few seconds of sustained contraction is usual, with fatigue after continued contraction. Muscle wasting is rare. Limb reflexes are decreased or absent in over 90% of cases. However, a potentiation of reflexes after maximal contraction of the involved muscle for 10 to 15 seconds may be present.

LABORATORY FINDINGS

Nerve conduction studies typically demonstrate low compound muscle action potential (CMAP) amplitudes of <50% the lower limit of normal, which increase with 20 to 50 Hz repetitive nerve stimulation or 10 seconds of maximum sustained voluntary muscle contraction (post-exercise facilitation of >100%) due to calcium accumulation in the presynaptic terminal with subsequent enhancement of ACh vesicle release. Sensory responses, nerve conduction velocities, and latencies are normal. Slow repetitive stimulation (2 Hz) produces a decremental response of the CMAP amplitude similar to MG. Antibodies to VGCCs can be tested in blood but their absence in early disease may give cause for repeat testing. The majority of patients with cancer-associated LEMS will have antibodies against SOX1.

TREATMENT

Treatment is directed at the responsible tumor or underlying autoimmune disorder. 3,4-diaminopyridine (3,4-DAP) and intravenous immunoglobulin (IVIg) have been demonstrated to improve muscle strength. 3,4-DAP inhibits voltage-gated $K+$ channels which prolongs the presynaptic action potential, thereby allowing more Ca^{2+} channels to open, resulting in increased $[Ca^{2+}]$ at the nerve terminal. 3,4-DAP doses range from 5 to 25 mg three times per day/ four times per day and there may be a synergistic effect with pyridostigmine (30–60 mg three times per day/ four times per day), which is an acetylcholinesterase inhibitor. IVIg and plasmapheresis may provide short-term improvement and serve as rescue therapy although responses tend to be less dramatic than with MG. If these treatments are ineffective then consideration of corticosteroids and/or steroid-sparing immunomodulators such as azathioprine, cyclosporine, and rituximab is warranted.

Prognosis for non-cancer-associated LEMS is good; however, life-long therapy is generally required. Prognosis of cancer-associated LEMS is largely related to prognosis of the underlying malignancy.

REFERENCES

Sanders, D. B., & Guptill, J. T. (2016). Disorders of neuromuscular transmission. In [eds], *Bradley's neurology in clinical practice*, Vol 2, ed 7 (pp. 1896–1914). Philadelphia: Elsevier.

Tarr, T. B., Wipf, P., & Meriney, S. D. (2015). Synaptic pathophysiology and treatment of Lambert-Eaton myasthenic syndrome. *Mol Neurobiol*, 52(1), 456–463.

LEARNING DISABILITIES

A learning disability (LD) is a neurological disorder presenting as difficulty in the acquisition and use of language, reading, mathematical abilities, or social skills in a patient with otherwise normal intelligence, that has persisted for at least 6 months, despite the provision of interventions that target those difficulties. The prevalence of LD is 5% to 15% among school-age children across different languages and cultures. Prevalence in adults is unknown but has been estimated as 4%.

Learning disabilities can also interfere with higher-level skills such as organization, time planning, abstract reasoning, long or short memory, and attention. It is important to realize that learning disabilities can affect an individual's life beyond academics and can impact relationships with family, friends, and in the workplace. Approximately 50% of children with LD have associated attention deficit hyperactivity disorder (predictive of worse mental health outcome), conduct disorder, anxiety disorders, and mood disorders. School dropout and co-occurring depressive symptoms increase the risk for poor mental health outcomes, including suicidality, whereas high levels of social or emotional support predict better mental health outcomes.

Dyslexia is the most common LD (80%). Dyslexia is a chronic condition in which there is impaired ability to break down words into their basic phonologic parts, resulting in difficulties in decoding and identifying the words. This will often present in a child having difficulty learning to read, and often persists into adulthood.

In pre-schoolers, LD usually becomes evident as language delay. A child who has no meaningful words by age 18 months, no meaningful phrases by age 24 months, or speech unintelligible to strangers by age 3 years should be evaluated for hearing loss and referred for speech therapy evaluation. In school-age children, LD usually becomes evident as unexpected school difficulty or failure. Manifestations may be behavioral (e.g., a reluctance to engage in learning; oppositional behavior); adults may avoid activities that demand arithmetic or reading. There is often a family history of learning problems. Prematurity or very low birth weight increase the risk for specific learning disorders, as does prenatal exposure to nicotine. Psychometric evaluation should be administered to children with school performance difficulties to verify normal intelligence and failure to achieve the expected level of performance. LD may not manifest fully until later school years, by which time learning demands have increased and exceed the individual's limited capacities.

In the United States, the clinician should assure parents that, under the Individuals with Disabilities Education Act, public schools are mandated to meet the educational needs of all developmentally disabled children. This act further mandates the proper assessment of educational needs (including psychometric testing) and enactment of an individual education plan (IEP). All of this assessment should be performed in a timely fashion.

Counseling for associated social, behavioral, and psychiatric symptoms should be tailored to the child's specific deficit. Parent support and consultation can help the family develop a supportive home environment and a behavioral reinforcement program.

REFERENCES

American Psychiatric Association. (2013). *Diagnostic and statistical manual of mental disorders,* ed 5. Washington, D.C.: APA.

Wolraich, M. L. (2003). *Development and learning,* ed 3. Decker: London, BC.

LIMBIC SYSTEM

The limbic system is a network of functionally and anatomically interconnected nuclei and cortical structures located in the telencephalon and diencephalon. These nuclei serve several functions; however most have to do with control of functions necessary for self-preservation and species preservation. They regulate autonomic and endocrine function, set the level of arousal, are involved in emotion, motivation, and reinforcing behaviors, and are critical to particular types of memory.

It should be noted that there is not universal agreement as to which structures should be considered part of the limbic system. The structures listed here are commonly accepted. Other structures are variably included, depending on the source.

Cortical regions involved in the limbic system include the hippocampus as well as areas of neocortex including the insular cortex, orbital frontal cortex, subcallosal gyrus, cingulate gyrus, and parahippocampal gyrus. This cortex has been termed the "limbic lobe" because it makes a rim surrounding the corpus callosum, following the lateral ventricle.

Subcortical portions of the limbic system include the hypothalamus, amygdala, septal nuclei.

Clinical significance of the limbic systems includes various neurodegenerative diseases (particularly Pick disease and Alzheimer disease), acquired lesions such as Klüver-Bucy syndrome or limbic encephalitis, developmental abnormalities such as septo-optic dysplasia, and various neuropsychiatric conditions.

REFERENCES

Sokolowski, K., & Corbin, J. G. (2012). Wired for behaviors: from development to function of innate limbic system circuitry. *Front Mol Neurosci, 5,* 55.

Vanderah, T., & Gould, D. J. (2016). *Nolte's the human brain: an introduction to its functional anatomy,* ed 7. Philadelphia: Elsevier.

LUMBOSACRAL PLEXOPATHY

The lumbosacral plexus comprises the anastomoses derived from the ventral primary rami of T12–S4 (Fig. 37).

ETIOLOGY

Lumbosacral dysfunction may be caused by neoplasms (cervix, prostate, bladder, colorectal, kidney, breast, ovary, and lymphoma), retroperitoneal hemorrhage, psoas abscess (from osteomyelitis), diabetes, inadvertent injections into the gluteal artery or umbilical artery, intravenous heroin, idiopathic retroperitoneal fibrosis, herpes zoster infections, pyelonephritis, appendicitis, retroperitoneal masses, aortic aneurysms, and trauma.

CLINICAL PRESENTATION

Pain, weakness, loss of deep tendon reflexes, and sensory changes may occur in the appropriate distribution (see also Dermatomes, Myotomes). Some variants of lumbar plexus disease are described:

I. Peripartum lumbosacral plexus neuropathy (less common than idiopathic brachial plexopathy): Occurs during labor and delivery when the descending fetal head may compress the lumbosacral trunk and S1 root at the point where they join and pass over the pelvic rim. It is characterized by a sudden onset of severe pain in the thigh or buttock, followed 5 to 10 days later by weakness in the distribution of the involved plexus and elevated erythrocyte sedimentation rate.

II. Radiation plexopathy: Usually occurs one to many years after radiation. Findings include unilateral or bilateral distal leg weakness, mild pain, and needle electromyography (EMG) showing myokymic discharges (50%).

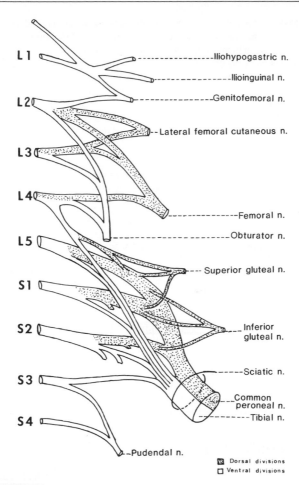

L

LUMBOSACRAL PLEXOPATHY

FIGURE 37

Lumbosacral plexus.

III. Human immunodeficiency virus (HIV) and acquired immunodeficiency syndrome (AIDS)-related lumbosacral polyradiculopathy: Sometimes associated with cytomegalovirus (CMV) infections, this is becoming a more common phenomenon. These radiculopathies occur in the late stages of the disease and include weakness, pain, paresthesias, and urinary retention.

IV. Idiopathic lumbar plexopathy and diabetic amyotrophy: Acute, severe pain in one lower limb, followed by subacutely developing ipsilateral weakness that spreads to the contralateral limb.

V. Neoplastic plexopathy: Severe pain that is worse while lying supine or straining, followed by subacute-chronic, progressive lower extremity weakness, numbness, and areflexia; commonly associated with abdominal/genitourinary malignancies, lymphomas, dural neoplasms. Paraneoplastic autoimmune may also lead to lumbosacral plexopathy as well.

DIAGNOSIS

EMG may be performed, and magnetic resonance imaging (MRI) is the imaging procedure of choice for visualizing the lumbosacral plexus.

TREATMENT

Treatment consists of identifying and treating the underlying cause. Steroids and intravenous immunoglobulin have been used in treatment of idiopathic lumbosacral plexopathy.

REFERENCES

Dyck, P. J., & Thaisetthawatkul, P. (2014). Lumbosacral plexopathy. *Continuum (Minneap Minn)*, *20*(5), 1343–1358

Robbins, N. M., Shah, V., & Benedetti, N. (2016). Magnetic resonance neurography in the diagnosis of neuropathies of the lumbosacral plexus: a pictorial review. *Clin Imaging*, *40*(6), 1118–1130.

LYME DISEASE, NEUROBORRELIOSIS

Lyme disease, also called Lyme borreliosis, is a systemic illness caused by a tick-transmitted spirochete, *Borrelia burgdorferi*. Blacklegged ticks, also known as deer ticks (*Ixodes scapularis* or *paficus*), are most commonly associated with Lyme disease in North America, while *Ixodes ricinus* occurs in Europe. Borrelia infections in Europe are associated with symptoms that vary from those seen in North America, probably due to other Borrelia species such as *B. garinii* or *B. afzelii*, although *B. burgdorferi* may occur.

CLINICAL PRESENTATION

For clinical purposes, Lyme disease is divided into three stages:

Stage I (3 days to 1 month): The early localized stage is characterized by an erythema migrans lesion manifest as a red macule or papule, expanding centrifugally to form an annular red lesion with central clearing (erythema chronicum migrans) (Fig. 38) in at least 80% of patients. The lesion occurs 7 to 14 days following the tick bite, although not all patients recall a tick bite. Systemic symptoms (malaise, myalgia, arthralgia, fever/chills, and headache) along with regional lymphadenopathy may also occur.

Stage II (up to 9 months): Hematogenous dissemination of *B. burgdorferi* occurs within days to weeks. Early Lyme neuroborreliosis occurs in about 15% of patients with untreated erythema migrans within 4 weeks. At this time, patients may develop multiple erythema migrans lesions as well as neurologic, cardiac, and rheumatologic disorders. The most common neurologic manifestations are cranial neuropathies (particularly facial nerve palsy),

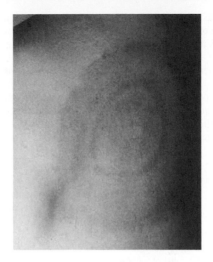

FIGURE 38

Erythema migrans.

lymphocytic meningitis, and radioculoneuritis—which often occur in combination. Facial paralysis is a common manifestation of Lyme neuroborreliosis; it can be bilateral in 25% of patients. Lyme meningitis can be acute or subacute, and typically presents with localized headache and mild neck stiffness. Cerebrospinal fluid (CSF) examination will show lymphocytic pleocytosis (100–200 white blood cells/mm^3 with >90% lymphocytes), moderately increased protein (100–300 mg/dL), and normal glucose. Lyme radiculoneuritis presents with severe, deep pain in the distribution of the affected nerves. Variations include mononeuritis, mononeuritis multiplex, brachial or lumbosacral plexopathy, and Guillain-Barré-like syndrome. Electrophysiologic testing usually points to axonal degeneration in distal nerves and roots. The most common cardiac abnormality is a fluctuating atrioventricular (AV) block.

Stage III (9 months and beyond): Late or persistent infection occurs months to years after initial infection. It manifests as Lyme arthritis, late Lyme neuroborreliosis, and acrodermatitis chronica atrophicans. Lyme arthritis presents about 6 months after disease onset as an asymmetric oligoarticular arthritis usually involving the knees. Acrodermatitis chronica atrophicans is a slowly progressive skin disorder involving the extensor surfaces of the extremities. Late Lyme neuroborreliosis occurs less frequently than the early disease. One of the late neurologic manifestations is a subtle encephalopathic syndrome affecting memory and cognition. In the peripheral nervous system, a chronic mononeuritis or polyneuritis may occur with electrophysiologic studies indicating a primarily axonal neuropathy.

Post-treatment Lyme disease syndrome (PTLDS) is also known as chronic Lyme disease: Defined as a documented episode of Lyme disease, treatment with an accepted antibiotic regimen, resolution/stabilization of the objective manifestations of Lyme disease, and persistent nonspecific symptoms for at least 6 months after treatment. No evidence exists that these patients benefit from additional antibiotic therapy.

European neuroborreliosis differs from North American disease. Erythema migrans is often slower spreading and subtler and less likely to be recalled. The most common presentation of European Lyme neuroborreliosis is the triad of **Banworth syndrome** (lymphocytic meningitis, cranial neuropathy, and painful radiculitis). Untreated infections caused by European Borrelia species can progress to chronic low-grade encephalitis.

DIAGNOSIS

There are two major categories of laboratory methods for the diagnosis of Lyme disease: direct methods that detect *B. burgdorferi,* and indirect methods that detect the immune response against it. Direct detection is difficult; culture is impractical, and polymerase chain reaction (PCR) sensitivity is low. Therefore, most tests performed are based on detection of the antibody responses against the spirochete in serum. Current Centers for Disease Control (CDC) recommendations consist of a two-tier approach using an initial sensitive enzyme immunoassay or indirect immunofluorescence assay, followed by separate immunoglobulin M (IgM) and immunoglobulin G (IgG) Western blots if the initial test is borderline or positive. The sensitivity of antibody-based tests increases with the duration of the infection, as a lag exists from infection to the time when serum contains enough antibodies to be detected. No current assays distinguish between active and inactive infection. Patients with erythema migrans should receive treatment based on the clinical diagnosis, as first-tier testing will be positive in <50% of these patients. In patients with neuroborreliosis, testing for *B. burgdorferi*-specific antibody synthesis in the CSF should be performed with a paired serum sample to measure the intrathecal antibody index.

TREATMENT

Lyme disease is successfully treated with antimicrobial therapy. Oral therapy is recommended for early and uncomplicated Lyme disease, including isolated CN VII palsy. Preferred oral agent: Doxycycline (100 mg PO BID × 14–28 days). Doxycycline is contraindicated in pregnancy and children less than 8 years old. Alternative oral agent: Amoxicillin (500 mg TID × 14–28 days). In early disease with meningitis or radiculoneuritis, or late disease, treatment with a parenteral regimen is recommended. Preferred IV agent: Ceftriaxone (2 g daily × 14–28 days). Alternative IV agent: Penicillin G (18–24 million units/day given in divided doses q4 hours × 14–28 days). There is little evidence for antibiotic effectiveness in chronic Lyme disease.

REFERENCES

Halperin, J. J. (2015). Nervous system Lyme disease. *Infect Dis Clin North Am*, *29*(2), 241–253.

Marques, A. R. (2015). Lyme neuroborreliosis. *Continuum*, *21*(6), 1729–1744.

M

MACROCEPHALY

Macrocephaly is defined as head circumference greater than 2 standard deviations above the normal distribution for age, gender, and gestation.

ETIOLOGY

Hydrocephalus (communicating or non-communicating), megalencephaly, thickening of the skull, cerebral edema, space-occupying lesions, hyperostosis, and hemorrhage into the subdural or epidural spaces may cause macrocephaly. Anatomic megalencephaly includes conditions in which the brain is enlarged because the number or size of cells increases. These children are macrocephalic at birth but have normal intracranial pressure. Children with metabolic megalencephaly are normocephalic at birth and develop megalencephaly during the neonatal period because of storage of abnormal substances or by producing cerebral edema (Table 80).

The causes of anatomic megalencephaly include genetic megalencephaly or megalencephaly (with gigantism, typical facial changes, and learning difficulties, as seen in Sotos syndrome or associated with mutations or deletions in the nuclear receptor-binding SET domain containing protein), neurocutaneous disorders (e.g., macrocephaly cutis marmorata telangiectatica congenital), or other neurologic disorders.

Examples of metabolic megalencephalies include leukodystrophies. Glutaric aciduria type I (glutaryl-CoA dehydrogenase deficiency) may present with macrocephaly before the individual goes on to develop severe leukoencephalopathy, at a potentially treatable stage. Megalencephalic leukoencephalopathy with subcortical cysts is a rare leukodystrophy characterized by macrocephaly and a slowly progressive clinical course marked by spasticity and cognitive decline. Macrocephaly is also frequently seen in autism, but its relationship to the pathogenesis is unclear.

EVALUATION

Evaluation involves review of prior head circumference measurements to assess rate of head growth (a rapidly growing head that is crossing percentile lines suggests hydrocephalus), assessment of head shape (frontal bossing is associated with hydrocephalus, lateral bulging with infantile subdural hematoma), measurement of head circumference of parents and siblings (benign familial megalencephaly), and computed tomography (CT) scan, magnetic resonance imaging (MRI), or ultrasound. If the infant is neurologically and developmentally normal, close observation may be all that is necessary.

A useful rule of thumb for normal rate of head growth follows:
- Premature infants: 1 cm/week
- 1 to 3 months: 2 cm/month

TABLE 80

CAUSES OF MACROCEPHALY

I. Hydrocephalus
- Noncommunicating
  - Arnold-Chiari malformation
  - Aqueductal stenosis
  - X-linked hydrocephalus with stenosis of the aqueduct of Sylvius (HSAS) syndrome (L1CAM)
  - Dandy-Walker malformation
  - Galenic vein aneurysm or malformation
  - Neoplasms, supratentorial, and infratentorial
  - Arachnoid cyst, infratentorial
  - Holoprosencephaly with dorsal interhemispheric sac
- Communicating
  - External or extraventricular obstructive hydrocephalus (dilated subarachnoid space)
- Arachnoid cyst, supratentorial
- Meningeal fibrosis/obstruction
  - Postinflammatory
  - Posthemorrhagic
  - Neoplastic infiltration
- Vascular
  - Arteriovenous malformation
  - Intracranial hemorrhage
  - Dural sinus thrombosis
- Choroid plexus papilloma
- Neurocutaneous syndromes
  - Incontinentia pigmenti
- Destructive lesions
  - Hydranencephaly
  - Porencephaly
- Familial, autosomal-dominant, autosomal-recessive, X-linked
II. Subdural Fluid
- Hematoma
- Hygroma
- Empyema
III. Brain Edema (Toxic-Metabolic)
- Intoxication
- Lead
- Vitamin A
- Tetracycline
- Endocrine (hypoparathyroidism, hypoadrenocorticism)
- Galactosemia
- Idiopathic (pseudotumorcerebri)
IV. Thick Skull or Scalp (Hyperostosis)
- Familial variation
- Anemia
- Osteoporosis, severe precocious autosomal-recessive osteoporosis (CLCN7, TCIRG1)
- Pycnodysostosis (CTSK)

Continued

TABLE 80

CAUSES OF MACROCEPHALY—CONT'D

- Craniometaphyseal dysplasia *(ANKH)*
- Craniodiaphyseal dysplasia
- Pyle dysplasia
- Sclerosteosis *(SOST)*
- Juvenile Paget disease
- Idiopathic hyperphosphatasia
- Familial osteoectasia
- Osteogenesis imperfecta
- Rickets
- Cleidocranial dysostosis
- Hyperostosis corticalis generalisata (van Buchem disease)
- Proteus syndrome

V. Megalencephaly and hemimegalencephaly

From Swaiman, K. F., Ashwal, S., et al. (2012). *Swaiman's pediatric neurology: principles and practice*, ed 5. Philadelphia: Elsevier.

- 3 to 6 months: 1 cm/month
- 6 to 12 months: 0.5 cm/month

REFERENCES

Daroff, R. B., Jankovic, J., & Mazziotta, J. C., et al. (Eds.), (2015). *Bradley's neurology in clinical practice*, ed 7. Elsevier.

Dulac, O., Lassonde, M., & Sarnat, H. B. (Eds.), (2013). *Pediatric neurology, Part I/II/III* (ed 1): Elsevier [Handbook of Clinical Neurology, vol. 111/112/113].

MAGNETIC RESONANCE IMAGING

Magnetic resonance imaging (MRI) creates images based on the behavior of various tissues exposed to strong magnetic fields, controlled magnetic field gradients, and radiofrequency (RF) pulses. Image intensity and contrast depends upon the concentration of unpaired protons, typically the motion of the hydrogen nuclei, nuclear magnetic relaxation parameters, and the type of sequence or acquisition being performed.

When tissue protons are placed in a magnetic field, they tend to align themselves either parallel in a low-energy state or antiparallel in a high-energy state to the vector of the imposed magnetic field, although they periodically flip between the two states. Because low-energy states are preferred, more protons align parallel than antiparallel at any given moment, creating a net magnetization vector. An RF pulse can then be applied, exciting the protons and changing them from longitudinal to transverse alignment. As these protons return to equilibrium within the magnetic field (i.e., longitudinal alignment), they emit energy (as an RF signal) that can be detected and converted into meaningful data—the image—by means of certain manipulations.

TECHNICAL PARAMETERS

Repetition time (TR) defines the duration of a cycle as the time between successive RF pulses.

Echo time (TE) defines a sampling interval during the cycle and is the time between giving the RF pulse and measuring the amount of RF signal being emitted by the tissue, the "echo." There may be single or multiple echoes sampled during a given cycle.

Relaxation time is the time it takes the protons to return to equilibrium within the magnetic field after an RF pulse has been given.

COMMON MAGNETIC RESONANCE IMAGING SEQUENCES

I. T_1 relaxation is based upon how fast protons return to equilibrium (longitudinal alignment) after being excited by an RF pulse. At any given time after the RF pulse is given TE, substances whose protons re-equilibrate fastest (lipids, for example, with the highest percentage of protons in the longitudinal position) appear brightest on T_1-weighted images (T1WI) where the T_1 characteristics are emphasized. Substances whose protons re-equilibrate slower (water, for example) will appear darker (Table 81). The shorter the TE, the greater the difference between various substances and tissues. At short TE, a large percentage of the lipid protons have regained their longitudinal position, whereas few water protons have done so. At longer TE, a greater percentage of both lipid and water protons have regained their longitudinal position. The greater the difference between the two substances (the shorter the TE), the greater the contrast on T1WI. Therefore, T1WI have both short TR and short TE.

II. T_2 relaxation is determined by how fast transverse magnetization decays. The longer transverse alignment is maintained, the stronger the signal that is emitted on T_2-weighted images (T2WI) (Table 82). At shorter TE, a higher percentage of both lipid and water protons are in transverse

---

TABLE 81

T_1-WEIGHTED IMAGE
DARK (LOW SIGNAL, LONG T_1)
Cerebrospinal fluid
Liquids
Cortical bone
Air
Edema
Most pathologic lesions
BRIGHT (HIGH SIGNAL, SHORT T_1)
Lipid
Gadolinium, other paramagnetic substances such as copper and manganese
Proteinaceous substances
Melanin

TABLE 82

T_2-WEIGHTED IMAGE

DARK (LOW SIGNAL, LONG T_2)

Cortical bone

Air

Melanin

Dense fibrous tissue

BRIGHT (HIGH SIGNAL, SHORT T_2)

Cerebrospinal fluid

Liquids

Edema

Most pathologic lesions

M

MAGNETIC RESONANCE IMAGING

alignment. At a longer TE, most of the lipid protons have lost their transverse magnetization (fast decay), whereas most of the water protons remain in transverse alignment (slow decay). Therefore, for greatest contrast on T2WI images, a longer TE should be chosen. Consequently, T2WI have long TE and long TR.

The degree of brightness or darkness on T1WI and T2WI can thus be determined by tissue content (Tables 81–83). In general, pathologic conditions are dark on T1WI, bright on T2WI, and bright on proton density images. The acquisition of data may be performed in a variety of patterns or sequences, which emphasize differences in tissue properties.

III. Spin echo (SE) sequence: an initial 90-degree pulse is given, and the echo is assessed at a predetermined point with an additional 180-degree pulse. The 180-degree pulse is necessary because of "dephasing" or spreading of the magnetic vectors of individual protons as they decay. If dephasing is not corrected, the vectors would eventually cancel each other out until the net vector becomes weak enough that the signal emitted would be undetectable. The 180-degree pulse "rephases" or brings back together

TABLE 83

INTRAPARENCHYMAL HEMATOMA

	T1WI	T2WI	Time Course	Type of Hemoglobin
Hyperacute	Isointense	Isointense or bright	Minutes to hours	Oxyhemoglobin
Acute	Isointense	Dark	Hours to days	Deoxyhemoglobin
Early	Bright	Dark	Days to weeks	Intracellular methemoglobin
Late	Bright	Bright	Several weeks	Extracellular methemoglobin
Chronic	Dark	Dark	Months	Hemosiderin

T1WI, T_1-weighted image; *T2WI*, T_2-weighted image.

the individual proton vectors so the echo emitted can be detected. T1WI images, T2WI images, and proton density images (PDIs) may be obtained with this sequence. PDIs emphasize tissue characteristics.

IV. Another frequently used acquisition sequence is the gradient echo (GRE), a relatively fast scanning technique. The sequence takes less scanning time and is useful for imaging flowing blood (flow-related enhancement), for detecting calcification or hemorrhage, and for moderate myelogram effect (white cerebrospinal fluid [CSF]) in the spinal canal. GRE images, like SE, may be either T_1-weighted or T_2-weighted, but usually only T2WI or PDIs are obtained.

V. Short tau inversion recovery (STIR) and fluid attenuated inversion recovery (FLAIR) are sequences where an inversion recovery preparation is used. A 180-degree RF pulse inverts the longitudinal magnetization, and then T1 recovery takes place. Depending on tissue, all longitudinal magnetization will have 0 magnitude in a specific time. If the excitation follows such time, the corresponding tissue is nulled: in STIR sequence, fat is dark; in FLAIR sequence, fluid (e.g. CSF) is dark.

VI. Perfusion-weighted images (PWIs) are useful in evaluating cerebral blood flow using a bolus-tracking method whereby repeated images are acquired at the same location during the passage of a high volume of intravenous gadolinium. These are T_2-weighted sequences and because gadolinium produces decreased signal intensity on T_2-weighted scans, areas of diminished blood flow are bright on PWI.

VII. Diffusion-weighted images (DWIs) are reflective of water motion in brain tissue. Areas with low diffusion appear bright. For example, DWI reveals cerebral infarcts as bright areas within 30 minutes of onset, with the increased signal intensity lasting 7 to 21 days.

VIII. Quantitative measurement using apparent diffusion coefficient (ADC) maps can be performed. ADC maps may be helpful in cases of suspected T_2 shine-through artifact on DWI, where bright signal on T_2 appears bright on DWI and ADC versus acute infarct (bright on DWI and dark in ADC).

IX. Susceptibility weighted imaging is a corrected GRE 3D high velocity MRI sequence, which is sensitive to detecting a very subtle amount of intracranial hemorrhage.

CLINICAL USES OF MRI

I. Vascular: Strokes appear earlier and in better detail on MRI (particularly DWI) than on computed tomography (CT). DWI and PWI images are vital in taking care of acute stroke patients. Combining both imaging sequences enables the clinician to identify the penumbra area, which represents potentially salvageable tissue. For vascular malformations, MRI and magnetic resonance angiography (MRA) are fine diagnostic tools. For aneurysms, MRA/computed tomography angiography (CTA) is excellent for screening, but a small aneurysm (<3 mm) could be missed. Conventional digital subtraction angiography is the gold standard for evaluating aneurysms. MR venography is superb for diagnosing dural venous sinus thrombosis. Although MRI can detect all types of hemorrhage, unenhanced CT is the appropriate screening examination due to quick exam time and easier access. In cases of suspected diffuse axonal injury, MRI may prove of diagnostic value, especially with the addition of a GRE pulse sequence.

II. Tumors: MRI is the procedure of choice to rule out small tumors or for tumor delineation. The ability to map the extent of a tumor (especially with the use of gadolinium) and the multiplanar capability of MRI make it very useful in surgical planning.

III. Infections: Cerebritis is well visualized with MRI. Abscess is well delineated with MRI (particularly DWI).

IV. Meningeal processes: MRI is more sensitive than CT for visualizing both infected and neoplasm-infiltrated meninges.

V. Trauma: MRI is not the examination of choice because of the lack of bony detail and the length of time needed. CT should be used.

VI. Demyelinating disease: MRI is the procedure of choice because of the excellent delineation of white matter disease. Active lesions of multiple sclerosis will enhance with gadolinium.

VII. Congenital/structural abnormalities: Multiplanar MRI is excellent for showing heterotopias and other anatomic abnormalities.

VIII. Spine imaging: Because the spinal cord is a thin, inherently low-contrast structure, MRI is the noninvasive examination of choice for the spine. Vertebral bone is well imaged on spinal MRI because it contains fatty marrow. However, small spinal column fractures are better seen on CT. MRI also allows good visualization of the soft tissue and ligaments.

IX. Pregnancy: The safety of MRI in pregnancy has yet to be determined; therefore, risk versus benefit must be considered. Gadolinium should not be administered during pregnancy.

ADVANTAGES OF MAGNETIC RESONANCE IMAGING

I. Multiplanar capability: The magnetic field can be adjusted to image in any plane without moving the patient.

II. No ionizing radiation.

III. Superior soft tissue contrast: Subtle differences in soft tissue proton relaxation characteristics enable visual distinction between soft tissues. This is considered "inherent" contrast of the soft tissue that can be significantly better appreciated with MRI than with any other modality.

IV. Vascular anatomy: Flowing blood has different characteristics than stationary soft tissue. Vessels can be imaged in detail with MRI. Magnetic resonance angiograms and magnetic resonance venograms can be reconstructed by subtracting out the background tissue signal.

V. MRI can easily image areas that are poorly visualized by CT (e.g., areas encased in thick bones, such as the posterior fossa and anterior temporal lobes).

M

MAGNETIC RESONANCE IMAGING

VI. Gadolinium is a paramagnetic IV contrast agent, which enhances tissues that are highly vascular or have a damaged blood–brain barrier. Unlike traditional contrast agents, gadolinium has very few contraindications. Adverse reactions are extremely rare. Contrast-enhanced MRI is generally obtained with T1WI, where gadolinium enhancement appears bright.

DISADVANTAGES AND LIMITATIONS OF MAGNETIC RESONANCE IMAGING

I. MRI has a longer imaging time than CT. This has improved markedly with newer generation machines.

II. Sensitivity to motion is very high, resulting in degraded image quality with patient movement. Chloral hydrate, benzodiazepines, barbiturates, or other medications can be used as a sedative, but timing and dosage and possible respiratory depression are important parameters to monitor.

III. Claustrophobia is often due to tighter confinement and longer imaging times than CT. Sedation may be necessary. Consider using an open MRI or benzodiazepine administration prior to the MRI.

IV. Metal and electronic devices, such as pacemakers, cochlear implants, and foreign bodies, often contraindicate MRI. A list may be obtained from the manufacturer, but it is becoming less problematic since the newest metal devices are being made MRI compatible.

V. Calcium is not well visualized. Dense cortical bone appears as a signal void. Therefore, bone signal is restricted to that given off by marrow fat. Areas of parenchymal calcification identified on CT may not be seen on MRI and, if seen, are often of variable signal intensity.

VI. Artifacts are common on MRI because of the complex interactions of several types of information, any of which can distort the final image.

INTRAOPERATIVE MAGNETIC RESONANCE IMAGING

The use of open MRI units in the operating room has contributed to an increased extent of tumor removal and a parallel improvement in survival times. In addition, preoperative MRI with the patient's head in a stereotactic frame or with fiducial markers can be used for surgical planning.

REFERENCES

Radue, E. W., et al. (2016). Introduction to magnetic resonance imaging for neurologists. *Continuum, 22*(5), 1379–1398.

MAGNETOENCEPHALOGRAPHY

Magnetoencephalography (MEG) records the extracranial magnetic fields produced by electrical current which is the basis of electroencephalogram (EEG), and measures vectors tangential to the cortical surface. MEG signal is very small, but it is not subject to distortion from dura, skull, or the scalp. MEG and EEG are complementary in obtaining cerebral electrical activity. MEG can assess the neural activity underlying cognitive processes in the brain and is widely used in neuropsychology research due to its excellent temporal resolution with good spatial resolution. In clinical neurology, MEG is used in localizing epileptiform activity in patients and in localizing eloquent areas of the cortex for surgical planning in patients with brain tumors or intractable epilepsy. The availability of MEG is limited by its cost and it is largely used in research settings.

REFERENCE

Gross, J., et al. (2013). Good practice for conducting and reporting MEG research. *Neuroimage, 65*, 349–363.

M

MARBURG DISEASE

MARBURG DISEASE

Approximately 7% of patients presenting with multiple sclerosis (MS) have radiographic features of fulminant disease. Among the recognized variants are Marburg variant and Balo concentric sclerosis. There is a great amount of clinical and radiological overlap among them, which makes a specific diagnosis challenging.

MARBURG VARIANT

Marburg first described a variant of MS in 1906, and most cases subsequently reported followed an aggressive course leading to death within 1 year. Lesions demonstrate significant mass effect and edema and may overlap with findings of acute disseminated encephalomyelitis. Marburg variant may be best thought of as an extreme end of the demyelinating disease spectrum and distinguishing it from other fulminant variants may be difficult in the clinical setting.

Balo Concentric Sclerosis

Presentation is usually monophasic, although it may follow a relapsing or progressive, and sometimes fulminant, course.

The characteristic feature is the development of alternating bands of demyelinated and myelinated white matter, which is seen on MRI as concentric rings, often described as "onion bulbs" due to their appearance, with rings of T2 hyperintensity surrounded by T2 hypointensity.

REFERENCES

Hu, W., & Lucchinetti, C. F. (2009). The pathological spectrum of CNS inflammatory demyelinating diseases. *Semin Immunopathol, 31*(4), 439–453.

Wattamwar, P. R., Baheti, N. N., Kesavadas, C., et al. (2010). Evolution and long-term outcome in patients presenting with large demyelinating lesions as their first clinical event. *J Neurol Sci, 297*(1-2), 29–35.

MECHANICAL THROMBECTOMY FOR ACUTE ISCHEMIC STROKE (See THROMBECTOMY)

Recent clinical advances established mechanical thrombectomy (MT) as the standard of care for acute ischemic stroke (AIS) secondary to large vessel occlusion (LVO) up to 24 hours of symptoms onset. Several clinical trials of endovascular treatment in AIS patients (MR CLEAN, ESCAPE, SWIFT PRIME, EXTEND-IA, and REVASCAT) demonstrated superior outcomes with endovascular therapy using second-generation MT devices (stent-retrievers) compared to intravenous recombinant tissue plasminogen activator (r-tPA) alone for patients with proximal LVO in the anterior circulation. Based on these data, the American Stroke Association/American Heart Association (ASA/AHA) in 2015 recommended MT as the standard of care (Class I, level of evidence A recommendation) for AIS patients who meet the following criteria:

(a) Pre-stroke modified Rankin score 0 to 1, (b) AIS receiving intravenous r-tPA within 4.5 hours of onset, (c) causative occlusion of the internal carotid artery or proximal middle cerebral artery (M1), (d) age $\geq$18 years, (e) National Institutes of Health Stroke Scale (NIHSS) score of $\geq$6, (f) ASPECTS of $\geq$6, and (g) treatment can be initiated (groin puncture) within 6 hours of symptom onset.

Furthermore, in 2017 and 2018 two hallmark trials (DAWN and DEFUSE 3) were published, extending the time windows up to 24 hours for AIS patients presenting with favorable imaging findings with small to moderate completed infarction and the presence of salvageable tissue on penumbra imaging. Based on these findings, the ASA/AHA updated their guidelines and recommended MT up to 16 hours (Class IA) and met both DEFUSE 3 and DAWN trials criteria of significant mismatch and small to moderate core volume, and up to 24 hours from symptoms onset (Class IB) if they met DAWN trial criteria of core infarct size less than 70 mL and significant mismatch.

The efficacy and safety of MT for patients who do not meet top-tier evidence criteria are under investigation. Patients with confirmed LVO on computed tomography angiography who did not meet top-tier evidence for MT—most commonly those with distal anterior circulation occlusion (M2, M3, or anterior cerebral artery [ACA] occlusions) or in the posterior circulation, NIHSS score <6, ASPECTS score <6, and pre-stroke baseline modified Rankin scale (mRS) score of >1—appear to have similarly high rates of good clinical outcome with no apparent increased risk. Given these results and the potential for devastating disability associated with emergent LVOs, when considering MT, clinicians should not defer sound clinical judgment in favor of a top-tier evidence-based checklist of inclusion/exclusion criteria. The suggested algorithm is below.

Minimizing the time to intervention is important to achieve the best possible outcomes and requires streamlined workflow, plus efficient triage and teamwork (Fig. 39). Treatment with intravenous r-tPA within 4.5 hours remains central to the management of patients with AIS; there is no evidence supporting bypassing it in favor of MT.

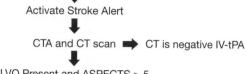

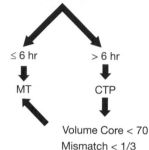

≤ 6 hr   > 6 hr

MT   CTP

Volume Core < 70
Mismatch < 1/3

FIGURE 39

Proposed acute ischemic stroke presenting within 24 hours triage algorithm.

REFERENCES

Powers, W. J., et al. (2015). American Heart Association/American Stroke Association focused update of the 2013 guidelines for the early management of patients with acute ischemic stroke regarding endovascular treatment: a Guideline for healthcare professionals from the American Heart Association/American Stroke Association. *Stroke, 46,* 3020–3035.

Powers, W. J., et al. (2018). Guidelines for the early management of patients with acute ischemic stroke: a guideline for healthcare professionals from the American Heart Association/American Stroke Association. *Stroke, 49*(3), e46–e110.

MELAS

Mitochondrial encephalopathy, lactic acidosis, and stroke-like episodes (MELAS) is a multisystem disorder that typically presents in childhood. It is a maternally inherited genetic syndrome caused by mutations in mitochondrial DNA, predominantly complex I of the electron transport chain. The most common mutation causing MELAS involves the A3243G gene (approximately 80%) which encodes for transfer RNA. In childhood, the first symptoms may manifest as developmental delay. This disease process manifests as encephalopathy which presents either as dementia or seizures, stroke-like episodes (appearing before the age of 40), recurrent vomiting, and headaches (typically recurring migraines). Other findings include ocular symptoms such as pigmentary retinopathy and ophthalmoplegia.

Due to the fact that it is a mitochondrial disorder, other diagnostic characteristics include other mitochondrial disorders such as myoclonic epilepsy with ragged red fibers on muscle biopsy (MERRF), elevated serum lactic acid, and with associated muscle weakness. Other non-neurologic signs include diabetes mellitus, renal disease, short stature, cardiomyopathy, and deafness. On magnetic resonance imaging (MRI) of the brain, lesions often are confined to the cortex (mainly occipital lobes) and are not localized to a vascular distribution. Discrete areas of lactic acidosis may be identified on magnetic resonance spectroscopy. Cerebrospinal fluid (CSF) protein is often elevated.

Therapeutic management includes supportive care and genetic counseling. Medication therapy includes anticonvulsants for seizures. Of note, in MELAS, use of valproic acid is associated with paradoxical convulsions, therefore, other medications should be used as an alternative for seizure prophylaxis. Physicians should refrain from statins, given their adverse effects of myopathy, when choosing a cholesterol-lowering medication. Other treatments include Coenzyme Q10 and other agents such as L-arginine and levocarnitine which decrease oxidative stress.

REFERENCES

Johnson, M. (2016). Encephalopathies; mitochondrial encephalopathies. In R. Kliegman, et al. (Eds.), *Nelson textbook of pediatrics,* ed 20, (p. 2901). Philadelphia: Elsevier.

Werring, D., Meschia, J., & Woo, D. (2016). Genetic basis of stroke occurrence, prevention and outcome. In J. Grotta, G. Albers, et al. (Eds.), *Stroke: pathophysiology, diagnosis, and management* (p. 271). Philadelphia: Elsevier.

MEMORY

Memory comprises the mental processes of registration, encoding, and storage of experiences and information. It has been traditionally divided into short-term or working memory (active holding and manipulation of information) and long-term memory (information stored for periods of minutes to decades). Memory systems can utilize a conscious awareness and recall (explicit, declarative) or unconscious awareness (implicit, nondeclarative). Episodic memory, for example, utilizes the explicit and declarative memory systems to narrate an experience or a story in our own context. Procedural memory of riding a motor bike or learning the sequence of numbers on a smartphone without conscious effort, on the other hand, utilizes implicit (nondeclarative) memory. Table 84 summarizes the features of some important memory systems.

The anatomy of memory involves many widely distributed neural structures. The medial temporal lobe memory system—comprising the hippocampus, the amygdala, and adjacent related entorhinal, perirhinal, and parahippocampal cortices and their connections to the neocortex—is involved in the processing and storage of long-term memory. Papez circuit plays a

TABLE 84

SELECTED MEMORY SYSTEMS, EXAMPLES AND MAJOR ANATOMICAL SUBSTRATES

Memory System	Examples	Awareness	Length of Storage	Major Anatomical Structures
Episodic memory	Remembering a short story, what you had for dinner last night, and what you did on your last birthday	Explicit Declarative	Minutes to years	Medial temporal lobe, anterior thalamic nucleus, mamillary body, fornix, prefrontal cortex
Semantic memory	Knowing who was the first US President, the color of a lion, and how a fork and comb are different	Explicit Declarative	Minutes to years	Inferior lateral temporal lobes
Procedural memory	Driving a standard transmission car, and learning the sequence of numbers on a touch-tone phone without trying	Implicit Nondeclarative	Minutes to years	Basal ganglia, cerebellum, supplementary motor area
Working memory	Phonological: keeping a phone number "in your head" before dialing Spatial: Mentally following a route, or rotating an object in your mind	Explicit Declarative	Seconds to minutes; information actively rehearsed or manipulated	Phonological: prefrontal cortex, Broca area, Wernicke area Spatial: Prefrontal cortex, visual association areas

Budson, A. E., & Kowall, N. W., eds. (2011). *The handbook of Alzheimer's disease and other dementias*, vol. 7. Chichester, UK: John Wiley & Sons.

M

MEMORY

critical role in the transfer of information into long-term memory and its emotional components.

Damage to basal forebrain structures (septum, nucleus basalis of Meynert, and orbitofrontal regions), as occurs in Alzheimer disease, is associated with memory disorder, which is often accompanied by other frontal lobe abnormalities. Damage to diencephalic structures—particularly dorsomedial and other thalamic nuclei, as in Korsakoff syndrome—leads to amnesia, possibly by the disconnection of cortical areas involved in memory processing. Bilateral damage of the limbic system causes severe memory disturbance. Bilateral damage to the amygdaloid region and anterior temporal lobes may produce the Klüver-Bucy syndrome, which is characterized by behavioral and cognitive deficits, placidity, apathy, hypersexuality, hyperorality, and visual and auditory agnosia.

Amnestic syndromes include retrograde or antegrade amnesia. Retrograde amnesia commonly follows head injury and involves loss of memory for a variable time before the event. Antegrade amnesia, the inability to incorporate ongoing experience into memory stores, is seen in head trauma, Wernicke-Korsakoff psychosis, or bilateral limbic lesions to the hippocampal-amygdala complex. The latter is usually due to occlusive vascular disease, hypoxic encephalopathy, or encephalitis. Total global retrograde amnesia, in which an individual loses all prior memory, is never due to organic dysfunction.

REFERENCES

Budson, A. E., & Kowall, N. W. (Eds.), (2011). *The handbook of Alzheimer's disease and other dementias,* vol. 7. West Sussex, UK: John Wiley & Sons.

Budson, A. E., & Price, B. H. (2007). Memory dysfunction in neurological practice. *Pract Neurol, 7*(1), 42–47.

MENINGITIS (See also NEUROLOGIC EMERGENCY APPENDIX)

DEFINITION

Meningitis is an infectious or inflammatory process that affects the leptomeninges. Most cases are secondary to a viral infection, while other causes include bacterial, fungal, and parasitic infections. In rare instances, meningitis can be secondary to chemical reactions or drug allergies.

CLINICAL PRESENTATION

Meningitis should be suspected in any patient with an acute onset of nuchal rigidity, headache, altered mental status, fever, emesis, and photophobia. Meningeal signs are often absent in infants younger than 6 months of age, elderly individuals, or immunosuppressed patients.

The classic triad includes fever, neck rigidity, and mental status changes. Physical examination can show evidence of meningismus—classic meningeal signs such as Brudzinski sign (spontaneous flexion of the hips during attempted passive flexion of the neck) or Kernig sign (the inability or reluctance to allow full extension of the knee when the hip is flexed 90 degrees).

DIAGNOSIS AND EVALUATION

If the diagnosis of acute bacterial meningitis is suspected, blood cultures and head computed tomography (CT) are obtained immediately. Antibiotic therapy should begin before the patient leaves the emergency room for the CT. A lumbar puncture should be performed with particular caution in patients with thrombocytopenia, raised intracranial pressure, mass effect on central nervous system imaging, clinical signs of impending herniation, or concomitant spinal epidural abscess. Antibiotics are chosen based on patient age, severity of clinical situation, and possible organisms (Table 85). If the CT result is normal, a cerebrospinal fluid (CSF) examination must be performed and sent for blood cell and differential cell counts, glucose and protein levels, and cultures (bacterial, viral, fungal, and mycobacterial, as appropriate). Organism-specific studies, including cryptococcal antigen studies and counterimmunoelectrophoresis specific for some strains of *Haemophilus influenzae, Neisseria meningitidis, Streptococcus pneumoniae,* fl-hemolytic streptococci, and *Escherichia coli* are often useful, especially if the results of the initial CSF cultures are negative (Table 86).

Laboratory evaluation of CSF includes a Gram stain and India ink examination of centrifuged CSF sediment. Cell counts greater than 100/mm, protein levels greater than 50 mg/dL, and glucose levels less than 30 mg/dL suggest bacterial infection. There is overlap with ranges more typical of fungal, tuberculous, and viral meningitis (see Cerebrospinal Fluid). A polymorphonuclear predominance is more common with bacterial meningitis and a lymphocytosis with aseptic meningitis. Approximately 10% of bacterial meningitides show a lymphocytosis. Hypoglycorrachia (low CSF glucose level) occurs in bacterial, tuberculous, fungal, carcinomatous, or chemical meningitis. In the subacute presentation (more than 24 hours of symptoms), unless mental status is impaired, a more detailed workup may be done before starting antibiotic therapy.

TABLE 85

WIDE-COVERAGE ANTIBIOTICS USED IN THE INITIAL TREATMENT OF ACUTE MENINGITIS BEFORE THE RETURN OF CULTURES

Patients	Antibiotic Therapy
Neonates	Ampicillin or penicillin G IV IM; aminoglycoside or ampicillin and cefotaxime; appropriate dosages depend on age and weight
Children 1–3 mo	Ampicillin 200 mg/kg/day IV divided q 6 hr and cefotaxime 200 mg/kg/day IV divided q 6 hr
Children >3 mo	Cefotaxime 200 mg/kg/day IV divided q 6 hr or ceftriaxone 100 mg/kg/day divided q 12 hr
Adults	Cefotaxime 1 g IV q 8 hr to 2 g IV q 4 hr or ceftriaxone 1 to 2 g IV q 12 hr

Note: For severe penicillin allergy consider giving chloramphenicol and trimethoprim-sulfamethoxazole. If methicillin-resistant Staphylococcus organisms are a consideration, vancomycin 1 g IV q 12 hr is recommended.

IM, Intramuscular; *IV,* intravenous.

TABLE 86

CAUSATIVE ORGANISMS IN MENINGITIS ACCORDING TO PATIENT
AGE AND CLINICAL SETTING

Infants <6 wk old: group B streptococci, *E. coli*, *S. pneumoniae*, *L. monocytogenes*,
  Salmonella organisms, *P. aeruginosa*, *S. aureus*, *H. influenzae*, Citrobacter
  organisms, herpes simplex 2

Children 6 wk to 15 yr old: *H. influenzae*, *S. pneumoniae*, *N. meningitidis*, *S. aureus*,
  viruses

Older children and young adults: *N. meningitidis*, *S. pneumoniae*, *H. influenzae*, *S.
  aureus*, viruses

Adults >40 yr old: *S. pneumoniae*, *N. meningitidis*, *S. aureus*, *L. monocytogenes*,
  gram-negative bacilli

Diabetes mellitus: *S. pneumoniae*, gram-negative bacilli, staphylococci, Cryptococcus
  organisms, Mucor

Alcoholism: *S. pneumoniae*

Sickle cell anemia: *S. pneumoniae*

Pneumonia or upper respiratory infection: *S. pneumoniae*, *N. meningitidis*, viruses, *H.
  influenzae*

AIDS or other abnormal cellular immunity: Toxoplasma, Cryptococcus, Coccidioides,
  and Candida organisms; *L. monocytogenes*, *M. tuberculosis*, and
  M. avium-intracellulare, *T. pallidum*, Histoplasma organisms, Nocardia,
  S. pneumoniae, gram-negative bacilli

Abnormal neutrophils: *P. aeruginosa*, *S. aureus*, Candida and Aspergillus organisms,
  Mucor

Immunoglobulin deficiency: *S. pneumoniae*, *N. meningitidis*, *H. influenzae*

Ventricular shunt infections: *S. epidermidis*, *S. aureus*, gram-negative bacilli

Penetrating head trauma, skin lesions, bacterial endocarditis or other heart disease,
  severe burns, IV drug abuse: *S. aureus*, streptococci, gram-negative bacilli

Closed head trauma, CSF leak, pericranial infections: *S. pneumoniae*, gram-negative
  bacilli

Following neurosurgical procedures: *S. aureus*, *S. epidermidis*, gram-negative bacilli

Tick bites: *B. burgdorferi*

Swimming in fresh water ponds: Naegleria organisms

Contact with water frequented by rodents or domestic animals: Leptospira organisms

Contact with hamsters or mice: Lymphocytic choriomeningitis virus

Exposure to pigeons: Cryptococcus organisms

Travel in southwestern United States: Coccidioides organisms

Modified from Mandell, G. L., et al. (1985). *Principles and practice of infectious diseases*, ed 2. New
York: John Wiley and Sons.
CSF, Cerebrospinal fluid; *IV*, intravenous.

Chronic meningitis is meningoencephalitis lasting for >4 weeks with a
persistently abnormal CSF study.

Recurrent meningitis describes repetitive episodes of meningitis with an
abnormal CSF followed by symptom-free periods and normal CSF (Table 87).

Mollaret meningitis is a benign recurrent aseptic meningitis associated with
herpes simplex virus, type 2, and may improve on administration of
prophylactic acyclovir.

TABLE 87

CAUSES OF ASEPTIC, CHRONIC (C), AND RECURRENT (R) MENINGITIS

INFECTIOUS

Actinomyces sp. (C)[a]

Amebas

Blastomyces sp. (C)[a]

Brucella sp. (C)

Borrelia sp. (C, R)

Candida sp. (C)

Coccidioides sp. (C)

Cryptococcus sp. (C)

Cysticercosis (C)[a]

Fungi (C, R)

Herpes simplex 1 and 2

Histoplasma sp. (C)

Human immunodeficiency virus (C)

Leptospira sp. (C, R)

Listeria sp.

Mycobacterium tuberculosis (C, R)

Mycoplasma sp.

Nocardia sp.[a]

Parameningeal suppurative foci (R)

Partially treated meningitis (R)

Rickettsia sp.

Treponema pallidum (C)

Toxoplasma sp. (C)[a]

NONINFECTIOUS

Behçet syndrome (C, R)

Chemical

Drugs (ibuprofen, isoniazide, sulindac, sulfamethoxazole)

Granulomatous angitis (C)

Lupus erythematosus (R)

Meningitis-migraine syndrome (R)

Mollaret meningitis (R)

Neoplasm (C, R)

Rupture of cyst (R)

Sarcoidosis (C, R)

Uremia

Uveomeningoencephalitis (C, R)

Viruses (R)

[a]More commonly cause brain abscess or focal lesion.

TREATMENT

Tailored to the underlying cause, initial broad-spectrum-wide coverage may include ceftriaxone 2 g q 24 hours, ampicillin 2 g IV q 4–6 hours, vancomycin 1 g q 12 hours, and metronidazole 500 mg IV q 6 hours. Glucocorticoid administration suppresses the inflammatory response, with resultant decreased brain edema and lowered intracranial pressure. Children with meningitis who receive treatment with dexamethasone 0.6 mg/kg/day in four divided doses for the initial 4 days of antibiotic therapy have lower rates of sensorineural hearing loss and neurologic sequelae.

Dexamethasone may reduce the rate of neurologic sequelae, such as seizures, focal neurologic deficits, and papilledema, particularly in patients with pneumococcal meningitis.

PROGNOSIS

The major complications from acute meningitis are seizure, stroke, abscess, hydrocephalus, and herniation with death (Fig. 40). Mortality rates for the different forms of meningitis are variable. The three most common bacterial meningitides (pneumococcal, meningococcal, and *H. influenzae*) have an average mortality rate of 10%; neurologic deficits occur in about 20% of survivors. The frequency of complications correlates with an increased duration of symptoms before treatment. Mental status changes, in particular agitation and confusion, are poor prognostic signs, as is an underlying malignancy, alcoholism, diabetes, or pneumonia. Common sequelae include hearing loss, vestibular dysfunction, cognitive and behavioral changes, and seizures.

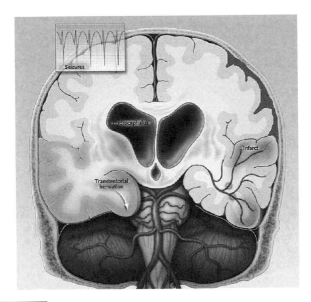

FIGURE 40

Cranial complications in bacterial meningitis. (Adapted van de Beek, D., et al. (2006). Community-acquired bacterial meningitis in adults. *N Engl J Med, 354*(1), 44–53.

REFERENCES

Brouwer, M. C., & van de Beek, D. (2017). Management of bacterial central nervous system infections. *Handb Clin Neurol*, *140*, 349–364.

Richie, M. B., & Josephson, S. A. (2015). A practical approach to meningitis and encephalitis. *Semin Neurol*, *35*(6), 611–620.

MENTAL STATUS TESTING

Routine clinical mental status examination should allow for quick screening of focal and global abnormalities. Elements of the mental status examination include state of awareness, attention, mood and affect, speech and language, memory, visual spatial function, executive functions (processing speed, attention, judgment, planning abstraction), praxis, and other aspects of cognition such as calculations and thought content. Patients who appear to have difficulties on unstructured testing during neurological examination should have a more detailed survey of their cognitive abilities, using short, standardized omnibus tests such as the Mini-Mental Status Examination or Montreal cognitive assessment (Fig. 41).

Interpretation of mental status testing cannot be performed in isolation. Widely used tests may not be valid for those with less than eight grades of education; norms may vary with race/ethnicity, education, and age. An inattentive patient may not perform well on memory tasks or language comprehension, but this is not indicative of primary language or memory disturbance. Aphasic patients may perform significantly worse than their functional status might suggest. Visual impairment may complicate constructional testing and naming. Fund of knowledge and proverb testing, although useful as a screening test, is highly dependent on educational level, socioeconomic status, and cultural background.

REFERENCES

Daffner, K. R., Gale, S. A., Barrett, A. M., et al. (2015). Improving clinical cognitive testing. Report of the AAN Behavioral Neurology Section Workgroup. *Neurology*, *85* (10), 910–918.

Tang-Wai, D. F., et al. (2003). Comparison of the short test of mental status and the mini-mental state examination in mild cognitive impairment. *Arch Neurol*, *60*, 1777–1781.

METABOLIC DISEASES OF CHILDHOOD

A metabolic disorder should be suspected under the following conditions: (1) neurologic disorder is replicated in sibling or close relative, (2) recurrent episodes of altered consciousness or unexplained vomiting in an infant, (3) recurrent unexplained ataxia or spasticity, (4) progressive central nervous system (CNS) degeneration, (5) mental deterioration in sibling or close relative, and (6) mental retardation in the absence of major congenital anomalies.

Actual	Possible	Orientation
_____	5	What is the date, year, month, day, season?
_____	5	Where are we: state, county, town, hospital, floor?

Registration

_____	3	Name three objects: 1 second to say each. Then ask the patient to name all three after you have said them. Give one point for each correct answer. Then repeat them until patient learns all three. Count trials and record. Trials _____

Attention and calculation

_____	5	Serial 7's. One point for each correct. Stop after five answers. As an alternative, spell "world" backwards.

Recall

_____	3	Ask for the names of the three objects repeated above. Give 1 point for each correct name.

Language

_____	2	Name a pencil and a watch.
_____	1	Repeat the phrase "No ifs, ands, or buts."
_____	3	Follow a three-stage command: "Take the paper in your right hand, fold it in half, and put it on the floor."
_____	1	Read and obey the following: "Close your eyes."
_____	1	Write a sentence.
_____	1	Copy the design shown here.

_____ **Total** (maximum score, 30)

Assess level of consciousness along the following continuum:

Alert   Drowsy   Stupor   Coma

FIGURE 41

Mini mental state examination (From Folstein, M. F., Folstein, S. E., & McHugh, P. R. (1975). "Mini-mental state." A practical method for grading the cognitive state of patients for the clinician. *Psychiatr Res, 12*(3), 189–198.)

The following procedures may be performed: (1) urine screen, (2) serum ammonia, fasting blood glucose, pH, P_{CO_2}, and lactic and pyruvic acid, (3) serum amino and organic acids, (4) x-ray, (5) serum lysosomal enzyme screen, (6) tissue biopsy for structural and biochemical alterations, and (7) CT or MRI.

CLASSIFICATION BY CLINICAL PRESENTATION

I. Acute encephalopathy presents shortly after birth or during early infancy with recurrent vomiting, lethargy, poor feeding, and dehydration. It initially affects the gray matter, and, hence, presents with cognitive impairment, seizures, or vision impairment. Course is rapidly progressive.

This presentation is usually caused by "small-molecule diseases" (amino acids, organic acids, and simple sugars) and represents an "intoxication" or toxic encephalopathy. Intoxications result from accumulation of toxic compounds proximal to the metabolic block. Serum lactate and ammonia, blood gas, and urine ketones permit classification of the metabolic disorders into those with (1) ketosis (maple syrup urine disease [MSUD]), (2) ketoacidosis and acidosis (organic acidurias), (3) lactic acidosis, (4) hyperammonemia with ketoacidosis (urea cycle disorders), and (5) no ketoacidosis or hyperammonemia (nonketotic hyperglycinemia, sulfite oxidase deficiency, and peroxisomal/lysosomal disorder) (Table 88).

II. Chronic or progressive encephalopathy manifests during late infancy, childhood, or adolescence. It initially affects white matter and presents with gradual onset of long-tract signs such as spasticity, ataxia, or hyperreflexia. Dementia may develop later. Liver, heart, muscle, or kidneys are frequently involved. This clinical presentation is caused by large-molecule (glycogen, glycoprotein, lipids, and mucopolysaccharides) or storage diseases and represents intoxication, energy deficiency, or both. Glycogen storage diseases, congenital lactic acidosis, fatty acid oxidation defects, mitochondrial respiratory disorders, and peroxisomal disorders belong to this group. Routine metabolic screening tests are seldom helpful. Neuroimaging and EEG, evoked potentials, electromyography and nerve conduction studies, and specialized genetic/metabolic testing are often necessary to elucidate the diagnosis.

The following metabolic disorders require early recognition and prompt treatment:

I. Phenylketonuria: autosomal recessive (AR); defect of phenylalanine hydroxylase; 2 months, vomiting and irritable; 4 to 9 months, mental retardation; later seizures, eczema, reduced hair pigmentation; early treatment with phenylalanine-restricted diet can preserve normal IQ.

II. MSUD: AR; defect in branched-chain amino acids (valine, leucine, isoleucine); first week, opisthotonos, intermittent hypertonia, feeding difficulties, and irregular breathing; 50% with hypoglycemia; sweet-smelling urine; if a diet restricted in branched-chain amino acids is started within first 2 weeks of life, normal or near-normal IQ may be achieved.

III. Homocystinuria: AR; cystathionine synthase defect; presents between 5 and 9 months; strokes, seizures, and psychiatric disturbances; ectopia lentis; sparse, blond, and brittle hair; treatment is methionine-restricted diet with or without pyridoxine 250 to 1200 mg/day. Cysteine-supplemented diet.

IV. Bassen-Kornzweig disease (abetalipoproteinemia): AR; first year, steatorrhea; second year, ataxia, retardation, retinitis pigmentosa; hypocholesterolemia, fat-soluble vitamin deficiencies, acanthocytosis; treat with vitamins E, A, and K.

V. Galactosemia: AR; defect in galactose-1-uridyl transferase; normal at birth and occur when milk feeding begins during first week; listless, jaundice, vomiting, diarrhea, and no weight gain; second week,

TABLE 88

DETECTION OF NEUROMETABOLIC DISORDERS: A PRACTICAL CLINICAL APPROACH

History (Early infancy)	Routine Laboratory Studies				Special Laboratory Studies			Enzyme Studies			Disorder
	Blood gases	Ketone	Lactic acid	Ammonia	Organic acids	Amino acids	Sulfites	WBC	Fibroblasts	Tissue	
Acute encephalopathy	−	+	−	−	+	+	−	+	+	+	Maple syrup urine disease
	+	+	−	−	+	−	−	+	+	−	Organic aciduria
	+	+	+	−	+	−	−	+	+	+	Lactic acidosis
	−	−	−	+	−	+	−	+	−	+	Urea cycle disorder
	−	−	−	−	−	+	−	−	+	−	Nonketotic hyperglycinemia
	−	−	−	−	−	−	+	+	+	−	Sulfite oxidase deficiency

History (Older child)	Urine MPS	Urine oligosaccharides	Lysosomal enzymes	VLCFA	inclusion bodies	WBC	Fibroblasts	Tissue	Disorder
Chronic encephalopathy	−	−	+	−	−	+	+	+	Sphingolipidosis
	+	−	+	−	−	+	+	+	Mucopolysaccharidoses
	−	+	+	−	−	+	+	+	Glycoprotein degradation disorder
	−	−	−	+	−	+	+	+	Peroxisomal disorder
	−	−	−	−	−	+	+	+	Fatty acid oxidation disorder
	−	−	−	−	+	−	−	−	Neuronal ceroid lipofuscinosis

hepatosplenomegaly; fourth week, cataracts; may be hypotonic and have pseudotumor cerebri; if untreated develops intellectual disability and motor retardation; treat with lactose-free diet; visual-perceptual deficits persist despite early treatment; susceptible to *Escherichia coli* sepsis.

VI. Hypothyroidism: post-term, macrosomia, jaundice, large posterior fontanel, mottled skin, big belly; second month, hypotonia, grunting cry, macrocephaly, coarse hair; later, developmental delay, deaf-mutism, and spasticity; if thyroid replacement not started within first 3 months of life, cerebellar and speech defects may persist.

VII. Pyridoxine deficiency: neonatal seizures and EEG abnormalities respond only to pyridoxine; requires lifelong treatment.

REFERENCES

Daroff, R. B., Jankovic, J., & Mazziotta, J. C., et al. (Eds.), (2015). *Bradley's neurology in clinical practice*, ed 7. Elsevier.

Dulac, O., Lassonde, M., & Sarnat, H. B. (Eds.), (2013). *Handbook of Clinical Neurology: vol. 111/112/113*. Pediatric neurology, Part I/II/III (ed 1): Elsevier.

M

MICROCEPHALY

MICROCEPHALY

Microcephaly refers to head circumference smaller than 2 standard deviations (SD) below the normal distribution for age and sex. It is important to note familial trends (measure the heads of both parents), as it can be a normal variant and normal intelligence and development are not uncommon. Head circumference smaller than 3 SD of age norms usually indicates later mental retardation. About 35 cm is the mean for head circumference at birth.

Microcephaly usually results from a small brain except in the case of craniosynostosis, in which premature closure of sutures occurs despite a normal brain (Fig. 42). Primary microcephaly refers to diminished brain size due to abnormal development early in the pregnancy.

Causes include inherited disorders (usually autosomal recessive), abnormal structural development (schizencephaly, lissencephaly, pachygyria, micropolygyria, agenesis of corpus collosum), and chromosomal abnormalities. Damage caused by irradiation or TORCH infections early in the pregnancy are also common causes. Secondary microcephaly implies that the brain was forming normally but a disease process impaired further growth. It usually occurs late in the pregnancy. Causes include intrauterine disorders (infection, toxins, vascular), perinatal brain injuries (hypoxic-ischemic encephalopathy, intracranial hemorrhage, encephalitis, stroke), and postnatal systemic diseases (chronic cardiopulmonary or renal disease, malnutrition).

Evaluation involves determining primary versus secondary causes, with special attention to identifying infectious causes (i.e., TORCH infections). Magnetic resonance imaging (MRI) is useful to distinguish the two forms, as secondary microcephaly often has identifiable abnormalities.

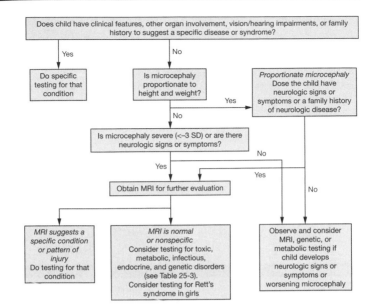

FIGURE 42

Algorithm for the diagnostic evaluation of the infant or child with postnatal-onset microcephaly. (Modified from Ashwal, S., et al. (2009). Practice parameter: evaluation of the child with microcephaly [an evidence-based review]: report of the Quality Standards Subcommittee of the American Academy of Neurology and the Practice Committee of the Child Neurology Society. *Neurology, 73*, 887–897.)

REFERENCES

Daroff, R. B., Jankovic, J., & Mazziotta, J. C., et al. (Eds.), (2015). *Bradley's neurology in clinical practice,* ed 7. Elsevier.

Dulac, O., Lassonde, M., & Sarnat, H. B. (Eds.), (2013). *Handbook of clinical neurology: vol. 111/112/113. Pediatric neurology, Part I/II/III.* (ed 1): Elsevier.

MITOCHONDRIAL DISORDERS

Mitochondrial diseases (MDs) are a clinically heterogeneous group of disorders that arise because of dysfunction of the mitochondrial respiratory chain as a result of nuclear or mitochondrial DNA (MDNA) mutation. MD may affect a single organ, but most involve multiple organ systems and often present with prominent neurologic and myopathic features. Because the sperm do not contribute mitochondria to the developing embryo, mitochondrial disorders involving MDNA mutations do not show male-to-male transmission. Nuclear

MD presents commonly in childhood and MDNA presents in late childhood or adult life.

CLINICAL FEATURES

Many MDs display a cluster of clinical features constituting a known clinical syndrome, such as the Kearns-Sayre syndrome, chronic progressive external ophthalmoplegia, mitochondrial encephalomyopathy with lactic acidosis and stroke-like episodes (MELAS), myoclonic epilepsy with ragged-red fibers (MERFF), neurogenic weakness with ataxia and retinitis pigmentosa, or Leigh syndrome (LS). However, the diagnostic criteria for many of these rare disorders have not been fully formalized. An alternative approach is to consider "red flags" for recognizing mitochondrial disorders.

Red-flag neurologic symptoms and red-flag symptoms in other organ systems include:

1. Stroke: Nonvascular distribution; on magnetic resonance imaging the apparent diffusion coefficient (ADC) map shows a mixture of hyperintensity and hypointensity
2. Basal ganglia lesions: Bilateral symmetric (characteristic of LS); also with brainstem lesions
3. Encephalopathy-hepatopathy: Precipitated by valproic acid exposure; associated hepatic failure epilepsy, epilepsia partialis continua, myoclonus, and status epilepticus
4. Cognitive decline: Regression with illness
5. Ataxia: Associated with epilepsy or other systemic symptoms; neuroimaging may show cerebellar atrophy, white matter lesions, and basal ganglia lesion
6. Ocular signs: Optic nerve atrophy, ophthalmoplegia, and ptosis; retinopathy
7. Sensorineural hearing loss: At early age, accompanied by other systemic symptoms
8. Cardiovascular: Hypertrophic cardiomyopathy with rhythm disturbance; unexplained heart block; cardiomyopathy with lactic acidosis; dilated cardiomyopathy with muscle weakness; Wolff-Parkinson-White arrhythmia
9. Ophthalmologic: Fluctuating, dysconjugate eye movements, sudden or insidious onset optic neuropathy/atrophy
10. Gastrointestinal (GI): Unexplained or valproate-induced liver failure; severe dysmotility; pseudo-obstructive episodes
11. Other: Unexplained hypotonia, weakness, failure to thrive, and a metabolic acidosis in infant or young child; exercise intolerance disproportional to weakness; hypersensitivity to general anesthesia; episodes of acute rhabdomyolysis; early onset diabetes mellitus

Symptoms can then be identified, family history obtained (note that clinical variability exists within families and many individuals do not fit neatly into one particular category), metabolic assessment (serum or cerebrospinal fluid [CSF] lactate and pyruvate, organic acids, carnitine, CoQ10), neuroimaging, muscle biopsy, and directed genetic testing can be obtained.

M

MITOCHONDRIAL DISORDERS

MANAGEMENT OF MITOCHONDRIAL DISORDERS

The management of MD is often multidisciplinary and presents some important challenges regarding diverse issues such as exercise and anesthesia, acute illnesses, genetic counselling, and supportive care. A major management issue is recognizing these disorders in a timely manner before organ damage or while symptoms can be prevented. More chronic management issues may include treatment of diabetes mellitus, cardiac pacing, ptosis correction, intraocular lens replacement for cataracts, and vision support services. Patients with mitochondrial cytopathies may benefit from oral administration of alpha lipoic acid and riboflavin and/or CoEnzyme Q10 (especially in CoQ10 deficiencies) but much of the data is anecdotal.

A special recommendation from a recent consensus document is the use of intravenous arginine hydrochloride to be administered urgently in the acute setting of a stroke-like episode associated with the MELAS m.3243 A>G mutation in the MTTL1 gene and considered in a stroke-like episode associated with other primary mitochondrial cytopathies, while other etiologies are being excluded.

REFERENCES

Parikh, S., et al. (2017). Patient care standards for primary mitochondrial disease: a consensus statement from the Mitochondrial Medicine Society. *Genet Med, 19*. https://doi.org/10.1038/gim.2017.107.

Schapira, A. H. (2006). Mitochondrial disease. *Lancet, 368*(9529), 70–82.

MOTOR NEURON DISEASE, AMYOTROPHIC LATERAL SCLEROSIS (See Also AAN GUIDELINE SUMMARIES APPENDIX)

AMYOTROPHIC LATERAL SCLEROSIS

Amyotrophic lateral sclerosis (ALS) is a progressive neurodegenerative disease primarily affecting the motor neurons. Annual incidence varies from 0.2 to 2.4 per 100,000. The majority of cases are sporadic. Five to 10 percent of cases are familial, with 20% of familial cases related to the mutation in the Cu/Zn superoxide dismutase (SOD1) gene located on chromosome 21. A combination of ALS, parkinsonism, and dementia occurs in several western Pacific islands, and may not have the same underlying pathogenesis as sporadic ALS. Onset of ALS is typically from age 55 to 75 years, but can occur at older and younger ages. Familial cases often have a younger age of onset. Male-female ratio is in the range of 1.4:1 to 2.5:1.

Clinical Presentation

Both upper motor neuron (UMN) and lower motor neuron (LMN) signs are present. Classic ALS accounts for the vast majority of cases, although onset is frequently initially limited to either the LMNs or UMNs, or to the bulbar muscles. Painless weakness and atrophy of distal muscles in the limbs are common symptoms. The distribution of weakness may be asymmetrical and over time progresses to adjacent myotomes in the same limb and the opposite limb. UMN complaints such as loss of fine movement and stiffness are also present. An

TABLE 89

CLASSIFICATION OF MOTOR NEURON DISEASE BY INITIAL PRESENTATION

Disease	Spinal Cord	Brainstem
Lower motor neuron (atrophic)	Spinal muscular atrophy	Progressive bulbar palsy
Upper motor neuron (spastic)	Primary lateral sclerosis	Progressive pseudobulbar palsy

initial bulbar onset occurs in 19% to 28% of all cases, resulting in dysarthria, dysphagia, and sialorrhea. In general, bulbar onset portends a worse prognosis. On clinical examination, patients with classic ALS have UMN signs (spasticity, increased tone, hyperreflexia) and LMN signs (muscle atrophy, weakness, and fasciculation) in bulbar or spinal innervated muscles or both (Table 89). Death is usually caused by respiratory insufficiency or aspiration pneumonia. Mean survival time from symptom onset to death is approximately 3 years, although roughly 10% of patients have a prolonged survival.

ALS subtypes include the very rare progressive bulbar palsy, in which involvement does not progress beyond the bulbar region at all. From 2% to 3.7% of all ALS cases present as primary lateral sclerosis, a condition involving only the UMN and progressing slowly over many years. Progressive muscular atrophy involves only the LMN. It occurs in approximately 2.4% of ALS patients and has a better prognosis than classic ALS.

Diagnosis

The Awaji-shima criteria are the most recent standard for diagnosis.

For diagnosis of ALS, these criteria require that all three of the following be present:

1. Evidence of LMN degeneration by clinical, electrophysiological, or neuropathological examination
2. Evidence of UMN degeneration by clinical examination
3. Progressive spread of symptoms or signs within one region or to other regions, as determined by history, physical examination, or electrophysiological tests

And that both of the following be absent:

1. Electrophysiological or pathological evidence of other disease processes that might explain the signs of LMN and/or UMN degeneration
2. Neuroimaging evidence of other disease processes that might explain the observed clinical and electrophysiological signs

Further, these criteria divide the neuraxis into bulbar, cervical, thoracic, and lumbar regions. "Clinically Definite ALS" requires UMN and LMN involvement in three regions. "Clinically Probable ALS" requires UMN and LMN signs in two regions with at least some UMN signs rostral to the LMN signs. "Clinically Possible ALS" is diagnosed if (1) UMN and LMN involvement are present in only one region, (2) UMN signs alone are present in two regions, or (3) UMN and LMN signs are present in two regions, but some LMN signs are rostral to the UMN signs.

M

MOTOR NEURON DISEASE

Finally, the Awaji-shima criteria require that other possible diagnoses must have been excluded by imaging and laboratory studies.

Differential Diagnosis

1. Diseases affecting the brain, including stroke, Parkinson disease, multiple system atrophy, and HIV infection;
2. Disorders affecting the brainstem and spinal cord, including cervical spondylosis, syringomyelia, multiple sclerosis, adrenomyeloneuropathy, vitamin B_{12} and copper deficiencies, familial spastic paraparesis, HTLV-1 infection, HIV infection;
3. Disorders affecting anterior horn cells, including adult-onset spinal muscular atrophy, Kennedy disease, hexosaminidase A deficiency, and infection with the polio and West Nile viruses;
4. Polyradiculopathies such as those caused by syphilis, CMV, and HIV, and neuropathies such as multifocal motor neuropathy (MMN), chronic inflammatory demyelinating polyradiculoneuropathy (CIDP), and POEMS syndrome;
5. Muscle diseases such as inclusion body myositis, myotonic dystrophy, and oculopharyngeal muscular atrophy; and
6. Rarely, systemic disorders such as hyperparathyroidism.

Laboratory Evaluation

Laboratory tests include CBC, ionized Ca, PO_4, Mg, CK, VDRL, ESR, TSH, vitamin B_{12}, and SPEP/UPEP. Testing for HIV may be indicated, as an ALS-like presentation has been reported to be treatable with antiretroviral therapy in at least one case. Anti-GM1 antibodies may be useful if a pure LMN presentation for possible MMN. Extensive electrodiagnostic evaluation is indicated in all cases. MRI of the neck and brain may be necessary to evaluate for cervical spondylosis and other structural lesions.

Management of ALS

I. Supportive management. Daytime sialorrhea can be treated with anticholinergic medications such as trihexyphenidyl, atropine, or glycopyrrolate. Botulinum toxin injection of the parotid gland may also be helpful. Depression and pain should be treated. Pseudobulbar affect is difficult to treat, but may respond to amitriptyline or dextromethorphan. Nutritional support is vital, particularly in patients with dysphagia. PEG tube placement may prolong survival by a few months, and should be done before the forced vital capacity (FVC) falls below 50% of normal. Serial pulmonary function tests can help in planning ahead. Bilevel positive airway pressure (BIPAP) should be offered when FVC falls to below 50% of normal. Dyspnea and progressive FVC decline predict poor prognosis, and the issue of resuscitation and whether the patient wishes to be on a mechanical ventilator should be discussed.

II. Medications. Riluzole 50 mg bid, when used early, slows ALS progression, and in bulbar onset group, prolongs survival by a few months. However, riluzole provides little benefit with more advanced disease and does not show any positive impact on patient's quality of life or muscle strength. Monthly follow-up of LFTs and CBC is necessary every 3 months.

Edaravone, a free-radical scavenger, is now approved by the Food and Drug Administration (FDA) and available as an IV infusion in the USA. As of the time this chapter was written, there is no evidence that it prolongs life, improves muscle strength, improves respiratory function, or improves quality of life. FDA approval for the drug was granted based on a single trial of a very specific subset of ALS patients. That study showed a decreased decline in rate of disease progression, as measured by the ALSFRS-R scale over 6 months.

ATYPICAL MOTOR NEURON DISEASES

ALS mimickers are disorders that primarily affect the motor system. These disorders are often referred to as atypical motor neuron diseases (Table 90). Most are distinguished from ALS clinically, while others have different

M

MOTOR NEURON DISEASE

TABLE 90

ATYPICAL MOTOR NEURON DISEASES

Immune-mediated motor neuropathies
   Multifocal motor neuropathy with conduction block
Nonimmune-mediated lower motor neuron syndromes
   Spinal muscular atrophy
   Distal spinal muscular atrophy
   X-linked bulbospinal muscular atrophy (Kennedy disease)
   Monomelic amyotrophy (benign focal amyotrophy)
   Fazio-Londe disease
Multiple system disorders with motor signs
   Adult hexosaminidase A deficiency
   Spinocerebellar degenerations
      Machado-Joseph disease (spinocerebellar ataxia type 3 [SCA III])
      Autosomal dominant cerebellar ataxia
Other multiple system disorders
   Shy-Drager syndrome
   Guamanian Parkinson-Amyotrophic lateral sclerosis-dementia complex
   Hallervorden-Spatz disease
   Creutzfeldt-Jakob disease
   Huntington disease
   Pick disease
Hyperparathyroidism
Electrical injury associated with motor neuron disease
Infectious/postinfectious
Retroviral-associated syndrome
Post-radiation motor neuron disease
Paraneoplastic disorders with motor neuron dysfunction (anti-Hu)
Toxins/drugs
Post-polio syndrome

laboratory, electrophysiologic, and pathologic characteristics. Clinical clues that may help differentiate these conditions from ALS include long duration of illness, lack of bulbar involvement after 1 year, onset before age 35 years, presence of family history (although familial ALS does occur), and absence of concurrent UMN and LMN signs in the same spinal segment. Absence of muscle wasting in chronically weak limbs may suggest that the weakness is a consequence of focal conduction block with preservation of motor axon, as seen in MMN. The presence of sensory involvement, bowel or bladder dysfunction, cerebellar or extrapyramidal dysfunction, extraocular muscle weakness, and involvement of other organ systems such as endocrine disorders should suggest ALS is not the diagnosis. A correct diagnosis is important to avoid missing a treatable disorder such as MMN or a familial disorder for which others are at risk.

REFERENCES

Al-Chalabi, A., et al. (2017). ENCALS statement on edaravone. *Amyotroph Lateral Scler Frontotemporal Degener*, *4*, 1–4. Epub ahead of print.
Hardiman, O., et al. (2017). Edaravone: a new treatment for ALS on the horizon? *Lancet Neurol*. *16*(7), 490–491.

MOYAMOYA DISEASE

Moyamoya disease was first described in 1957 by Takeuchi and Shimizu as "hypogenesis of bilateral internal carotid arteries." In 1969, Suzuki and Takaku gave the Japanese name "moyamoya," meaning "puff of smoke," to the disease based on the angiographic appearance of fine, collateral blood vessels arising from the large vessels at the base of the brain.

EPIDEMIOLOGY

Moyamoya disease mainly affects people of Asian descent, but it is seen worldwide. Mean age of diagnosis is bimodal (largest peak 10 to 14 years of age and smaller peak in the 40s), and there is female preponderance (1.8:1 female-male ratio).

PATHOGENESIS

A chronic cerebral vasculopathy results in the gradual occlusion of large intracranial arteries arising from the circle of Willis. Over time, a sprouting of myriad, thin, fragile collateral vessels distal to the stenotic arteries occurs (Fig. 43). These collaterals are highly susceptible to rupture, resulting in intracranial hemorrhage. The genetic and environmental factors involved in the moyamoya disease process are unknown. Moyamoya may be a heterogeneous disease, as similar findings may be seen in patients with sickle cell disease, Down syndrome, neurocutaneous syndromes, Fanconi anemia, cyanotic congenital heart disease, cranial irradiation, and other vasculitides.

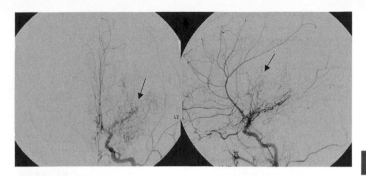

FIGURE 43

Moyamoya disease: Biplane angiography demonstrating the occlusion of the middle cerebral artery with fine sprouting of collaterals (arrows) indicating the puff of smoke.

M

MOYAMOYA DISEASE

CLINICAL PRESENTATION

Based on a study of 34 US adult patients with angiographically proven idiopathic moyamoya disease, the following initial clinical presentations were observed: ischemic stroke (15, 44%), hemorrhagic stroke (7, 20%), TIAs (9, 26%), asymptomatic (3, 9%). There was bilateral vascular involvement in 22 (65%) and unilateral involvement in 12 (35%). The median age of presentation in this group was 42 years (range 20 to 79 years). The initial clinical diagnosis in patients with Asian ethnicity is likely different than in this population. Based on a study of moyamoya patients in Hawaii, in which most patients had Asian ancestry, 29% had intracranial hemorrhage as their initial clinical presentation. In general, it is thought that moyamoya presents more often with ischemic stroke in children and hemorrhagic stroke in adults.

DIAGNOSIS

Radiographic diagnosis of moyamoya disease requires cerebral angiography; however, magnetic resonance angiogram (MRA) or computed tomography angiogram (CTA) may be used as noninvasive alternatives. The angiography must demonstrate stenosis or occlusion at the terminal portions of the intracranial internal carotid artery (ICA), and at the proximal portions of the anterior and middle cerebral arteries. There should also be a characteristic abnormal network of fine collateral vessels stemming from the circle of Willis. Occasionally, there may be only unilateral carotid involvement. There is a high association of aneurysms and arteriovenous malformations with moyamoya disease. The moyamoya classification established by Suzuki in 1989 is the most commonly used one: Stage 1: Narrowing of carotid fork. Stage 2: Initiation of the "Moyamoya vessels," dilatation of the intracerebral main arteries. Stage 3: Intensification of the "Moyamoya vessels," non-filling of the anterior and middle cerebral arteries. 3a: partial non-filling of the anterior and middle cerebral arteries. 3b: partial preservation of the anterior and middle cerebral arteries. 3c: complete lack of the anterior and middle cerebral arteries. Stage 4: Minimization of the "Moyamoya vessels," disappearance of the posterior cerebral artery.

MANAGEMENT

Surgical treatment is generally preferred and in some cases has improved cerebral blood flow and allowed resolution of the affected collateral vessels. More widely used surgical procedures are encephaloduroarteriosynangiosis (EDAS) and encephaloduralmyosynandiosis. EDAS involves rerouting a branch of the external carotid (EC) artery intradurally through non-anastomotic means. This allows for the development of more stable intracranial collateral circulation. Other surgical procedures including extracranial-intracranial (EC-IC) bypass have been used, but EDAS is the most common for treating moyamoya. The complication rate of EDAS has been cited at 4%.

Medical management of moyamoya has included antiplatelets, pentoxifylline, and calcium channel blockers, but no definitive data is available. Dehydration and hypotension should probably be avoided because of the precarious blood supply. Anticoagulants are not generally used because of the association of moyamoya with intracranial hemorrhage. There are no studies comparing medical to surgical management.

PROGNOSIS

The stroke recurrence rate based on the previously mentioned study of 34 US adult patients diagnosed with moyamoya was assessed in medically managed and surgically managed groups. The risk varies from 65% in unilateral cases to 82% in bilateral involvement over 5 years in medically managed cases. In surgically managed cases, the risk was 17% inclusive of perioperative or subsequent strokes or death. There are many predictors to understand long-term outcome including age of onset, timing of surgical procedure, and post-surgical cerebral hemodynamics. Intellectual impairment affecting independence has been noticed in 20% to 40% of the pediatric population with ischemic strokes even after surgical revascularization over 5 years.

REFERENCES

Scott, R. M., & Smith, E. R. (2009). Moyamoya disease and moyamoya syndrome. *N Engl J Med, 360*(12), 1226–1237.

Thines, L., Petyt, G., Aguettaz, P., et al. (2015). Surgical management of moyamoya disease and syndrome: current concepts and personal experience. *Rev Neurol (Paris), 171*(1), 31–44.

MULTIPLE SCLEROSIS (See also AAN GUIDELINE SUMMARIES AND THERAPEUTIC APPENDICES)

EPIDEMIOLOGY

Multiple sclerosis (MS) is the most common demyelinating disease, affecting 250,000 to 350,000 people in the United States and over 1 million people worldwide. Onset of the disease is usually between the ages of 10 and

60 years, with peak age between 20 and 30. The cause remains unknown but is generally considered to be autoimmune. The incidence of MS increases with latitude in temperate climates. Risk for development of the disease correlates with the latitude at which one lived before the age of 15 years. There is a familial predisposition for its development; women are more affected than men and whites more than blacks or Asians. Approximately 80% of patients will have relapsing-remitting MS, while 20% follow a primary progressive course. Of the patients with relapsing-remitting disease, 50% will develop secondary progressive MS (Fig. 44).

CLINICAL PRESENTATION
Symptomatology is related to the location of lesions. A wide variety of symptoms may occur: Optic neuritis (most common initial symptom), fatigue, limb weakness, spasticity, hyperreflexia, paresthesias, Lhermitte sign (sensation of "electricity" down the back associated with neck flexion), ataxia, tremor, nystagmus, internuclear ophthalmoplegia, diplopia, vertigo, bowel or bladder dysfunction, impotence, depression, emotional lability, and cognitive abnormalities. The Uhthoff phenomenon is the worsening of a sign or symptom

M

MULTIPLE SCLEROSIS

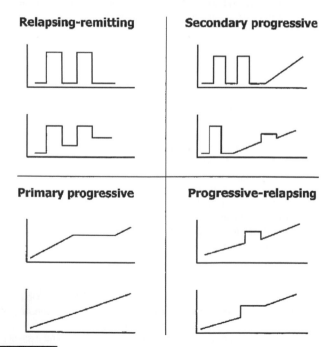

Clinical classification of multiple sclerosis.

with exercise or increased temperature (increased temperature slows axon conductance of action potentials).

DIAGNOSIS

MS is a clinical diagnosis that aims at proving dissemination in space and in time. For diagnostic purposes, symptomatic attacks should have objective dysfunction lasting at least 24 hours and occurring in different central nervous system (CNS) locations involving primarily white matter and should be separated by a period of at least 1 month (separated by space and time). Various sets of diagnostic criteria have been used since the 1960s and rely on clinical characteristics and laboratory studies such as cerebrospinal fluid (CSF) evaluation and evoked potentials, and then CT and MRI as they developed from the 1970s and 1980s. Most recently, the McDonald criteria—formulated by the international panel on MS diagnosis in 2001 and revised most recently in 2010—are intended to replace the older Poser criteria and Schumacher criteria, incorporating MRI with clinical evaluation and laboratory studies (Table 91). These criteria help in the early diagnosis of MS even after the first clinical event. The true onset of MS is now believed to be long before the onset of clinical symptoms, and axonal damage usually occurs early in MS. Earlier diagnosis allows earlier treatment with disease-modifying drugs and should lead to better outcomes.

Radiologic and laboratory studies support the clinical diagnosis. CT results are usually normal but can show areas of decreased attenuation in the white matter, areas of contrast enhancement, or both. MRI is far more sensitive than CT for detecting MS plaques and is the imaging procedure of choice. Enhancement with gadolinium is considered evidence of an "active" plaque. T_2 weighted imaging frequently demonstrates finger-like extensions along the small or medium-sized blood vessels ("Dawson fingers") radiating perpendicular to the longitudinal axis of the lateral ventricles. T_1 weighted imaging may reveal areas of decreased signal "black holes."

CSF shows normal to mildly elevated protein, normal glucose, moderate lymphocytic pleocytosis (5 to 20 cells/mm^3), elevated IgG index, and oligoclonal IgG bands in 90% of cases. Free kappa light chains or myelin basic protein are elevated during flares. Visual, auditory, and somatosensory evoked potentials may reveal abnormalities in their respective pathways. Cystometry may show an uninhibited, spastic, or flaccid bladder or detrusor-sphincter dyssynergy.

TREATMENT

General management includes making the diagnosis based on available evidence, treatment of disease flares, avoidance of heat, and excessive fatigue. A small, spastic bladder can be treated with oxybutynin, propantheline, imipramine, or tolterodine (long acting). Sphincter dyssynergy and a spastic bladder often coexist and are treated with phenoxybenzamine, diazepam, or both. A large, flaccid bladder is treated with Valsalva or Credé maneuvers,

TABLE 91

2010 REVISED MCDONALD DIAGNOSTIC CRITERIA FOR MULTIPLE SCLEROSIS

Clinical (Attacks)	Lesions	Additional Data Needed for MS Diagnosis
Two or more attacks[a]	Objective clinical evidence of two or more lesions or objective clinical evidence of one lesion with reasonable historical evidence of a prior attack[b]	None[c]
Two or more attacks[a]	Clinical evidence of one lesion	DIS, demonstrated by: one or more T2 lesions in at least 2 of 4 MS-typical regions of the CNS (periventricular, juxtacortical, infratentorial, spinal cord)[d] or await further clinical attack[a] implicating a different CNS site
One attack[a]	Objective clinical evidence of two or more lesions	DIT, demonstrated by: two or more lesions concurrent asymptomatic gadolinium-enhancing and non-enhancing lesions—a new T2 or enhancing lesion(s) on follow-up MRI or await a second attack[a]
One attack	Objective clinical evidence of one lesion	Dissemination in space, demonstrated by ≥ one T2 lesion in at least two MS typical CNS regions (periventricular, juxtacortical, infratentorial, spinal cord); OR await further clinical attack implicating a different CNS site AND dissemination in time, demonstrated by simultaneous asymptomatic contrast-enhancing and non-enhancing lesions at any time; OR a new T2 and/or contrast-enhancing lesions(s) on follow-up MRI, irrespective of its timing; OR await a second clinical attack
0 (Primary progression from onset)		One year of disease progression (retrospective or prospective) AND at least 2 out of 3 criteria—dissemination in

Continued

TABLE 91

2010 REVISED MCDONALD DIAGNOSTIC CRITERIA FOR MULTIPLE SCLEROSIS—CONT'D

Clinical (Attacks)	Lesions	Additional Data Needed for MS Diagnosis
		space in the brain based on one T2 lesion in periventricular, juxtacortical, or infratentorial regions—dissemination in space in the spinal cord based on two T2 lesions; OR positive CSF

[a]An attack is defined as an episode of neurological disturbance in the absence of fever or infection for which causative lesions are likely to be inflammatory and demyelinating in nature with subjective report (backed up by objective findings) or objective observation that the event lasts ≥ 24 hr.

[b]Clinical diagnosis based on objective clinical findings for two attacks is most secure. Reasonable historical evidence for one past attack, in the absence of a documented neuro exam, can include historical events with symptoms and evolution characteristics for a prior inflammatory demyelinating event.

[c]No additional tests required, but it is desirable that any MS diagnosis is made with access to imaging based on these criteria. If imaging or other tests (CSF) are negative, alternative diagnoses must be considered. There must be no better explanation for the clinical presentation, and objective evidence must be present to support a diagnosis of MS.

[d]Gadolinium-enhancing lesions are not required; symptomatic lesions are excluded from consideration in subjects with brainstem or spinal cord syndromes.

1—If criteria indicated are fulfilled and there is no better explanation for the clinical presentation, the Dx is "MS."

2—If suspicious, but the criteria are not completely met, the Dx is "possible MS."

3—If another Dx arises during the evaluation that better explains the entire clinical presentation, the Dx is "not MS."

CNS, Central nervous system; CSF, cerebrospinal fluid; DIS, dissemination in space; DIT, dissemination in time; MRI, magnetic resonance imaging.

Treatment: See chapter on MS Treatments.

Modified from Polman, C. H., Reingold, S. C., Banwell, B., et al. (2011). Diagnostic criteria for multiple sclerosis: 2010 revisions to the McDonald criteria. Ann Neurol, 69(2), 292–302.

catheterization (intermittent or permanent), or pharmacologic agents such as bethanechol and phenoxybenzamine. Spasticity is treated most commonly with baclofen at doses of 40 to 80 mg/day or tizanidine in doses up to 36 mg/day with diazepam or dantrolene as needed to control spasms. Chronic pain or neuralgia is treated with carbamazepine, gabapentin, phenytoin, or amitriptyline. Depression is treated with selective serotonin reuptake inhibitors and fatigue with modafinil or amphetamine/dextroamphetamine. Muscle fatigue can be alleviated with dalfampridine.

REFERENCES

Montalban, X., et al. (2017). N Engl J Med, 376, 209.

Tramacere, I., et al. (2015). Cochrane Databse Syst Rev CD011381. .

MUSCLE DISEASES AND TESTING

Bedside examination of the muscles involves assessment of bulk, tone, strength, and the presence or absence of fasciculations, myokymia, or cramping. In certain neuromuscular diseases, fatigue of muscle strength or improvement of strength with exercise may be important.

Assessment of muscle strength is most frequently done by manual muscle testing of specific muscle groups (Table 92), and this gives a rough impression of motor power. Subtle weakness may not be demonstrated by action against resistance but may be revealed with provocative postures or movement, such as pronator drift or arm-rolling. More quantitative measures, like grip dynamometry, can provide a more precise measurement of change in motor strength over time. It is also helpful to follow the assessments made by the patient's physical and occupational therapists. Location of muscle weakness may provide invaluable information about the underlying disease and pathophysiology (Table 93).

In any suspected neuromuscular disorder, electrodiagnostic testing—that is, electromyography (EMG) and nerve conduction studies—should be considered. Electrodiagnostic testing is widely available, repeatable, objective, and can provide considerable information about the patient's condition, including markers of chronicity and severity. It can provide clues to help localize the condition to muscle, neuromuscular junction, or peripheral neural structures. Nerve conduction studies can help distinguish between demyelinating and axonal neuropathies. Refer to the chapter on EMG and nerve conduction studies for more information.

There are three different types of muscle fibers (Table 94), and different muscles in the body contain different proportions of these fiber types.

In cases of suspected muscle disease, muscle biopsy of an affected muscle, with histochemical and immunohistochemical staining, is helpful for

M
MUSCLE DISEASES AND TESTING

TABLE 92

GRADING OF MUSCLE STRENGTH

Grade	Strength
0	No perceptible contraction.
1	Trace contraction is observed, but no movement is achieved.
2	Movement is achieved in horizontal plane but not against gravity.
3	Movement is achieved against gravity but not against additional resistance.
4−	Movement is achieved against slight resistance.
4	Movement is achieved against moderate resistance.
4+	Movement is achieved against large resistance but is less than expected, given patient age and fitness.
5	Intact strength.

From *Aids to the examination of the peripheral nervous system*, ed 3. East Sussex: Baillière Tindall, 1986.

TABLE 93

POSSIBLE DIAGNOSES OF MUSCLE WEAKNESS

Predominant Weakness	Differential Diagnosis and Localization
Ocular	Brainstem and motor cranial nerve pathology, Horner syndrome, oculopharyngeal muscular dystrophy, Kearns-Sayre syndrome, Graves disease, and congenital myasthenia
Bulbar	Brainstem and multiple cranial nerve pathology, motor neuron disease, obstructive lesion of the nasal and oropharynx
Lateralized limb weakness	Stroke, peripheral nerve or root lesion

DISTAL EXTREMITY	
Arm	Distal myopathies
Leg	Peroneal neuropathy or L5 radiculopathy
Isolated respiratory	Acid maltase deficiency, myotonic dystrophy, polymyositis, motor neuron disease, Lambert-Eaton myasthenic syndrome
Isolated neck	Motor neuron disease, inflammatory myopathy, paraspinous myopathy

Modified from Kaminski, H. (2002). Myasthenia gravis. In B. Katirji et al. (Eds), *Neuromuscular diseases in clinical practice.* Boston: Butterworth-Heinemann.

TABLE 94

CHARACTERISTICS OF MUSCLE FIBER TYPES

Characteristic	Type 1	Type 2a	Type 2b
Speed	Slow	Fast	Fast
Metabolism	Oxidative	Oxidative-glycolytic	Glycolytic
Fatigue resistance	+	+	−

confirming the presence of myopathy and further characterizing the muscle disease (Table 95). Characteristics of myopathic tissue include rounded fibers, the presence of larger and smaller muscle fibers, and movement of myofiber nuclei toward the center of the fiber. Necrotic fibers, inflammation, vacuoles, and inclusions may also be present and aid in diagnosis.

REFERENCES

Miles, J. D., & Cohen, M. L. (2011). Skeletal muscle and peripheral nerve disorders. In R. A. Prayson (Ed.), *Neuropathology,* ed 2. Philadelphia: Elsevier.

Miles, J. D., & Cohen, M. L. (2013). Nerve and muscle biopsies. In B. Katirji et al. (Eds.), *Neuromuscular disorders,* ed 2. New York: Springer.

TABLE 95

SYNDROMIC CLASSIFICATION OF MUSCLE DISEASE

I. Acute (evolving in days) or subacute (weeks) paretic or paralytic disorders of muscle
   A. Rarely fulminant myasthenia gravis or myasthenic syndrome from a "mycin" antibiotic or hypokalemia
   B. Idiopathic polymyositis and dermatomyositis
   C. Viral polymyositis
   D. Acute paroxysmal myoglobinuria
   E. "Alcoholic" polymyopathy
   F. Familial (malignant) hyperpyrexia precipitated by anesthetic agents
   G. Neuroleptic malignant syndrome
   H. First attack of episodic weakness may enter into differential diagnosis (see below)
   I. Botulism
   J. Organophosphate poisoning
II. Chronic (i.e., months to years) weakness or paralysis of muscle, usually with severe atrophy
   A. Progressive muscular dystrophy
      1. Sex-linked recessive
         a. Duchenne
         b. Becker
         c. Benign with early contractures (Dreifuss-Emery)
         d. Scapuloperoneal
      2. Autosomal recessive
         a. Scapulohumeral (limb-girdle)
         b. Autosomal recessive dystrophy of childhood (Erb)
         c. Congenital
   B. Normokalemic or hyperkalemic familial periodic paralysis
   C. Paramyotonia congenita (von Eulenberg)
   D. Nonfamilial hyperkalemic and hypokalemic periodic paralysis (including primary hyperaldosteronism)
   E. Acute thyrotoxic myopathy (also thyrotoxic periodic paralysis)
      3. Autosomal dominant
         a. Facioscapulohumeral (Landouzy-Dejerine)
         b. Scapuloperoneal
         c. Late-onset recessive (Erb)
         d. Distal—adult onset
         e. Distal—childhood onset
         f. Ocular (Hutchinson-Fachs)
         g. Oculopharyngeal (Victor-Hayes-Adams)
         h. Myotonic dystrophy
   B. Chronic polymyositis or dermatomyositis (may be subacute)
      1. Idiopathic
      2. With connective tissue disease
      3. With occult neoplasm
      4. Inclusion body myositis
   C. Chronic thyrotoxic and other endocrine myopathies
   D. Chronic, slowly progressive, or relatively stationary polymyopathies
      1. Central core and multicore diseases
      2. Rod-body and related polymyopathies
      3. Mitochondrial and centronuclear polymyopathies
      4. Other congenital myopathies (reducing-body, fingerprint, zebra-body, fiber-type atrophies, and disproportions)
      5. Glycogen storage disease
      6. Lipid myopathies (carnitine deficiency myopathy and undefined lipid myopathies)
III. Episodic weakness of muscle
   A. Familial (hypokalemic) periodic paralysis
   B. Myopathy resulting from myophosphorylase deficiency (McArdle disease), phosphofructokinase deficiency, and other forms of contracture
   C. Contracture with Addison disease
   D. Idiopathic cramp syndromes
   E. Myokymia and syndromes of continuous muscle activity

M

MUSCLE DISEASES AND TESTING

Continued

TABLE 95

SYNDROMIC CLASSIFICATION OF MUSCLE DISEASE—CONT'D

F. Conditions in which weakness fluctuates
1. Myasthenia gravis, immunologic type
2. Myasthenia associated with
   a. Lupus erythematosus
   b. Polymyositis
   c. Rheumatoid arthritis
   d. Nonthymic carcinoma
3. Familial and sporadic myasthenia
4. Myasthenia resulting from antibiotics and other drugs
5. Lambert-Eaton syndrome

G. Exercise intolerance
1. Myoadenylate deaminase deficiency
2. Ca-adenosine triphosphate deficiency
3. Hypothyroidism
4. "Fibromyositis" syndrome
5. Hypoparathyroidism
6. Glycogenosis (debranching enzyme deficiency)

IV. Disorders of muscle presenting with myotonia, stiffness, spasm, and cramp
A. Myotonic dystrophy, congenital myotonia (Thomsen disease), paramyotonia congenita, and Schwartz-Jampel syndrome.
B. Hypothyroidism with pseudomyotonia (Debré-Sémélaigne and Hoffman syndromes)
C. Tetany
D. Tetanus
E. Black widow spider bite

V. Myalgic states
A. Connective tissue diseases (rheumatoid arthritis, mixed connective tissue disease, Sjögren syndrome, lupus erythematosus, polyarteritis nodosa, scleroderma, polymyositis)
B. Localized multifocal fibrositis (myogelosis)
C. Trichinosis
D. Myopathy of myoglobinuria and nonimmunologic types of McArdle disease
E. Myopathy with hypoglycemia
F. Bornholm disease and other forms of viral polymyositis
G. Anterior tibial syndrome
H. Other
1. Hypophosphatemia
2. Hypothyroidism
3. Psychiatric illness (hysteria, depression)

VI. Localized muscle mass(es)
A. Rupture of a muscle
B. Muscle hemorrhage
C. Muscle tumor
1. Rhabdomyosarcoma
2. Desmoid
3. Angioma
4. Metastatic nodules
D. Monomyositis multiplex
1. Eosinophilic type
2. Other
E. Localized and generalized myositis ossificans
F. Fibrositis (fibromyalgia)
G. Granulomatous infections
1. Sarcoidosis
2. Tuberculosis
3. Wegener granulomatosis
H. Pyogenic abscess
I. Infarction of muscle in the diabetic

From Adams, R. A., & Victor, M. (1993). *Principles of neurology*, ed 5. New York: McGraw-Hill.

MUSCULAR DYSTROPHY

INTRODUCTION

The muscular dystrophies (MDs) are a group of hereditary, degenerative myopathies that cause progressive weakness. Although clinical and pathologic criteria have been used in the past, most criteria are now classified based on genetics.

Myotonic Dystrophy

Myotonic dystrophy is the most common MD but is reviewed in the section on myotonia.

Dystrophinopathies

The dystrophinopathies are X-linked, recessive (XLR) disorders that are consequent to mutations in the gene for dystrophin, Duchenne muscular dystrophy *(DMD),* the largest in the human genome. Dystrophin is a subunit of the dystrophin glycoprotein complex, which mechanically links the sarcomere to the extracellular matrix. Dystrophinopathy should be suspected in any male patient with progressive, limb-girdle weakness, particularly when there is a substantially elevated serum creatine kinase, cardiomyopathy, or a positive family history. The most common forms are DMD and Becker muscular dystrophy (BMD).

Clinical features: The incidence of DMD is approximately 1:3500 to 1:5000 male births, and BMD is approximately {1/10} that rate. Boys with DMD typically present between 3 and 5 years of age with delayed motor milestones, falls, and difficulty running and jumping. Upon examination, there is pseudohypertrophy of the calves, a mildly lordotic posture, and a waddling gait. The *Gowers maneuver* is characteristic. BMD is a milder form of DM. If a boy stops walking by 12 years of age, he is considered to have DMD, and if he is between 12 and 16 years of age, he is considered to have an intermediate phenotype. If the boy can walk past 16 years, he is considered to have BMD. Female carriers may be asymptomatic or may manifest milder weakness with onset in the third decade or later but are still at risk of cardiac disease. Any first-degree female relative of a patient with DMD or BMD should undergo genetic evaluation. If positive, follow-up evaluation for weakness or cardiac disease is recommended. Cognitive dysfunction is common in DMD (50% have intellectual disability) and less so in BMD. Joint contractures generally begin in the ankles while patients are still ambulatory and later affect the hips, knees, elbows, and wrists. Cardiac and pulmonary involvement are common and patients should be followed by cardiology (arrhythmia, dilated cardiomyopathy) and pulmonology (spirometry should be monitored). Death usually occurs in the third decade due to respiratory insufficiency or cardiomyopathy.

Evaluation: CK levels may be as high has 10 to 200 times the upper limit of normal. Aspartate and alanine aminotransferases and myoglobin are other muscle enzymes that may be elevated. Patients with BMD or female carriers may present with less striking clinical manifestations, and the diagnostic evaluation may be more involved. Serum CK levels are elevated in 50% to 70% of female carriers. ECG abnormalities are present in 80%. Electromyography (EMG) can demonstrate myopathic motor units and may reveal muscle membrane instability. DNA analysis of the *DMD* gene is often diagnostic. Multiplex PCR, or multiplex ligation-dependent probe amplification, is used for evaluation of deletions or duplications. If this is unrevealing, gene sequencing can be performed. In some cases, muscle biopsy may be performed prior to genetic testing or to clarify the likely pathogenicity of variants of unknown significance. Biopsy typically reveals marked variability of fiber size, scattered hypercontracted muscle fibers, and proliferation of endomysial connective tissue. Immunostaining for dystrophin demonstrates decreased or absent dystrophin-positive fibers.

Treatment: Glucocorticoids should be offered to all boys with DMD and have been demonstrated to prolong walking, improve strength and slow muscle degradation, improve pulmonary function, and may improve cardiac and cognitive function. The optimal age at which to initiate glucocorticoids and what regimen to use are unclear, but most initiate treatment between 5 and 7 years of age before patients begin to lose milestones. Prednisone 0.75 mg/kg/day or deflazacort 0.9 mg/kg/day are commonly used. Physical therapy, nighttime splinting, stretching, and standing boards can delay contractures. Achilles tendon release or surgical correction of scoliosis may be indicated.

Facioscapulohumeral Muscular Dystrophy

Facioscapulohumeral muscular dystrophy (FSHD) is an autosomal dominant (AD) condition with high penetrance but variable expression. Between 70% and 90% of patients inherit the disorder from an affected parent; up to 30% arise de novo.

Clinical features: As the name suggests, FSHD affects the facial, periscapular, biceps, and triceps muscles and typically progresses rostrocaudally (i.e., the facial muscles are first affected, then the scapular muscles, arms, and finally the legs). In contrast to the other MDs, asymmetry is common in FSHD and some patients may not have the full pattern or weakness. Ninety percent of patients show signs of FSHD by 20 years of age but usually do not present until the upper extremities become weak, because facial weakness is rarely functionally limiting. On examination, facial weakness manifests with inability to bury the eyelashes, widened palpebral fissures, lip pursing weakness, or a transverse smile. A prominent axillary crease may be present due to pectoral muscle wasting, and scapular winging is common. The "triple hump sign" (deltoid, acromion process, and high-riding scapula) with arm abduction is characteristic. Foot dorsiflexion weakness may be observed with foot-slapping gait, and later in the course, the proximal leg muscles may also weaken. Hearing loss and retinal vascular abnormalities are present in a majority of patients and are generally subclinical in adults but problematic in infantile-onset FSHD. Cardiac arrhythmias may occur but are generally asymptomatic. Life expectancy is normal, but approximately 20% of patients will eventually require a wheelchair.

Evaluation: When the disease is fully developed, the diagnosis can be made on history and examination alone. Serum CK is mildly elevated in 75% of patients and ranges from normal to 1000 U/L. EMG demonstrates myopathic changes. Muscle biopsy shows inflammatory changes in up to 30% of patients. Genetic testing is 95% sensitive for FSHD. In almost all patients, FSHD results from a reduced number of tandem repeats (D4Z4) on chromosome 4q35.

Treatment: There is no specific treatment for FSHD. Conservative management with nonsteroid antiinflammatory drugs, range of motion exercises, and gentle stretching exercises may help with discomfort and pain in the shoulder and back. In carefully selected patients with relatively good deltoid function, surgical fixation of the scapula to the rib cage can improve arm function and enable the patient to carry or lift objects. The procedure is usually done unilaterally.

Emery-Dreifuss Muscular Dystrophy

Emery-Dreifuss muscular dystrophy (EDMD), also known as humeroperoneal MD, is a genetically heterogeneous disorder. It includes XLR (EDMD1 and EDMD6), AD (EDMD2, EDMD4, and EDMD5), or autosomal recessive (AR; EDMD3) inheritance patterns.

Clinical features: The cardinal features of EDMD are flexion contractures at the elbows and ankles with early spine disease, humeroperoneal weakness that begins in childhood, cardiac disease with arrhythmias, conduction block, and cardiomyopathy. The inability to fully extend the elbows and toe walking are early signs of the diagnosis. Sudden cardiac death related to arrhythmia is the major mortality concern. Female carriers of the X-linked forms may develop weakness and are at risk of cardiac disease and should be evaluated by a cardiologist.

Evaluation: CK may be normal or mildly elevated but is rarely greater than 2000 U/L. EMG reveals myopathy, usually without evidence of irritability. Six different genetic mutations can cause EDMD; all function at the inner nuclear membrane, but the precise mechanisms of injury are unknown. Most common is *LMNA* mutation (AD; ~33% of all) followed by *EMD* (XLR; ~17% of all); others include *SYNE1*, *SYNE2*, *TMEM43* (all AD), and *FHL1* (XLR).

Treatment: There is no specific treatment. Early contractures can be managed by physical therapy and surgical release. All patients should be seen followed by a cardiologist, and annual cardiac evaluation (ECG, Holter monitor) is required. Placement of combined pacemaker/internal defibrillator should be strongly considered.

Limb-Girdle Muscular Dystrophies

The limb-girdle muscular dystrophies (LGMDs) are genetic muscle diseases with postnatal onset of proximal upper and lower extremity weakness and atrophy. Although the phenotypic pattern of LGMDs is relatively conserved, there is both phenotypic and genetic heterogeneity; more than 25 different

M

MUSCULAR DYSTROPHY

genetic muscle disorders are considered within the LGMD spectrum. Dysfunction of proteins involved in a variety of muscle fiber functions can cause LGMD, including those involved in cellular signal transduction and trafficking, intracellular and extracellular structural proteins, proteins of the sarcomere, sarcoplasm, sarcolemma, and proteins involved in sarcolemma repair. The LGMDs are categorized based on pattern of inheritance (type 1 for AD and type 2 for AR) and order of discovery (A, B, etc.). The spectrum of LGMDs is beyond the scope of this review, but a few of the most common forms are explored. In approaching a patient with predominantly proximal muscle weakness, the clinician should bear in mind that other etiologies, such as the dystrophinopathies, myasthenia gravis, spinal muscular atrophy, and acquired muscle disorders (toxic, metabolic, and autoimmune myopathies), are more common than the LGMDs. Therefore these should be considered and excluded early in the evaluation, and dystrophin mutation analysis should be offered to males and considered in females.

Calpainopathies (LGMD2A) are responsible for approximately 30% of all AR LGMDs in the United States. Calpain is a calcium-activated protease that binds to titin. Most patients present in their teens with weakness in the lower extremities, more striking than in the shoulder girdle. Weakness of the hip extensors, adductors, and knee flexors is especially severe. CK levels average approximately 4000 but can be greater than 20,000 U/L. Cardiac disease and pulmonary involvement are uncommon, and intelligence is normal.

Dysferlinopathies (LGMD2B) can manifest as Myoshi distal myopathy (which prominently involves the calves) or as LGMD, accounting for 5% to 35% of LGMDs. They are more common in patients of Asian or Mediterranean descent. Dysferlin functions in membrane trafficking, fusion, and repair, including mitochondrial. Most patients present between 15 and 30 years of age, usually with predominant weakness in the lower extremities. CK may be strikingly elevated to as much as 40,000 U/L. Muscle biopsy may demonstrate endomysial or perimysial infiltration that can be mistaken for myositis. Cardiopulmonary involvement is very rare.

Sarcoglycanopathies (LGMD2C-F) are responsible for 15% to 20% of LGMDs, with higher prevalence in those of North African or Brazilian descent. The sarcoglycans form a complex with dystrophin, sarcospan, and dystroglycans that anchors the cytoskeleton and the contractile proteins of the sarcomere to the extracellular basement membrane. The clinical manifestations span the spectrum from severe DMD-like phenotypes to asymptomatic hyperCKemia. Cardiopulmonary involvement is common and can be severe. CK values range from 1000 to 25,000 U/L.

Fukutin-related proteinopathies (LGMD2I) account for approximately 15% of LGMDs, and they predominantly affect those of Northern European descent. The affected protein normally functions in the glycosylation of alpha-dystroglycan. Weakness in the pelvic and femoral muscles, and later the legs and proximal arms, develops over a broad age range but most often before the third decade. Calf and tongue hypertrophy are common, as is lordosis of the lumbar spine. CK may be elevated in the range of 500 to greater than 10,000 U/L, and cardiopulmonary involvement is common.

Oculopharyngeal Muscular Dystrophy

Oculopharyngeal muscular dystrophy (OPMD) is caused by a $(GCN)_{12-17}$ expansion in the poly(A)-binding protein 2 gene (PABPN1). The normal number of repeats is 10. Although initially described as a $(GCG)_{8-13}$ polyalanine disease, it is now recognized that both GCG/alanine and GCA/alanine repeats are involved. The repeat size is stable, and anticipation does not occur. OPMD has a worldwide distribution but is more prevalent in those of French-Canadian descent.

Clinical features: OPMD is unusual in that it presents later in life—usually in the fifth or sixth decade—with ptosis as the initial manifestation. Affected individuals eventually develop extraocular muscle dysfunction, especially in upward gaze, but progression is slow enough that most do not report diplopia. Dysphagia may be the first manifestation but more often follows ptosis by several years, and it is the major cause of morbidity and mortality. Tongue atrophy is seen in 82%, vocal changes in 67%, and facial weakness in 43%. Seventy-one percent and 38% percent of patients eventually develop slowly progressive lower extremity weakness or upper extremity weakness, respectively. Cognitive dysfunction may develop in homozygous patients, and subtle executive dysfunction can cause heterozygotes.

Evaluation: Diagnosis is clinically established with genetic confirmation. The differential diagnosis includes myasthenia gravis (ptosis and other signs are variable/fatigable), mitochondrial myopathy (maternally inherited and may present with seizures, deafness, diabetes, neuropathy, cardiomyopathy), and myotonic dystrophy (temporal wasting, "Christmas tree" cataracts, percussion/grip myotonia). CK is usually normal and, when elevated, rarely rises to greater than 1000 U/L. Muscle biopsy is not needed but may reveal rimmed vacuoles on light microscopy and filamentous intranuclear inclusions on electron microscopy.

Treatment: There is no specific treatment for OPMD, but management of dysphagia is important given the risk of aspiration, anorexia, and cachexia. Cricopharyngeal myotomy, upper esophageal sphincter dilation, or gastrostomy or jejunostomy tube placement may be necessary. Ptosis can also be surgically corrected.

Distal Myopathies

Distal myopathies are characterized exclusively or predominantly by distal weakness in the extremities. The advances in molecular genetics have expanded the list of distinct distal myopathies to more than 20 different entities, and a clinical classification scheme has been developed. Patients are first sorted by age of onset and inheritance pattern, then magnetic resonance imaging (MRI) of the distal legs further sorts patients into those with anterior compartment, posterior compartment, and mixed patterns. Another system involves morphologic categorization. A comprehensive review of these

M

MUSCULAR DYSTROPHY

categories is not within the scope of this chapter, but the following provides a limited discussion.

Late-Adult-Onset Autosomal Dominant Forms
The late-adult-onset distal myopathies include Welander myopathy, tibial MD (Udd myopathy), distal myotilinopathy, ZASPopathy (Markesbery-Griggs), Matrin3 distal myopathy (VCPDM, MPD2), VCP-mutated distal myopathy, and alpha-B crystallin–mutated distal myopathy. Welander myopathy usually begins in the fifth to sixth decade with weakness in the distal upper extremities and progresses slowly. Life expectancy is normal, and CK is slightly elevated. Rimmed vacuoles may be present on muscle biopsy with nuclear filaments on EM. Udd myopathy is a titinopathy linked to chromosome 2q31 that typically begins in the fourth to fifth decade. Foot drop is typically the first sign, followed by variable involvement of the finger and wrist extensors. CK is slightly elevated and muscle biopsy shows rimmed vacuoles.

Adult-Onset Autosomal Dominant Distal Myopathies
The adult-onset AD distal myopathies include desminopathy (DES mutation), distal ABD-filaminopathy (FLNC mutation), Finnish-MPD3, Italian 19p13-linked distal myopathy, US-Polish family, and oculopharyngeal distal myopathy (reviewed previously).

Early-Onset Autosomal Dominant Distal Myopathies
The early-onset AD distal myopathies include Laing distal myopathy (MPD1 mutation) and KLHL9-mutated distal myopathy (KLHL9 mutation).

Early-Onset Autosomal Recessive Distal Myopathy
The only form known to date is distal nebulin myopathy, resulting from NEBl mutation.

Early-Adult-Onset Autosomal Recessive Distal Myopathies
Miyoshi myopathy (DYSF mutation), distal anoctaminopathy (ANO5 mutation), distal myopathy with rimmed vacuoles (GNE mutation, AKA Nanoka myopathy), and oculopharyngeal distal myopathy are included in this category. In Miyoshi distal myopathy, weakness characteristically begins in the calf muscles between 15 and 25 years of age and the proximal leg muscles are eventually affected. Nonaka myopathy presents with weakness of the ankle dorsiflexors and toe extensors in the second to third decade of life. Proximal weakness may eventually occur, but the quadriceps are spared.

Adult-Onset Autosomal Recessive Distal Myopathy
Calf myopathy non-DYSF/ANO5 is in this category.

Congenital Myopathies

The congenital myopathies are a rare group of genetically and phenotypically diverse, heritable skeletal muscle disorders that typically present with early infantile or childhood weakness, hypotonia, and developmental delay. Most are slowly progressive or static. They are broadly divided into three pathologic categories: the core myopathies (myofibers with areas of absent oxidative enzymes), centronuclear or myotubular myopathies (internally located myonuclei), and the nemaline myopathies (myofibers contain electron dense nemaline bodies or rods). More than 20 genes have been associated with congenital myopathy. In approaching the diagnostic evaluation, the history and physical examination are most important. Clues to the diagnosis include family history, early onset of weakness, atrophy, slow or static course, myopathic facies, bulbar involvement, and orthopedic complications. CK is usually normal or slightly elevated. Electromyography and nerve conduction studies (EMG/NCS) reveal normal nerve conduction studies apart from compound muscle action potentials (CMAPs), which may have reduced amplitude. Needle examination typically reveals myopathic recruitment but may have neurogenic findings related to atrophy and occasionally increased jitter or electrodecrement in some conditions. Muscle MRI can help to determine patterns of myopathy, especially early in the illness. The differential diagnosis in hypotonic infants also includes congenital MD, myasthenic syndromes, neuropathies, spinal muscular atrophy, glycogen storage disease, and metabolic etiologies, including botulinum intoxication. Treatment is primarily supportive and orthopedic complications may require surgery. Many cases require cardiac and/or pulmonary monitoring. Some are at risk of malignant hyperthermia.

Core Myopathies

The core myopathies are among the most common forms of congenital myopathy and include central core and multiminicore myopathies. Areas within the myofibers that lack evidence of oxidative activity are devoid of mitochondria. The most common causes include mutations in the skeletal ryanodine receptor (RYR1; AD or AR) and selenoprotein N-1 (*SEPN1*; AR). Less often, mutations in skeletal muscle alpha-actin or titin can cause core myopathy. Most patients present in infancy with hypotonia and prominent, proximal muscle weakness. Ptosis, ophthalmoplegia, dysphagia, and respiratory insufficiency suggest against the diagnosis. Patients with central core myopathy caused by RYR1 mutations are at risk for malignant hyperthermia, which can be a fatal complication of volatile anesthetics or muscle relaxants. Those with multiminicore usually have AR mutations in *SEPN1,* and no cases of malignant hyperthermia have been reported.

Centronuclear Myopathies

The centronuclear myopathies are a heterogeneous group of conditions with at least eight genes implicated in their pathogenesis. Inheritance patterns include XLR: *MTM1*, AD: *DNM2, BIN1, CCDC78,* and AR *BIN1, MTMR14, TTN,* and *SPEG. DNM2* is the most common and usually presents in early adulthood with a relatively mild distal myopathy. Most boys (XLR) with neonatal *MTM1* mutations have severe weakness and approximately 40% die within a year, despite supportive therapy; 80% of those who live beyond a year are ventilator dependent. Those with later-onset *MTM1* mutations present with a milder form of exercise intolerance and fatigue and may be at risk of cardiomyopathy.

Nemaline Myopathies

The nemaline myopathies are distinguished pathologically by threadlike or rodlike inclusions that are dark red on Gomori trichrome stain. At least 10 genes have been associated with nemaline myopathy, including AD: *ACTA1,* AR: *NEB, CFL2, TNNT1, TPM2, TPM3, KLHL40, KLHL41,* and *KBTBD13.* The clinical spectrum of nemaline myopathies is broad, ranging from severe neonatal forms to relatively mild axial/limb-girdle myopathy that progresses to involve the distal extremities. The common pattern of weakness includes the facial muscles and flexors of the neck and trunk, with prominent weakness in the foot dorsiflexors and toe extensors. The most common cause of nemaline myopathy is *NEB* mutation, which phenotypically ranges from severe neonatal forms to later onset, milder forms.

REFERENCES

Brandsema, J. F., & Darras, B. T. (2015). Dystrophinopathies. *Semin Neurol, 35*(4), 369–384.

Mah, J. K., & Joseph, J. T. (2016). An overview of congenital myopathies. *Continuum (Minneap Minn), 22,* 1932–1953.

MYASTHENIA GRAVIS

Myasthenia gravis (MG) is a disorder in which autoantibodies cause dysfunction of signal transmission across the neuromuscular junction (NMJ), characterized by muscle fatigue and fluctuating weakness. Autoantibodies against acetylcholine receptors (AChRs) in the postsynaptic membrane of the NMJ can result in one or more of these: blocking the binding of acetylcholine to AChR; causing complement-mediated destruction of the receptors; or causing cross-linking of AChRs resulting in their internalization. Anti-AChR antibodies (binding, blocking, or modulating) are found in 85% of generalized and 50% of ocular MG cases. Fifty percent of the seronegative generalized MG patients have other antibodies (e.g., anti-muscle specific kinase [MUSK] antibodies that reduce AChR clustering on endplates). Antibodies against low-density lipoprotein receptor-related protein 4, agrin, etc., are recent discoveries. Congenital myasthenia, which can be presynaptic or postsynaptic, can present in infancy or early childhood with fatigable weakness and positive family history.

The prevalence of MG is 1 per 5000 people. Women are more likely to develop MG between age 10 and 40 years; men are more likely to develop MG after age 50 years. Neonatal myasthenia occurs due to transplacental transmission of autoantibodies in ~15% of babies born to mothers with MG. Ocular myasthenia is more prevalent in older men and MUSK-related MG is more common in women.

CLINICAL FEATURES

MG classically presents with fluctuating muscle fatigue and weakness that worsens with exertion and varies through the day. Ocular weakness (eyelid droop) is the initial manifestation of the disease in about half of the cases and is eventually involved in 90% of the cases. Isolated ocular MG (~15%) can progress later to generalized MG. Weakness of bulbar muscles, including muscles of facial expression, mastication, swallowing, and speech, is also common. Sustained or repeated activity exacerbates weakness, which improves after rest. There is no muscle atrophy, and deep tendon reflexes are intact. Ptosis and/or diplopia can be induced by having patients look up for several minutes. Fatigability is revealed by repetitively testing the proximal limb or neck muscles. Applying an icepack over the drooped eyelid reduces acetyl choline breakdown in the NMJ and reverses ptosis (icepack test). Dysphagia and dysarthria, weakness of neck muscles, and inability to count to 20 in a single breath are serious signs of pharyngeal and respiratory muscle weakness.

DIAGNOSIS

Diagnosis is made on clinical grounds, with confirmation by the following diagnostic investigations:

I. Tensilon test. This is an old test in which IV edrophonium (Tensilon), an ultra-short-acting cholinesterase inhibitor, is used to assess rapid improvement particularly of ptosis. Antibody testing and better electrophysiological evaluations have rendered this obsolete.

II. Serum anti-AChR antibody titers have a specificity of ~99% in generalized MG. Antibodies have lower sensitivity in ocular MG. About half of the anti-AChR negative cases have anti-MUSK antibodies. Titers do not correlate with disease severity. Suspected paraneoplastic cases should be evaluated for Lambert-Eaton myasthenic syndrome with anti-voltage-gated calcium channel antibodies.

III. Electromyography (EMG) examination. Routine nerve conduction studies and needle EMG examination are normal in MG, which helps to differentiate MG from myopathic and neurogenic disorders. On 2 to 3 Hz slow repetitive stimulation of a proximal nerve, the presynaptic acetyl choline stores are depleted and a decrement of $\geq 10\%$ in compound muscle action potential amplitude is observed in 50% to 70% of the patients with generalized MG. Proximal muscles such as orbicularis oculi muscles (facial nerve stimulation) and the trapezius (spinal accessory n.) have higher yields due to being proximal.

IV. Single-fiber EMG (SF-EMG). Due to reduced AChRs in MG, muscle depolarization is delayed, which can cause variation in the firing times of

M

MYASTHENIA GRAVIS

two adjacent muscle fibers of the same motor unit. SF-EMG detects this variation in the form of increased "jitter" in 95% to 99% of the patients with generalized MG. If the muscle depolarization fails, it is detected as "blocking." Single-fiber EMG can also be abnormal in several other neuropathic and myopathic diseases and is not specific to NMJ disorders. Hence clinical context is important in interpreting its results.

V. Additional testing. CT of the chest to evaluate for thymoma. Tests of thyroid function, erythrocyte sedimentation rate, antinuclear antibody titers, and vitamin B_{12} level can help in evaluating concurrent disease and other autoimmune diseases. Serial pulmonary function testing, especially negative inspiratory force, is important in following the course of myasthenic exacerbation.

TREATMENT

I. Cholinesterase inhibitors (e.g., pyridostigmine [Mestinon]) increase the amount of acetylcholine available at the NMJ to bind the postsynaptic AChR. Initial dose is 30 to 60 mg every 3 to 4 hours and titrated to a range of 60 to 120 mg every 3 to 6 hours based on response. Doses greater than 480 mg/day are unlikely to be beneficial. It is available as a 60 mg tablet, a 12 mg/mL syrup, and a 180 mg sustained-release preparation for bedtime use. Adverse muscarinic side effects include excess salivation, abdominal cramping, and secretory diarrhea. Diarrhea can be controlled with anticholinergic medications. Cholinergic crises due to medication excess should be suspected in patients who have been on high dosage of pyridostigmine if they present with respiratory failure, miosis, sialorrhea, diarrhea, bronchorrhea, cramps, and fasciculations. Treatment is supportive in addition to withdrawal of anticholinesterases.

II. Corticosteroids are helpful in all types of MG. Prednisone, started at a low dose of 0.75 to 1 mg/kg/day, is gradually titrated up to 1 to 1.5 mg/kg/day. This dose should be maintained until remission, and then switched to alternate-day dosing. If strength fluctuates between "on" and "off" days, a small dose may be added to "off" days. Maximal benefit may take months (3–6) to achieve. Anticholinesterases should be tapered first to verify remission. Steroids are then tapered over 6 to 12 months. If the patient relapses, tapering is stopped and the dose is adjusted appropriately. Hypertension, hyperglycemia, weight gain, and osteoporosis should be considered when titrating steroids. Steroids possess NMJ blocking properties and may worsen MG crises acutely.

III. Long-term immunosuppression. Azathioprine at 2 to 3 mg/kg with prednisone is the recommended first-line combination for long-term immunosuppression in generalized MG. Its effect is delayed by 6 to 15 months. Close monitoring of hepatic transaminases and leukocyte counts is needed. Cyclosporine is a second-line option. In refractory cases, rituximab, a B-cell-depleting monoclonal antibody, has been tried with success, especially in anti-MUSK myasthenia.

IV. Plasma exchange (PLEX) and intravenous immunoglobulin (IVIg) are used as short-term treatments in patients with MG with life-threatening signs such as respiratory insufficiency or dysphagia; in preparation for surgery in patients with significant bulbar dysfunction; when a rapid response to treatment is needed; when other treatments are insufficiently effective; and prior to beginning corticosteroids if deemed necessary to prevent or minimize exacerbations. PLEX has higher efficacy than IVIg in some published series.

V. Thymectomy should be done if thymoma is present. In non-thymomatous MG, thymectomy may help minimize the dose or duration of immunotherapy in the long run, or if patients fail to respond to immunotherapy. It is generally safe in juvenile MG. The patient's status should be optimized by PLEX before thymectomy.

VI. Myasthenic crisis. Patients with severe weakness, bulbar signs, and symptoms of respiratory compromise need to be hospitalized, their respiratory status closely monitored, and intubated if needed. Cholinergic crisis should be considered in those who are on high-dose anticholinesterases (see above). Precipitating causes of myasthenic crisis (e.g., medications, infections) should be searched for and treated. Drugs that affect transmission across NMJ include quinine and curare, antiarrhythmic drugs quinidine, procainamide, and propranolol; quinolones and aminoglycoside antibiotics; d-penicillamine and magnesium-containing drugs. IVIg and PLEX are the mainstay of treatment in crisis and they take 2 to 5 days for peak effect. Steroids and nonsteroidal immunosuppressants can be started when beneficial effects of IVIg or PLEX start to show. PLEX works quicker but the choice of IVIg or PLEX is dependent on comorbidities.

VII. MG in pregnancy. Prednisone and oral pyridostigmine, as well as PLEX and IVIg, are safe in pregnancy. Azathioprine is relatively safe per recent international guidelines, but should be reserved for cases resistant to pyridostigmine and steroids. Thymectomy can often be postponed until after pregnancy.

REFERENCES

Sanders, D. B., Wolfe, G. I., Benatar, M., et al. (2016). International consensus guidance for management of myasthenia gravis: executive summary. *Neurol, 87*, 419–425.

Wolfe, G. I., Kaminski, H. J., Sonnett, J. R., et al. (2016). Randomized trial of thymectomy in myasthenia gravis. *NEJM, 375*, 511–522.

MYELOGRAPHY

Traditionally, myelography was an imaging technique that combined conventional x-ray of the spine with injection of contrast into the subarachnoid space with indications including spinal cord and root compression. Currently, Computerized tomography (CT) myelography is performed after conventional plane films have been obtained. Contrast material is injected intrathecally to highlight the contour of spinal subarachnoid space in relation to the surrounding bones and soft tissue. A block in cerebrospinal fluid (CSF) flow is indicative of narrowing of the spinal canal and potential compression of the cord, whereas extradural collection of contrast is indicative of CSF leak. Despite the use of CT along with conventional plain films, magnetic resonance imaging (MRI) has largely supplanted the role previously played by myelography. However, in cases in which MRI is equivocal, especially in assessing the nerve roots or in determining if a fluid collection communicates with the CSF, CT myelography is still useful. It is still a critical technique for indications such as spinal stenosis, brachial plexus injury, and radiation therapy treatment planning. In addition, when MRI of the spine is contraindicated such as when the patient has a pacemaker or other MRI-incompatible metallic device, CT myelography would be the next-best diagnostic tool.

REFERENCES

Klein, J. P. (2015). A practical approach to spine imaging. *Continuum (Minneap Minn)*, *21*(1 Spinal Cord Disorders), 36–51.

Pomerantz, S. R. (2016). Myelography: modern technique and indications. *Handb Clin Neurol, 135*, 193–208.

MYOCLONUS

Myoclonus is defined as brief arrhythmic or repetitive muscular contractions of cortical, reticular, or spinal origin. It can be focal, segmental, or generalized; rhythmic or irregular; spontaneous or induced by action; stable or progressive. Clonus refers to monophasic rhythmic contractions and relaxations of a group of muscles (compare with Tremors).

CLINICAL PRESENTATION

The clinical presentation falls into two broad categories: (1) primary, and (2) secondary or symptomatic. Primary is further classified into (1) physiologic, (2) essential, and (3) epileptic (15%). Myoclonus is usually symptomatic/ secondary origin (75%) and related to post-hypoxia, toxic-metabolic disorders, reactions to drugs, storage disease, and neurodegenerative disorders. The assessment of myoclonus includes an initial screening for those causes that are common or easily corrected. Precipitants of myoclonus include sensory stimuli, physical contact, and anxiety, which may modulate the intensity of the myoclonus.

Origin of myoclonus: Cortical, sub-cortical, spinal (segmental or propriospinal), or peripheral; best differentiated by electro-physiologic techniques.

Palatal myoclonus: Rhythmic, synchronous contractions of the palate at an average rate of 120 to 130/minute; it can be either bilateral or unilateral and may be associated with contractions of extraocular muscles, larynx, neck, diaphragm, trunk, or limb. Palatal myoclonus persists during sleep. There is hypertrophic degeneration of the contralateral inferior olivary nucleus if the myoclonus is unilateral. The lesion can be anywhere within the Guillain-Mollaret triangle—red nucleus, inferior olivary nucleus, and contralateral dentate nucleus—and the connecting pathways (central tegmental tract and crossing dentato-olivary pathway). The movements disappear after damage to the pathways of corticobulbar or corticospinal motor neurons. Palatal myoclonus is seen in cerebrovascular disease, multiple sclerosis, and encephalitis, and occasionally it is idiopathic.

CLASSIFICATION

I. Physiologic (in persons with normal health)
  A. Sleep jerks (hypnic jerks)
  B. Anxiety induced
  C. Exercise induced
  D. Hiccough (singultus)
  E. Benign infantile myoclonus with feeding
II. Essential myoclonus (no known cause and no other gross neurologic deficit)
  A. Hereditary (autosomal dominant)
  B. Sporadic
III. Epileptic myoclonus (seizures predominate, and encephalopathy is absent, at least initially)
  A. Fragments of epilepsy
    1. Isolated epileptic myoclonic jerks
    2. Epilepsia partialis continua
    3. Idiopathic stimulus-sensitive myoclonus
    4. Photosensitive myoclonus
    5. Myoclonic absences in petit mal
  B. Childhood myoclonic epilepsies
    1. Infantile spasms (West syndrome)
    2. Myoclonic astatic epilepsy (Lennox-Gastaut syndrome)
    3. Juvenile myoclonic epilepsy (Janz)
  C. Benign familial myoclonic epilepsy
  D. Progressive myoclonus epilepsy
    1. Baltic myoclonus (Unverricht-Lundborg)
    2. Lafora disease
    3. Myoclonic epilepsy with ragged red fibers (MERRF)
IV. Symptomatic myoclonus (progressive or static encephalopathy dominates)
  A. Storage diseases
    1. Lipidoses (such as GM2 gangliosidosis, Tay–Sachs disease, and Krabbe disease)
    2. Ceroid lipofuscinosis (Batten disease and Kufs disease)
    3. Sialidosis
  B. Spinocerebellar degenerations
    1. Ramsay–Hunt syndrome
    2. Friedreich ataxia
    3. Ataxia-telangiectasia

C. Basal ganglia degenerations
   1. Wilson disease
   2. Torsion dystonia
   3. Hallervorden-Spatz disease
   4. Progressive supranuclear palsy
   5. Huntington disease
   6. Parkinson disease
D. Dementias
   1. Creutzfeldt-Jakob disease
   2. Alzheimer disease
E. Viral encephalitides
   1. Subacute sclerosing panencephalitis
   2. Encephalitis lethargica
   3. Arboviral encephalitis
   4. Herpes simplex encephalitis
V. Postinfectious encephalomyelitis
   F. Metabolic
      1. Hepatic failure
      2. Renal failure
      3. Dialysis syndrome
      4. Hypoglycemia
      5. Infantile myoclonic encephalopathy (polymyoclonus) (with or without neuroblastoma)
      6. Nonketotic hyperglycemia
      7. Multiple carboxylase deficiency
      8. Biotin deficiency
      9. MERRF
   G. Toxic encephalopathies
      1. Bismuth
      2. Heavy metal poisonings
      3. Methyl bromide and dichlorodiphenyltrichloroethane
      4. Drugs (levodopa, amantadine, penicillin, amitriptyline, imipramine, morphine, meperidine, l-tryptophan plus monoamine oxidase inhibitor, lithium, and phenytoin)
   H. Physical encephalopathies
      1. After hypoxia (Lance-Adams syndrome)
      2. Post-traumatic
      3. Heat stroke
      4. Electric shock
      5. Decompression injury
   I. Focal central nervous system damage
      1. After stroke
      2. After thalamotomy
      3. Tumor
      4. Trauma
      5. Palatal myoclonus

Diagnostic studies helpful in differentiating myoclonus from tics, myokymia, and psychogenic disorders, and in determining the origin include: surface electromyography (EMG), electroencephalogram (EEG), EEG-EMG back averaging and somatosensory-evoked potentials. Psychogenic jerks often have Bereitschaftspotential, which is a slow, negative EEG potential that begins 1 to 2.5 seconds before EMG onset and is indicative of movement preparation.

TREATMENT

Treatment of myoclonus depends on the underlying pathology; however, the degree of disability determines whether treatment is warranted. The following drugs have been helpful:

I. Treat or remove the underlying cause (drug, etc.).
II. Clonazepam 1 to 1.5 mg/day is given in divided doses, with a gradual increase if necessary.
III. Valproic acid is the drug of choice for many of the myoclonic epilepsies but is also used to treat essential myoclonus, post-hypoxic myoclonus, and other secondary myoclonic conditions such as Huntington disease with myoclonus. Initial dosage is 250 mg/day, increasing up to a usual therapeutic dosage of 1200 to 1500 mg/day. Levetiracetam (1000 to 3000 mg/day) is also a first-line agent. Topiramate and zonisamide are second-line agents.
IV. 5-Hydroxytryptophan 100 mg/day is given in divided doses, increasing by 200 mg every 2 to 3 days up to a total of 1000 to 4000 mg/day; carbidopa, 75 to 150 mg/day, may be given to prevent extra-cerebral decarboxylation of 5-hydroxytryptophan to serotonin. This regimen is reported to help many patients with post-hypoxic myoclonus and some with progressive myoclonic epilepsy.
V. Many other medications have been used, mostly anecdotally, including alcohol, estrogens, botulinum toxin (palatal myoclonus), tetrabenazine, trihexyphenidyl, and benztropine, baclofen, and N-acetylcysteine.
VI. Phenytoin, carbamazepine, and lamotrigine might worsen cortical myoclonus.

REFERENCES

Avanzini, G., Shibasaki, H., Rubboli, G., Canafoglia, L., Panzica, F., Franceschetti, S., et al. (2016). Neurophysiology of myoclonus and progressive myoclonus epilepsies. *Epileptic Disord*, *1*(S2), 11–27 18.
Eberhardt, O., & Topka, H. (2017). Myoclonic disorders. *Brain Sci*, *7*(8), 103.

MYOGLOBINURIA, RHABDOMYOLYSIS, CREATINE KINASE

Myoglobinuria (myoglobin in the urine) is the result of rhabdomyolysis that occurs within several hours of acute muscle injury and necrosis.

CLASSIFICATION

I. Hereditary myoglobinuria
  A. Enzyme deficiency known
    1. Phosphorylase deficiency (McArdle disease)
    2. Phosphofructokinase deficiency (Tarui disease)
    3. Carnitine palmitoyltransferase deficiency
  B. Incompletely characterized syndromes
    1. Excess lactate production (Larsson syndrome)
  C. Uncharacterized
    1. Familial, no clear biochemical abnormality
    2. Familial susceptibility to succinylcholine or general anesthesia ("malignant hyperthermia")
    3. Repeated attacks in an individual; no known biochemical abnormality
II. Sporadic myoglobinuria
  A. Exertional myoglobinuria in untrained individuals
    1. Squat-jump and related syndromes, including "march myoglobinuria"
    2. Anterior tibial syndrome
    3. Convulsions, high-voltage electric shock
  B. Crush syndrome
    1. Compression by fallen weights
    2. Compression in prolonged coma
  C. Ischemic myoglobinuria
    1. Arterial occlusion
    2. Ischemic element in compression and anterior tibial syndrome
  D. Metabolic abnormalities
    1. Metabolic depression
      a. Barbiturate, carbon monoxide, narcotic coma
      b. Diabetic acidosis
      c. General anesthesia
      d. Hypothermia
    2. Exogenous toxins and drugs
      a. Haff disease (toxin unknown; associated with fish consumption)
      b. Heroin, cocaine
      c. Alcoholism
      d. Toluene
      e. Malayan sea-snake bite poison
      f. Malignant neuroleptic syndrome
      g. Plasmocid (anti-malarial drug)
      h. Fluphenazine
      i. Succinylcholine, halothane
      j. Glycyrrhizate, carbenoxolone, amphotericin B
    3. Other disorders
      a. Chronic hypokalemia
      b. Heat stroke

      c. Toxic shock syndrome
  E. Myoglobinuria with progressive muscle disease
  F. Myoglobinuria resulting from unknown cause

DIAGNOSIS

Diagnosis depends on further characterization of pigmenturia (myoglobin, hemoglobin, and porphyrins) by urinalysis, including dipstick and microscopic evaluation. Spectrophotometry, electrophoresis, or immunoprecipitation may be utilized if urinalysis fails to characterize the pigment. Myalgia or fever and malaise, or both, may be present. Serum muscle enzyme levels are elevated. Complications include acute tubular necrosis with oliguria and azotemia, hyperkalemia, hypercalcemia, hyperuricemia, and uncommonly, respiratory failure and death.

TREATMENT

Myoglobinuria is life-threatening only if there is renal injury, which should be treated vigorously with intravenous fluid hydration using normal saline. Aggressive diuresis with mannitol and/or alkalinization of urine by adding sodium bicarbonate to the fluids is controversial and has not proven to provide additional benefits to using normal saline alone.

CREATINE KINASE

Creatine kinase (CK) is an enzyme located on the inner mitochondrial membrane, on myofibrils, and in the muscle cytoplasm that catalyzes the reversible conversion of ADP and phosphocreatine into ATP and creatine. It is the most sensitive indicator of muscle injury, and is the best measure of the course of muscle injury. CK is a dimer molecule and occurs in three distinct isoenzyme forms, termed MM, MB, and BB. Normal skeletal muscle CK is more than 99% MM with small amounts of MB. A serum CK level of more than 1000 U/L helps to distinguish muscle disease from neurogenic causes of weakness.

Causes of Elevation in Creatine Kinase

  I. Diseases affecting muscle or causing excessive muscle breakdown
    A. Inflammatory myopathies
      1. CK can approach 100 times the normal value.
      2. In dermatomyositis or polymyositis CK generally normalizes 4 to 6 weeks after the initiation of corticosteroid therapy. Failure to respond suggests an alternative diagnosis. CK is used to monitor for relapse of disease.
    B. Inclusion body myositis: CK may be normal but usually elevated two- to five-fold. CK elevations (<10 times normal) occur in about 80% of patients. CK does not normalize with steroids.
    C. Connective tissue diseases: CK is reported to be low in 40% of patients with rheumatologic disease. An inverse correlation has also been reported between the level of inflammation and the level of CK. CK elevation may suggest a subclinical myositis, drug-induced myopathy

(e.g., chloroquine), or an overlap syndrome with polymyositis/dermatomyositis.

D. Dystrophinopathies: CK levels are elevated in Duchenne and Becker muscular dystrophy from the newborn period, reaching levels that are 50 to 100 times normal. A child or adult with a normal CK level does not have a dystrophinopathy.

E. Limb-girdle dystrophies: CK is usually 4 to 25 times the normal range in dominantly inherited types and higher (10–80 times the normal range) in the recessively inherited types.

F. Other inherited/metabolic myopathies

1. Deficiency of myophosphorylase, phosphorylase kinase, phosphofructokinase, phosphoglycerate kinase, phosphoglycerate mutase, lactate dehydrogenase, carnitine palmitoyltransferase, short- and long-chain acyl-CoA dehydrogenase and myoadenylate deaminase present with episodic muscle damage severe enough to cause rhabdomyolysis.

2. Miyoshi distal myopathy also may present with CK elevation >100 times normal.

G. Rhabdomyolysis: An acute rise in CK level more than five times the normal range is due to many causes as listed above. A CK level above 1600 IU/dL predicts renal failure in around 60% of patients with rhabdomyolysis. With adequate treatment, CK should normalize within 1 week (half-life of 1 to 3 days) unless there is an underlying or ongoing muscle injury.

H. Medication-induced myopathy: Elevated CK is seen with colchicine, antimalarials, statins, gemfibrozil, nicotinic acid, clofibrate, cocaine, heroin, methadone, D-lysergic acid diethylamide (LSD), alcohol, nondepolarizing muscle blocking agents, selective serotonin reuptake inhibitors, zidovudine, colchicine, lithium, and high-dose corticosteroids. Drug-induced myopathies may unmask a preexisting muscle abnormality.

I. Exposure to toxins: metabolic poisons (e.g., carbon monoxide), snake and insect venoms, mushroom poisoning, Haff disease (rhabdomyolysis after fish ingestion)

J. Infectious myopathies: HIV, other viruses (HTLV1, coxsackie, influenza), bacteria (TB, Lyme disease, Mycoplasma, Legionella, tularemia, Streptococcus and Salmonella, *Escherichia coli*, leptospirosis, *Coxiella burnetii*, and staphylococcal infection), fungi, and parasites (trypanosomiasis, cysticercosis) can cause myositis with CK up to 1000 times normal.

K. Malignant hyperthermia: Fever, generalized muscular contraction and rigidity, metabolic acidosis, and rhabdomyolysis (with CK rising to 100 times normal) may occur in susceptible individuals and may be familial. CK may be elevated at baseline when asymptomatic. Elevated CK also has been reported in neuroleptic malignant syndrome and drowning/hypothermia.

II. Elevated muscle enzyme in the absence of muscle disease
   A. Exercise: Serum CK concentrations reach peak levels at 8 to 24 hours after exercise, begin to decrease by 24 to 48 hours, and return to baseline levels by 72 hours. Massive elevation of CK may arise with marked physical exertion, particularly when one or more of the following risk factors is present: individual is physically untrained; extremely hot, humid conditions; use of anticholinergic medications (impairment of sweating), sickle cell trait, and hypokalemia.
   B. Iatrogenic muscle injury: Intramuscular injection, falls, major surgery, electromyography, muscle biopsy, high-voltage electrical injury, compartment syndrome, crush injuries, and extensive third-degree burns are among the possible causes.
   C. Pathologic hyperkinetic states; for example, generalized tonic-clonic seizures, delirium tremens, psychotic agitation, and amphetamine overdose.
   D. Motor neuron disease: In amyotrophic lateral sclerosis CK may be elevated up to approximately 1000 U/L on the basis of denervation. No elevation of CK is noted in other neuropathies.
   E. Endocrine causes
      1. Hypothyroidism, complicated diabetes mellitus, and hypoparathyroidism can cause a small elevation in CK.
      2. Cushing disease can cause a myopathy, but the CK level is usually normal.
   F. Idiopathic: Idiopathic myopathy occurs more frequently in males and in people of African ethnic descent.
   G. CK-immunoglobulin complexes: Macro CK-1 is a complex formed between the creatine kinase dimer, CK-BB, and immunoglobulin-G, and is detected on electrophoresis. It is present in 1% to 2% of the normal healthy population.
III. Low serum CK levels are seen in chronic end-stage diseases in which muscle mass is reduced, corticosteroid treatment, hyperthyroidism, and rheumatologic diseases.

REFERENCES

Giannoglou, G. D., Chatzizisis, Y. S., & Misirli, G. (2007). The syndrome of rhabdo-myolysis: pathophysiology and diagnosis. *Eur J Intern Med*, *18*(2), 90–100.

Khan, F. Y. (2009). Rhabdomyolysis: a review of the literature. *Neth J Med*, *67*(9), 272–283.

MYOPATHY

Myopathy is a general term meaning a disorder of muscle. All specific myopathies are rare. However, as there are many subtypes of myopathy, any neurologist can expect to encounter patients with myopathies in the clinic or hospital setting. The major categories of myopathies are discussed below, with some specific examples given.

MAJOR CATEGORIES
Inflammatory
Infectious
Endocrine
Toxic
Metabolic
Congenital
Muscular dystrophies (see Muscular Dystrophy)
Myotonic disorders (see Myotonia)
Periodic paralysis (see Periodic Paralysis)

INFLAMMATORY MYOPATHIES
Dermatomyositis (DM) and polymyositis (PM) are the two most common inflammatory myopathies. T cells and macrophages predominate in PM compared to B cells in DM. As DM and PM are associated with an increased risk of neoplasm, a thorough workup for malignancy is required for all patients.
- Polymyositis presents as subacute to chronic painless symmetrical progressive weakness of the proximal limb (hip and thigh more than shoulder and neck) and trunk muscles without dermatitis. In general, presentation develops between the third and sixth decades of life with a female predominance. Sudden death may result from necrosis of myocardial fibers leading to cardiac abnormalities; interstitial lung disease may develop as well. Physical therapy is recommended to prevent fibrous contractures.
- Dermatomyositis: presentation is similar to PM with the addition of variable skin findings that may precede weakness. Skin changes may include localized/diffuse erythema, maculopapular eruption, scaling eczematoid dermatitis, and exfoliative dermatitis. Other findings include pink–purple patches of scaly roughness over extensor surfaces (Gottron papules, considered pathognomonic for DM) and heliotrope over the eyelid, the bridge of the nose, the cheek and the forehead. The disease is more common in females.
- Diagnosis:
    - Blood work may show elevated creatine kinase (CK) and aldolase, with normal to mildly elevated erythrocyte sedimentation rate (ESR). About 20% of patients have antibodies against cellular components of muscle such as cytoplasmic transfer ribonucleic acid synthetase (anti-Jo1); other associated antibodies include cytoplasmic ribonucleoprotein complex (signal recognition particle [SRP]) and nuclear helicase (Mi-2).
    - Electromyography (EMG) can be normal or may show findings typical of myopathy: abnormally short, low amplitude, polyphasic motor unit action potentials. There also may be numerous fibrillation potentials and myotonic activity.

M

MYOPATHY

- Biopsy: samples from multiple sites or multiple samples of one site can increase sensitivity.
  - Idiopathic PM: destruction of single muscle fiber segments via phagocytosis of muscle fibers by mononuclear cells and lymphocytic infiltration with evidence of regeneration.
  - DM: perifascicular atrophy is a key diagnostic feature on biopsy; muscle fibers are disproportionately atrophic where the muscle fascicle and perimysium meet. Inflammation of small blood vessels in the skin and muscle—the underlying cause of the skin and muscle changes—are visible on biopsy. In addition, there may be microvascular changes including endothelial alterations (tubular aggregate in endothelial cytoplasm) and occlusion of vessels by fibrin thrombi with infarction.
- Treatment: May start with prednisone at 1 mg/kg, and strength and CK are monitored for effectiveness. Once CK has normalized, prednisone can be decreased slowly, no more than 5 mg every 2 weeks until 20 mg daily.
  - For acute or severe case: methylprednisolone 1 g/day for 3 to 5 days
  - Intravenous immunoglobulin (IVIG) or plasma exchange can be used in addition to steroids.
  - Other immune suppressants, including methotrexate or azathioprine are often used in conjunction with prednisone
- Prognosis is favorable except if it is associated with malignancy. The degree of recovery varies and may depend on the acuteness and severity upon initial presentation as well as duration of disease prior to the initiation of therapy.

Inclusion Body Myositis (IBM): Most common inflammatory myopathy in those older than 50 years of age. Unlike DM, males are affected more commonly than females. IBM is characterized by intracytoplasmic and intranuclear inclusions. Sporadic inclusion body myositis can be differentiated from hereditary inclusion body myopathy.

- Presentation: steadily progressive painless weakness and atrophy in distal arms and proximal and distal legs. There may be selective weakness of flexor pollicis longus, isolated quadriceps weakness, or neck extensor weakness. Deltoids are often spared. Dysphagia is common. Compared to DM and PM, there may be early loss of reflexes. Many patients also have a superimposed peripheral polyneuropathy.
- Diagnosis: CK may be normal or only mildly elevated. EMG findings may be similar to DM and PM as noted above. The co-occurrence of both large (neuropathic) and small (myopathic) motor unit action potentials on needle EMG should raise suspicion for IBM.
  - Biopsy: intracytoplasmic subsarcolemmal vacuoles (rimmed by basophilic granular material) and eosinophilic inclusions in cytoplasm and nuclei of degenerating muscle fibers. May also stain for beta amyloid. Overall, inflammatory changes are less severe compared to PM.
  - Cytosolic antibodies (anti-cN1; NT5C1A) are found in two-thirds of IBM patients.

- Treatment: At this time, there is no clinically effective treatment.
- **Sarcoid myopathy** is characterized by noncaseating granulomata in muscle as well as other organs. About 50% of sarcoid patients have muscle involvement on biopsy, and most of those are asymptomatic. Chronic, proximal myopathy is the most common clinical muscle presentation. Women are affected four times as often as men. Corticosteroid therapy is the treatment of choice.
- **Polymyalgia rheumatica** is characterized by muscle pain and stiffness that worsen with rest and abate with continued exercise. There is no muscle weakness. Onset is after the age of 55 years, and twice as many women as men are affected. Shoulder muscles are most commonly involved. Temporal arteritis may develop in 55% to 75% of patients. ESR is elevated, and anemia is often present. The level of CK, the EMG results, and the muscle biopsy specimens are usually normal. Treat with prednisone 30–50 mg/day if with associated temporal arteritis or 10–20 mg/day if isolated polymyalgia rheumatica, then taper. Clinical response and ESR must be followed up during the taper.

INFECTIOUS MYOPATHIES
Parasitic
Trichinosis: resulting from infection with nematode, *Trichinella spiralis*

- Other than skeletal muscle, may also carry a predilection for ocular muscles resulting in strabismus and diplopia, tongue resulting in dysarthria and masseter, and pharyngeal muscles with impaired chewing and swallowing. Other affected sites include the diaphragm and myocardium. Patient may present with conjunctival, orbital, and facial edema with subconjunctival and subungual splinter hemorrhages.
- Prognosis: infection may be asymptomatic and complete recovery can be achieved once trichinae become encysted. On the other hand, significant diaphragmatic and cardiac involvement may be fatal.
- Diagnosis: blood work may show eosinophilia with normal ESR and moderately elevated CK. ELISA blood test becomes positive after 1 to 2 weeks. Muscle biopsy may demonstrate muscle fibers undergoing segmental necrosis with interstitial inflammatory infiltrates including eosinophils. Profuse fibrillation potentials may be present on EMG.
- Treatment: for most patients no treatment is necessary. Thiabendazole 25–50 mg/kg daily with prednisone 40–60 mg/day for 5 to 10 days can be used if severe pain an issue.

Toxoplasmosis: Toxoplasma gondii
- Usually not symptomatic in immunocompetent patients. In the immunocompromised, toxoplasmosis may manifest with multisystem involvement including brain. Myopathy generally occurs in the setting of lymphopenia and organ failure resulting in weakness, wasting, myalgia, and elevated CK.
- Treatment: sulfadiazine with pyrimethamine or trisulfapyrimidine.

Other notable parasitic etiologies of infectious myopathy include cysticercosis *(Taenia solium)*, which may present with dramatic pseudohypertrophy of the thigh and calf. In coenurosis (*Taenia multiceps* and *T. serialis*) and sparganosis (genus Spirometra), movable lumps in the rectus abdominis, thigh, calf, and pectoralis may be palpated.

Viral
HIV and human T-lymphotropic virus type I: unclear pathogenesis of associated myopathy as direct infection of muscle fibers is rarely observed with a pathology specimen. Patients generally present with painless weakness of girdle and proximal limb muscles. CK is elevated, and on EMG, there is evidence of active myopathy with fibrillations, brief polyphasic motor units and complex repetitive discharges. Differential may also include zidovudine induced myopathy for patients compliant with highly active antiretroviral therapy (HAART). Presentation is usually dose dependent with higher risk in those receiving 1200 mg daily for at least 1 year. Biopsy shows ragged red fibers suggestive of mitochondrial toxicity.

M

MYOPATHY

ENDOCRINE MYOPATHIES
Myopathies can be seen in disorders involving the thyroid, parathyroid, adrenal glands, growth hormone (slowly progressive proximal myopathy in acromegaly), gonadal (testosterone deficiency), diabetes (myonecrosis), and carcinoid syndrome.

Thyroid
- Hypothyroid: may present with mild proximal weakness, muscle fatigue, and muscle cramps. Delayed relaxation of reflex may rarely be seen. Serum CK can be elevated in overt hypothyroidism. EMG is often normal. Biopsy shows type 2 fiber atrophy and type 1 fiber hypertrophy.
- Hyperthyroidism: may present with slow progressive weakness; in thyroid storm, presentation may be more acute and rapidly progressive.
- Thyroid ophthalmopathy (Graves disease): the inferior and medial recti are most commonly affected and may lead to compression of the optic nerve. Steroids, cyclosporine and orbital radiation therapy may be used.
- Thyrotoxic periodic paralysis: characterized by proximal more than distal weakness, hypotonia, and hyporeflexia, occurring in the hyperthyroid state, especially in Asian males. Attacks may last from minutes to days that are separated by weeks or months, and may be triggered by hypokalemia. Treatment is by correcting hypokalemia, addressing thyroid abnormalities, and initiating beta blockers.

Parathyroid
- Hypercalcemia and hypomagnesemia: nonnecrotizing myopathy with limb girdle weakness
- Hypophosphatemia: necrotizing myopathy with rhabdomyolysis

Critical illness myopathy: limb girdle and axial weakness; difficult to wean from artificial ventilation. On biopsy, severe type 2 fiber atrophy and loss of myosin heavy chain can be seen.

TOXIN-INDUCED MYOPATHIES

- Statins:
    - Toxic necrotizing myopathy: appears soon after initiating statin with gradual improvement months after discontinuation.
    - Necrotizing immune myopathy: In some cases, patients do not improve even several months after withdrawal of statin medications. Many of these patients have antibodies against HMG-CoA reductase.
- Amiodarone: onset after months to years
- Antiretroviral: zalcitabine, didanosine, lamivudine
- Chloroquine and hydroxychloroquine: rimmed vacuoles may be seen on biopsy.
- Colchicine
- Alcohol: can be slowly progressive, though binge drinking or acute intoxication may trigger acute necrotizing myopathy.

METABOLIC MYOPATHIES

Glycogen storage diseases (GSD): disorders of glycolysis or glycogenolysis

- Genetics: autosomal recessive except for two X-linked recessive disorders, phosphorylase b kinase deficiency (GSD 9) and phosphoglycerate kinase 1 deficiency
- Presentation: most come to clinical attention in the second and third decades of life with muscle cramps/myalgia with power/sprint sports; may present later due to learned lifestyle modification. Pigmenturia may be present post-exercise due to myoglobin from rhabdomyolysis. Exam may be normal between exercise, though untreated aldolase A deficiency (GSD 12) may present with fixed muscle weakness. There may be increased incidence of gout due to myogenic hyperuricemia.
- Diagnosis:
    - Forearm exercise test: isometric rhythmic exercise for 1 min and compare lactate and ammonia pre- and post-exercise. Diagnostic of glycogen storage disorder if lactate increases less than three times the baseline. Failure of ammonia to increase is suggestive of suboptimal effort versus AMPD1 polymorphism. A negative forearm exercise test rules out all GSD except for phosphorylase b kinase, which can be further evaluated with an aerobic cycling exercise test.
    - EMG and nerve conduction studies can be normal.
    - Genetic testing
    - Muscle biopsy is recommended only if genetic testing is negative and suspicion remains high. Typical findings include high glycogen, absent phosphorylase or phosphofructokinase.
- Treatment: lifestyle adjustment including avoiding high intensity exercise and starting with low intensity activities.

McArdle disease (GSD 5): most common metabolic myopathy
- Gene: PYGM gene defect affects myophosphorylase, such that glycogenolysis cannot be initiated. The most common disease mutation is R49X in which no protein is expressed due to nonsense-mediated mRNA decay. A secondary deficiency of pyridoxine (vitamin B6) may also be present.
- Presentation: muscle pain and contracture develop shortly after exercise initiation. A "second wind phenomenon" may be seen in which patients perceive less effort needed after a few minutes of exercise due to delivery of blood-borne substrate; this is not present with glycolytic defects. Patients are less symptomatic after a high carbohydrate meal, which is also different from phosphofructokinase glycolytic defects (Tarui disease), where patients generally feel better with fasting.
- Diagnosis: CK is chronically elevated.
- Treatment: low-dose creatine monohydrate, sucrose or glucose 5 to 10 minutes prior to exercise and possibly a high carbohydrate diet though no randomized control trials have been conducted.

Fatty Acid Oxidation Defects
- Autosomal recessive
- Three most common are carnitine palmitoyltransferase II deficiency, trifunctional protein deficiency, and very long chain acyl-CoA dehydrogenase deficiency.
- Presentation: myalgia precipitated by long duration exercise (compared to GSD), fasting, or superimposed metabolic stress such as fever or infection; are more symptomatic in males.
- Diagnosis:
  - The most sensitive and specific test is the acylcarnitine profile obtained via liquid chromatography-tandem mass spectrometry. Yield may be increased with fasting.
  - Urine organic acid analysis: elevation of specific dicarboxylic acid
  - Genetic testing
- Treatment: lifestyle modification to avoid triggers, consume high carbohydrate food immediately before and during long endurance exercise and a low fat (<30%) high carbohydrate diet can be considered. Other recommendations include progressive exercise training and L-carnitine replacement if deficient; triheptanoin (odd chain free fatty acid) has been shown to reduce hospitalization and to improve exercise capacity.

Mitochondrial Myopathies:
- Genetics: maternally inherited. Homoplasmy (all copies of mtDNA affected) versus heteroplasmy (variable proportion of wild type to mutant) results in heterogeneous presentation.
- Key syndromes: MELAS (mitochondrial encephalomyopathy, lactic acidosis, and stroke-like episodes); Leber hereditary optic neuropathy; Kearns–Sayre syndrome

M

MYOPATHY

- Presentation: shortness of breath due to low VO_{2max}, premature fatigue; exertional nausea and vomiting, and rhabdomyolysis are rarer compared to fatty acid oxidation defects and GSD. Often systemic manifestations predominate, including seizure, encephalopathy, and cardiomyopathy.
- Diagnosis: ragged red fibers and cytochrome C oxidase-negative fibers may be seen with muscle biopsy; genetic testing should be considered.
- Treatment: exercise modification, endurance, and resistance exercise training as well as combination of coenzyme Q_{10} or idebenone, α-lipoic acid, vitamin E, and creatine monohydrate.

Congenital Myopathies

- Presentation: "floppy infant" with hypotonia, decreased deep tendon reflexes, decreased spontaneous movement, and muscular weakness. Associated anomalies are variable and include scoliosis, high-arched palate, elongated facies, ophthalmoplegia, and pectus excavatum.
- Diagnosis: biopsy for classification
- *Central core disease*: hypotonia, proximal weakness, delayed motor milestones; bulbar musculature is relatively spared. Biopsies show a well-circumscribed circular region in the center of muscle fibers and a predominance of type I fibers.
- *Nemaline myopathy*: dysmorphic features and bulbar involvement (poor suck-and-swallow reflexes with a weak cry). The severe congenital type can result in respiratory failure and death. Biopsy specimens show a predominance of type I fibers and dark-staining rods originating from Z lines.

REFERENCES

Katzberg, H. D., & Kassardjian, C. D. (2016). Toxic and endocrine myopathies. *Continuum (Minneap Minn)*, *22*(6, Muscle and Neuromuscular Junction Disorders), 1815–1828.

Tarnopolsky, M. A. (2016). Metabolic myopathies. *Continuum (Minneap Minn)*, *22*(6, Muscle and Neuromuscular Junction Disorders), 1829–1851.

MYOTOMES

Myotomes are discussed in Table 96.

REFERENCE

Aids to the examination of the peripheral nervous system, ed 5. St Louis: Elsevier, 2010.

TABLE 96

MYOTOMES

Muscle	Nerve	Root	How to Test
Trapezius	Spinal accessory, C3, 4	C3, 4	Elevation of shoulder AR
Teres major	Subscapular	C5, 6, 7	Adduction of elevated upper arm AR
Levator scapulae	C3, 4, and dorsal scapular	C3, 4, 5	Resting the palms of the hand on the back and pushing the shoulder AR
Rhomboids (major and minor)	Dorsal scapular	C4, 5	Resting the palms of the hand on the back and pushing the shoulder AR
Supraspinatus	Suprascapular	C5, 6	First 30 ∞ of shoulder abduction
Infraspinatus	Suprascapular	C5, 6	External rotation of upper arm to shoulder AR
Deltoid	Axillary	C5, 6	Abduction of upper arm at 90 ∞ AR
Biceps brachii	Musculocutaneous	C5, 6	Flexion of supinated forearm AR
Brachioradialis	Radial	C5, 6	Flexion of forearm AR between pronation and supination
Supinator	Radial	C5, 6	Supination of forearm ≤ AR with forearm extended
Flexor carpi radialis	Median	C6, 7	Flexion and abduction of hand (at the wrist) AR
Pronator teres	Median	C6, 7	Pronation of forearm AR
Serratus anterior	Long thoracic	C5, 6, 7	Push against the wall with the palms of the outstretched hands
Latissimus dorsi	Thoracodorsal	C6, 7, 8	Adduction AR with upper arm horizontal
Pectoralis major	Lateral pectoral	C5, 6	Push forward AR with clavicular head upper arm above horizontal
Sternal head	Medial pectoral	C6, 7, 8	Adduction of upper arm AR
Triceps brachii	Radial	C6, 7, 8	Extension of forearm (at the elbow) AR
Extensor carpi	Radial	C5, 6, 7, 8	Extension and abduction radialis longus of the hand (at the wrist) AR
Anconeus	Radial	C7, 8	Elbow extension AR
Extensor digitorum	Radial	C7, 8	Extension of metacarpophalangeal joints AR

M

MYOTOMES

Continued

TABLE 96

MYOTOMES—CONT'D

Muscle	Nerve	Root	How to Test
Extensor carpi ulnaris	Radial	C7, 8	Extension and adduction of the hand (at the wrist) AR
Extensor indicis	Radial	C7, 8	Extension of the index finger AR
Palmaris longus	Median	C7, 8, T1	
Flexor pollicis longus	Median	C8, T1	Flexion of distal IP joint of thumb against resistance with proximal phalanx fixed
Flexor carpi ulnaris	Ulnar	C7, 8, T1	Abduction of little finger AR: flexion and adduction of the hand (at the wrist) AR
Flexor digitorum superficialis	Median	C8, T1	Flexion of proximal IP joint AR with proximal phalanx fixed
Flexor digitorum profundus	I and II: median	C8, T1	Flexion of distal IP joint III and IV: ulnar AR with middle phalanx fixed
Pronator quadratus	Median	C7, 8	Pronation of forearm AR
Abductor pollicis brevis	Median	C8, T1	Abduction of thumb to palm AR
Opponens pollicis	Median	C8, T1	Touch base of little finger with thumb AR
Flexor pollicis brevis	Median	C8, T1	
Lumbricals I and II	Median	C8, T1	Extension of IP joint AR with MCP joint hyperextended and fixed
First dorsal interosseous	Ulnar	C8, T1	Abduction of index finger AR
Abductor digiti minimi	Ulnar	C8, T1	Abduction of little finger AR
Iliopsoas	Femoral	L2, 3, 4	Flexion of thigh at hip AR with knee and hip flexed
Adductor longus	Obturator	L2, 3, 4	Adduction of limb AR with knee extended
Gracilis	Obturator	L2, 3, 4	Adduction of limb with knee extended
Quadriceps femoris	Femoral	L2, 3, 4	Extension of leg AR with hip and knee flexed
Tibialis anterior	Deep peroneal	L4, 5	Dorsiflexion of foot AR

Continued

TABLE 96

MYOTOMES—CONT'D

Muscle	Nerve	Root	How to Test
Extensor hallucis longus	Deep peroneal	L4, 5	Dorsiflexion of distal IP joint of big toe AR
Extensor digitorum longus	Deep peroneal	L4, 5	Dorsiflexion of toes AR
Extensor digitorum brevis	Deep peroneal	L4, 5, S1	Dorsiflexion of proximal IP joint of toes AR
Peroneus longus	Superficial peroneal	L5, S1	Foot eversion AR
Internal hamstrings	Sciatic	L4, 5, S1	Lying on back, flexion of knee AR with hip flexed
External hamstrings	Sciatic	L5, S1	Lying on face, flexion of knee AR
Gluteus medius	Superior gluteal	L4, 5, S1	Internal rotation of thigh AR with limb, knee, and hip flexed
Gluteus maximus	Inferior gluteal	L5, S1, 2	Extension of limb at hip AR with knee extended
Tibialis posterior	Tibial	L5, S1	Foot inversion AR
Flexor digitorum longus	Tibial	L5, S1	Flexion of toes AR
Abductor hallucis brevis	Tibial (medial plantar)	L5, S1, 2	Usually not tested
Abductor digiti pedis	Tibial (lateral plantar)	S1, 2	Usually not tested
Gastrocnemius (lateral)	Tibial	L5, S1, 2	Usually not tested
Gastrocnemius (medial)	Tibial	S1, 2	Plantar flexion of foot AR with leg extended
Soleus	Tibial	S1, 2	Plantar flexion of foot AR with hip and knee flexed

AR, Against resistance; *IP*, interphalangeal; *MCP*, metacarpophalangeal.

M

MYOTONIA, MYOTONIC DYSTROPHY

MYOTONIA, MYOTONIC DYSTROPHY

Myotonia

Myotonia is the repetitive firing of muscle action potential causing prolonged muscle contractions even after mechanical stimulation to the muscle has ceased. This results in a delay in muscle relaxation demonstrated after voluntary action (such as hand grip or forced eye closure) or percussion of a muscle such as the thenar or wrist extensor muscles (percussion myotonia). EMG shows repetitive discharges with waxing and waning amplitude and frequency, giving a characteristic "dive bomber" sound. In common myotonic disorders, myotonia results from hyperexcitability of muscle membrane caused by different channelopathies: (1) reduced chloride conductance in muscle membrane, and (2), abnormal inactivation of sodium channels.

Diagnostic approach to a patient with myotonia:

I. Confirm myotonia by evaluating for grip myotonia or percussion myotonia.
II. Evaluate for presence of muscle atrophy or weakness, which is indicative of myotonic dystrophy types 1 or 2 (DM1 or DM2); these are absent in other myotonic disorders.
III. Evaluate for paramyotonia—myotonia occurring in cold environment or with exercise.
IV. Needle EMG may show insertion myotonia (bursts of action potentials elicited by needle electrode insertion).
V. Slit lamp examination for cataract. Check fasting blood sugar, hemoglobin A_{1c}, immunoglobulin levels, serum CPK if DM1 or DM2 is suspected.
VI. Consider appropriate genetic studies for confirmation and counseling.

The following diseases present with myotonia:

I. Myotonic dystrophy type 1 (dystrophia myotonica type 1, DM1)
II. Myotonic dystrophy type 2 (DM2)
III. Myotonia congenita (Thomsen disease)
IV. Autosomal recessive generalized myotonia (Becker type)
V. Paramyotonia congenita (Eulenberg disease)
VI. Hyperkalemic periodic paralysis
VII. Myotonia fluctuans
VIII. Pompe disease (glycogen storage disease type II)
IX. Chondrodystrophic myotonia (Schwartz-Jampel syndrome), abnormality at the neuromuscular junction, and not a channelopathy

Myotonia Treatment: Myotonia can be treated with membrane-stabilizing drugs such as quinine, procainamide, phenytoin, or tocainide. If potassium sensitivity is demonstrated, acetazolamide may be used. These medications treat myotonia with variable success but are often unable to improve associated weakness.

Myotonic dystrophy

Myotonic dystrophy is the most common adult-onset muscular dystrophy (1:7500 persons). DM1 is more common than DM2 (Table 97). Inheritance is autosomal dominant. "Anticipation," or earlier onset of more severe disease in successive generations, has been linked to an increasing number of repetitions of an unstable DNA sequence on chromosome 19 found in offspring of patients.

Weakness occurs in excess of myotonia, particularly involving the face and distal limbs. Atrophy of the temporalis and masseter muscles causes the jaw to hang open, producing a characteristic so-called "hatchet-head" and "fish-mouth" appearance. Frontal balding, ptosis, and neck muscle atrophy add to this appearance. Muscle biopsy shows internalized nuclei, type I fiber atrophy, and ring fibers. Other neurologic features include hypersomnia, dysarthria, dysphagia with nasal regurgitation, and cognitive dysfunction.

Systemic features of myotonic dystrophy include cardiac conduction defects, impaired gastric motility, testicular atrophy, insulin resistance,

TABLE 97

CLINICAL AND GENETIC ABNORMALITIES OF MYOTONIC DYSTROPHY 1 (DM1) VERSUS MYOTONIC DYSTROPHY 2 (DM2)

	Myotonic Dystrophy 1	Myotonic Dystrophy 2
Myotonia	+	+
Cataract	+	+
Muscle weakness	+ (distal muscles)	+ (proximal muscles)
Muscle pain	−	+
Cardiac arrhythmia	++	++
Muscle enzyme elevation	+	+
Cognitive dysfunction	+	+
Inheritance	Autosomal dominant	Autosomal dominant
Chromosome locus	19q 13.3	3q 21.3
Genetic abnormality	(CTG)n expansion	(CCTG)n expansion

hypoadrenalism, hypothyroidism, early subcapsular cataracts, hypogammaglobulinemia (particularly IgG and IgM), and increased risk associated with general anesthesia.

The course is slowly progressive; death typically occurs in the sixth decade of life as a result of cardiac or respiratory complications.

Management revolves around managing the weakness, myotonia, and systemic manifestations. Physical and occupational therapy can help preserve or increase strength and flexibility in muscles and provide techniques to compensate for loss of strength and dexterity. Systemic management includes ophthalmology referral for cataracts and ptosis (upper lid blepharoplasty), cardiology referral for pacemaker placement as indicated, treatment of diabetes mellitus, hypothyroidism, hypogonadism, excessive daytime sleepiness, and sleep apnea.

Congenital myotonic dystrophy is a rare disorder in which myotonia is a late feature. It is associated with maternal inheritance and presents with hypotonia and bulbar and respiratory weakness in neonates. Affected children may have distinctive facial features and club feet, and 70% have developmental delay. Treatment is symptomatic for adult and congenital forms of disease.

Myotonia congenita (*Thomsen disease* is the autosomal dominant form; *Becker disease* is the autosomal recessive form) patients typically complain of diffuse myotonic muscle stiffness *after resting* which improves with exercise.

In paramyotonia congenita (*Eulenberg disease*) the stiffness is often induced by cold and *worsened by exercise*. Muscles of the face and distal upper extremities are most often involved. It is most often caused by mutations in the sodium channel SCN4A gene, although other channels have been implicated, as have mutations in a large number of genes.

Table 98 delineates the clinical features of the myotonias and myotonic dystrophies.

REFERENCES

Kurihara, T. (2005). *Intern Med*, 44(10), 1027–1032.
Machuca-Tzili, L., & Brook, D. (2005). *Muscle Nerve*, 32, 1–18.

MYOTONIA, MYOTONIC DYSTROPHY

M

TABLE 98

CHARACTERISTICS OF THE MYOTONIAS

| Feature | Myotonic Dystrophy | Myotonia Congenita | | Paramyotonia Congenita | Hyperkalemic Periodic Paralysis |
		Thomsen Disease	Becker Disease		
Inheritance	AD	AD	AR	AD	AD
Defect	Protein kinase	Chloride channel	Chloride channel	Sodium channel	Sodium channel
Common gene locus	19q	7q	7q	17q	17q
Age of onset	Teens to twenties	Infancy to childhood	Childhood	Infancy	Childhood
Course	Slowly progressive	Nonprogressive	Rarely progressive	Variable weakness	Variable weakness
Presenting complaint	Distal weakness	Stiffness	Stiffness/weakness	Cold-induced stiffness	Episodic weakness

N

NEGLECT

Neglect is the failure to report, respond to, or orient to novel and meaningful stimuli presented to the side opposite a brain lesion when this failure cannot be attributed to either sensory or motor dysfunction. Components of neglect include inattention or sensory neglect, motor neglect, spatial neglect, personal neglect, allesthesia (perception of sensation of a stimulus in a location different from where the stimulus was applied; e.g., the contralateral limb), and anosognosia. Bedside tests for neglect include visual confrontation, double simultaneous stimulation, letter or figure cancellation, figure drawing, and line bisection. Lesions associated with neglect correlate with the type of neglect syndrome. Attention system defects with sensory neglect are associated with right parietal lobe lesions. Motor neglect with varying degrees of akinesia and motor impersistence can be seen in frontal lesions. Defects in the representational system are often associated with right hemisphere lesions because the right hemisphere is important as an attention system for both the left and right hemispace, whereas the left hemisphere is primarily important only for attention to the right hemispace. Another explanation posits a bihemispheric network of attention systems, which is overrepresented in the right hemisphere.

REFERENCE

Heilman, K. H. (2012). In E. Valenstein (Ed.), *Clinical neuropsychology*, ed 5. New York: Oxford University Press.

NEUROCUTANEOUS SYNDROMES

Neurocutaneous syndromes, or phakomatoses, are congenital or heritable disorders that produce characteristic integumentary and neurologic lesions. While advances in molecular genetics have improved our understanding of some phakomatoses, a grasp of the clinical features (generally summarized by the clinical diagnostic criteria) is necessary in order to recognize and treat these conditions. Treatment remains largely focused on the management of complications and on preventative screening.

AUTOSOMAL DOMINANT

Neurofibromatosis-1 (NF1, von Recklinghausen disease) is an autosomal dominant (AD) syndrome that results from a mutation in the *NF1* gene on chromosome 17q11.2; with an incidence of ~1/3000 people, NF1 is the most common phakomatosis. The diagnosis requires at least two of the following: ≥6 of café au lait spots larger than 5 mm in diameter; axillary or inguinal freckles, two neurofibromas of any type or one or more plexiform neurofibromas; optic nerve or chiasmatic glioma; ≥2 Lisch nodules (pigmented hamartomas of the iris); first-degree relative with NF1; bony abnormalities, such as thinning of the cortical long bone or sphenoid dysplasia. Genetic confirmation is available. Spontaneous mutations account for ~50% of new cases, hence family history is often negative. Mosaicism is not uncommon. Neurofibromas are benign peripheral nerve tumors composed predominantly of Schwann cells and fibroblasts that can develop at any age. Plexiform neurofibromas have a 5% to 13% lifetime risk of malignant transformation into malignant peripheral nerve sheath tumors, which are associated with a poor 5-year survival. Optic nerve gliomas are the most common tumors in NF1. Given the complications associated with NF1, expert guidelines recommend annual evaluation to monitor blood pressure and developmental milestones (up to 18 years of age), as well as skin, musculoskeletal, and neurologic examinations.

Neurofibromatosis-2 (NF2) is an AD disease caused by a mutation on chromosome 22 of the *NF2* gene, which produces a protein called merlin, a novel regulator of the tuberous sclerosis complex (TSC)/mTORC1 signaling pathway. It occurs in approximately 1 in 50,000 people. Onset occurs most often in the late teens or early adulthood and rarely in childhood. Patients with NF2 generally have fewer cutaneous findings and more central nervous system (CNS) tumors. The diagnostic criteria include: bilateral eighth nerve tumors (vestibular schwannomas); unilateral eighth nerve tumor and a first-degree relative with NF2; a first-degree relative with NF2 and two of the following: glioma, schwannoma, presenile posterior cataract, astrocytoma, neurofibroma of another type, plexiform neurofibroma, or retinal hamartoma. The MISME mnemonic is helpful: *m*ultiple *i*nherited *S*chwannomas, *m*eningiomas and *e*pendymomas. Genetic confirmation is available and spontaneous mutations are common, so family history is often negative. As with NF1, mosaicism is not uncommon. Given the role of merlin in mTOR signaling, rapamycin is being investigated for the treatment of tumors related to NF2, but malignant degeneration is exceedingly rare.

Schwannomatosis is the third form of neurofibromatosis and is clinically and genetically distinct from NF1 and NF2. Most cases are likely related to inactivated mutations in the tumor suppressor genes *SMARCB1* and *LZTR1*. Schwannomatosis typically presents in young adulthood with pain and multiple noncutaneous schwannomas, without vestibular schwannomas. The incidence is similar to NF2. Diagnostic categories include definite, possible, and segmental schwannomatosis.

Tuberous sclerosis complex is an AD disorder with variable penetrance related to defective cellular differentiation and proliferation, which affects the brain, skin, heart, kidneys, lungs, and other organs. Genetic diagnostic criteria were updated in 2012 and require only the identification of a pathogenic mutation in *TSC1* or *TSC2* located on chromosome 9 q34. Conventional genetic testing will fail to identify 10% to 25% of patients with TSC, and clinical expression is highly variable. Definite clinical diagnosis requires two major, or one major and two or more minor features. **Major criteria** include ≥3 hypomelanotic macules, at least 5 mm in diameter; ≥3 angiofibromas or fibrous cephalic plaques; ≥2 nail ungual fibromas; Shagreen skin raised patch;

multiple retinal hamartomas; cortical dysplasias including tubers and cerebral white matter radial migration lines; subependymal nodules; subependymal giant cell astrocytoma; cardiac rhabdomyoma; lymphangioleiomyomatosis; ≥ 2 angiomyolipomas. **Minor criteria** include confetti skin lesions; ≥ 3 dental enamel pits; ≥ 2 intraoral fibromas; retinal achromic patch; multiple renal cysts; nonrenal hamartomas. Infants often present with seizures and cardiac involvement, while adults may present with more subtle findings. Common neurologic manifestations include seizures (in 80% to 90%), intellectual disability, and behavioral abnormalities. Cortical/subcortical tubers and calcified subependymal nodules can be seen on imaging, and 6% to 14% of patients will develop subependymal giant cell astrocytomas, which may lead to hydrocephalus. Roughly 60% will have a cardiac rhabdomyoma.

Von Hippel–Landau (VHL) disease is an AD syndrome with a prevalence of 1/40,000, caused by a mutation of the *VHL* gene on chromosome 3p25-26. VHL is characterized by hemangioblastomas of the retina and CNS, and visceral cysts and tumors of the kidney, pancreas, liver, islet cell, and epididymis, as well as pheochromocytoma. Diagnostic criteria include hemangioblastoma of the CNS (most commonly found in the cerebellum, medulla, spinal cord, or cerebral hemispheres) or retina, and one additional characteristic lesion or a direct relative with the disease. Careful screening of affected patients is the most important aspect of management and includes annual examination/urinalysis (including 24-hour collection for vanillylmandelic acid); direct ophthalmoscopy with vascular imaging (retinal hemangioblastoma); renal ultrasound; brain magnetic resonance imaging (MRI) or computed tomography (CT) every 3 years until age 50, then every 5 years thereafter, and abdominal CT every 3 years. There are also screening protocols for at-risk relatives.

Hereditary hemorrhagic telangiectasias (HHT; Osler-Weber-Rendu syndrome) is an AD disorder with high penetrance, which causes telangiectasias of the skin, mucous membranes, lungs, liver, and other organs as a result of mutations in either the *HHT1* or the *HHT2* gene on chromosome 12 ALK1. Neurologic manifestations are common and include headaches, vertigo, and seizures. Intraparenchymal hemorrhage is a feared complication, and screening with MRI and angiography generally occurs every 5 years. Treatment of cerebral arteriovenous malformations (AVMs) with embolization, resection, or radioablation may be necessary. Antibiotic prophylaxis is recommended for dental work given some risk of brain abscess related to occult pulmonary AVM.

AUTOSOMAL RECESSIVE
Ataxia-telangiectasia is a progressive neurodegenerative autosomal recessive (AR) disease caused by mutation of the *ATM* gene located on chromosome 11q22.3, which normally produces a protein involved in regulating cell division and DNA damage repair. Affected individuals present in childhood with slowly progressive cerebellar ataxia and tremor, abnormal eye movements (e.g., oculomotor apraxia), impaired smooth pursuit, and eventually dystonia

and chorea. Telangiectasias of the conjunctivae, ears, and flexor surfaces appear later. Systemic manifestations include immunodeficiency (decreased immunoglobulin [Ig]A, IgE, or IgG are seen in 80%), increased alpha-fetoprotein, recurrent pulmonary infections, sensitivity to ionizing radiation, and the development of lymphoid malignancies (10% to 15% by early adulthood). Early diagnosis helps to initiate screening for malignancies. Antioxidants such as vitamin E, alpha-lipoic acid, and folic acid are sometimes recommended, but it is unknown whether these are effective in slowing progression.

Xeroderma pigmentosa is a group of uncommon AR phakomatoses that result from a mutation in one of several genes involved in DNA repair (*DDB2, ERCC1, ERCC2, ERCC3, ERCC4, ERCC5, POLH, XPA,* or *XPC*). Cutaneous and ocular manifestations occur consequent to damage incurred by ultraviolet light exposure and generally develop in the first year or two of life. Blistering, persistent erythema with minimal sun exposure and marked freckling are common. Sunlight-induced keratitis and lid atrophy occur. Roughly half of all affected individuals will develop skin cancer. Approximately 25% of affected individuals develop neurologic manifestations including microcephaly, progressive dementia that begins in childhood, sensorineural hearing loss, ataxia, choreoathetosis, and absent deep tendon reflexes. Treatment of premalignant and malignant skin lesions, along with appropriate surveillance, is important; skin cancer, neurodegeneration, and visceral cancers are the most common causes of death.

OTHER PHAKOMATOSES

Hypomelanosis of Ito is the third most common phakomatosis after NF1 and TSC, and is usually spontaneous. A variety of genetic aberrations occur, including aneuploidy, unbalanced translocations, ring chromosome 22, 18/X translocation, and mosaic trisomy 18 among others. Patients present with hypopigmented whorls, streaks, and patches that follow the lines of Blaschko in two-thirds of those affected. There are other skin manifestations, such as café au lait spots, focal hypertrichosis, trichorrhexis, and nail dystrophy. Of those with cutaneous findings, 50% to 80% have neurologic abnormalities, including seizures (50%) and intellectual disability. Structural pathology can include macrocephaly, cortical migration abnormalities, lissencephaly, and periventricular white matter lesions. From 50% to 70% will have other systemic signs that include ocular abnormalities, musculoskeletal anomalies, cardiac defects, and both renal and endocrine disorders.

Sturge-Weber syndrome (meningofacial angiomatosis with gyriform cerebral calcifications) is a sporadic syndrome characterized by facial cutaneous angioma (port-wine nevus) and ipsilateral leptomeningeal and brain angioma. Somatic mutations in *GNAQ* on chromosome 9 have been identified in some patients. Neurologic manifestations include seizures (72% to 80% with unilateral lesions; 93% when bilateral), intellectual disability, and focal neurologic deficits referable to the intracranial vascular lesion (often vision loss related to occipital lobe lesions). On neuroimaging, CT can demonstrate gyriform calcifications, and contrasted MRI reveals focal areas of calcification, atrophy, and vascular malformation. However, only 10% to 20% of children with port-wine nevus have a leptomeningeal angioma. Surgical resection of vascular lesions may help improve seizure control, but patient selection and timing of surgery is an area of debate. Functional imaging may help in lesion selection. Hemispherectomy or corpus callosotomy may be necessary in some cases.

Neurocutaneous melanosis is a rare congenital disorder of melanocyte development, which is characterized by large, pigmented, hairy nevi, intracranial melanoma, and intracranial hemorrhage. Leptomeningeal melanosis occurs in most patients and predominantly affects the base of the brain and the upper spinal cord, and can lead to obstructive hydrocephalus. Cerebrospinal fluid may demonstrate mild pleocytosis with cytopathology, consisting of round cells with small, ovoid nuclei, and abundant cytoplasm containing melanin granules. MRI demonstrates T1 hyperintense lesions in the cerebellum, anterior temporal lobes, and basilar meninges, as well as possible leptomeningeal contrast enhancement.

Incontinentia pigmenti is a rare X-linked disease (XLD) resulting from mutations in the *NF-κB* essential modulator (NEMO), which consists of skin (characteristic lesions that evolve from blisters to verrucous, then linear/pigmented, and eventually atrophic and hypopigmented), ocular, and CNS pathology. The skin lesions also tend to follow the lines of Blaschko, but should not be confused with hypomelanosis of Ito. Neurologic involvement has been historically overestimated, but a higher incidence of seizures has been noted, and while affected females are of normal intelligence, most males do not survive; however, those with mosaicism do survive, but usually have developmental delay and immunodeficiency.

Fabry disease (papular eruption, painful sensory neuropathy, and stroke)

Linear nevus syndrome (linear yellow papules, developmental disability, and seizures)

Klippel-Trenaunay-Weber syndrome (limb hypertrophy and hemangiomas)

Wyburn-Mason syndrome (facial angioma, retinal AVMs, cerebrovascular anomalies, and seizures)

REFERENCES

Fusco, F., Conte, M. I., Diociaiuti, A., Bigoni, S., Branda, M. F., & Ferlini, A. (2017). Unusual father-to-daughter transmission of incontinentia pigmenti due to mosaicism in IP males. *Pediatrics*, *140*(3), 1–7.

Smith, M. J., Bowers, N. L., Bulman, M., Gokhale, C., Wallace, A. J., & King, A. T. (2017). Revisiting neurofibromatosis type 2 diagnostic criteria to exclude LZTR1-related schwannomatosis. *Neurology*, *88*(1), 87–92.

NEUROLEPTIC MALIGNANT SYNDROME

Neuroleptic malignant syndrome (NMS) is a clinical syndrome consisting of a tetrad of rigidity, autonomic instability, hyperthermia, and mental status change occurring in the setting of the use of dopamine-blocking agents or the withdrawal of dopamine-enhancing medications. The underlying pathophysiologic mechanism of NMS remains unclear; however it is likely related to the marked and sudden reduction in central dopaminergic activity following D2 dopamine receptor blockade within the nigrostriatal, hypothalamic, and mesolimbic/cortical pathways.

PRESENTATION

NMS symptoms typically evolve over 24 to 72 hours. The first recognized symptom (often due to under recognition of subtle parkinsonism) is mental status change in the form of agitated delirium with confusion rather than psychosis; catatonic signs and mutism may be prominent. Concurrently, patients often begin to develop generalized muscular rigidity, increased tone or "lead pipe rigidity" with superimposed tremor; less commonly akinesia, bradykinesia, dystonia, opisthotonus, trismus, chorea, and other dyskinesias. Next, temperatures begin to rise above 38°C, and if untreated may rapidly escalate above 40°C. Autonomic instability typically follows in the form of tachycardia, tachypnea, and diaphoresis. The clinical course lasts around 7 to 10 days, with a longer time for depot neuroleptics due to slower clearance. In individuals with Parkinson disease who have been on dopamine agonists, NMS can occur in the setting of a sudden withdrawal of the agonist agent, dosage change, or medication change.

Characteristic laboratory findings include elevated CPK (200 to 10,000 IU/L) due to rhabdomyolysis, leukocytosis (10,000 to 40,000 cells/μL), metabolic acidosis, and iron deficiency. Cerebrospinal fluid and imaging studies are usually normal, but an electroencephalogram (EEG) may show non-generalized slowing. Toxicology screening is recommended.

RISK FACTORS

The main risk factors for developing NMS are the initiation or increase in dose of a neuroleptic medication, or less likely, the abrupt cessation or reduction in dose of dopaminergic medications. Other risk factors include genetic factors, males under 40 years old, postpartum women, dementia with Lewy bodies, dehydration, physical exhaustion, exposure to heat, hyponatremia, iron deficiency, malnutrition, trauma, thyrotoxicosis, alcohol, psychoactive substances, and presence of a structural or functional brain disorder.

DIFFERENTIAL DIAGNOSIS

Many medical conditions can mimic the presentation of NMS, with some of the more common being heat stroke, central nervous system (CNS) infections, toxic encephalopathies, agitated delirium, status epilepticus, or drug-induced extrapyramidal symptoms. Other mimickers include infectious (brain abscess, encephalitis meningitis, rabies, septic shock, tetanus, delirium, lethal catatonia, nonconvulsive status epilepticus), pharmacological (anticholinergic delirium, drug-drug interaction, drug withdrawal, extrapyramidal side effects, malignant hyperthermia, serotonin syndrome), toxic exposure (heavy metals, lithium, salicylates, substances of abuse), or endocrine abnormalities (pheochromocytoma, thyrotoxicosis).

TABLE 99

MEDICATIONS ASSOCIATED WITH THE DEVELOPMENT OF NEUROLEPTIC MALIGNANT SYNDROME

- Neuroleptics
  - Typical antipsychotics:
    - Haloperidol**
    - Fluphenazine
    - Chlorpromazine
    - Prochlorperazine
    - Trifluoperazine
    - Thioridazine
    - Thiothixene
    - Loxapine
    - Perphenazine
    - Bromperidol
    - Clopenthixol
    - Promazine
  - Atypical antipsychotics:
    - Clozapine
    - Risperidone
    - Olanzapine
    - Quetiapine
    - Ziprasidone
    - Aripiprazole
- Nonneuroleptics with antidopaminergic activity
  - Metoclopramide
  - Promethazine
  - Tetrabenazine
  - Reserpine
  - Droperidol
  - Amoxapine
  - Diatrizoate
  - Phenelzine
- Dopaminergics (withdrawal)
  - Levodopa
  - COMT inhibitors
    - Tolcapone
    - Entacapone
  - Dopamine agonists
    - Bromocriptine
    - Pergolide
    - Ropinirole
    - Pramipexole
    - Cabergoline
    - Apomorphine
    - Amantadine
- Others (rare)
  - Tricyclic and selective serotonin reuptake inhibitor (SSRI) antidepressants (carbamazepine, desipramine, trimipramine)
  - Tramadol

Continued

Both serotonin syndrome and malignant hypothermia share s
features of NMS and need to be distinguished from NMS, althoug,
management may overlap as well. Intercurrent conditions such as
myxedema, or other causes of catatonia may complicate NMS.

MANAGEMENT/TREATMENT

Initial treatment of patients with suspected NMS is to immediately disco
the suspected offending agent(s) (Table 99) given that morbidity and mor
risk associated outweighs the risk of untreated psychosis and agitation. 1
opposite is true for the discontinuation of pro-dopaminergic medications i
which case they should be restarted as quickly as possible.

Supportive care is essential given the complications associated with NMS
Such measures include the removal of restraints, reducing elevated room
temperature, cooling blankets, antipyretics, careful monitoring of cardiovascular
functions, intravenous (IV) fluid resuscitation, and electrolyte correction.

Treatment of NMS is mainly empirical and few prospective studies of this
rare condition have been done. NMS overlaps with other syndromes such as
Malignant Hyperthermia and Serotonin syndrome and treatments for those
syndromes follows similar patterns of medication usage. Treatment by stage
and severity has been proposed in (Table 100). First-line pharmacologic
therapy includes benzodiazepines, bromocriptine, and dantrolene. Long-
acting benzodiazepines (e.g., lorazepam, diazepam, and clonazepam) are
often used to reverse the hypofunctioning GABAergic system and clinically as
a sedative. Bromocriptine is often used to counteract parkinsonian features
of NMS. Given oral formulation, it is typically administered via feeding tube.
Bromocriptine may cause dose-related hypotension, necessitating upward
titration over several days. Dantrolene is the drug of choice for treatment of
malignant hyperthermia and has been widely used in NMS treatment.
Dantrolene is typically weaned over several days to avoid recurrence of NMS.
Adjunctive agents include amantadine and electroconvulsive therapy (ECT).
Amantadine can be used as an adjunctive or replacement of bromocriptine in
moderate to severe cases. ECT has been shown to be successful following
the failure of multiple medications. Administration is started immediately and
continued for 10 days after the resolution of symptoms. Pharmacotherapy
shortens the clinical course of NMS.

REFERENCE

Oruch, R., Pryme, I. F., Engelsen, B. A., & Lund, A. (2017). Neuroleptic malignant
syndrome: an easily overlooked neurologic emergency. *Neuropsychiatr Dis Treat*, *13*,
161–175.

NEUROLEPTICS

Neuroleptics include several classes of compounds whose primary common
feature is blockade of dopamine receptors, although all of them have other
effects at other receptors, such as anticholinergic activity. An exception is
clozapine and other "atypical antipsychotics" (olanzapine, quetiapine), which
block serotonin receptors and have little dopamine receptor blockade. The

TABLE 99

MEDICATIONS ASSOCIATED WITH THE DEVELOPMENT OF NEUROLEPTIC MALIGNANT SYNDROME—CONT'D

- Diatrizoate
- Lithium
- Cocaine
- Amphetamines

**most common.

primary clinical use of neuroleptics is in the treatment of psychosis and agitation. Neuroleptics are also used for control of hyperkinetic movement disorders (chorea, tics, and dystonia), for suppressing nausea, for control of vertigo, neuralgic pain, and acute and refractory migraines, and for treating the abdominal pain of porphyric crises.

Aliphatic phenothiazines such as chlorpromazine (Thorazine) are strongly sedating. Potent α-adrenergic antagonism results in postural hypotension. Antiemetic and anticholinergic effects are significant. Extrapyramidal and dystonic symptoms occur with medium frequency.

Piperidine phenothiazines such as thioridazine (Mellaril) and mesoridazine (Serentil) have a relative potency similar to that of the aliphatic compounds. Sedative and α-adrenergic antagonism are less than with aliphatic compounds. Antiemetic effects are negligible. This class has a low incidence of extrapyramidal and dystonic side effects.

Piperazine phenothiazines, such as prochlorperazine (Compazine), trifluoperazine (Stelazine), perphenazine (Trilafon), and fluphenazine (Prolixin), have the highest relative potency and the strongest antiemetic effects. They also have the highest incidence of extrapyramidal and dystonic symptoms. Sedation and α-adrenergic antagonism are minimal.

The pharmacologic features of butyrophenones such as haloperidol (Haldol) closely resemble those of the piperazines. They have strong dopaminergic-blocking effects and a high incidence of extrapyramidal and dystonic symptoms. Relatively less orthostatic hypotension and sedation occur than with lower potency neuroleptics.

Pimozide (Orap), a diphenylbutylpiperidine, is similar in effect to haloperidol and is used in the United States primarily for the treatment of Tourette syndrome.

The thioxanthenes resemble the phenothiazines. Thiothixene (Navane) resembles the piperazines, with greater dystonic and extrapyramidal side effects.

Atypical antipsychotics differ from typical psychotics in their "limbic-specific" dopamine (D4) receptor binding and high ratio of serotonin type 2 (5-HT2)-receptor binding to D2 binding. These include clozapine, olanzapine, risperidone, quetiapine, and ziprasidone. Clozapine use has fallen due to agranulocytosis in 1% to 2% of patients and significant lowering of seizure threshold. Complete blood counts must be closely monitored if clozapine is

TABLE 100

NMS TREATMENT BY STAGE AND SEVERITY

Stage (Woodbury Classification)	Clinical features	General Measures	Primary Medication	Secondary Medication	Other Considerations
1. Drug Induced Parkinsonism	Tremor and Rigidity	Stop suspected etiological drug	Anticholinergics	—	Follow up observation
2. Catatonia	Psychomotor retardation; Rigidity; decreased speech; Tremor variable	Maintain hydration and Nutrition	Lorazepam 1–2 mg po/IM/IV every 4–6 hours	Diazepam or Clonazepam	Manage risk factors
3. Early NMS	Rigidity, confusion T<38°C; Pulse <100 beats per minute(bpm)	As above anc monitor vital signs and labs	Lorazepam 1–2 mg IV/IM every 4–6 hours	Diazepam 10 mg IV every 8 hours	Follow serum Creatine kinase (CK)
4. Moderate NMS	Moderate rigidity, catatonia, decreased speech, encephalopathy T 38–40°C; Pulse 100–120 bpm	Hydration and maintain electrolytes; Maintain normothermia with cooling	Lorazepam OR Diazepam as above AND Bromocriptine 2.5–5 mg po	Amantadine 100 mg po every 8 hours as alternative to Bromocriptine	Consider EEG and Neuroimaging; consider ICU placement Follow CK; check for myoglobinuria; maintain hydration
5. Severe NMS	Severe rigidity; dysautonomia; Encephalopathy or coma T ≥ 40°C; Pulse ≥ 120 bpm	ICU care	Dantrolene 1–2.5 mg/kg every 6 hours or continuous infusion for 48 hours AND Bromocriptine 2.5–5mg enterally	Lorazepam Amantadine as alternative to Bromocriptine	Follow mental status carefully; Every 2 hour neurochecks; Continual vital sign monitoring; treat agitation

Adapted from Woodbury MM, Woodbury MA (1992). Case Study: Neuroleptic-Induced Catatonia as a Stage in the Progression toward Neuroleptic Malignant Syndrome. Journal of the American Academy of Child & Adolescent Psychiatry 31:1161–1164.

used. These medications can be sedating and associated with weight gain and anticholinergic side effects.

EXTRAPYRAMIDAL SIDE EFFECTS

Dystonia may occur early (1 to 3 weeks) in the course of neuroleptic therapy or after a single parenteral injection. It may consist of generalized torsion dystonia, opisthotonos, torticollis, retrocollis, oculogyric crisis, trismus, or focal appendicular dystonia. Dystonia is more common in younger patients, especially children or adolescents, and in black males. It usually resolves spontaneously within 24 hours of stopping use of the drug but may be terminated within minutes with benztropine (Cogentin) 1 mg intramuscular (IM) or intravenous (IV), or diphenhydramine (Benadryl) 50 mg IV, or benzodiazepines; oral therapy may be continued for 24 to 48 hours.

Parkinsonian symptoms of stiffness, "cog-wheeling," tremor, and shuffling gait are dose related and may begin as early as a few days to 4 weeks after starting therapy. The neuroleptic dosage should be decreased or an anticholinergic agent may be added. Anticholinergic agents in use include benztropine 0.5 to 1 mg bid, biperiden (Akineton) 2 mg qd to tid, and trihexyphenidyl (Artane) 1 to 5 mg tid. Anticholinergics carry the risk of precipitating anticholinergic delirium, which may mimic psychotic symptoms; therefore, prophylactic use should be limited to patients at high risk for extrapyramidal symptoms.

Akathisia is a subjective sensation of motor restlessness with an urge to move around that generally occurs within several weeks of starting neuroleptic therapy. It improves on decreasing the dose of neuroleptic or adding beta blockers or benzodiazepines. Neuroleptic dose should not be increased to treat this form of "agitation," which may mimic the initial psychotic symptoms.

Tardive dyskinesia, consisting of oral-lingual-facial-buccal movements or other choreoathetoid or ballistic movements, may occur after prolonged neuroleptic therapy. Its incidence may be decreased by using neuroleptics only when indicated, keeping doses as low as possible and duration of therapy as short as possible, and early detection through careful monitoring. The more advanced the dyskinesia, the less likely is resolution. Withdrawing or changing the neuroleptic is common practice, but there is insufficient data in the literature to determine if it is helpful. There is no strong evidence for any effective treatment for tardive dyskinesia. In their review of available evidence, the American Academy of Neurology recommends clonazepam or that gingko biloba be considered as treatment, and that amantadine and tetrabenazine might be considered. While many other medications are often used, there is little evidence regarding their efficacy. Risperidone, diltiazem, galantamine, and eicosapentaenoic acid are not recommended.

A withdrawal syndrome, seen particularly in children and consisting of choreiform movements, may occur when long-term administration of neuroleptics is suddenly stopped. The syndrome usually resolves within

6 to 12 weeks but can be avoided by restarting the drug therapy and tapering more slowly.

The neuroleptic malignant syndrome is rare but often (20% to 30%) fatal. Hyperthermia, hypertonia of skeletal muscles, fluctuating consciousness, and autonomic instability are characteristic. Laboratory findings include elevated creatine kinase level, leukocytosis, and liver function abnormalities. The differential diagnosis includes heat stroke (neuroleptics may potentiate by decreasing sweating), malignant hyperthermia associated with anesthesia, idiopathic acute lethal catatonia, drug interactions with monoamine oxidase inhibitors, serotonin syndrome, and central anticholinergic syndromes. Treatment begins with discontinuing the neuroleptic and providing cooling blankets, antipyretics, and IV hydration. Dantrolene 1 to 2 mg/kg IV, amantadine 100 mg PO, and bromocriptine 2.5 mg Q6-8H PO have been used.

Neuroleptics lower the seizure threshold and may precipitate seizures. Their use in patients with epilepsy is not contraindicated unless seizure control is a significant problem.

REFERENCES

Bhidayasiri, R., Fahn, S., Weiner, W., et al. (2013). Evidence-based guideline: treatment of tardive syndromes: report of the Guideline Development Subcommittee of the American Academy of Neurology. *Neurology*, *81*, 463–469.

Horn, S. (2004). Drug-induced movement disorders. *Continuum*, *10*(3), 142–153.

NEUROPATHY (See Also AAN GUIDELINE SUMMARIES APPENDIX)

CLINICAL CLASSIFICATION OF NEUROPATHY

I. Polyneuropathies
   A. Acute predominantly motor neuropathy with variable sensory involvement
      1. Acute inflammatory demyelinating polyradiculoneuropathy (AIDP) (Guillain-Barré syndrome [GBS])
      2. Polyneuropathy associated with
         a. Diphtheria
         b. Porphyria
         c. AIDS
         d. Thallium
         e. Triorthocresyl phosphate, dapsone
   B. Acute motor neuropathy
      1. Diabetic multiple mononeuropathy (asymmetrical proximal diabetic neuropathy, diabetic amyotrophy)
   C. Acute asymmetrical sensorimotor polyneuropathy (multiple mononeuropathy or mononeuritis multiplex)
      1. Polyarteritis nodosa
      2. Wegener granulomatosis
      3. Diabetes
      4. AIDS
      5. Other angiopathies, vasculitides

D. Subacute symmetrical sensorimotor neuropathy
   1. Toxic
      a. Heavy metals—arsenic, mercury, thallium
      b. Drugs
         i. Antibiotics—clioquinol, ethambutol, isoniazid, nitrofurantoin, streptomycin
         ii. Antineoplastic—vinca alkaloids, cisplatin, chlorambucil, methotrexate, daunorubicin
         iii. Cardiovascular—clofibrate, disopyramide, hydralazine
         iv. Other—gold salts, colchicine, phenylbutazone, methaqualone, penicillamine, chloroquine, disulfiram, cyclosporine A
      c. Industrial chemicals—triorthocresyl phosphate, acrylamide, methyl bromide, n-hexane, methyl-n-butyl ketone
   2. Nutritional deficiency—vitamin B12, niacin (pellagra), thiamine (B1, beriberi/Wernicke-Korsakoff syndrome), pyridoxine (B6), vitamin E
   3. Uremia
   4. Chronic alcoholism (nutritional deficiency)
   5. Early chronic relapsing demyelinating polyneuropathy
E. Subacute to chronic, predominantly sensory neuropathy
   1. Diabetes
   2. Drugs—chlorambucil, metronidazole, ethambutol, pyridoxine, phenytoin (rare), propylthiouracil
   3. Sjögren syndrome
   4. Leprosy
   5. Paraneoplastic disease
   6. AIDS
   7. Idiopathic nonmalignant inflammatory sensory polyganglionopathy
   8. Vitamin deficiency: vitamins B12 and E
F. Subacute to chronic, predominantly motor neuropathy
   1. Diabetes—proximal diabetic motor neuropathy ("amyotrophy")
   2. Lead
G. Chronic sensory motor neuropathy
   1. Diabetes—mixed sensorimotor-autonomic neuropathy
   2. Associated with multiple myeloma
   3. Other dysproteinemias—macroglobulinemia, cryoglobulinemia, ataxia-telangiectasia
   4. POEMS syndrome—polyneuropathy, organomegaly (lymphadenopathy, splenomegaly, or hepatomegaly), endocrinopathy (usually hypogonadism or hypothyroidism), monoclonal gammopathy, and skin changes
   5. Paraneoplastic disease
   6. Uremia
   7. Leprosy

8. Amyloidosis
9. Chronic inflammatory demyelinating polyneuropathy (CIDP)
10. Sarcoidosis

H. Hereditary motor and sensory neuropathies, types I to IV
I. Hereditary sensory neuropathies, types I to IV
J. Hereditary neuropathies with known or suspected metabolic defects
   1. Fabry disease (alpha-galactosidase deficiency, X-linked)
   2. Metachromatic leukodystrophy (aryl sulfatase A deficiency, autosomal recessive)
   3. Refsum disease (phytanic oxidase deficiency, autosomal recessive)
   4. Adrenomyeloneuropathy (X-linked)
   5. Tangier disease (hypo-alpha-lipoproteinemia, autosomal recessive)
   6. Krabbe disease (globoid cell leukodystrophy, galactosyl ceramidase deficiency, autosomal recessive)
K. Other hereditary neuropathies
   1. Familial amyloid neuropathy
   2. Hereditary predisposition to pressure palsies
   3. Giant axonal neuropathy
   4. Friedreich ataxia

II. Mononeuropathies
   A. Trauma—fractures and dislocations, penetrating injuries, and pressure palsies
      1. Brachial plexus—fracture of clavicle or humerus, birth trauma, traction injuries
      2. Axillary nerve—as for brachial plexus, also intramuscular (IM) injections, shoulder subluxation
      3. Radial nerve—fracture of head of humerus, compression at the radial groove ("Saturday palsy" and "bridegroom palsy")
      4. Ulnar nerve—fracture of radius or ulna
      5. Median nerve—carpal tunnel syndrome, anterior interosseous syndrome
      6. Sciatic nerve—fracture of pelvis (sacroiliac joint), fracture of acetabulum, IM gluteal injections
      7. Femoral nerve—fracture of femur, lithotomy position, renal transplants
      8. Lateral femoral cutaneous nerve (meralgia paresthetica)
      9. Tibial nerve—fracture of tibia or fibula
      10. Common or superficial peroneal nerve—pressure palsy at fibular head from crossed legs or after weight loss
   B. Entrapment (see Carpal Tunnel Syndrome, Ulnar Neuropathy)
   C. Carcinomatous infiltration
   D. Vasculitis
   E. Leprosy

CLINICAL FEATURES OF SELECTED NEUROPATHIES
HMSN (Charcot-Marie-Tooth Disease), Types I to IV

Hereditary neuropathies are common and may occur in subtle forms. Family history and examination of family members (including foot examination for pes cavus and electromyography [EMG]) are important.

Differential diagnosis of HMSN types include Friedreich ataxia, hereditary distal spinal muscular atrophy, and chronic inflammatory demyelinating polyneuropathy (CIDP), which has slight asymmetries in the involvement of different peripheral nerves, as opposed to the hereditary types, which demonstrate uniform involvement.

I. CMT I: Hypertrophic form of Charcot-Marie-Tooth (CMT) (peroneal muscular atrophy, Roussy-Levy syndrome).

   A. Inheritance: Autosomal dominant with variable penetrance, rarely autosomal recessive.

   B. Onset usually occurs in the second decade but may appear later. Many patients have subtle findings and are undiagnosed. There is slowly progressive distal weakness and atrophy with little sensory loss. The lower extremities are more involved than the upper. Palpably thickened nerves occur in 50% of cases. Total areflexia is common. Foot deformity (pes cavus, calluses, hammertoes) result from unopposed flexor action of the posterior compartment muscles and may be the only clinical finding.

   C. Laboratory tests: Nerve conduction velocities are decreased by 40% to 75%. EMG reveals dispersed compound muscle action potentials with low amplitude, due to chronic denervation. EMG abnormalities may precede and be more extensive than clinical involvement. The cerebrospinal fluid (CSF) is usually normal.

   D. Pathologically, there are hypertrophic ("onion bulb") changes and myelinated axon loss due to chronic demyelination and remyelination. Genetic testing for subtypes of CMT I showed that CMT1-A subtype is linked to chromosome 17p11.2-12 duplication, and CMT1-B subtype is linked to chromosome 1q22-23 point mutations. The linkage of CMT1-C is still undetermined.

   E. Prognosis: Life span is usually normal, with only rare wheelchair confinement.

II. CMT II: Neuronal form (peroneal muscular atrophy).

   A. Inheritance is as in CMT I, except that onset occurs slightly later. CMT2-A subtype is linked to chromosome 1p36, CMT2-B subtype is linked to chromosome 3q-22, and CMT2-D subtype is linked to chromosome 7p14. The CMT2-C subtype linkage is undetermined. CMT II is distinguished from CMT I by the absence of hypertrophic changes, later age of onset, slower progression, less involvement of upper extremities, and greater involvement of lower extremities (atrophy of ankle flexors, inverted champagne bottle).

   B. Laboratory tests: Nerve conduction velocities are normal or slightly slowed, but amplitudes are severely diminished. EMG reveals spontaneous activity and denervation changes. CSF is usually normal.

C. Pathologically: No hypertrophic changes are seen and demyelination is mild; axonal number is decreased in distal myelinated nerves.

III. CMT III: Dejerine-Sottas disease (hypertrophic neuropathy of childhood, congenital hypomyelination neuropathy). Inheritance is autosomal recessive. Onset is congenital or in infancy. The congenital form is more severe. Motor milestones are initially delayed and then lost. Walking occurs after 15 months and as late as 3 to 4 years. Best motor performance occurs late in the first, or early in the second, decade. Patients are confined to a wheelchair by the end of the second decade. Severe, progressive weakness and atrophy are initially distal but eventually affect proximal muscles. There is severe sensory loss and sensory ataxia. Skeletal deformities (short stature, kyphoscoliosis, hand and foot deformities) are more severe and frequent than in CMT I or II. Motor nerve conduction velocities are extremely slow, and sensory nerve action potentials are unrecordable. CSF protein is elevated. Pathologically, in addition to hypertrophic changes, myelin sheaths are thin or absent. Linkage studies show that CMT3-A subtype is linked to chromosome 17p11.2-12 duplication, and CMT3-B subtype is linked to chromosome 1q22-23 point mutation.

IV. CMT IV
   A. Inheritance is autosomal recessive. CMT4 subtype is linked to chromosome 8q13 21.1.
   B. Clinically: Early onset occurs in childhood and progressive weakness leads to inability to walk in adolescence.
   C. Laboratory tests: Nerve conduction studies (NCS) are slow and CSF protein is normal. Nerve biopsy shows loss of myelinated fibers, hypomyelination, and onion bulbs.

V. X-linked CMT: X-linked CMT is clinically similar to CMT type I, but shows an X-linked pattern of inheritance (chromosome Xq13.3 point mutation). There is no male-to-male transmission. Symptoms usually start between ages 5 and 15.

There are other complex, poorly characterized forms of CMT, which show pyramidal tract signs, optic atrophy, spinocerebellar degeneration, or deafness, in addition to neuropathy.

Hereditary Sensory and Autonomic Neuropathies (HSAN), Types I to IV

I. HSAN I: Dominantly inherited sensory neuropathy (hereditary sensory neuropathy of Denny-Brown).
   A. Inheritance is autosomal dominant.
   B. Clinically, onset occurs in the second to third decade. There is progressive, distal lower-extremity, dissociated sensory loss; pain and temperature are relatively more involved. There is distal hyporeflexia. Autonomic function is normal, except for impaired distal sweating. Painless ulcerations and foot deformities may be present. Mild distal lower extremity weakness and atrophy are late findings. Upper extremity sensory loss is mild. Life expectancy is normal. NCS of the lower extremity reveal decreased sensory amplitudes

and normal or mildly decreased sensory conduction velocities; motor NCS are normal.

    C. Pathologically, axonal degeneration causes decreased numbers of small myelinated fibers and unmyelinated fibers. Differential diagnosis includes diabetic neuropathy, hereditary amyloidosis (prominent autonomic dysfunction), and syringomyelia.

II. HSAN II: Infantile and congenital sensory neuropathy (Morvan disease).

    A. Inheritance is autosomal recessive.

    B. Clinically HSAN II is similar to HSAN I except that onset occurs in infancy, and involvement of all sensory modalities is equal, severe, and proximal, as well as distal. The lips and tongue may be affected. Strength is normal. Painless ulcerations and fractures are common. There is distal areflexia.

    C. Laboratory tests: Sensory nerve action potentials are unrecordable; motor NCS are normal.

    D. Pathologically, myelinated axons are severely decreased, with moderately decreased numbers of unmyelinated fibers and some segmental demyelination and remyelination.

III. HSAN III: Familial dysautonomia (Riley-Day syndrome).

    A. Inheritance is autosomal recessive, and it occurs primarily in Ashkenazi Jews.

    B. Clinically, onset of symptoms usually occurs shortly after birth with episodic cyanosis, vomiting, unexplained fever, poor suck, and an increased susceptibility to infection. There is characteristic blotching of the skin and no fungiform papilla on the tongue. Autonomic symptoms include decreased lacrimation, hyperhidrosis, fluctuating body temperature, and episodic postural hypotension. There is a dissociated sensory loss with predominant involvement of pain and temperature, causing corneal ulcerations, painless skin lesions, and deformed joints. Areflexia is generalized. Strength, sweating, and sphincter function are normal. Intelligence is usually normal.

    C. Laboratory tests: Sensory nerve action potentials are diminished; motor NCS may be mildly abnormal. Peripheral nerves show marked depletion of unmyelinated fibers.

    D. Prognosis is generally poor, but occasionally individuals survive to middle age.

IV. HSAN IV: Congenital sensory neuropathy. Inheritance is autosomal recessive. This very rare disorder is characterized by congenital anhidrosis, generalized insensitivity to pain and temperature, mental retardation, and episodic pyrexia.

DIABETIC NEUROPATHY

This clinical or subclinical disorder of the somatic or autonomic peripheral nervous system occurs in patients with diabetes mellitus without other causes for peripheral neuropathy. Proposed etiologic factors include localized endoneurial hypoxia, chronic hyperglycemia, episodic hypoglycemia, polyol accumulation, myoinositol deficiency, and impaired axonal transport. Microangiopathy and infarction have been proposed as the mechanism for diabetic multiple mononeuropathies. The following diabetic neuropathy syndromes are recognized:

I. Symmetrical polyneuropathies
   A. Distal sensory polyneuropathy is the most common.
      1. Clinically, onset is usually insidious, but it may occur acutely following an episode of diabetic coma or hypoglycemia. Usually, clinical manifestations reflect involvement of all fiber types. However, occasionally a large or small fiber pattern is more prominent. The large fiber pattern presents with paresthesias in the feet and loss of distal reflexes, position sensation, and vibratory sensation. The small fiber pattern is loss of thermal and pinprick sensation, associated with burning pain. Autonomic neuropathy often accompanies the small fiber pattern.
      2. Laboratory tests: NCS show reduced sensory action potential amplitude and variable slowing of motor nerve conduction velocity (related to degree of demyelination). EMG shows denervation, despite little or no weakness.
      3. Pathologically, there is distal axonal loss with variable degrees of segmental demyelination.
   B. Autonomic neuropathy. Clinical features include abnormal pupillary reaction, postural hypotension, abnormalities of heart rate, peripheral edema, anhidrosis, abnormalities of reflex vasoconstriction, abnormal gastrointestinal motility, diarrhea, atonic bladder, and impotence. Sudden death may occur from lack of reaction to hypoglycemia or cardiorespiratory arrest.
   C. Symmetrical proximal lower extremity motor neuropathy ("amyotrophy")
      1. Clinically, there is slowly progressive, symmetrical weakness, which is distinct from asymmetrical "amyotrophy," which is discussed under the focal diabetic neuropathies. Initial manifestations include lower back and proximal lower extremity pain, which is followed by progressive proximal weakness, loss of patellar reflexes, and atrophy. Sensation is spared, but a distal sensory polyneuropathy may coexist.
      2. Laboratory tests: Initial EMG shows reduced motor unit recruitment, while evidence of denervation appears later.
      3. Prognosis for recovery varies, but is generally worse with insidious onset of symptoms. Control of hyperglycemia may promote recovery.

II. Focal and multifocal diabetic neuropathies
   A. Trunk and limb mononeuropathy (including mononeuropathy multiplex)
      1. Clinically, disease occurs acutely, most often in the ulnar, median, radial, femoral, lateral cutaneous, thoracic, and peroneal nerves. These lesions often occur at the same sites as entrapment neuropathics. It is important to exclude other causes, such as

radiculopathy. It may not be possible to distinguish between a diabetic mononeuropathy and an entrapment syndrome.
2. Prognosis for recovery is good.
B. Cranial neuropathies most commonly affect the extraocular muscles (see Ophthalmoplegia) and may be associated with facial pain or headache. Third nerve lesions show rapid onset and pupillary sparing, whereas aneurysmal compression typically has an unresponsive pupil.
C. Asymmetrical proximal lower limb motor neuropathy is the unilateral form of "amyotrophy." Onset of unilateral pain and proximal weakness is sudden, progressing over 1 to 2 weeks. The patellar reflex is lost, and proximal atrophy eventually develops. Although the cause remains uncertain, prognosis is good. There have been reports of successful treatment with steroids, plasma exchange, and intravenous gamma globulins.

Inflammatory Demyelinating Polyneuropathies

I. GBS (Guillain-Barré-Strohl syndrome, AIDP) is probably immunologically mediated, involving both cellular and humoral responses, but no single autoantigen has been identified (see AAN Guideline Summaries).
   A. Clinical presentation: Paresthesias in the distal extremities are followed by lower extremity weakness. The weakness then ascends to involve the arms and face. Bilateral sciatica is common. Initial examination shows symmetrical limb weakness, absent or greatly diminished deep tendon reflexes, and minimal sensory loss. Progression to involve respiration, eye movements, swallowing, and autonomic function occurs in severe cases. Weakness progresses for 1 to 3 weeks before stabilizing and recovering. Severity of symptoms varies among individuals. In severe cases, complications of pneumonia, sepsis, adult respiratory distress syndrome, pulmonary embolus, and cardiac arrest are responsible for most severe illness and even death.
   B. Risk factors: GBS is often preceded by an infection, usually viral. Important associated infections include human immunodeficiency virus (HIV), Epstein-Barr virus, cytomegalovirus, influenza virus, and *Campylobacter jejuni* enteritis. Underlying systemic diseases, such as systemic lupus erythematosus (SLE), Hodgkin disease, and sarcoidosis are occasionally associated with GBS. Surgery and vaccinations may also precede GBS.
   C. Evaluation: Lumbar puncture (LP) shows CSF protein greater than 55 mg/dL with little or no pleocytosis (albuminocytologic dissociation) starting about 1 week after onset of symptoms. CSF protein is often normal during the first few days of the illness. NCS show signs of demyelination early, before CSF protein changes, with loss of F and H waves and nerve conduction block (>dissociation) starting about 1.
   D. Differential diagnosis includes spinal cord disease, myasthenia gravis, neoplastic meningitis, vasculitic neuropathy, paraneoplastic

neuropathy, botulism, diphtheria, heavy-metal intoxication, poliomyelitis, and porphyria.

E. GBS variants: These share signs of diminished reflexes, demyelination pattern on NCS, and elevated CSF protein. Variant syndromes include Miller-Fisher syndrome (ophthalmoplegia, ataxia, and areflexia with little associated weakness, + GQ1b Ab), acute motor axonal neuropathy, Bickerstaff encephalitis pharyngeal-cervical-brachial weakness, paraparesis, pure sensory and pure ataxia.

F. Treatment: Monitor for respiratory failure and dysautonomia. Intubation might be indicated in a patient with FVC < 20 mL/kg or MIP < 30 cmH_2O. Dysautonomia is a major cause of morbidity and should be treated aggressively with hydration, vasoactive drugs, and pacemakers if needed.

Plasma exchange significantly alters the progression and severity of GBS, decreasing the need for mechanical ventilation by approximately 50%. The efficacy of intravenous immunoglobulin treatment (IVIG) is probably comparable with plasmapheresis. IVIG given daily at 0.4 g/kg/day for 5 days is the preferred treatment in unstable patients; recent literature suggests a better response for IVIG in anti-GM1b-positive GBS (axonal variant). Corticosteroids are not efficacious in GBS.

II. CIDP, or chronic relapsing dysimmune polyneuropathy

A. Clinical presentation: CIDP is similar to GBS but shows a protracted, often relapsing course, pronounced sensory involvement, response to corticosteroid treatment, and greater association with systemic disease. Worsening of symptoms for longer than 2 months, with subacute onset and fluctuation of symptoms over years, is characteristic of CIDP. Sensory involvement often accompanies proximal extremity and neck flexor weakness and diminished reflexes. Laboratory findings are similar to CSF and EMG findings of GBS, with more chronic changes on EMG and NCS.

B. Differential diagnosis includes monoclonal gammopathies, lymphoma, connective tissue disease (polyarteritis nodosa, cryoglobulinemia, SLE), anti-MAG-associated polyneuropathies, Lyme disease, HIV infection, and sarcoidosis.

C. Treatment: Prednisone 100 mg/day for 4 weeks, tapering gradually over 1 year to 10 to 20 mg qod. Plasma exchange is usually given in 3 to 5 exchanges over 1 to 2 weeks. Plasmapheresis with lower dose prednisone may be tried as initial therapy. IVIG given at 0.4 g/kg/day for 5 days is efficacious according to some but not all studies. Immunosuppressive drugs are used in refractory cases.

GENERAL PRINCIPLES OF TREATMENT OF NEUROPATHIES

I. Patient education and counseling

II. Genetic counseling

III. Withdrawal of medications suspected of causing neuropathy

IV. Withdrawal from toxic exposure
V. Correction of nutritional and vitamin deficiencies
VI. Treatment of alcoholism
VII. Blood glucose control in diabetic neuropathies
VIII. Specific drug therapies
    A. Chelating agents in lead neuropathy
    B. Hematin infusions in acute intermittent porphyria
    C. Long-term prednisone or other immune-modifying regimens in CIDP
    D. Phytanic acid (reduced) diet in Refsum disease
IX. Plasmapheresis in AIDP and other autoimmune disorders
X. Pain control
    A. Improve blood glucose control in diabetic neuropathies
    B. Simple analgesics—aspirin and acetaminophen
    C. Gabapentin, phenytoin, and carbamazepine—achieve anticonvulsant levels
    D. Tricyclic drugs—amitriptyline and imipramine
    E. Transcutaneous electrical nerve stimulation
XI. Meticulous foot care
XII. Orthotic devices and splints
XIII. Surgical correction of entrapment neuropathies
XIV. Physical and occupational therapy

REFERENCES

Watson, J. C., & Dyck, P. J. (2015). Peripheral neuropathy: a practical approach to diagnosis and symptom management. *Mayo Clin Proc*, *90*(7), 940–951.
Wijdicks, E. F., & Klein, C. J. (2017). Guillain-Barré syndrome. *Mayo Clin Proc*, *92*(3), 467–479.

NUTRITIONAL DEFICIENCY SYNDROMES

Table 101 discusses nutritional deficiency syndromes.

REFERENCE

Goodman, B. P. (2015). Neurologic complications of nutritional disorders.
    In K. D. Flemming, & L. K. Jones (Eds.), *Mayo Clinic neurology board review: clinical neurology for initial certification and MOC* (pp. 747–752). New York: Oxford University Press.

NYSTAGMUS

Nystagmus is a biphasic ocular oscillation in which at least one phase is slow. The nystagmus direction is defined as the direction of the fast component. The direction may be horizontal, vertical, diagonal, or rotational. There are two general types, jerk, and pendular. If the second phase is a fast eye movement, the nystagmus is termed "jerk." If the second phase is a slow eye movement, the nystagmus is termed "pendular." Jerk nystagmus usually reflects acquired disease of the brainstem but may also occur congenitally. Pendular nystagmus may be acquired or congenital.

TABLE 101

NUTRITIONAL DEFICIENCY SYNDROMES

Type	Source	Etiology of Deficiency	Neurologic Manifestations	Symptoms	Diagnostic Testing	Treatment	Prognosis
Vitamin B$_1$ (thiamine)	Grains Rice (fortified) Cereals Pork Organ meats	Alcoholism Malnutrition Pregnancy Malignancy Hemodialysis Refeeding syndrome	1. Beriberi (sensorimotor, peripheral neuropathy, cardiomyopathy) 2. Wernicke syndrome (encephalopathy, ophthalmoplegia, gait ataxia) 3. Korsakoff syndrome (anterograde and retrograde amnesia, confabulation)	Paresthesias Distal muscle weakness with foot drop Pain in muscles Subacute confus on Ophthalmoplegia (esp. lateral recti) Nystagmus Truncal ataxia Profound memory impairment, usually after symptoms of Wernicke's subside	Clinical diagnosis MRI may show T2 and FLAIR signal abnormalities in periaqueductal regions, medial thalami, and bilateral mamillary bodies; lesions may be enhancing Serum thiamine and RBC transketolase activity may be decreased	Immediate treatment with thiamine 100 mg IV should be given before D50 to avoid worsening of symptoms of Wernicke syndrome Continue IV thiamine for about 5 days, then continue PO 50–100 mg daily, indefinitely	Sensorimotor (thiamine) neuropathy in beriberi gradually improves with thiamine over weeks to months; in severe cases, recovery is incomplete
Vitamin B$_6$ (pyridoxine)	Chicken, fish Fruits Vegetables Grains	Isoniazid therapy Hydralazine Penicillamine Alcoholism	1. Peripheral neuropathy (adults) 2. Intractable seizures (infants)	Paresthesias: burning and tingling usually feet first; may proceed	Mainly a clinical diagnosis Urinary 4-pyridoxic acid Serum PLP	Discontinue offending medication 50 mg pyridoxine	Variable Convulsions respond to treatment Long-term functional outcome variable

Nutrient	Sources / Causes	Clinical	Diagnosis	Treatment	Prognosis
	GI diseases End-stage renal disease on hemodialysis Malnutrition in infancy	proximally Confusion Convulsions (infants) Exaggerated auditory startle (infants) Hyperirritability	(active form of pyridoxine) RBC aspartate aminotransferase Clinical diagnosis (infants) by history of convulsions, response of seizures to pyridoxine	daily for several weeks, then 2 mg daily In infants, 10 mg IV push to terminate seizures, then 75 mg daily for life	
Vitamin B$_{12}$	Meat Fish Legumes Malabsorption Gastrectomy Pernicious anemia Small bowel resection Poor intake	1. Peripheral neuropathy (vibration and JPS especially) 2. Myelopathy 3. Subacute combined (rare) (posterior columns + corticospinal tract dysfunction) 4. Dementia 5. Optic neuropathy Paresthesias: mainly hands and feet Unsteady gait Weakness Mental slowing Depression GI symptoms Encephalopathy Dementia Lhermitte sign Decreased vibration and JPS Variable reflexes Visual defects	Vitamin B$_{12}$ level, MMA homocysteine levels, folate CBC with peripheral smear (hypersegmented neutrophils) Delusions factor antibodies Schilling test MRI brain and spinal cord (lateral and posterior columns) EMG/NCS (decreased sural in 80%)	Vitamin B$_{12}$: 1000 mg IM daily × 7 days, then 1000 mg IM weekly × 4 weeks, then 1000 mg IM monthly for life Parietal cell and intrinsic	At least partial improvement with treatment is likely; most in first 6 months, but can take up to a year Myelopathy is least likely to recover

Continued

TABLE 101

NUTRITIONAL DEFICIENCY SYNDROMES—CONT'D

Type	Source	Etiology of Deficiency	Neurologic Manifestations	Symptoms	Diagnostic Testing	Treatment	Prognosis
Copper	Shellfish, Oysters Whole grain	Excessive zinc ingestion Gastric surgery Chronic GI dz	Myelopathy Myeloneuropathy	Sensory ataxia	Serum copper Ceruloplasmin 24-h urinary copper Serum zinc	Oral elemental copper 8 mg daily in wk 1 6 mg daily in wk 2 4 mg daily in wk 3 2 mg daily thereafter	Variable w/residual neuro deficits
Vitamin D	Milk (fortified) Fatty fish and fish oils Sunlight	Hyperparathyroidism Hypophosphatemia Chronic renal failure Anticonvulsants Dietary deficiency Inadequate sunlight	1. Osteomalacia—bone weakness and proximal muscle weakness with waddling gait (pelvic girdle muscles weak) 2. Rickets	Muscle weakness Waddling gait Pain (bone fractures)	Elevated alkaline phosphatase Low or normal serum calcium and phosphorus Mildly elevated CK EMG may show myopathic pattern X-rays may show osteoporosis	Ergocalciferol 800–4000 IU daily for 8 weeks, then 400 IU/day until precipitating factor resolved Monitor serum calcium levels	Responsive to treatment over months
Vitamin E	Vegetable oils	GI disease (biliary atresia,	1. Spinocerebellar dysfunction	Gait ataxia Areflexia	Serum vitamin E level	For pure vitamin E deficiency:	Variable

	Nuts Green leafy vegetables Cereal (fortified)	chronic cholestasis, Crohn disease, celiac disease) Cystic fibrosis Hereditary (abetalipoprotein-emia)	2. Peripheral neuropathy (vibration and JPS) 3. Retinopathy of prematurity	Mild to moderate weakness Severely decreased vibration and JPS sense Ptosis Nystagmus Retinal pigmentation	CBC with smear (acanthocytes) MRI spinal cord (posterior columns abnormal T_2 in some) NCS/EMG (mild axonal neuropathy)	alpha-tocopherol 800–1200 mg daily For abetalipoproteinemia alpha-tocopherol 5000–7000 mg daily	Unclear
Folate	Grains	Alcoholism Small bowel disease (sprue, Crohn, Ulcerative colitis Pregnancy Drugs: anticonvulsants, methotrexate, others	1. Usually no symptoms 2. Cognitive impairment 3. Subacute combined degeneration Fetal neural tube defects	Mild cognitive impairment Depression associate Increased stroke risk (hyperhomocy-steinemia)	RBC folate (better test than plasma folate) homocysteine Vitamin B_{12} level (r/o B_{12} deficiency)	Folic acid 1 mg daily May need to initially give parenterally Adequate nutrition	

Continued

TABLE 101

NUTRITIONAL DEFICIENCY SYNDROMES—CONT'D

Type	Source	Etiology of Deficiency	Neurologic Manifestations	Symptoms	Diagnostic Testing	Treatment	Prognosis
Nicotinic acid (niacin, vitamin B₃)	Bread	Dietary deficiency (underdeveloped populations where maize is a staple) Diarrhea Cirrhosis Alcoholism Isoniazid therapy Carcinoid tumor	1. Pellagra (endemic area) (dementia, diarrhea, dermatitis) 2. Chronic unexplained encephalopathy may resemble Wernicke 3. Spina bifida and neural tube defects in fetal development	Neuropsychiatric (irritability, apathy, depression, memory loss) Stupor or coma Spasticity Babinski sign Startle myoclonus Gegenhalten	Mainly a clinical diagnosis Decreased urinary NMN (N- methylnicotina-mide) secretion	Parenteral nicotinic acid 100 mg IV daily × 5–7 days Or Oral nicotinic acid 50 mg 10 times daily × 3 weeks	Excellent if treated appropriately

MMA, Methylmalonic acid; *JPS,* joint position sense.

When examining a patient with nystagmus, observe changes in amplitude and frequency with change in gaze direction. Nystagmus may indicate dysfunction somewhere in the posterior fossa, that is, vestibular system (and end organ), brainstem, or cerebellum. Table 102 provides a clinical classification of nystagmus.

Congenital nystagmus is noted within 6 months of birth. Its waveform may be pendular, jerk, or a combination of both. It may be found in the presence of ophthalmic disorders that diminish vision (sensory form) or may be related to an isolated manifestation (motor form). The principal causes of vision loss in the sensory form of congenital nystagmus are corneal and lens opacities, albinism, aniridia, achromatopsia, Leber's congenital amaurosis, and optic neuropathy.

The distinguishing features of congenital nystagmus can be remembered by using the mnemonic CONGENITAL: Convergence and eye closure dampen the nystagmus; Oscillopsia is usually absent; Null zone is present; Gaze position does not change the direction of nystagmus; Equal amplitude and frequency of nystagmus in each eye; Near acuity is good (convergence dampens the nystagmus); Inversion of optokinetic nystagmus occurs; Turning of head or abnormal head posture to allow eyes to enter a null zone leads to better visual acuity; Absent nystagmus during sleep; Latent nystagmus occurs.

ASSESSMENT OF NYSTAGMUS

First, one needs to determine whether nystagmus is congenital or acquired. In congenital nystagmus, visual loss often occurs early on and patients do not usually complain of oscillopsia. In acquired nystagmus, visual acuity is typically degraded but not severely affected. Second, the eye movement should be assessed in the following manner: (1) primary gaze position–esotropia, exotropia, or orthotropia; (2) perform pursued and saccade eye movement at extreme gaze and describe nystagmus in terms of its amplitude, frequency, and waveform; (3) complete other neurologic examinations to augment the localization of the lesion; (4) MRI of brain or cervical spine if necessary.

TREATMENT

Treatment of symptomatic nystagmus relies on physical and pharmacologic methods. Congenital nystagmus can be treated with prisms, surgery, and contact lenses. Baclofen may benefit acquired periodic alternating nystagmus. Gabapentin (tapered slowly to doses as high as 300 mg po four times daily) may be useful for pendular nystagmus. GABAergic medications including clonazepam, valproate, isoniazid, and baclofen have been somewhat effective in treating downbeat nystagmus. Surgical decompression of Arnold-Chiari malformation may reduce downbeat nystagmus.

REFERENCES

Biousse, V., & Newman, N. J. (2015). *Neuro-ophthalmology illustrated,* ed 2. New York: Thieme Medical Publishers, Inc.

Leigh, J. R., & Zee, D. (Eds.). (2006). *The neurology of eye movements*, ed 4. New York: Oxford University Press.

TABLE 102

CLINICAL CLASSIFICATION OF NYSTAGMUS

Types	Definition	Significance	Associated Condition
Optokinetic nystagmus	Composed of an initial slow pursuit eye movement and a compensatory fast eye movement (saccade, quick phase). Often can be elicited by looking at a spinning drum.	Physiologic response unless there is unequal or reduced amplitude in two eyes which would signify deep parietal lobe lesion or subtle internuclear ophthalmoplegia.	Internuclear ophthalmoplegia
Caloric nystagmus	Nystagmus induced by instilling either cold or warm water. Cold water results in fast phase beating away from irrigated side; warm water results in fast phase beating toward the irrigated side: COWS.	Physiologic response if vestibulo-ocular connection, cranial nerve III/VI and PPRF are intact.	Both structural and metabolic coma can result in diminished fast phase of nystagmus, and if severe, slow phase can also be eliminated
Nystagmus due to peripheral vestibular imbalance	Due to imbalance of the peripheral vestibular system, which will manifest as either purely horizontal or mixed—horizontal-torsional with the fast phase directed away from the side of the lesion.	Peripheral vestibulopathy	Labyrinthitis or vestibular neuritis
Latent nystagmus	Congenital jerk nystagmus induced by monocular occlusion of either eye. Patient develops bilateral jerk nystagmus with the fast phase toward the open, fixating eye when one eye is closed.	Pathologic	Often associated with infantile esotropia, amblyopia, or strabismus

Spasmus nutans	Triad of head tilt, head nodding, and nystagmus that is monocular or markedly asymmetrical. The nystagmus is pendular, rapid, and of small amplitude.	Often benign. Onset between ages 4 and 14 months and usually disappears by 5 years of age. However, it may be pathologic. MRI is indicated to rule out perichiasmal pathology.	May be associated with chiasmal glioma, third ventricular tumor, or degenerative disorder
Internuclear ophthalmoplegia	Nystagmus of the abduction eye.	Lesion at MLF	Often associated with demyelinating disease such as multiple sclerosis
Downbeat nystagmus	Nystagmus in the primary position of gaze with the fast phase beating in a downward direction.	Often involved in cervicomedullary junction disorder. MRI is often indicated to examine cervicomedullary junction.	Arnold-Chiari malformation, spinocerebellar degeneration, anticonvulsant intoxication, magnesium deficiency, brainstem encephalitis, lithium use, alcoholic cerebellar degeneration
Upbeat nystagmus	Nystagmus in the primary position of gaze with the fast phase beating in an upward direction.	Always a sign of acquired disease of the brainstem, anywhere from midbrain to the medulla, or of the cerebellum. MRI is indicated to examine brainstem and cerebellar disease.	Tumors, stroke, intoxication, inflammation, and degeneration
Periodic alternating nystagmus	Horizontal jerk nystagmus which periodically changes direction. Usually consists of 90 s of nystagmus in one direction and 10 to 15 s of no nystagmus in primary position followed by nystagmus in the opposite direction.	May be congenital or may be due to craniocervical junction abnormalities or brainstem and cerebellar disease. MRI of the head is needed.	Arnold-Chiari malformation, multiple sclerosis, cerebellar pathology, brainstem infarction, and anticonvulsant use

Continued

N

NYSTAGMUS

TABLE 102

CLINICAL CLASSIFICATION OF NYSTAGMUS—CONT'D

Types	Definition	Significance	Associated Condition
Convergence-retraction nystagmus	Cocontraction of the extraocular muscles on attempted convergence or upgaze.	Often associated with papillary light-near dissociation and bilateral lid retraction. Lesion localized at dorsal rostral midbrain.	Pineal gland tumor in Parinaud syndrome
Seesaw nystagmus	Characterized by alternate elevation and depression of one eye accompanied by a similar movement in the other eye but in the opposite direction.	Often secondary to large parasellar lesion expanding to the third ventricle. Need to look for bitemporal hemianopia MRI of the brain with attention to parasellar area.	Pituitary tumor
Gaze-evoked nystagmus	Nystagmus induced by moving the eyes into an eccentric position.	Physiologic if it is unsustained. Pathologic if it is sustained and sustained and indicates dysfunctional neural integrator system.	Cerebral or brainstem process or a weak extraocular muscle if there is a paresis of gaze
Nystagmus in MG	Manifests as a gaze-evoked nystagmus in any direction with asymmetry between the two eyes especially after prolonged eccentric gaze.	Signifies fatigability of the ocular muscle. Also referred to as "pseudointernuclear ophthalmoplegia."	MG

COWS indicates for direction of fast nystagmus—cold water = opposite direction and warm water = same direction; *MG*, myasthenia gravis; *MLF*, medial longitudinal fasciculus; *PPRF*, paramedian pontine reticular formation.

O

OCCIPITAL LOBE

The occipital lobe extends from the parieto-occipital fissure on the medial surface of the brain to the lateral surface, where it merges with the parietal and temporal lobes. The calcarine sulcus divides the occipital lobe into lingula and cuneus, and it marks the boundary of the primary visual area (Brodmann area 17). The rest of the occipital lobe constitutes the visual association cortex (Brodmann areas 18 and 19). Its function is mainly concerned with visual perception and interpretation. Clinical symptoms associated with occipital lesions include visual field defects, cortical blindness, visual agnosias, achromatopsia, metamorphopsias, illusions, and hallucinations. Visual symptoms occur commonly in migraine. Occipital lobe is commonly involved in the posterior reversible encephalopathy syndrome secondary to medications or hypertension. Occipital lobe epilepsy may present with visual phenomena, as well as postictal blindness. Some of the clinical syndromes in the occipital lobe lesion include the following:

1. Anton syndrome (visual anosognosia or cortical blindness): A patient's lack of awareness of their defect, associated with bilateral lesions.
2. Balint syndrome: Seen with bilateral occipital and parieto-occipital infarctions, consisting of optic ataxia, paralysis of gaze and disturbance of visual attention, and simultanagnosia.

REFERENCES

Andersen, R. A., Andersen, K. N., Hwang, E. J., & Hauschild, M. (2014). Optic ataxia: from Balint's syndrome to the parietal reach region. *Neuron, 81*(5), 967–983.

Martinaud, O. (2017). Visual agnosia and focal brain injury. *Rev Neurol (Paris), 173*(7–8), 451–460.

OCULAR OSCILLATIONS

The following abnormal oscillatory eye movements are distinct from nystagmus because of waveform differences (e.g., no distinct slow and fast phases characteristic of nystagmus):

I. Ocular bobbing consists of intermittent downward jerks of both eyes, followed by a slow drift to primary position. It is seen with destructive lesions of the pons but also occurs with pontine compression, obstructive hydrocephalus, and metabolic encephalopathy. Reflex eye movements are usually not brought out in this situation.

II. Ocular dipping is an inverse movement (slow downward, fast upward) with unreliable localization.

III. Ping-pong gaze denotes slow, horizontal, conjugate drift of the eyes that alternates every few seconds and is seen with bilateral hemispheric dysfunction.

IV. Ocular myoclonus refers to pendular vertical oscillations seen with brainstem lesions often accompanied by rhythmic palatal movements. It typically occurs with lesions between the red nucleus, inferior olive, and dentate nucleus.

The term saccadic oscillation includes several specific entities:

I. Saccadic dysmetria can produce oscillation when overshooting saccades are followed by one or more corrective saccades.

II. Square wave jerks are seen most prominently in cerebellar disorders and progressive supranuclear palsy; saccades interrupt fixation with normal intersaccadic intervals.

III. Macro square wave jerks are seen in multiple sclerosis and olivopontocerebellar atrophy.

IV. Ocular flutter and opsoclonus produce flurries of rapid eye movements without an intersaccadic interval; movements may be purely horizontal (flutter) or multidirectional (opsoclonus). Both can be secondary to viral infection, drug effects, tumor, or paraneoplastic syndromes such as neuroblastoma in children or with anti-Purkinje cell antibodies in adults (mostly women with gynecologic tumors).

Superior oblique myokymia is a monocular torsional oscillation of small amplitude, high-frequency contractions of a monocular superior oblique muscle. It causes oscillopsia, diplopia, or visual blurring. Although sometimes seen with brainstem disease, it is usually idiopathic and may respond to carbamazepine therapy.

Spasmus nutans is an ocular oscillation accompanied by head nodding and torticollis. It appears before 18 months of age and remits spontaneously, usually by age 3 years. The abnormal eye movements are usually dysconjugate and vary in direction. Although usually benign, this entity must not be confused with signs of intracranial tumor; the presence of poor feeding, optic atrophy, or raised intracranial pressure should be investigated by neuroimaging studies.

REFERENCES

Biousse, V., & Newman, N. J. (2015). *Neuro-ophthalmology illustrated,* ed 2. New York: Thieme Medical Publishers, Inc.

Leigh, J. R., & Zee, D. (Eds.). (2006). *The neurology of eye movements*, ed 4. New York: Oxford University Press.

OLFACTION

The sense of smell is mediated by the first cranial nerve. It is the only sensory modality without a thalamic relay before synapsing in the cortex. Deficits in olfaction include anosmia, hyposmia, parosmia, or loss of appreciation of flavors in food.

Smell is tested clinically using non-irritating, aromatic compounds such as oil of wintergreen, cloves, coffee, almond oil, or lemon oil. The stimulus is presented to one nostril with the other occluded. The ability to appreciate the presence of a substance, even if not properly identified, is evidence that anosmia is not present. Unilateral anosmia is more often due to a structural lesion rather than a diffuse process. More detailed olfactory testing using the University of Pennsylvania Smell Identification Test can distinguish hyposmia, anosmia, or malingering.

Causes of anosmia or hyposmia include the following:

I. Infection: URI (most frequent cause of olfactory dysfunction), rhinitis, sinusitis, basilar meningitis, frontal abscess, osteomyelitis (frontal, ethmoidal), viral hepatitis, syphilis, influenza.

II. Toxic or metabolic disorders: pernicious anemia, zinc deficiency, lead and calcium intoxication, diabetes mellitus, hypothyroidism, medication effects.

III. Neoplasms: frontal tumor, olfactory groove or sphenoid meningioma, radiation therapy.

IV. Head trauma, including trauma to cribriform plate.

V. Congenital: olfactory agenesis (Kallmann syndrome) and septo-optic dysplasia (De Morsier syndrome).

VI. Others: hydrocephalus, amphetamine and cocaine abuse, smoking, trigeminal lesions (causing mucosal atrophy), anterior cerebral artery disease, Sheehan syndrome, nasal polyps, multiple sclerosis, sarcoidosis, aging, Alzheimer disease, Parkinson disease (hyposmia commonly presents years before disease onset).

Anosmia most commonly occurs secondary to head trauma, and may not be noticed until several weeks or months after the injury. A third of the cases spontaneously resolve within a year.

Hyperosmia is seen in somatization disorders, migraine, hyperemesis gravidarum, cystic fibrosis, Addison disease, and strychnine poisoning. Multiple chemical sensitivity syndrome is a vague disorder associated with unexplained odor sensitivity and excitability to multiple chemical and environmental stimuli.

Olfactory hallucinations are a feature of mesial temporal lobe seizures ("uncinate fits"), which may be triggered or even arrested by olfactory stimulation. Anosmia is not present in such cases. They may also be seen in psychiatric disease (olfactory reference syndrome) and neoplasms or vascular disease involving the inferomedial temporal lobe.

There is no current effective medical treatment for most cases of olfactory loss; however, systemic steroids can be tried in post-viral, conductive, and idiopathic olfactory loss. Removal of offending agents (drugs, etc.) and treatment of underlying cause may also help improve olfaction.

O

OLFACTION

REFERENCES

Cho, S. H. (2014). Clinical diagnosis and treatment of olfactory dysfunction. *Hanyang Med Rev, 34*, 107–115.

Dawes, P. J. (1998). Clinical tests of olfaction. *Clin Otolaryngol Allied Sci, 23*(6), 484–490. https://doi.org/10.1046/j.1365-2273.1998.2360484.x.

OPALSKI SYNDROME

Opalski syndrome refers to lateral medullary syndrome (Wallenberg syndrome), *plus ipsilateral hemiplegia.* Lesion is usually located lower than that in Wallenberg syndrome, involving the corticospinal fibers caudal to the pyramidal decussation. The syndrome is usually caused by vertebral artery occlusion. A related syndrome is Babinski-Nageotte syndrome, which manifests contralateral hemiparesis due to hemimedullary infarct before the pyramidal tract decussation.

REFERENCES

Katsumata, M., Oki, K., Nakahara, J., Izawa, Y., Abe, T., & Takahashi, S. (2015). Ipsilateral facial tactile hypesthesia in a patient with lateral medullary syndrome. *J Stroke Cerebrovasc Dis, 24*(11), e315–e317.

Uemura, M., Naritomi, H., Uno, H., et al. (2016). Ipsilateral hemiparesis in lateral medullary infarction: clinical investigation of the lesion location on magnetic resonance imaging. *J Neurol Sci, 365*, 40–45.

OPHTHALMOPLEGIA

If a patient complains of diplopia or if extraocular muscle testing reveals misalignment of the visual axes, first determine whether this is due to nerve palsy or some other causes of impaired motility.

I. Causes of impaired ocular motility other than nerve palsy
   A. Concomitant strabismus
   B. Graves ophthalmopathy (most commonly inferior and medial recti muscles)
   C. Myasthenia gravis (and other pharmacologic or toxic causes of neuromuscular blockade)
   D. Convergence spasm
   E. Blowout fracture of the orbit with entrapment myopathy
   F. Restrictive ophthalmopathy (Brown's superior oblique tendon sheath syndrome)
   G. Orbital inflammatory disease (orbital pseudotumor)
   H. Orbital masses, neoplasms
   I. Orbital infections
   J. Brainstem disorders causing abnormal prenuclear inputs (internuclear ophthalmoplegia [INO], skew deviation)

K. Ocular myopathies
L. Chronic progressive external ophthalmoplegia (CPEO; Kearns-Sayre and related mitochondrial syndromes)
M. Congenital syndromes

II. Causes of abducens nerve (CN VI) palsies
  A. Nuclear (associated with ipsilateral horizontal gaze palsy)
    1. Developmental anomalies (*Möbius*, *Duane* syndromes)
    2. Infarction
    3. Tumor (pontine glioma, cerebellar tumors)
    4. Wernicke-Korsakoff syndrome
  B. Fascicular
    1. Infarction
    2. Demyelination
    3. Tumor
  C. Subarachnoid space lesions
    1. Aneurysm or anomalous vessels (anterior inferior cerebellar artery, basilar artery)
    2. Subarachnoid hemorrhage
    3. Meningitis (infectious, neoplastic)
    4. Sarcoidosis
    5. Cerebellopontine angle tumor (acoustic neuroma, meningioma)
    6. Clivus tumor (chordoma, nasopharyngeal carcinoma)
    7. Trauma
    8. Surgical complication
    9. Postinfectious
  D. Petrous
    1. Infection or inflammation of mastoid or petrous tip
    2. Trauma (petrous fracture)
    3. Thrombosis of inferior petrosal sinus
    4. Increased intracranial pressure (idiopathic intracranial hypertension, supratentorial mass)
    5. Following lumbar puncture
    6. Aneurysm
    7. Persistent trigeminal artery
    8. Trigeminal schwannoma
  E. Cavernous sinus and superior orbital fissure
    1. Aneurysm
    2. Cavernous sinus thrombosis
    3. Carotid cavernous fistula
    4. Dural arteriovenous malformation
    5. Tumor (pituitary adenoma, meningioma, nasopharyngeal carcinoma, metastasis)
    6. Pituitary apoplexy
    7. Sphenoid sinusitis (mucormycosis)

      8. Herpes zoster
      9. Granulomatous inflammation (sarcoidosis, *Tolosa-Hunt* syndrome)
  F. Orbital
    1. Tumor
    2. Infection
    3. Trauma
  G. Uncertain localization
    1. Nerve infarction (diabetes, hypertension, arteritis)
    2. Migraine

III. Causes of trochlear nerve (CN IV) palsies
  A. Nuclear and fascicular
    1. Developmental anomalies
    2. Hemorrhage
    3. Infarction
    4. Trauma
    5. Demyelination
    6. Surgical complications
  B. Subarachnoid
    1. Trauma
    2. Tumor (pineal, tentorial meningioma, trochlear schwannoma, ependymoma, metastases)
    3. Surgical complication
    4. Meningitis (infectious, neoplastic)
    5. Mastoiditis
  C. Cavernous sinus and superior orbital fissure
    1. As for CN VI palsies
  D. Orbital
    1. Trauma
    2. Ethmoiditis
    3. Ethmoidectomy
  E. Uncertain localization
    1. Infarction (diabetes, hypertension, arteritis)

IV. Causes of oculomotor nerve (CN III) palsies
  A. Nuclear and fascicular
    1. Developmental anomaly
    2. Infarction
    3. Tumor
  B. Subarachnoid
    1. Aneurysm (posterior communicating artery)
    2. Meningitis (infectious, syphilitic, neoplastic)
    3. Infarction
    4. Tumor
    5. Surgical complication

C. Tentorial edge
1. Increased intracranial pressure (uncal herniation, idiopathic intracranial hypertension)
2. Trauma
D. Cavernous sinus and superior orbital fissure
1. As for CN IV and VI palsies
2. Infarction
E. Orbital
1. Trauma
2. Tumor
3. Infection
F. Uncertain localization
1. Mononucleosis and other viral infections
2. Following immunization
3. Migraine
4. Cyclic oculomotor palsy of childhood
5. Guillain-Barré and Miller-Fisher syndromes
6. Sjögren and Behçet syndromes

Combined ophthalmoparesis (third, fourth, and sixth cranial nerve involvement) most commonly occurs with base of skull infiltrations, cavernous sinus or superior orbital fissure lesions, and generalized neuropathies. Proptosis, chemosis, and vascular engorgement suggest orbital or cavernous sinus involvement. Base of skull problems include extension of nasopharyngeal carcinoma, sarcoidosis, lymphoma, clivus chordoma, pituitary apoplexy, meningeal carcinoma, and cavernous sinus thrombosis.

CPEO is a slowly progressive, painless, symmetrical ophthalmoplegia, without fluctuations or remissions. Saccades are slow, usually with no diplopia. Ptosis and orbicularis oculi weakness usually accompany the external ophthalmoplegia. The pupils are spared, and there are no orbital signs. Fibrotic changes of the extraocular muscles may occur over time, causing a superimposed restrictive ophthalmopathy. CPEO has multiple causes. Mitochondrial cytopathy (*Kearns-Sayre* syndrome) is one cause. Painful ophthalmoplegias may be due to diabetes, aneurysm, tumors (primary and metastatic), *Tolosa-Hunt* syndrome (granulomatous inflammatory process affecting the cavernous sinus and surrounding structures), herpes zoster, cavernous sinus thrombosis, carotid cavernous fistula, ophthalmoplegic migraine, arteritis, carcinomatous meningitis, or fungal infection.

INO is characterized by (1) slow, incomplete adduction of the eye or complete inability to adduct past midline (convergence movements may be preserved) and (2) dissociated nystagmus of the opposite abducting eye. Skew deviation (hypertropia on the lesion site) is often present. INO is caused by a lesion of the medial longitudinal fasciculus (MLF) between mid-pons and the oculomotor nucleus ipsilateral to the side of impaired adduction. Subtle defects are best solicited by observing the fast phases of optokinetic nystagmus. In bilateral INOs, gaze-evoked vertical nystagmus, impaired vertical pursuit, and decreased vertical vestibular responses are often present. The most frequent cause of INO in young adults (especially when bilateral) is multiple sclerosis. Vascular causes are more common in older patients. Other causes include intra- or extra-axial brainstem tumors, hydrocephalus, subdural hematoma, infection, nutritional and metabolic disorders, and drug intoxication. Myasthenia gravis and Miller-Fisher syndrome could cause similar appearing "pseudo-INO."

One-and-a-half syndrome refers to ipsilateral horizontal gaze palsy and INO (see Gaze palsy). This results from combined lesions of the MLF and the more ventral, ipsilateral abducens nucleus or paramedian pontine reticular formation (PPRF). The only intact horizontal movement is abduction of the contralateral eye. Acutely, the patient may appear exotropic, with nystagmus in the deviated eye. Vergence and vertical movements may be spared. Causes include brainstem ischemia (most common), multiple sclerosis, tumor, or hemorrhage. As with INO, myasthenia must be considered if there are no long tract or sensory signs. There is also a vertical one-and-a-half syndrome due to a dorsal midbrain lesion.

REFERENCES

Leigh, J. R., & Zee, D. (Eds.). (2006). *The neurology of eye movements*, ed 4. New York: Oxford University Press.

Şahlı, E., & Gündüz, K. (2017). Thyroid-associated ophthalmopathy. *Turk J Ophthalmol*, *47*(2), 94–105.

OPTIC NERVE

The optic nerve (CN II) forms from the axons of the corresponding ipsilateral retinal ganglion cells and transmits visual information posteriorly to the optic chiasm. Anatomically, the optic nerve has four major portions: (1) intraocular (1 mm); (2) intraorbital (~25 mm); (3) intracanalicular (~9 mm); and (4) intracranial (~16 mm). As each optic nerve contains information from the ipsilateral retina, an optic nerve lesion will produce a visual field defect referable to the retinal field of the affected eye.

The symptoms of optic nerve dysfunction may include blurry vision, a decreased sense of brightness, and color desaturation in the affected eye. Eye pain or headache may occur, depending on the cause.

The signs of optic nerve dysfunction include diminished visual acuity, color desaturation, and characteristic visual field defects—central, centrocecal, arcuate, or altitudinal scotomas. An afferent pupillary defect may be observed. This is demonstrated by the "swinging flashlight test," in which a light source is moved from one eye to the other, and the direct and consensual light responses on each side are observed. With a damaged optic nerve, the direct pupillary light response on the dysfunctional side will be abnormal owing to an impaired afferent limb (CN II), but the indirect response will remain intact. Consequently, swinging the light source from the affected eye to the normal eye will produce bilateral pupillary constriction as expected, but when swinging the light source from the normal eye to the affected eye, one will observe paradoxic bilateral pupillary dilation despite the presence of the light.

Funduscopic examination may reveal findings that may be helpful in diagnosing the optic nerve dysfunction, including papilledema, papillitis, or optic atrophy:

I. Papilledema is disk swelling caused by increased intracranial pressure (ICP). The ICP is transmitted to the optic nerve, causing stasis of axoplasmic transport resulting in intra-axonal edema. Initially, disk hyperemia and slightly blurred disk margins may be seen, as well as absent venous pulsations. This may develop into a grossly elevated optic disk with obliterated disk margins, venous congestion, peripapillary hemorrhages, exudates, and cotton-wool spots. Over months, the swelling resolves and the disk becomes gray or pale, representing optic atrophy. Papilledema is usually bilateral. However, unilateral papilledema may be seen with some subfrontal masses such as meningioma in the Foster-Kennedy syndrome of anosmia, unilateral optic atrophy, and contralateral papilledema. Papilledema may not be seen acutely, as it takes hours to days to develop. Furthermore, vision is usually not affected in the acute setting of papilledema, unless the inciting factor is directly injuring the optic nerve. A characteristic enlargement of the blind spot may occur in chronic elevated ICP. There may also be a constriction of visual fields due to selective involvement of damage to axons involving peripheral vision. Arcuate defects may be due to specific nerve fiber infarcts related to elevated ICP.

II. Papillitis refers to infarction or inflammation of the most anterior region of the optic nerve. The differential diagnosis includes demyelinating disease, ischemia from branch or complete retinal artery occlusion, giant cell arteritis, syphilis, Lyme disease, systemic lupus erythematosus (SLE), and sarcoidosis.

III. Retrobulbar neuritis affects the intraorbital portion of the optic nerve and is usually the result of demyelinating disease. Idiopathic causes are more common here than in papillitis. The disk usually appears normal in the acute setting. Rapid loss of vision and pain on movement of the affected eye are typical in this case.

IV. Optic atrophy is a chronic finding seen in diseases that damage the axons of the optic nerve. Funduscopy shows that the optic disk appears pale. Atrophy may include part of or the entire disk, depending on the cause. The differential diagnosis may include anterior ischemic optic

O

OPTIC NERVE

neuropathy (AION), nonischemic optic neuropathy, optic neuritis, trauma, and other inflammatory disorders (sarcoidosis, SLE, Lyme disease).

V. Optic neuritis is inflammation of the optic nerve. In two thirds of the patients, the site of inflammation is retrobulbar. It is most common between 15 and 45 years of age, is seen more commonly in women, and presents as an acute unilateral visual loss, with increased periorbital pain with eye movement. Disk swelling occurs in 50% of affected adults. Visual acuity usually returns to near normal levels within several months. Most cases are idiopathic or associated with multiple sclerosis. About 30% of patients with an episode of idiopathic optic neuritis will be diagnosed with multiple sclerosis within 5 years, and 50% in 15 years. The risk for neuromyelitis optica is unclear, but can be suggested by more severe, recurrent, and bilateral attacks of optic neuritis. Other causes of optic neuritis include viral or postviral syndromes, sinusitis or meningitis, sarcoidosis, tuberculosis, syphilis, and paraneoplastic disease.

Treatment: One protocol that was successfully used in the Optic Neuritis Treatment Trial (ONTT) and was shown to hasten recovery in young patients (ages 18 to 46 years) with acute optic neuritis is the following: intravenous (IV) methylprednisolone 1000 mg per day for 3 days, followed by oral prednisone dosed at 1 mg/kg for 11 days. The risk of recurrent episodes of optic neuritis was lower in these patients than for patients treated with oral prednisone alone, but the long-term (5-year) risk of developing multiple sclerosis was not significantly different between the groups.

VI. AION is caused by infarction of the optic nerve. AION usually presents as acute unilateral visual loss and is painless in about 90% of cases. It usually affects the papillae region, but the retrobulbar region is rarely affected. AION occurs more frequently in the elderly than optic neuritis. The recovery of vision is usually poor. Funduscopic examination may reveal disk swelling and pallor.

Treatment: The common "idiopathic" form is associated with hypertension and diabetes mellitus, a normal erythrocyte sedimentation rate (ESR), and steroid unresponsiveness. The rarer "arteritic" form is related to giant cell arteritis. Symptoms include headaches, weight loss, fever, arthralgias, myalgias, jaw claudication, scalp tenderness, an elevated ESR, and steroid responsiveness.

VII. Toxic, nutritional, neoplastic, and infectious optic neuropathies present as painless, slowly progressive bilateral visual deficits. They are usually retrobulbar. Pallor is more often in the temporal quadrant. Causes include drugs (e.g., ethambutol, isoniazid, chloramphenicol, and streptomycin), toxins (lead and methanol), and vitamin deficiencies (vitamin B_{12}, thiamine, niacin, and riboflavin). A tobacco-alcohol amblyopia is seen with heavy tobacco and alcohol abusers (thought to be nutritional). Optic neuropathy may be caused by tumors such as a compressive meningioma or astrocytoma, a primary optic nerve tumor (optic nerve gliomas, schwannomas), infiltrative tumors (such as lymphomas, plasmacytomas, histiocytomas), or carcinomatous meningitis. Other forms are radiation induced (may be delayed for years), infectious (Lyme disease, syphilis, and fungal infection), inflammatory (SLE, vasculitis, and sarcoidosis), or hereditary (Leber's hereditary optic neuropathy, mitochondrial mutation). Trauma may also lead to optic atrophy.

REFERENCES

Bradley, W. G., Daroff, R. B., Fenichel, G. M., & Jankovic, J. (Eds.). (2004). *Neurology in clinical practice,* ed 4. Boston: Butterworth-Heinemann.
Pirko, I., Blauwet, L. A., Lesnick, T. G., et al. (2004). The natural history of recurrent optic neuritis. *Arch Neurol, 61*(9), 1401.

OPTOKINETIC NYSTAGMUS

The optokinetic system is an oculomotor subsystem that enhances the ability to stabilize images on the retina when the head remains stationary, thus enhancing visual acuity. When the head moves for an extended period, the vestibular response diminishes due to the mechanical properties of the labyrinthine sense organs. Only retinal information remains, thus producing the input resulting in compensatory eye movements. Optokinetic nystagmus (OKN) is the term given to the involuntary eye movement in which a moving visual field produces rhythmic oscillation of the eye.

OKN is generated when the appropriate conditions are reproduced in the laboratory through the motion of the entire visual environment. This phenomenon consists of slow components of nystagmus that match the rapidity of the eye's movement with the speed of movement of the visual environment.

At bedside, a true optokinetic stimulus is generally impossible. Stimulation using handheld moving stripes induces nystagmus, which reveals the smooth-pursuit eye movement function (slow components) and the saccadic system integrity (fast components). Saccades are rapid eye movements in which the gaze is shifted to direct the fovea toward objects of visual interest to allow exploration of the visual world.

An alternative technique for examination is the use of the optokinetic drum, which allows the combined testing of smooth pursuit movements and saccades in both horizontal and vertical directions. This technique is effective with uncooperative or drowsy patients or children.

During the diagnostic procedure, the examiner evaluates for the presence of the components of nystagmus and symmetry in both the horizontal and vertical directions. The presence of these components indicates the unhindered function of the midbrain and the pons. Some clinical conditions become very apparent through the observation of the bedside OKN response:

I. The presence of optokinetic nystagmus proves that visual function is at least partially intact and is effective in examining infants and in patients with suspected psychogenic blindness or complex visual impairment (parietal and occipital lesions).

II. Frontal lobe lesions often produce abnormalities in the saccades while sparing pursuit. The eyes tonically deviate in the direction of the moving target, and the fast phases may be absent or impaired when the target moves toward the side of the lesion. Progressive supranuclear palsy causes an early loss of OKN quick phases that manifest into saccadic gaze palsies. Typically, excessive square wave jerks are present, and the slowing of both upward and downward saccades is common.

III. Deep parietal lesions may impair pursuit toward the side of the lesion, causing an abnormal slow component of OKN when the target moves toward the side of the lesion. There may be an amplitude asymmetry between the two directions.

IV. Extensive hemispheric lesions may impair both pursuit and saccades. Movement of the target toward the side of the lesion may produce deficits in both slow and fast components.

V. In occipital or temporal lesions OKN response is asymmetrical; deep parietal involvement is probable.

VI. Moving the OKN target away from the field of action of an individual eye muscle prompts saccades in the appropriate direction and may help define a muscle paresis. Evaluate for differences between paired muscles. For example, compare the left lateral rectus and the right medial rectus. In this case, the paretic eye moves more slowly than the other.

VII. Internuclear ophthalmoplegia may be demonstrated by horizontal movement of the target, resulting in dysconjugate saccades when fast components of OKN require action of the affected medial rectus muscle.

VIII. Downward movement of the OKN target may help demonstrate convergence retraction nystagmus (see Nystagmus).

IX. Congenital nystagmus may be accompanied by OKN, in which the fast components are in the direction of target's movement.

REFERENCES

Leigh, J. R., & Zee, D. (Eds.). (2015). *The neurology of eye movements*, ed 5. New York: Oxford University.

Lloyd-Smith Sequeira, A., Rizzo, J.-R., & Rucker, J. C. (2017). Clinical approach to supranuclear brainstem saccadic gaze palsies. *Front Neurol*, *8*, 429. https://doi.org/10.3389/fneur.2017.0042.

P

DEFINITION AND EPIDEMIOLOGY

Paget disease of the bone, also known as osteitis deformans, is the most common bone disorder after osteoporosis. It affects about 3% of the population in the United States, has no gender preference, and increases in incidence after age 50.

PATHOPHYSIOLOGY

Abnormal osteoclastic, and later osteoblastic, activity results in sclerotic, trabecular bone remodeling, which weakens the skeleton, most commonly in axial locations. Etiology may be related to stimulation of the immune system via viral antigens, particularly measles, but family history is also present 40% of the time, suggesting a possible genetic predisposition. A genetic mutation in the valosin containing protein (VCP) or RIN3 gene combines Paget disease, frontotemporal dementia and familial inclusion body myositis.

CLINICAL PRESENTATION

Because pain is usually a late complication, many people, perhaps as many as 70%, may be asymptomatic. Primary bone pain is described as dull, deep, and predominantly nocturnal. Pain secondary to complications is more frequent than primary pain, especially due to the neurological entrapment or joint deformities. Bone pain typically increases with rest and weight bearing, as well as with limb warming and at night. The neurologic complications are usually the result of osseous overgrowth causing nerve compression, resulting in deafness, radiculopathy, and spinal stenosis, as well as cranial neuropathy and brainstem compression. Neurological symptoms may also be related to a vascular steal syndrome. These are overshadowed, however, by the potential for malignant transformation to osteosarcoma and high-output cardiac heart failure due to hypervascularization of the bone marrow.

EVALUATION

X-ray findings are specific, showing early lytic or late sclerotic changes, but are not very sensitive. Bone scans can increase sensitivity but are less specific. Biochemical markers, including bone-specific alkaline phosphatase and urinary pyridinoline, have replaced urinary hydroxyproline as a more accurate marker of disease activity and severity.

TREATMENT

Bisphosphonates or, less commonly, calcitonin is typically started on symptomatic patients, asymptomatic patients with involvement of weight-bearing regions, or when serum alkaline phosphatase levels rise above 125%

of normal. Pain usually responds to nonsteroidal anti-inflammatory medications. Suspicion of osteosarcoma requires oncology consultation.

REFERENCE

Alonso, N., Calero-Paniagua, I., & Del Pino-Montes, J. (2017). Clinical and genetic advances in Paget's disease of bone: a review. *Clin Rev Bone Miner Metab, 15,* 37–48. https://doi.org/10.1007/s12018-016-9226-0.

PAIN

Pain is the most common reason Americans seek medical care. The International Association for the Study of Pain has defined pain as "an unpleasant sensory and emotional experience associated with actual or potential tissue damage, or described in terms of tissue damage, or both." The pain experienced by a patient is dependent upon not only any physical source of pain, but also on the patient's physiological and psychological milieu.

There are neural mechanisms that modify the transmission of pain and the emotional reaction to it.

Pain can be nociceptive or neuropathic. The sensation of nociceptive pain is produced physiologically, generated by the stimulation of peripheral nociceptors or afferent nerve fibers in response to a noxious stimulus. An example would be the pain felt in a tissue injury. Neuropathic pain arises from a lesion or dysfunction of neural structures, such as the burning one feels in diabetic polyneuropathy.

Physiologic pain sensations are carried by multiple anatomical pathways. The spinothalamic tract is a major pain pathway: cutaneous afferent nociceptive fibers enter the dorsal horn of the spinal cord, where they may ascend or descend one to two segments as Lissauer tract. Primary afferents terminate in the superficial layers of the dorsal horn in an area known as the substantia gelatinosa. Second-order neurons decussate and ascend rostrally as the lateral and anterior spinothalamic tracts. The spinothalamic tract projects to the ventral posterolateral nucleus of the thalamus, which then sends its projections to other diencephalic structures, the brainstem reticular activating system, the limbic system, and the primary somatosensory cortex. In addition to the ascending pain system, there is a descending modulation system with origins in the brainstem periaqueductal gray and projections to the raphe nucleus. Projections from the raphe nucleus project directly to the ventral and dorsal horns of the spinal cord, including the substantia gelatinosa, and act to inhibit nociception. Serotonin is the main transmitter in this system. The locus ceruleus also acts as a descending modulating system, using norepinephrine as its transmitter. Prominent within the pain-modulating systems are the opiate receptor system and endogenous opioid peptides, which exist throughout the nervous system, particularly in the periaqueductal gray and raphe nucleus.

Acute pain follows an injury and generally resolves with healing. It has a well-defined temporal onset and is often associated with objective physical signs of autonomic activity such as tachycardia, hypertension, and diaphoresis.

Chronic pain persists beyond expected healing time and often cannot be related to a specific injury. It may not have a well-defined onset, may not respond to treatments aimed at the presumed origin or cause, and may not be associated with signs of autonomic activity; the patients do not "look" like they are in pain.

Complex regional pain syndrome (CRPS) and phantom limb pain are unique chronic pain syndromes. CRPS is characterized by burning pain, hyperesthesia, swelling, hyperhidrosis, and trophic skin and bone changes. It is treated with sympathetic denervation and aggressive physical therapy. (For more information, refer to the chapter on "Complex Regional Pain Syndrome.") Phantom limb pain differs from the usual nonpainful sensory illusion that the lost limb is still present. Phantom limb pain is refractory to most treatments. Many treatments have been suggested, including mirror therapy and local anesthetic injections, but to date there is insufficient evidence to support any treatment as first line.

Chronic (noncancer) pain requires an integrated multidisciplinary approach directed at both physical and psychological rehabilitation. The goal is to control the factors that increase pain. All therapies, especially drugs, should be given on a time-contingent basis, not as necessary (prn). The patient thus is not rewarded for having pain by getting medication. This approach serves to reduce the total amount of drug required daily. Each drug must be given an adequate trial. Start with simple analgesics, increase the dose or frequency before changing drugs, and when changing, use equianalgesic doses. Avoid excessive sedation.

Pharmacologic management of pain utilizes treatment directed at specific sites along the pain pathways. Peripherally, aspirin and nonsteroidal anti-inflammatory agents produce analgesia by preventing the formation of prostaglandin from arachidonic acid metabolism (inhibition of cyclooxygenase). Prostaglandin sensitizes tissues to the pain-producing effects of bradykinin and other substances resulting from tissue injury. These medications are effective in treatment of mild to moderate pain, especially bone pain. These substances also potentiate the effects of narcotic analgesics. Capsaicin, a derivative of hot peppers, acts by depleting nociceptors of substance P, rendering the skin insensitive to pain. A treatment trial requires 2 to 4 weeks of daily topical application, three to four times per day, to the affected area.

Tricyclic antidepressants (TCAs) act via influencing the biogenic amine system, affecting levels of serotonin, norepinephrine, and dopamine. Patients with pain are often locked into a pain-depression-insomnia cycle, and TCAs can affect each of these aspects of pain. The TCAs are effective in a variety of chronic pain conditions, including chronic low back pain, headache, neuropathy, and neuralgias. Anticonvulsants act to suppress spontaneous neuronal firing. They are useful in the management of chronic pain states such as trigeminal neuralgia, postherpetic neuralgia, diabetic neuropathy, and postamputation pain. Venlafaxine, which increases levels of both serotonin and norepinephrine, is emerging as a relatively nonsedating but effective medication for treating neuropathic pain.

Narcotic analgesics are used to treat severe, acute pain and chronic pain. When using narcotics, start with the lowest dose needed to obtain analgesia and titrate to pain relief or to the appearance of unacceptable side effects. Whereas prn dosing for several days allows for the determination of total daily dose, thereafter narcotic analgesics are given on a fixed dosing schedule. Add non-narcotic drugs to increase analgesia. Tolerance to narcotics usually becomes evident as a reduction in duration of analgesia and the need for higher doses. Treat this situation by increasing the dose or by using an alternative drug (start with one half of the equianalgesic dose). The narcotic conversion nomograms can guide conversion between narcotics (Figs. 45 and 46). For example, 30 mg of oral methadone is equivalent to approximately 20 mg of parenteral morphine. Physical dependence occurs if the patient receives prolonged therapy in high doses, and patients experience withdrawal symptoms with abrupt narcotic

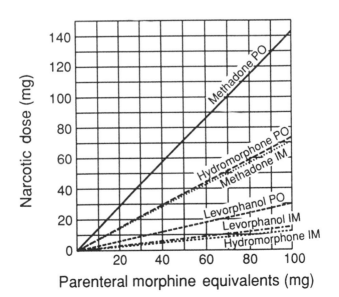

FIGURE 45

Narcotic conversion nomogram: high-potency narcotics. (From Grossman, S. A., & Sheidler, V. R. (1987). An aid to prescribing narcotics for relief of cancer pain. *World Health Forum*, 8(4), 525–529.)

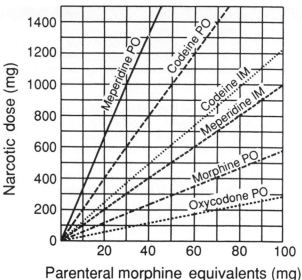

FIGURE 46

Narcotic conversion nomogram: low-potency narcotics. (From Grossman, S. A., & Sheidler, V. R. (1987). An aid to prescribing narcotics for relief of cancer pain. *World Health Forum, 8*(4), 525–529.)

cessation. Physical dependence is not to be confused with psychological dependence, which is a behavioral syndrome of drug craving.

Other pharmacologic interventions include the use of corticosteroids in the treatment of cancer, especially when cancer is due to bony metastasis; neuroleptics, venlafaxine, or gabapentin in dysesthetic pain; and dextroamphetamine for potentiating narcotic analgesia and reducing narcotic-induced sedation. Antihistamines (hydroxyzine) and neuroleptics can also be used to decrease nausea associated with narcotic use.

Other treatment modalities used in pain management include trigger-point injections; epidural, intrathecal, and sympathetic blockade; ganglionolysis; cordotomy; transcutaneous and percutaneous electrical stimulation; dorsal column stimulation; and relaxation techniques, including biofeedback and hypnosis.

REFERENCES

Richardson, C., & Kulkarni, J. (2017). A review of the management of phantom limb pain: challenges and solutions. *J Pain Res, 10*, 1861–1870.

Vanderah, T., & Gould, D. (2016). *Nolte's the human brain: an introduction to its functional anatomy*, ed 7. Philadelphia: Elsevier.

PARANEOPLASTIC NEUROLOGIC SYNDROMES

Paraneoplastic neurologic syndromes (PNS) are autoimmune, remote effects of cancer that are not caused by metastatic complications of a systemic cancer. Autoantibodies have been identified in several types of PNS and are summarized in Table 103. Less than 60% of PNS are associated with anti-neuronal antibodies, and neurologic symptoms precede the identification of cancer in only 50% of cases.

Clinical features that suggest PNS include (1) subacute onset; (2) severe neurologic disability; (3) inflammatory cerebrospinal fluid (CSF) with increased cells, elevated protein, and oligoclonal bands; (4) clinical syndrome that predominantly affects one specific portion of the nervous system; and (5) stereotypical presentation.

There are two main groups: (1) "classic" PNS, in which antibodies when detected almost always indicate that the disorder is paraneoplastic, T-cell mediated with no direct pathologic role of the antibodies targeting intracellular epitopes that are also expressed by the cancer (Lambert-Eaton myasthenic syndrome [LEMS], subacute cerebellar degeneration [SACD], opsoclonus/myoclonus in children), and (2) PNS that can be associated with cancer or appear in the absence of a neoplasm with cell dysfunction directly mediated by antibodies directed at cell surface/synapse epitopes (limbic encephalitis, polymyositis, polyneuropathy). The presence of autoantibodies helps confirm the clinical diagnosis and focuses the search for an underlying malignancy. The mainstays of PNS treatment are immunotherapy and direct tumor therapy. PNS associated with antibodies, directed at intracellular antigens (onconeuronal antibodies), generally respond poorly to treatment; early treatment offers the best chance of recovery. On the contrary, PNS associated with antibodies targeting surface antigens are usually highly responsive to treatments.

PNS includes the following:
I. Brain and cranial nerves: SACD, opsoclonus-myoclonus, limbic encephalitis and other autoimmune encephalitis, paraneoplastic cerebellar degeneration, optic neuritis, photoreceptor degeneration;
II. Spinal cord and dorsal root ganglia: myelitis, necrotizing myelopathy, sensory neuronopathy, subacute motor neuronopathy, motor neuron disease;
III. Peripheral nerves: subacute or chronic sensorimotor peripheral neuropathy, acute inflammatory demyelinating neuropathy, mononeuritis multiplex and vasculitic neuropathy, brachial neuritis, autonomic neuropathy, peripheral neuropathy with islet-cell tumors or paraproteinemias;
IV. Neuromuscular junction and muscle: LEMS, myasthenia gravis, dermatomyositis or polymyositis, acute necrotizing myopathy, carcinoid myopathy, myotonia, cachectic myopathy, neuromyopathy;
V. Multiple levels of central and peripheral nervous system or unknown site: encephalomyelitis, neuromyopathy, stiff-person syndrome.

TABLE 103

ANTINEURONAL ANTIBODY-ASSOCIATED PARANEOPLASTIC SYNDROMES

Antibody	Associated Cancer	Syndrome
Anti-Hu (ANNA-1)	SCLC, neuroblastoma	Encephalomyelitis, sensory neuronopathy
Anti-Yo (PCA-1)	Gynecologic, breast	Cerebellar degeneration
Anti-Ri (ANNA-2)	Breast, gynecologic, SCLC	Cerebellar ataxia, opsoclonus
Anti-amphiphysin	Breast	Stiff-person, encephalomyelitis
Anti-VGCC	SCLC	LEMS
Anti-MYsB	SCLC	LEMS
Anti-Ma	Multiple	Cerebellar, brainstem dysfunction
Anti-Ta	Testicular	Limbic encephalitis, brainstem dysfunction
Anti-Tr	Hodgkin lymphoma	Cerebellar degeneration
Anti-CAR	SCLC, others	Photoreceptor degeneration
Anti-CV2/CRMP5	SCLC, others	Encephalomyelitis, cerebellar degeneration
Anti-NMDAR	Ovarian teratoma	Anti-NMDAR encephalitis
Anti-GAD	Neuroendocrine, thymoma, small cell lung carcinoma	Limbic encephalitis, cerebellar ataxia, stiff-person syndrome
Anti-AMPAR	Lung, breast, thymus	Limbic encephalitis
Anti-LGI1	Usually none	Faciobrachial dystonic seizures, myoclonus, encephalitis
Anti-Caspr2	Thymoma	Neuromyotonia, encephalitis, or Morvan syndrome
Anti-mGluR5	Hodgkin lymphoma	Ophelia syndrome
Anti-α-GlyR	Hodgkin lymphoma	Stiff-person syndrome, progressive encephalomyelitis with rigidity and myoclonus
Anti-AchR	Thymoma	Myasthenia gravis
Anti-GABA-A	Hodgkin lymphoma	Refractory status epilepticus or epilepsia partialis continua

AchR, acetylcholine receptor; *ANNA-1*, antineuronal nuclear antibody type 1; *ANNA-2*, antineuronal nuclear antibody type 2; *Caspr2*, contactin-associated protein-like 2; *CRMP-5*, collapsin response mediator protein-5; *DNER*, delta/notch-like epidermal growth factor-related receptor; *GABA*, gamma aminobutyric acid A; *GAD*, glutamic acid decarboxylase; *GlyR*, glycine receptor; *LEMS*, Lambert-Eaton myasthenic syndrome; *LGI1*, leucine-rich glioma-inactivated 1; *mGluR5*, metabotropic glutamate receptor 5; *NMDAR*, anti-N-methyl-D-aspartate receptor; *PCA-1*, Purkinje cell antibody-1; *PCA-2*, Purkinje cell antibody-2; *SCLC*, small cell lung cancer; *VGCC*, voltage-gated calcium channels.

P

PARANEOPLASTIC NEUROLOGIC SYNDROMES

REFERENCES

Cui, D., Xu, L., Li, W. Y., & Qian, W. D. (2017). Anti-Yo positive and late-onset paraneoplastic cerebellar degeneration associated with ovarian carcinoma: a case report. *Medicine (Baltimore)*, 96(32), e7362.

Lancaster, E. (2015). Paraneoplastic disorders. *Continuum (Minneap Minn)*, 21(2), 453–475.

PARIETAL LOBE

The parietal lobe is located posterior to the central sulcus, superior to the sylvian fissure, and anterior to the parieto-occipital sulcus on the medial surface. The parietal lobe functions primarily in sensory integration of visual, auditory, and somatosensory inputs.

It contains two major sulci: the postcentral sulcus, which marks the posterior boundary of the somatosensory cortex, and the intraparietal sulcus. Extending from the postcentral sulcus dorsally, the intraparietal sulcus separates the parietal cortex into superior (Brodmann area 5 and 7) and inferior parietal lobules, the latter of which contains the supramarginal (Brodmann area 40), and angular gyri (Brodmann area 39) as well as Wernicke area (Brodmann area 22) in the dominant hemisphere.

The postcentral gyrus serves as the primary somatosensory cortex receiving input from the ventral posterior thalamic nucleus and projects to the somatosensory association cortex located in superior parietal lobule (Brodmann area 5).

CLINICAL PRESENTATION OF PARIETAL LOBE LESIONS

Unilateral parietal lesion can cause:

- Corticosensory syndromes such as astereognosis and agraphesthesia, sensory extinction, neglect (more commonly seen with right parietal lobe lesions)
- Homonymous hemianopia or inferior quadrantanopia

Dominant (usually left) parietal lesion may also cause:

- Alexia, apraxia
- Gerstmann syndrome: dysgraphia, dyscalculia, finger agnosia, right-left confusion

Bilateral parietal lesions cause Balint syndrome, which is characterized by simultanagnosia (inability to perceive more than one object at a time), optic apraxia (difficulty with directing gaze), and optic ataxia.

REFERENCE

Ropper, A. H., Samuels, M. A., & Klein, J. P. (2014). Neurologic disorders caused by lesions in specific parts of the cerebrum. In A. H. Ropper, M. A. Samuels, & J. P. Klein (Eds.), *Adam and Victor's principles of neurology*, ed 10 (pp 455–485). China: McGraw-Hill Education.

PARKINSON DISEASE

PRESENTATION/DIAGNOSIS

Parkinson disease (PD) very rarely occurs before age 30. Symptoms are usually gradual and progressive and include motor and nonmotor symptoms. The nonmotor symptoms include cognitive changes, behavioral/neuropsychiatric changes, and symptoms related to autonomic nervous system dysfunction.

The cardinal symptoms of PD can be remembered using the mnemonic TRAP:

- **T**remor at rest (4 to 6 Hz, typically pill-rolling of the hands)
- **R**igidity (cogwheel or lead pipe)
- **A**kinesia/Bradykinesia (slowness, difficulty initiating or fatiguing of movement)
- **P**ostural instability (stooped posture/shuffling gait accompanied by poor or absent arm swing)

Symptoms are often asymmetric, and may begin unilaterally, eventually progressing to bilateral involvement. Resting tremor is the presenting symptom in over 70% of patients. Later in the disease course, patients will likely display postural instability.

Other motor symptoms include micrographia (small tapering writing), diminished facial expression (masked facies), hypophonia, stooped posture, shuffling gait accompanied by poor or absent arm swing, and diminished blink rate.

A prodrome of non-motor features may precede motor symptoms of PD by many years. These include: constipation, hyposmia (altered sense of smell), REM-sleep behavior disorder, restless leg syndrome, periodic limb movements of sleep, autonomic dysfunction (e.g., orthostasis and hyperhidrosis, erectile dysfunction), neurobehavioral disorders (depression, anxiety), and urinary urge incontinence.

Differential diagnosis is challenging, given the fact that the classic PD symptoms may be present in other neurodegenerative disorders. Careful history-taking and astute physical assessment coupled with initial medical therapy are necessary to distinguish idiopathic PD from essential tremor, dementia with Lewy bodies, corticobasal degeneration, multiple system atrophy, progressive supranuclear palsy, or secondary parkinsonism (see Parkinsonism chapter).

Neurological imaging may help distinguish PD from vascular parkinsonism, essential tremor, multiple system atrophy (MSA), and progressive supranuclear palsy (PSP) but there are no pathognomonic radiographic findings to identify idiopathic PD itself.

Diagnostic criteria have been adopted by the Movement Disorders Society to determine if a patient has "clinically established PD" or "clinically probable PD." A required feature for either diagnosis is the presence of parkinsonism, defined as bradykinesia plus either tremor or rigidity.

Absolute exclusion criteria include: Unequivocal cerebellar abnormalities; downward vertical gaze palsy; diagnosis of probable frontotemporal dementia or primary progressive aphasia within the first 5 years of disease; parkinsonian features restricted to the lower limbs for more than 3 years; history of medication use consistent with drug-induced parkinsonism; absence of observable response to high-dose levodopa despite at least moderate severity of disease; cortical sensory loss; normal functional neuroimaging of the presynaptic dopaminergic system; presence of an alternative condition likely to produce the patient's symptoms. If any of these are present, neither "clinically established PD" nor "clinically probable PD" can be diagnosed.

The criteria have also established a set of 10 "red flags" which suggest that the patient may not have PD but are not absolute exclusions. These include: wheelchair dependence within 5 years of onset; complete absence of progression of motor findings over 5 years (unless this can be attributed to treatment); early bulbar dysfunction; inspiratory respiratory dysfunction; severe autonomic failure in the first 5 years; recurrent falls because of impaired balance within 3 years of onset; disproportionate anterocollis or contractures within the first 10 years; absence of any common non-motor features of disease despite 5 years' disease duration; unexplained pyramidal tract signs; bilateral symmetric parkinsonism. If there are more than 2 red flags, neither "clinically established PD" nor "clinically probable PD" can be diagnosed.

Criteria that support the diagnosis include: Clear and dramatic beneficial response to dopaminergic therapy; presence of levodopa-induced dyskinesia; rest tremor of a limb; the presence of either olfactory loss or cardiac sympathetic denervation on metaiodobenzylguanidine (MIBG) scintigraphy.

If the patient has parkinsonism, has no absolute exclusion criteria, has no red flags, and has at least 2 supportive criteria, then the diagnosis of clinically established PD can be made.

If the patient has parkinsonism, has no absolute exclusion criteria, has 2 or fewer red flags, and the number of red flags is equal to or less than the number of supportive criteria, then the diagnosis of clinically probable PD can be made.

PATHOPHYSIOLOGY

The pathological definition of PD is loss or degeneration of the dopaminergic (dopamine-producing) neurons in the substantia nigra and development of Lewy bodies (a pathologic hallmark) in dopaminergic neurons. Accordingly, dopamine replenishment therapy dominates the therapeutic strategies available for PD patients.

TREATMENT/MANAGEMENT

There is no cure for PD, and there is no treatment that can slow or reverse its progress. The central objective for the use of medications in PD is management of the symptoms, both motor and non-motor. All anti-PD medications ameliorate symptoms, rather than change the course of the disease. Thus, dosage and intervals should be titrated to the individual patient's symptomatic need. The following categories of medications are used to treat PD motor symptoms:

- Levodopa
- Dopamine agonists

- MAO-B inhibitors
- COMT-inhibitors
- Amantadine
- Anticholinergics

These medications, dosages, treatment regiments, indications, and side effects are discussed in detail in Table 104. Clinical management of PD is individually tailored to a patient's needs with the goal of minimizing "off-time" and extending "on-time." "Off-time" refers to periods of the day when the medication is not working well, causing worsening of symptoms, whereas "on-time" refers to periods of adequate control of PD symptoms. The following are guidelines helpful in management:

- Initial Management
  a. If no functional impairment exists, consider disease monitoring and delaying onset of pharmacological management.
  b. Carbidopa/levodopa is used effectively as initial monotherapy for management of PD. Concomitant intake of large amino acid loads (protein load particularly in dairy products) will competitively inhibit the transport of levodopa into the brain. COMT-inhibitors extend the benefit of levodopa by reducing "off" symptoms between doses and reducing therapeutic dose beneficial for preventing the nausea that can be caused by levodopa alone.
  c. Dopamine agonists are used effectively as a monotherapy in early PD or in combination with carbidopa/levodopa for persistent symptoms. Use is complicated by side effects including compulsive, aggression, and hallucinations. Unadvised for use in the elderly.
  d. Anticholinergics agents are used in young people with tremor-predominant PD, though side effects may limit their usefulness. Unadvised for use in the elderly.
  e. MAO-B inhibitors used effectively for modest symptom control in early PD or in combination with other medications to reduce "off-time" and extend "on-time". Drug interactions of medication weaning limit effect utility.
- Regiment Modification
  a. Gradual decline in responsiveness to levodopa is inevitable. The appearance of motor fluctuations ("wearing-off") and involuntary movements (dyskinesia) prompts regiment modification.
  b. Declining responsiveness to medication initially managed by fractionating levodopa therapy by amount and timing of doses.
  c. *Increasing motor fluctuations* managed by decreasing levodopa therapy and substituting a controlled/slow release carbidopa/levodopa or additional MAO-I.
  d. *Diphasic dyskinesias* managed with increasing the dose of levodopa or switching to a dopamine agonist with a lower dose of levodopa.
  e. Amantadine is beneficial in PD patients with prominent tremor or bothersome levodopa-induced dyskinesia.

P

PARKINSON DISEASE

TABLE 104

MEDICATIONS FOR THE TREATMENT OF PARKINSON DISEASE

Medication	Dosages in Milligrams (mg)	Typical Treatment Regimens	Potential Side Effects	Indications for Usage
LEVODOPA				
Carbidopa/levodopa immediate-release (Sinemet)	10/100, 25/100, 25/250	150–1000 mg of levodopa total daily dose (divided 3–4 times)	Low blood pressure, nausea, confusion, dyskinesia	*Monotherapy or combination therapy* for slowness, stiffness, and tremor
Carbidopa/levodopa oral disintegrating (Parcopa)	10/100, 25/100, 25/250	150–1000 mg of levodopa total daily dose (divided 3–4 times)	Same as above	Same as above, plus need for dissolvable medication in mouth especially if swallowing is impaired
Carbidopa/levodopa extended-release (Sinemet CR)	25/100, 50/200	150–1000 mg of levodopa in divided doses, depending on daily need	Same as above	*Monotherapy or combination therapy* for slowness, stiffness, and tremor
Carbidopa/ levodopa/ entacapone (Stalevo) [see COMT-inhibitors below]	12.5/50/200, 18.75/75/ 200, 25/100/200, 31.25/125/200, 37.5/ 150/200, 50/200/200	150–1000 mg of levodopa total daily dose, depending on daily need	Same as above, plus diarrhea and discolored urine (due to entacapone)	*Replacement for carbidopa/ levodopa,* for motor fluctuations (benefit of entacapone)

Carbidopa/levodopa extended-release capsules (Rytary)	23.75/95, 36.25/145, 48.75/195, 61.25/245	285–2450 mg of levodopa total daily dose	Same as above	*Monotherapy or adjunct therapy* for slowness, stiffness, and tremor. **Note that dosages of Rytary are not interchangeable with other carbidopa/levodopa products.**
Carbidopa/levodopa enteral solution (duopa)	Clinician-determined	Up to 2000 mg of levodopa over 16 hours	Same as above	For the treatment of motor fluctuations in patients with advanced Parkinson disease
DOPAMINE AGONISTS				
Ropinirole (Requip)	0.25, 0.5, 1, 2, 3, 4, 5	9–24 mg total daily dose (divided 3–4 times)	Low blood pressure, nausea, leg swelling and discoloration, confusion, sleep attacks, compulsive behaviors, somnolence	*Monotherapy or combination therapy* for slowness, stiffness, and tremor. Effective in decreasing the required dose of L-dopa and delaying the adverse motor fluctuations
Ropinirole XL (Requip XL)	2, 4, 6, 8, 12,	8–24 mg once/day	Same as above	Same as above
Pramipexole (Mirapex)	0.125, 0.25, 0.5, 0.75, 1, 1.5	1.5–4.5 mg total daily dose (divided 3–4 times)	Same as above	Same as above
Pramipexole eR (Mirapex eR)	0.375, 0.75, 1.5, 2.25, 3, 3.75, 4.5	1.5–4.5 mg once/day	Same as above	Same as above

Continued

P

PARKINSON DISEASE

TABLE 104

MEDICATIONS FOR THE TREATMENT OF PARKINSON DISEASE—CONT'D

Medication	Dosages in Milligrams (mg)	Typical Treatment Regimens	Potential Side Effects	Indications for Usage
Rotigotine (Neupro)	1, 2, 3, 4, 6, 8 patch	4–8 mg once/day	Same as above	Same as above; patch delivery an advantage for some
Apomorphine (apokyn)	30 mg/3 mL vial	2–6 mg	Significant nausea; must take anti-nausea medication with dose, especially when starting therapy	*Adjunct therapy for sudden wearing off; the only injectable, fast-acting dopaminergic drug*
Bromocriptine (Parlodel)	—	—	Cognitive deficit and hallucination tendencies may be exacerbated, and adverse gastrointestinal symptoms and hypotension are not uncommon. Heart valve abnormalities in minority of patients	*The Food and Drug Administration determined that the risk outweighed the benefit, and removed it from the U.S. market for use in PD in March 200*
Pergolide (Permax)	—	—	Same as above	Same as above
MAO-B INHIBITORS				
Selegiline (l-deprenyl, eldepryl)	5	5 mg once or twice a day	Nausea, dry mouth, light-headedness, constipation; may worsen dyskinesia; possible rare interaction with antidepressants and other drug classes	*Monotherapy for slowness, stiffness, and tremor; adjunct therapy for motor fluctuations. Delay and decrease the need for L-dopa*

Rasagiline (azilect)	0.5, 1.0	1 mg once/day	Same as above	Same as above
Zydis selegiline HCL Oral disintegrating (Zelapar)	1.25, 2.5	1.25–2.5 mg once/day	Same as above	Same as above, plus need for dissolvable medication in mouth (absorbed in mouth)
COMT-INHIBITORS				
Entacapone (Comtan)	200	200 mg 4–8 times daily (with each levodopa dose)	Diarrhea, discolored urine, plus enhancing side effects of levodopa, especially dyskinesia confusion, liver failure	*Combination therapy with levodopa* for motor fluctuations. Recommended in advanced PD patients who require greater than 600 mg of L-dopa daily
Tolcapone (Tasmar)	100, 200	100 mg up to 3 times daily	Same as above plus increased risk of liver inflammation	Same as above (second-line due to side effects)
OTHER ANTIPARKINSON MEDICATIONS				
Amantadine (Symmetrel)	100 mg capsules; 50 mg/5 mL syrup	100 mg 2–3 times daily	Nausea, confusion, leg discoloration (livedo reticularis), mild anticholinergic effects (see below)	*Monotherapy* for slowness, stiffness, and tremor; *combination therapy* with levodopa for levodopa-induced motor fluctuations; especially helpful for suppressing dyskinesia

Continued

P

PARKINSON DISEASE

TABLE 104

MEDICATIONS FOR THE TREATMENT OF PARKINSON DISEASE—CONT'D

Medication	Dosages in Milligrams (mg)	Typical Treatment Regimens	Potential Side Effects	Indications for Usage
ANTICHOLINERGICS				
Trihexyphenidyl (formerly artane)	2, 5 mg tablets; 2 mg/5 mL elixir	1–2 mg 2 or 3 times daily—lowering doses (to bid, last dose before 3 PM) is recommended in the elderly	Confusion, memory issues, hallucinations, dry mouth, blurry vision, urinary retention, livedo reticularis	*Monotherapy or combination therapy,* predominantly for tremor in younger people; should be avoided in elderly. Utilized mainly for refractory tremor and sialorrhea
Benztropine (Cogentin)	0.5, 1, 2	0.5–2 mg once daily, or divided over 2 doses	Same as above	Same as above

PD, Parkinson disease.

f. Surgical interventions such as deep brain stimulation (DBS) can be an effective treatment for appropriate patients. These treatments are used in addition to medication.
- Non-Motor Symptom Management
    a. Depression in PD is best treated with a combination of psychotherapy, antidepressants, and therapeutic physical and mental exercise.
    b. Botulinum toxin A can be an effective treatment for severe drooling, although oral and transdermal medications should be tried first in the interest of cost saving.
    c. Urinary complaints in PD are typically not responsive to dopaminergic medications but can be remedied by drugs that relax the bladder and allow it to fill to a greater capacity.

SURGICAL OPTIONS

Surgical therapies are usually reserved for PD patients who are experiencing decreased effects of medical dopamine therapy over time.

- DBS is the most frequently performed surgical therapy for PD. In DBS, an electrode is surgically implanted in the subthalamic nucleus, globus pallidus, or ventral intermediate nucleus of the thalamus, providing continuous high-frequency electrical stimulation. Generally, DBS response is best for patients who have had good preoperative response to levodopa and report shorter disease duration (<16 years). If effective, DBS can help reduce tremor, stiffness, bradykinesia, and effective medication dose.
- Surgical lesions for PD include posteroventral pallidotomy (attenuation of bradykinesia, akinesia, rigidity, tremor and long-term improvement of dyskinesia and fluctuations), ventroinferomedial thalamotomy (attenuation of resting tremor, dyskinesia, dystonia, and rigidity) and subthalamic nucleus (attenuation akinetic symptoms).

REFERENCES

Elbaz, A., Carcaillon, L., Kab, S., et al. (2016). Epidemiology of Parkinson's disease. *Revue Neurologique*, *172*(1), 14–26.

Postuma, R. B., Berg, D., Stern, M., et al. (2015). MDS clinical diagnostic criteria for Parkinson's disease. *Mov Disord*, *30*(12), 1591–1601.

PARKINSONISM

Parkinsonism is a general term that refers to a group of neurological disorders that cause movement problems similar to those of Parkinson disease (PD), but distinguished by a known precipitant, atypical presentation, or additional neurologic symptoms. Parkinsonism-plus syndromes may also be seen in a group of heterogeneous degenerative neurological disorders, which differ from classical idiopathic PD in some associated clinical features, poor response to levodopa, distinctive pathological characteristics, and poor prognosis. Parkinsonism-plus syndromes are often misdiagnosed, given subtle clinical differences that require autopsy confirmation.

PROGRESSIVE SUPRANUCLEAR PALSY (PSP)

Progressive supranuclear palsy (PSP) is the second most common neurodegenerative cause of parkinsonism after PD. PSP is classically recognized as a combination of downgaze palsy, progressive rigidity, and imbalance that leads to falls. The distinguishing feature of PSP is the complaint of early onset, postural instability, and frequent falls within the first year that are uncharacteristic of PD. On examination, vertical, slow saccades may be the earliest sign. Ophthalmoplegia is vertical in the majority of patients and upward gaze is affected more than downward, although downward gaze is much more specific because upward gaze restriction is more common in the elderly. Over time, symptoms worsen to include supranuclear ophthalmoplegia, pseudobulbar palsy, axial rigidity, dysphagia, dysarthria, mild dementia, and parkinsonism.

MRI is the modality of choice for imaging patients with suspected PSP. MRI demonstrates atrophy of the dorsal mesencephalon and a widening of the aqueduct, with a decrease in the midbrain-to-pons area ratio, reduction of anteroposterior midline midbrain diameter (e.g., Mickey Mouse sign), lateral margin of the tegmentum of midbrain (e.g., morning glory sign), and a flattening or concave of the midbrain (e.g., hummingbird sign).

There is no specific drug therapy. In the early stages, mild to moderate improvement in symptoms may occur with levodopa or dopamine agonists, but without sustainability. Median survival time is about 5 to 6 years.

MULTIPLE SYSTEM ATROPHY

Multiple system atrophy (MSA) is an adult-onset, fatal neurodegenerative disease characterized by progressive autonomic failure, parkinsonian features, and cerebellar and pyramidal features in various combinations. Given variability of clinical presentation, MSA was initially divided between three patterns: Shy-Drager syndrome (autonomic symptoms predominant), striatonigral degeneration (parkinsonian features predominant), and olivopontocerebellar atrophy (cerebellar dysfunction predominant). However, since 2007, MSA has been divided clinically into two MSA-C (cerebellar predominant) and MSA-P (parkinsonism predominant) subtypes.

Like PD, MSA has a prodromal premotor phase, including sexual dysfunction, urinary urge incontinence or retention, orthostatic hypotension, inspiratory stridor, and a rapid-eye-movement sleep behavior disorder that appear months to years before the first motor symptoms. However, unlike PD, as motor features begin to emerge, patients develop disabling dysautonomia, postural hypotension, erectile disturbances, bladder and bowel dysfunction, and hypohidrosis. Patients with the MSA-C generally present with late-onset cerebellar ataxia, while MSA-P may be indistinguishable from PD early in the disease progression. Definitive diagnosis is confirmed only with pathology.

MRI is the modality of choice for imaging patients with suspected MSA. MSA-C subtype typically shows disproportionate atrophy of the cerebellum and brainstem, and MRI T2 hyperintensities typically present in the pontocerebellar tracts (e.g., hot cross bun sign). MSA-P subtype will typically show reduced volume in the putamen with an abnormally high T2 linear rim surrounding the putamen (e.g., putaminal rim sign).

The management of patients with MSA is usually complex. Parkinsonism may respond markedly to levodopa in the early stages, but the response is usually incomplete and short-lived. Patients with MSA have a median survival of 6 years.

CORTICOBASAL GANGLIONIC DEGENERATION

Corticobasal ganglionic degeneration (CBGD) is a neurodegenerative disease that is clinically, genetically, and pathologically similar to frontotemporal dementia. It is defined by asymmetric cortical atrophy, most predominantly in the superior parietal lobule and frontoparietal. Other features include atrophy of corpus callosum, substantia nigra, and bilateral basal ganglia. CBGD is distinguishable from PD by the presence of asymmetrical cortical symptoms and signs.

Onset typically occurs in the sixth decade or later with asymmetrical focal reflex myoclonus and its highly characteristic stiff, dystonic, jerky movements. Patients often present with parkinsonism signs, such as asymmetry dystonia, apraxia, alien limb, and ideomotor apraxia. Other symptoms may include gradual development of aphasia, loss of cortical sensory functions, depression, obsessive-compulsive neurosis, and late onset dementia. Clinically and pathologically, CBGD can present with anterior cortical predominance, manifesting as frontotemporal dementia, or lateral dominant frontal lobe, manifesting as primary progressive aphasia.

MRI is the modality of choice for assessing CBGD. CGBD progresses slowly over the course of 6 to 8 years, and it is often resistant to symptomatic therapy. Death is generally caused by pneumonia or other complications.

DIFFUSE LEWY BODY DISEASE

Diffuse Lewy body (DLB) is a particular dementia syndrome with features of parkinsonism. Cognitive deficits may emerge in the course of PD; however, DLB is defined by cognitive impairment with later emergence of parkinsonism. Keys to diagnosis include cognitive fluctuation, visual hallucination, and marked neuroleptic sensitivity.

Management of DLB is difficult. If motor symptoms are prominent, these are best managed with small doses of L-dopa; anticholinergic and neuroleptic drugs should be avoided.

DRUG-INDUCED PARKINSONISM

Drug-induced parkinsonism (DIP) is the second most common cause of parkinsonism in the elderly after PD. Many patients with DIP are misdiagnosed with PD because the clinical features of these two conditions are indistinguishable. Moreover, neurological deficits in patients with DIP may be severe enough to affect daily activities and persist for long periods after cessation of the offending agent. In addition to typical antipsychotics, DIP may be caused by gastrointestinal prokinetics (e.g., metoclopramide), calcium channel blockers (e.g., cinnarizine and flunarizine), atypical antipsychotics, MAO inhibitors (reserpine and tetrabenazine), and antiepileptic drugs. Other agents that rarely induce parkinsonism include selective serotonin reuptake inhibitors (SSRIs), lithium, valproate, antiarrhythmics, and diazepam.

VASCULAR PARKINSONISM
Vascular or "multi-infarct" parkinsonism is a form of parkinsonism that presents following small strokes. Accounting for less than 5% of parkinsonism cases, patients with vascular parkinsonism often present with sudden onset, asymmetric parkinsonism. This predominantly includes lower body involvement, postural instability, falls, dementia, corticospinal findings, incontinence, or emotional lability.

SECONDARY PARKINSONISM
Secondary parkinsonism refers to disorders that are secondarily associated with an akinetic rigid syndrome, which includes postencephalitis, hydrocephalus, hypoxia, trauma, metabolic imbalance (parathyroid), and toxins (manganese, carbon monoxide, 1-methyl-4-phenyl-1,2,3,6-tetrahydropyridine [MPTP], and cyanide). Other diseases with parkinsonism include Hallervorden-Spatz disease, Huntington disease, Lubag disease, Wilson disease, sporadic pallidal degeneration, bilateral striatopallidodentate calcinosis, neuroacanthocytosis, and mitochondrial cytopathies with striatal necrosis. Treatment is symptomatic and consists of elimination of the primary cause.

REFERENCES
Boxer, A. L., Yu, J. T., Golbe, L. I., Litvan, I., Lang, A. E., & Höglinger, G. U. (2017). Advances in progressive supranuclear palsy: new diagnostic criteria, biomarkers, and therapeutic approaches. *Lancet Neurol, 16*(7), 552–563.

Glasmacher, S. A., Leigh, P. N., & Saha, R. A. (2017). Predictors of survival in progressive supranuclear palsy and multiple system atrophy: a systematic review and meta-analysis. *J Neurol Neurosurg Psychiatry, 88*(5), 402–411.

PERIODIC PARALYSIS (See MYOTONIA)
Periodic paralysis is a neuromuscular disorder characterized by recurrent episodes of flaccid, painless weakness. Clinical presentation is correlated according to the serum potassium concentration, either high or low, during the attack. However, the episodes can occur based on the sensitivity to potassium and changes in its level rather than by its absolute value. They can be primary familial (autosomal dominant) forms or can result from other causes which affect serum potassium levels. Genetic forms of periodic paralysis are

channelopathies associated with mutations in the α-subunit of the skeletal muscle sodium channel protein (more commonly hyperkalemic periodic paralysis) or voltage-gated calcium channels (predominantly hypokalemic periodic paralysis). Other channelopathies with mutations in potassium channels can also cause attacks of periodic paralysis; for example, *Andersen-Tawii* syndrome. In this syndrome, weakness can occur due to low, normal, or high levels of extracellular potassium. Other findings include dysmorphic features and cardiac abnormalities. Table 105 reviews clinical features of the primary familial kalemic periodic paralysis.

Secondary hypokalemic periodic paralysis occurs in illnesses with potassium depletion, including hyperaldosteronism, chronic diarrhea, or chronic use of potassium-depleting diuretics. Thyrotoxicosis is another cause of secondary hypokalemic periodic paralysis with a high frequency in Asian men.

P

PERIODIC PARALYSIS

TABLE 105		
PRIMARY FAMILIAL KALEMIC PERIODIC PARALYSIS		
Characteristic	Hypokalemic	Hyperkalemic
Gene	CACL1A3 (type1) SCN4A (type 2)	SCN4A
Chromosome	1q31-32 (type1) 17q24 (type 2)	17q23
Prevalence	1:100,000	1:100,000
Age of onset	Any age, predominantly 2nd decade	Infancy/childhood
Inheritance	Autosomal dominant	Autosomal dominant
Clinical presentation	Often occurs in the early morning. Begins with back or lower extremity weakness followed by involvement of proximal muscles, and spreads distally. Usually spares respiratory muscles.	In infancy, can present as a change or an abnormal cry. Proximal > distal weakness, spreads over minutes, associated with myotonia of face, eyes, and hands. Can have respiratory involvement, but not common.
Duration of attack	Hours to days	Minutes to hours
Frequency of attack	7–9 episodes monthly	~16 attacks monthly
Precipitating factors	Heavy carbohydrate meal, exercise followed by rest, sleep, or alcohol	Rest after exercise, anesthesia, sleep, cold
Provocative tests	Glucose ± insulin	Oral potassium chloride (KCl)
Electrocardiogram (ECG) changes	ECG changes of hypokalemia	ECG changes of hyperkalemia
Electromyography (EMG)	EMG silent during attack	EMG silent during attack
Treatment	KCl, acetazolamide, dichlorphenamide, potassium-sparing diuretic	Acetazolamide, dichlorphenamide, thiazide diuretic

Secondary hyperkalemic periodic paralysis is seen with very high potassium levels, and can occur with excessive potassium supplementation, renal insufficiency, potassium-sparing diuretics, and adrenal insufficiency.

All forms of periodic paralysis may respond to carbonic anhydrase inhibitors such as dichlorphenamide and acetazolamide. Other kaliuretic diuretics (such as thiazides) may also be effective. Aside from medications, other treatment includes dietary modification with attention to potassium contents as well as avoiding provoking factors.

REFERENCES

Amato, A. (2016). Disorders of skeletal muscle. In [Eds], *Bradley's neurology in clinical practice,* ed 7 (pp. 1915–1955). Philadelphia: Elsevier.

Barohn, R., & Jeffrey, M. (2013). Muscle channelopathies: the nondystrophic myotonias and periodic paralyses. *Continuum Life Long Learn Neurol*, *19*(6), 1598–1611.

PERIPHERAL NERVE DISEASE (See also NEUROPATHY)

This outline lists clinical clues that may be helpful in the diagnosis of focal peripheral nerve disease:

UPPER EXTREMITY

1. Terminal branches of the posterior cord include the radial and axillary nerve
   a. Radial nerve (C5-T1): travels from the axilla through the spiral grove into the forearm. It innervates the triceps, anconeus, supinator, as well as the extensor muscle groups in the forearm and hand. Within the forearm, the nerve branches into the posterior interosseous nerve (motor) and the superficial radial nerve (sensory).
   b. Axillary (C5, C6) innervates the deltoids.
   c. When evaluating wrist drop, place the wrist angle to the neutral position before testing finger flexors and extensors:
      i. In an isolated posterior interosseous mononeuropathy, the brachioradialis and triceps are spared and there is no sensory loss.
      ii. If only the triceps is spared, the radial nerve lesion is at the spiral groove.
      iii. If the triceps is weak, the radial nerve lesion is at the axilla.
   d. A posterior cord brachial plexopathy occurs when both the triceps and deltoid are weak.
2. Terminal branches of the lateral cord include the musculocutaneous nerve as well as the median nerve (also contains fibers from the medial cord).
   a. The musculocutaneous nerve (C5-C7) supplies innervation to the coracobrachialis, biceps, and brachialis.
      i. With marked differences in strength between biceps and brachioradialis (C5-C6 roots, upper trunk), think of:
         1. A lesion of the lateral cord or musculocutaneous nerve (if biceps is weaker).

       2. A lesion of the posterior cord or radial nerve (if brachioradialis is weaker).

    ii. With marked differences in strength between biceps and deltoid, think of:

       1. A lesion of the lateral cord or musculocutaneous nerve (if biceps is weaker).

       2. A lesion of the posterior cord or axillary nerve (if deltoid is weaker).

b. The median nerve (C6-T1) supplies primarily forearm flexors except for FCU and gives off the anterior interosseous nerve. It enters the hand through the carpel tunnel where it can become easily compressed.

    i. The median nerve sensory fibers to the hand pass via the upper brachial plexus, originating from:

       1. The C6 root to the thumb.

       2. The C6 and C7 roots to the index finger.

       3. The C7 root to the middle finger.

c. The ulnar nerve (C8, T1) is the terminal branch of the medial cord.

    i. It is not possible to differentiate C8 from T1 radiculopathy because all intrinsic muscles of the hand are innervated by both roots.

    ii. With an ulnar nerve lesion of the arm, elbow, or upper forearm, sensory loss usually involves palmar and dorsal aspects of the little and ring fingers. With an ulnar nerve lesion of the distal forearm or wrist, sensory loss involves only the palmar aspect of these fingers (due to sparing of the dorsal ulnar sensory branch that arises 6 to 7 cm above the wrist).

    iii. With ulnar neuropathy, sensory loss is isolated below the wrist. However, in a C8-T1 radiculopathy or lower trunk plexopathy, sensory loss can occur along the medial aspect of the upper limb, following the distribution of the medial cutaneous nerves of the forearm and arm (both arising from the lower trunk).

    iv. With weakness or atrophy of the thenar and hypothenar eminences, think of:

       1. C8-T1 radiculopathy or a lower trunk brachial plexopathy.

       2. The presence of Horner syndrome is supportive evidence of a C8 from T1 radiculopathy/plexopathy.

d. Concomitant ulnar and median mononeuropathy (e.g., carpal tunnel syndrome and ulnar neuropathy at the elbow). In this case, flexor pollicis longus should be intact (flexor of the distal phalanx of the thumb, located in the forearm, and innervated by the anterior interosseus branch of the median nerve).

3. In the case of scapular winging, the winging is caused by:

a. Serratus anterior (long thoracic nerve, C5-C7) weakness if:

    i. There is considerable winging at rest with medial translocation of the scapula (vertebral border closer to the midline).

    ii. The shoulder appears lower on the affected side.

    iii. Winging is accentuated by forward flexion of the humerus.

   b. Trapezius weakness if:
      i. There is less winging at rest with lateral translocation of the scapula.
      ii. The shoulder is definitely lower on the affected side.
      iii. Winging is decreased by forward flexion of the humerus and increased by abduction of the humerus.

LOWER EXTREMITY
1. Femoral nerve (L2-L4) supplies innervation to primarily muscles in the anterior thigh compartment including the quadriceps.
   a. It is not possible to differentiate L2 from L3 radiculopathy because quadriceps, iliopsoas, and adductor muscles are innervated by L2 and L3 roots.
   b. The testing of thigh adductors (L2-L4, obturator nerve) is essential in differentiating "pure" femoral neuropathy from root or lumbar plexus involvement.
   c. In proximal weakness of the lower extremity(ies), compare quadriceps and thigh adductors with thigh abductors. If the weakness is significantly different, think of a selective root-plexus involvement rather than a myopathy.
2. Sciatic nerve supplies innervation to muscles primarily in the posterior thigh and divides into the common peroneal and tibial nerves.
   a. When evaluating foot drop (complete or incomplete), testing inversion of the ankle (tibialis posterior) and flexion of the toes (flexor digitorum longus) is very important. These muscles are innervated by L5 (and to a lesser extent S1) nerve roots via the tibial nerve. They are spared with peroneal neuropathy but are weak with L5 radiculopathy. Remember to correct the angle of the foot back to 90 degrees before testing eversion and inversion.
   b. The only L4-innervated muscle below the knee is the tibialis anterior (L4-5, dorsiflexor of the ankle).
   Peripheral innervation is shown in Figs. 47 to 54.

REFERENCES
Chad, A. (2016). Disorders of nerve roots and plexuses. In R. Daroff, et al. (Ed.), *Bradley's neurology in clinical practice*, ed 7. London: Elsevier.
Katirji, B. (2016). Disorders of peripheral nerves. In R. Daroff, et al. (Ed.), *Bradley's neurology in clinical practice*, ed 7. London: Elsevier.

PET AND SPECT

Both positron emission tomography (PET) and single-photon emission computed tomography (SPECT) are based on cross-sectional reconstruction of images derived from the distribution of administered radionuclides. Spatial resolution is significantly lower than that obtained with CT or MRI. However, several types of PET scanners are operating in 3D mode with enhanced sensitivity, improved signal-to-noise ratio, and increased spatial resolution. PET

P

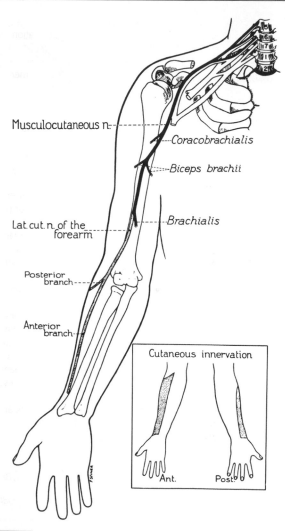

FIGURE 47

Musculocutaneous nerve. (From Haymaker, W., & Woodhall, B. (1953). *Peripheral nerve injuries: principles of diagnosis.* Philadelphia: WB Saunders).

methodology provides both qualitative and quantitative data (the latter require an arterial line for serial blood sampling), whereas SPECT provides only qualitative data. Both methods are noninvasive, and actual radiation exposure is less than or equal to that received in many other routine radiologic procedures.

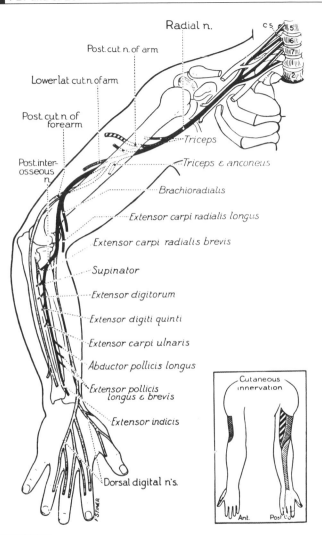

Radial nerve. (From Haymaker, W., & Woodhall, B. (1953). *Peripheral nerve injuries: principles of diagnosis.* Philadelphia: WB Saunders).

PET uses positron-emitting radionuclides such as oxygen-15, fluorine-18, carbon-11, and nitrogen-13, which are produced in a cyclotron. They have a short half-life that enables administration of relatively high doses of radioactivity but within safe limits of radiation exposure. These radionuclides

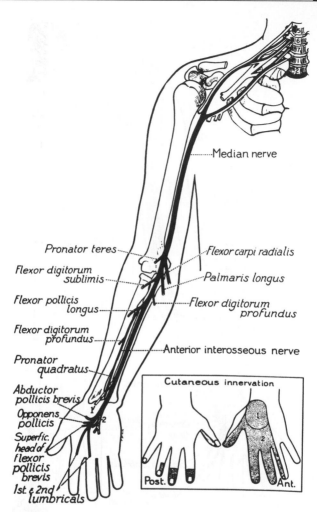

FIGURE 49

Median nerve. (From Haymaker, W., & Woodhall, B. (1953). *Peripheral nerve injuries: principles of diagnosis*. Philadelphia: WB Saunders).

can be incorporated into biologically active compounds to investigate metabolism, receptor binding, and alterations in regional blood flow. Deoxyglucose labeled with fluorine-18 (fluorodeoxyglucose) is used to measure brain glucose metabolism. Compounds labeled with oxygen-15 are

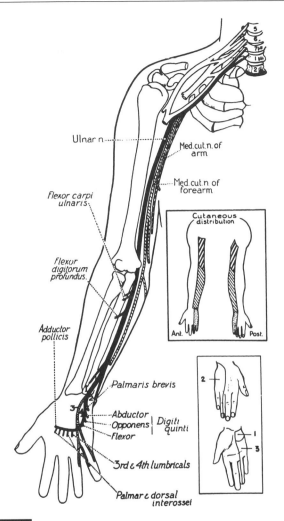

FIGURE 50

Ulnar and medial cutaneous nerves. (From Haymaker, W., & Woodhall, B. (1953). *Peripheral nerve injuries: principles of diagnosis*. Philadelphia: WB Saunders).

used to measure regional cerebral blood flow and volume, as well as cerebral metabolic rates.

In clinical situations, PET has utility in the *inter-ictal evaluation* of patients with refractory seizures of presumed focal origin. *Gliomas* can also be evaluated

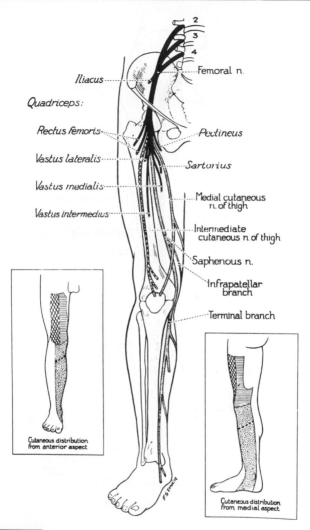

FIGURE 51

Femoral nerve. (From Haymaker, W., & Woodhall, B. (1953). *Peripheral nerve injuries: principles of diagnosis*. Philadelphia: WB Saunders).

for malignant potential based on their metabolism, including high-grade tumors that demonstrate hypermetabolism and low-grade tumors that demonstrate hypometabolism. FDG uptake patterns can differentiate *radiation necrosis* (no or low activity) from tumor recurrence (increased activity). PET is

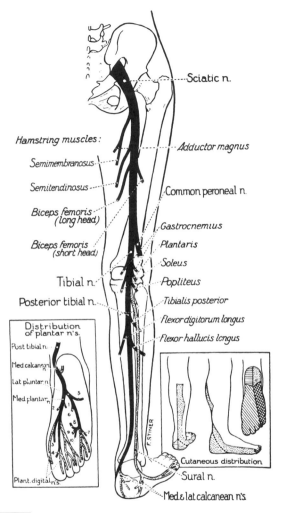

FIGURE 52

Sciatic, tibial, posterior tibial, and plantar nerves. (From Haymaker, W., & Woodhall, B. (1953). *Peripheral nerve injuries: principles of diagnosis*. Philadelphia: WB Saunders).

also being used in ischemia and dementia. For evaluation of dementia, PET has been approved to differentiate *Alzheimer disease* (hypometabolism in bilateral temporoparietal lobes) from *frontotemporal dementia* (hypometabolism in frontotemporal lobes). Dopamine labeled tracer uptake

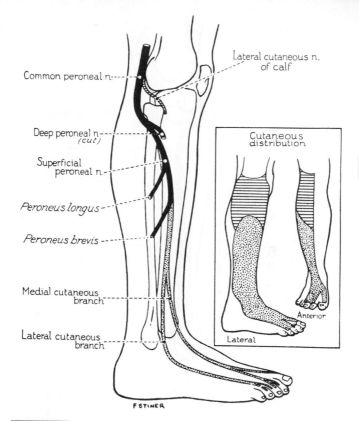

Common peroneal n.

Lateral cutaneous n.
of calf

Deep peroneal n.
(cut)

Superficial
peroneal n.

Peroneus longus

Peroneus brevis

Medial cutaneous
branch

Lateral cutaneous
branch

Cutaneous
distribution

Anterior

Lateral

F STINER

P

PET AND SPECT

FIGURE 53

Superficial peroneal nerve. (From Haymaker, W., & Woodhall, B. (1953). *Peripheral nerve injuries: principles of diagnosis*. Philadelphia: WB Saunders).

can be assessed in patients with early *Parkinson disease*. Other uses for PET have been limited to research studies due to high cost, invasiveness, and need for extremely sophisticated technology.

SPECT utilizes gamma emitters, such as Iodine-123, Iodine-131, or technetium-99, attached to highly lipophilic substances that easily pass the blood-brain barrier by simple diffusion. Thus, uptake, as measured by gamma camera, is proportional to regional blood flow. Gamma emitters have also been successfully labeled to various neurotransmitter analogues, allowing for localization and evaluation of receptor densities. Indications for studies are similar to those for PET. In contrast to PET, however, SPECT technology is widely available, with lower cost.

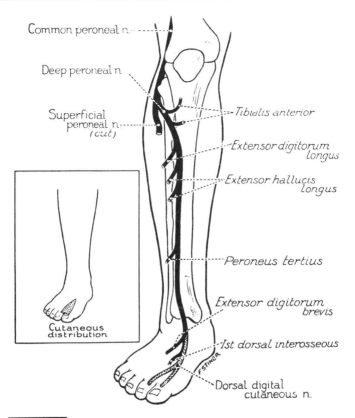

Common peroneal n.

Deep peroneal n.

Superficial peroneal n. (cut)

Tibialis anterior

Extensor digitorum longus

Extensor hallucis longus

Peroneus tertius

Extensor digitorum brevis

1st dorsal interosseous

Dorsal digital cutaneous n.

Cutaneous distribution

FIGURE 54

Deep peroneal nerve. (From Haymaker, W., & Woodhall, B. (1953). *Peripheral nerve injuries: principles of diagnosis.* Philadelphia: WB Saunders).

REFERENCES

Szyszko, T. A., & Cook, G. J. R. (2018). PET/CT and PET/MRI in head and neck malignancy. *Clin Radiol, 73*(1), 60–69.

Yang, M., Sun, J., Bai, H. X., Tao, Y., Tang, X., States, L. J., et al. (2017). Diagnostic accuracy of SPECT, PET, and MRS for primary central nervous system lymphoma in HIV patients: a systematic review and meta-analysis. *Medicine (Baltimore), 96*(19), e6676.

PITUITARY DISORDERS (PITUITARY ADENOMA, HYPO- AND HYPERPITUITARISM, APOPLEXY)

The anterior pituitary gland produces thyrotropin, prolactin, corticotropin, growth hormone (GH), luteinizing hormone (LH), and follicle-stimulating hormone (FSH); it is supplied by the superior and inferior hypophysial arteries. The posterior pituitary gland produces vasopressin (antidiuretic hormone, ADH) and regulates oxytocin secretion; it is supplied by the inferior hypophysial arteries.

PITUITARY ADENOMAS

Pituitary adenomas account for 15% of all intracranial tumors. They may cause isolated endocrine symptoms if smaller than 10 mm (microadenoma). Tumors > 10 mm (macroadenomas) can also produce visual symptoms, headache, or both via mass effect. Management includes multidisciplinary approach incorporating surgery, neurology, endocrinology, ophthalmology, radiology, and/or radiation therapy. While some pituitary adenomas are nonsecreting (nonfunctional), approximately 30% to 50% are hormone-secreting (functional) as follows:

PROLACTINOMAS (30% TO 50%)
Symptoms
Occur more frequently in females (3:1). Amenorrhea, galactorrhea, or both in females and decreased libido and impotence in males. Galactorrhea may also occur in males. May rapidly expand during pregnancy.

Diagnosis
Serum prolactin levels > 250 µg/mL. MRI scan with postcontrast gradient echo (GRE) supports the diagnosis. However, because microadenomas are sometimes undetected by MRI, endocrinologic testing is needed to confirm the diagnosis of small, hormone-secreting pituitary tumors if they are suspected on clinical examination.

Treatment
Medical: Symptomatic prolactinoma treatment often consists of bromocriptine (2.5 to 7.5 mg PO daily) or cabergoline (initially 0.25 mg PO twice a week up to 1mg PO twice a week after cardiovascular evaluation). Cabergoline (D2 receptor-specific) preferred as initial treatment due to greater efficacy and fewer adverse effects. Dopamine agonist therapy may be tapered to cessation after 2 years with absence of adenoma on imaging and serum prolactin levels normalized. Dopamine agonists should be avoided during pregnancy due to increased rate of obstetric complications.

Surgical resection: For refractory cases to medical treatment or intolerance of side effects (3% to 12%). Biochemical remission can be achieved in up to 72% of patients. In patients with life expectancy > 10 years, surgical approach may be cost-effective. May be a treatment option for pregnant patients.

Radiation: Biochemical remission in 17% to 26%.

GROWTH HORMONE-SECRETING ADENOMAS (10%)

Symptoms

Male to female ratio 3:2. Gigantism and acromegaly before and after epiphyseal growth plate closure, respectively. Associated with entrapment neuropathies, such as carpal tunnel syndrome, and diabetes.

Diagnosis

Elevated serum IGF-1 for confirmation of acromegaly. If IGF-1 level is equivocal, oral glucose tolerance test performed and lack of GH suppression to < 1 μg/L is diagnostic. Postcontrast GRE MR used to assess size and location.

Treatment

Surgical: First-line therapy with biochemical remission up to 70% of pts.

Medical: Second-line therapy. Somatostatin analogs used to inhibit GH-secreting pituitary somatotroph cells. These include octreotide and lanreotide administered monthly. Adverse side effects include GI symptoms, including gallstones. For refractory cases, daily dosing of pegvisomant (GH-receptor antagonist); adverse side effects include hepatotoxicity.

Radiation: May become second-line alternative after surgical therapy. Hypopituitarism may occur in 85% of patients.

ACTH-SECRETING ADENOMAS (5%)

Symptoms

Female to male ratio is 3:1. Cushing disease, including central obesity, DM, hypertension, mental status changes, personality changes, and myopathy. High circulating levels of cortisol cause potent effects even when < 1 cm diameter.

Diagnosis

Once endogenous hypercortisolism identified, diagnosis of Cushing disease is made with confirmation of a pituitary source and exclusion of ectopic adrenocorticotropic hormone (ACTH)-secreting tumors. Elevated ACTH can rule out an adrenocortical tumor. Adenomas often small with mean size ~6 mm; inferior petrosal sinus sampling may be required to identify source of ACTH hypersecretion (pituitary vs. ectopic).

Treatment

Surgical: first line

Radiation: Considered in patients with persistent symptoms s/p resection or unresectable disease (i.e., within cavernous sinus).

Medical: alternative approach to nonsurgical candidates or failed surgical treatment. Includes steroidogenesis inhibitors (ketoconazole w/possible side effects of hepatotoxicity, etomidate, metyrapone), corticotroph-directed agents (pasireotide with possible side effect of hyperglycemia), glucocorticoid receptor blockers (mifepristone). Studies currently underway for utilization of temozolomide for treatment-resistant adenomas.

THYROTROPIN SECRETING ADENOMAS (1% TO 2%)

May present with symptoms of hyperthyroidism, including palpitations, goiter, eye symptoms. Management and outcome not clearly defined yet. Surgical resection usually first-line treatment. Recurrence is frequent and long-term follow up is necessary.

GONADOTROPH-SECRETING ADENOMAS (<1%)

FSH/LH secreting adenomas make up majority of nonfunctional lesions. Functional gonadotroph-secreting tumors are rare. Present with oligo- or amenorrhea, infertility, or galactorrhea in female. Diagnosis made by imaging and clinical features and elevated serum levels. Resection is first-line approach. Medical treatment largely unsuccessful. Management and outcome not clearly defined yet.

Special Syndromes

I. **Hypopituitarism** from primary disease or as a complication of treatment requires supplementation of essential hormones. GH deficiency can lead to growth failure. Prolactin deficits can cause infertility and inability to breastfeed. LH/FSH problems cause delayed puberty, infertility, impotence, and amenorrhea. Hypothyroidism can be caused by thyrotropin deficiency, and corticotropin failure causes hypoadrenalism. Low ADH causes problems of fluid/electrolyte homeostasis in the form of diabetes insipidus (please see "Diabetes Insipidus"), while oxytocin is involved in lactation/labor difficulties. Oxytocin also mediates social attachment between mother and child, but may also apply in adults. Critical hormones of ADH, thyroid stimulating hormone (TSH), and ACTH can be exogenously supplemented with 1-deamino-8-D-arginine vasopressin (desmopressin), l-thyroxine, and cortisone, respectively. Testosterone/estrogen (LH/FSH deficiency) and synthetic GH are also administered for their respective disorders. There is no current therapy for prolactin deficits. Simmonds syndrome is the eponym given to panhypopituitarism. Sheehan syndrome is a pituitary infarction secondary to postpartum infarction. It presents with headache and visual symptoms and may cause circulatory collapse and coma.

II. **Pituitary apoplexy** refers to the sudden expansion of the pituitary gland, usually the result of hemorrhage into a preexisting adenoma. Sudden severe headache, variable ocular motor palsies, rapid loss of vision (chiasmal or optic nerve), evidence of hypopituitarism, and subarachnoid hemorrhage with associated changes in mental status including coma may be present.

P

PITUITARY DISORDERS

Features helpful in the difficult clinical distinction from aneurysmal subarachnoid hemorrhage are the presence of mixed oculomotor palsies or bilateral ophthalmoplegias and the presence of an afferent pupillary defect or chiasmal patterns of field loss. Diagnostic procedures include CT and MRI, which may show a pituitary mass containing blood; angiography to exclude an intracavernous aneurysm; and lumbar puncture. Baseline hormonal levels should be obtained before treatment for subsequent determination of endocrine dysfunction. Treatment includes immediate high-dose IV corticosteroid therapy and prompt transsphenoidal decompression to prevent further vision loss if needed.

III. **Empty sella syndrome** is the major cause of asymptomatic sellar enlargement. The subarachnoid space extends into the sella through an incompetent diaphragm with flattening of the gland inferiorly and posteriorly. Empty sella syndrome may accompany idiopathic intracranial hypertension, spontaneous regressive changes of pituitary adenomas, and surgery. Although usually asymptomatic, symptoms may include headache, occasional mild endocrine abnormalities, CSF rhinorrhea, and rarely, visual disturbances. If symptoms are present, pituitary tumor should be excluded with endocrine and neuro-ophthalmic evaluations and MRI. Differential diagnosis of an enlarged sella turcica in the absence of endocrinopathy includes nonsecreting adenoma, empty sella syndrome, and craniopharyngioma. Hypopituitarism, diabetes insipidus, and visual field defects are much less common in empty sella syndrome. A ballooned sella without erosion is more characteristic of craniopharyngioma.

IV. Syndrome of inappropriate antidiuretic hormone secretion (SIADH) is defined as excessive secretion of ADH, resulting in excess of water reabsorption, resulting in hypervolemia and dilutional hyponatremia. Can also occur from ectopic ADH secretion from small-cell carcinoma of lung. Treatment includes fluid restriction and treatment of underlying etiology. Care must be taken to correct hyponatremia to avoid central pontine myelinolysis by correction < 12 mEq/L/day.

DIFFERENTIAL DIAGNOSIS OF SELLAR MASS LESIONS

1. Sellar masses: dermoids, teratomas, arachnoid cysts, and rare tumors of the neurohypophysis. Meningiomas, metastases, and cholesteatomas may occur in any location around the sella.
2. Suprasellar masses: craniopharyngiomas, optic gliomas, chondromas, hypothalamic gliomas, supraclinoid carotid artery aneurysms, choroid plexus papillomas, and colloid cysts of the third ventricle.
3. Parasellar lesions: cavernous carotid aneurysms, temporal lobe neoplasms, and gasserian ganglion neuromas.
4. Retrosellar region: chordomas and basilar artery aneurysms.
5. Infrasellar lesions: sphenoid sinus mucoceles, carcinomas, granulomas, and other nasopharyngeal tumors.

REFERENCES

Cooper, P. E., & Stan, H. M. (2016). Neuroendocrinology. In R. B. Daroff, & J. Jankovic (Eds.), *Bradley's neurology in clinical practice: principles of diagnosis and management: Vol. 1*, ed 7 (pp. 703–711). Philadelphia: Elsevier Health Sciences.

Mehta, G. U., & Lonser, R. (2017). Management of hormone-secreting pituitary adenomas. *Neuro-Oncol, 19*(6), 762–763.

PORPHYRIA

The porphyrias are rare disorders of heme biosynthesis with neurologic, cutaneous, and other organ manifestations. They are classified as hepatic and erythropoietic. Neurologic symptoms occur in the hepatic porphyrias: acute intermittent porphyria (AIP), variegate porphyria (VP), hereditary coproporphyria (HC), and Doss porphyria (DP). These disorders (except DP, which is inherited as an autosomal recessive) are autosomal dominant enzymatic defects of the pathways of heme biosynthesis in the liver, resulting in elevations and excess excretion of the porphyrins and the porphyrin precursors (Fig. 55). Although the enzymatic defects are well characterized, the pathogenesis of neurologic dysfunction is not known. It has been postulated that the delta-aminolevulinic acid (ALA) and porphobilinogen (PBG) are directly neurotoxic. Other possibilities include abnormalities of heme metabolism in neurons or interference with serotonergic metabolism.

The first step in the pathway catalyzed by ALA synthase results in the formation of ALA, and it is the rate-limiting step. Heme exerts control at this step via three different mechanisms: (1) repression of synthesis of new enzyme, (2) interference of transfer of the enzyme from cytosol to mitochondria, and (3) direct inhibition of enzyme activity. Processes that deplete the regulatory pool of heme by inducing cytochrome P450 or increasing the turnover of hemoglobin will drive the heme synthesis pathway. For example, phenytoin induces the cytochrome P450 system, and starvation increases the turnover of hemoglobin. Both processes deplete the heme pool, thereby removing repression of ALA synthetase.

Depending on the specific enzyme deficiency, there will be an excess of intermediates from preceding steps in the pathway excreted in urine and stool; it is the pattern of porphyrin precursors in the urine, feces, and serum that characterizes the type of porphyria. Diagnosis is complicated by the variable intensity of porphyrin excretion in affected individuals and drug-induced porphyrinuria in some normal individuals leading to occasional false-positive results (Table 106). Lead poisoning can lead to elevation of ALA and porphyrins. Special handling of specimens obtained for porphyria is necessary. Twenty-four-hour urine collections should be kept refrigerated in a dark container. Twenty-four-hour stool collections must be kept frozen and in a light-free container.

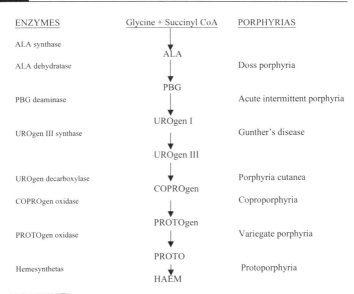

ENZYMES   Glycine + Succinyl CoA   PORPHYRIAS

ALA synthase

                 ALA

ALA dehydratase   Doss porphyria

                 PBG

PBG deaminase   Acute intermittent porphyria

                 UROgen I

UROgen III synthase   Gunther's disease

                 UROgen III

UROgen decarboxylase   Porphyria cutanea

                 COPROgen

COPROgen oxidase   Coproporphyria

                 PROTOgen

PROTOgen oxidase   Variegate porphyria

                 PROTO

Hemesynthetas   Protoporphyria

                 HAEM

FIGURE 55

The heme synthetase pathway. Enzymes involved in porphyrias: *ALA*, Delta aminolevulinic acid; *COPROgen*, coproporphyrinogen; *PBG*, porphobilinogen; *PROTO*, protoporphyrin; *PROTOgen*, protoporphyrinogen; *URO*, uroporphyrin; *UROgen*, uroporphyrinogen.

The most common of these rare disorders is AIP. Prevalence is estimated at 5 to 10 per 100,000 in the United States. Up to 90% of people with the enzyme deficiency (50% of normal activity) are asymptomatic. During the acute attacks, large amounts of PBG and ALA (20- to 200-fold elevated above normal levels) are excreted. About one-third of clinically asymptomatic carriers show an abnormal excretion of PBG (two to fivefold above the normal level), whereas the rest show normal excretion of this precursor. AIP lacks cutaneous manifestations; the PBG is not a porphyrin.

VP occurs mainly in South Africa but has occurred worldwide; HC and DP are very rare. HC and VP have neurologic and cutaneous manifestations such as photosensitive skin and blistering with excessive sun exposure or mild trauma.

Clinical manifestations include the following:

I. Dysautonomia presenting as abdominal pain (95%) out of proportion to clinical findings, nausea, vomiting (90%), diarrhea or constipation (85%), tachycardia (70%), orthostatic hypotension, hypertension (36%), diaphoresis, and urinary retention.

II. A motor more than sensory polyneuropathy often occurs (10% to 40%); rare cases have mononeuritis multiplex as well as ascending flaccid

TABLE 106

HEPATIC PORPHYRIAS: BIOCHEMICAL FEATURES

Type of Porphyria	Enzyme Defect	Erythrocyte Porphyrins	Urine	Feces
Acute intermittent porphyria	PBG deaminase	None	↑ALA, PBG	None
Variegate porphyria (VP)	Protoporphyrinogen oxidase	None	↑ALA, PBG, COPRO	↑COPRO, PROTO
Hereditary coproporphyria (HC)	Coproporphyrinogen oxidase	None	↑↑COPRO	↑↑COPRO
ALA dehydratase deficiency	ALA dehydratase	Protoporphyrin	ALA	None

ALA, Aminolevulinic acid; *COPRO*, coproporphyrin; *PBG*, porphobilinogen; *PROTO*, protoporphyrin.

paralysis (2%) resembling Guillain-Barré syndrome, which may result in fatal respiratory failure. Cranial nerves are often involved as well.

III. Headaches.

IV. Seizures in adults (15%) and in children (30%).

V. Psychiatric symptoms (25%): depression, delirium, psychosis, or agitation.

VI. Myalgia (72%).

Definitive diagnosis requires measuring PBG deaminase activity in erythrocytes. Screening for the porphyrias is accomplished by measuring stool porphyrins and urinary ALA and PBG concentration.

The differential diagnosis of the porphyrias is broad and should include:

I. Guillain-Barré syndrome in the setting of ascending motor and sensory neuropathy. Recurrent attacks without albuminocytologic dissociation are more suggestive of a porphyria.

II. Heavy metal toxicity, such as lead, which can cause similar hematopoietic derangements and peripheral neuropathy.

III. Vasculitis

IV. Poliomyelitis

V. Mental illness. A disproportionally large percentage of porphyria patients relative to the general population are misdiagnosed as schizophrenic.

Hyponatremia is common during porphyria attacks, and may contribute to the observed central nervous system manifestations, such as encephalopathy and seizures. Early MRI changes have documented a posterior-reversible encephalopathy syndrome-like appearance along with documented reversible vasoconstriction.

Treatment consists of avoiding precipitating factors, such as drugs that activate heme biosynthesis (Table 107), weight loss, or skipping meals. Other prophylactic measures include a high carbohydrate diet and propranolol. Acute attacks are treated initially with hemin 3 to 4 mg/kg body weight for 3 to 4 days. High doses of glucose and supportive care can be used in mild cases or as a stop gap when hemin is unavailable acutely. Urinary ALA and PBG decrease dramatically after 2 to 3 days of therapy. Hematin should not be used in

P

PORPHYRIA

TABLE 107	
DRUGS AND ACUTE PORPHYRIA	
DRUGS THAT MAY PRECIPITATE AN ATTACK OF ACUTE INTERMITTENT PORPHYRIA	
Alcohol	Meprobamate
Barbiturates	Methsuximide
Carisoprodol	Methyldopa
Chloramphenicol	Methyprylon
Chlordiazepoxide	Pentazocine
Chloroquine	Phenylbutazone
Dichloralphenazone	Phenytoin
Ergots	Progesterones
Estrogens	Pyralones
Eucalyptol	Sulfonamides
Glutethimide	Sylfonal
Griseofulvin	Testosterones
Imipramine	Tolbutamide
	Trional
	Tramadol
DRUGS THAT DO NOT EXACERBATE ACUTE INTERMITTENT PORPHYRIA	
Ascorbic acid	Neostigmine
Aspirin	Nitrofurantoin
Atropine	Opiates (excluding tramadol)
B vitamins	Penicillins
Chloral hydrate	Phenothiazines
Corticosteroids	Promethazine
Digoxin	Propranolol
Diphenhydramine	Rauwolfia alkaloids
Guanethidine	Scopolamine
Levetiracetam	Streptomycin
Meclizine	Tetracyclines
Methenamine mandelate	Tetraethylammonium bromide

conjunction with anticoagulant therapy because of its side effects, such as coagulopathy and phlebitis (the vein for infusion has to be changed each day). Women with cyclic perimenstrual acute attacks have benefited from luteinizing hormone releasing hormone agonists. Psychiatric symptoms may be treated with phenothiazines. Abdominal symptoms respond to chlorpromazine. Opiates are used for treatment of pain, but tramadol should not be used. Treatment of seizures is perplexing because many anticonvulsants are porphyrinogenic, although benzodiazepines may be less likely to induce porphyria. Gabapentin and levetiracetam, which are not metabolized by the liver, may be useful in this clinical setting. The safety of other new antiepileptic drugs is unknown.

REFERENCES

Simon, N. G., & Herkes, G. K. (2011). The neurologic manifestations of the acute porphyrias. *J Clin Neurosci*, *18*(9), 1147–1153.

Stein, P. E., Badminton, M. N., & Rees, D. C. (2017). Update review of the acute porphyrias. *Br J Haematol, 176*, 527–538. https://doi.org/10.1111/bjh.14459.

POSTERIOR REVERSIBLE ENCEPHALOPATHY SYNDROME (PRES), See also HYPERTENSIVE ENCEPHALOPATHY

Posterior reversible encephalopathy syndrome (PRES) is a well distinguished clinic-radiological syndrome commonly encountered in neurology practice with the hallmark of encephalopathic presentation, and posterior more than anterior bilateral confluent magnetic resonance imaging (MRI) vasogenic edema changes.

Clinically, it is commonly present with headache, seizure, change in mental status, and visual symptoms. The most common precipitating factor is hypertension, eclampsia/pre-eclampsia. Other commonly encountered etiologies are: acute or chronic renal disease, transplant patients, immunosuppressive agents and chemotherapy, vasoactive drugs, sympathomimetics, illicit drugs, and electrolytes/osmotic imbalance.

MRI or computed tomography (CT) scan of the head usually has three distinguishing bilateral vasogenic edema features: (1) superior frontal sulcus pattern, (2) holo-hemispheric patchy watershed pattern, and (3) dominant posterior parietal-occipital pattern. Many patients may also have mixed pattern.

Differential diagnosis may include progressive multifocal leukoencephalopathy (PML), cerebral autosomal dominant arteriopathy with subcortical infarcts and leukoencephalopathy, central nervous system (CNS) vasculitis, and mitochondrial myopathy encephalopathy lactic acidosis and stroke like episodes.

The pathophysiology is related to blood-brain barrier (BBB) dysfunction with either loss of autoregulation or impaired endothelium leading to cerebral edema.

Treatment: Symptomatic and supportive care, slow control of the blood pressure versus rapid is very important as well as slow reversal of metabolic aberrancies and discontinuation of potential medications that may be contributing to PRES and BBB injury. Hydration, treatment of underlying infection, and seizure control are key elements in the supportive care for PRES patients.

Prognosis: Depends on the underlying etiology; however in the majority of the cases mild to moderate disability is seen. Mortality is less than 15%.

REFERENCE

Granata, G., Greco, A., Iannella, G., et al. (2015). Posterior reversible encephalopathy syndrome–insight into pathogenesis, clinical variants and treatment approaches. *Autoimmun Rev, 14*(9), 830–836.

PREGNANCY

Underlying neurologic conditions may initially present during, or be altered by, pregnancy. Moreover, the course of pregnancy can be influenced by the presence of a neurologic disease. This section describes a variety of neurologic disorders that may affect, or may be affected by, pregnancy.

I. Peripheral nerve disorders and muscle disease
  A. Mononeuropathies:
    1. Bell palsy may have a more severe course in pregnant women, who are more likely to present with complete facial paralysis (a poor prognostic factor). Incidence of Bell palsy increases threefold during pregnancy, with the majority of cases occurring in the third trimester and the first puerperal weeks. No clear evidence-based guidelines have been published for treating Bell palsy in pregnant women. Supportive care is recommended with nutritional and vitamin support; steroid may be considered. Recurrence is rare.
    2. Carpal tunnel syndrome is common during pregnancy, and usually resolves in the postpartum period; management is conservative.
    3. Meralgia paresthetica is a sensory mononeuropathy occurring from lateral femoral cutaneous nerve injury. It presents with paresthesias and sensory loss along the anterolateral thigh that worsens with walking and hip flexion or extension. Deep tendon reflexes and strength are intact. Most cases resolve within several months of delivery, and management is symptomatic (avoiding tight clothing, excessive weight gain, etc.).
  B. Plexopathies:
    1. Neuralgic amyotrophy (also known as Parsonage-Turner syndrome or brachial neuritis) has hereditary and idiopathic forms; both may occur postpartum. The upper trunk of the brachial plexus is usually affected. It presents with attacks of neuropathic pain in the shoulder, followed by upper limb weakness and atrophy. The hereditary form is related to mutations in the SEPT9 gene on chromosome 17q25. Treatment with steroid may be considered, but no proven therapy.
    2. Lumbosacral plexopathies occur during the third trimester or delivery. Malpresentation and fetal macrosomia are risk factors. Muscles innervated by L4/L5 are most often affected. Patients present with pelvic and proximal leg weakness and pain with associated weakness in ankle inversion, eversion, and dorsiflexion. The S1 deep tendon reflex is usually spared. Management is conservative.
  C. Polyneuropathies:
    1. Guillain-Barré syndrome: Incidence and course are unaffected by pregnancy. Treatment is either a course of plasma exchange or intravenous immunoglobulin (IVIG); there have been no reported treatment-related complications in pregnancy. In general, acute inflammatory demyelinating polyneuropathy (AIDP) does not

affect uterine contractility, and operative delivery can be reserved for obstetric indications.

2. Chronic inflammatory demyelinating polyradiculopathy relapse rate is three times greater during pregnancy, mostly occurring during the third trimester and postpartum period. Studies are limited due to peak incidence between 40 and 60 years of age.

3. Diabetic polyneuropathy has several autonomic manifestations that can complicate pregnancy. Gastroparesis exacerbates nausea and vomiting in pregnancy, leading to malnutrition and poor blood glucose control; patients may benefit from metoclopramide or erythromycin (Category B).

4. Polyneuropathy related to nutritional deficiencies can present during pregnancy, especially in association with hyperemesis gravidarum. The most common nutritional deficiencies are thiamine, pyridoxine, and cobalamin. Cobalamin deficiency may also present with ophthalmoparesis, nystagmus, or other features of Wernicke encephalopathy. To diagnose a nutritional deficiency, serum B_6 and whole blood thiamine can be accurately measured; however, serum B_{12} studies should be accompanied by methylmalonic acid and homocysteine levels to increase diagnostic yield. B_6 supplementation has been used to treat emesis during pregnancy, and B_6 toxicity may also be a cause of polyneuropathy.

5. Acute intermittent porphyria: Pregnancy may induce crisis in some patients. Most relapses occur early; the most serious (15%) occur in the second and third trimester or are complicated by hypertension, hyperemesis, eclampsia, and preexisting renal disease. These cases are associated with prematurity and high fetal and maternal mortality.

6. Charcot-Marie-Tooth (CMT) disease may worsen during pregnancy. However, retrospective data on pregnancy outcomes in CMT are usually favorable.

D. Myotonic dystrophy disability remains the same or worsens during pregnancy, especially the third trimester. Regional anesthesia is preferred, and depolarizing muscle relaxants are contraindicated. Polyhydramnios suggests fetal myotonia.

II. Movement disorders

A. Chorea gravidarum (chorea arising during pregnancy) occurs in slightly more than 1 in 100,000 pregnancies. It is closely linked to connective tissue disorders, but the most common cause is likely drug-induced. The chorea usually begins in the first trimester, and spontaneously resolves before delivery in one-third, and after delivery in the remainder of patients. It recurs with subsequent pregnancies in about 20%. Symptomatic treatment is reserved for situations in which the patient (or fetus) would be adversely affected by the continuation of the chorea. Haloperidol and chlorpromazine are helpful in the second and third trimesters and are safe in low doses.

B. Restless leg syndrome (RLS) is the most common movement disorder in pregnancy. It can occur for the first time during pregnancy, and it usually resolves after delivery. The majority of women with pre-existing RLS will experience worsening of symptoms during pregnancy. There is an increased prevalence of RLS in the pregnant population, which may be due to iron or folate deficiency (known RLS risk factors).

III. Autoimmune disorders

A. Multiple sclerosis (MS): There is a decreased annualized relapse rate during pregnancy, with the lowest point in the third trimester, compared to the year before pregnancy. However, in the 3 months postpartum, there is an increased relapse rate. Available evidence suggests that breastfeeding is safe for MS patients. Glatiramer acetate has the most favorable data regarding pregnancy. Breastfeeding does not preclude the use of glatiramer acetate or interferon-β. Teriflunomide is pregnancy category X, requiring washout with elimination procedure.

B. The disease course of myasthenia gravis (MG) is unpredictably altered by pregnancy. MG may initially present during pregnancy or the postpartum period. The disease is worsened or unmasked in about one-third of patients during their pregnancy, and immediate postpartum exacerbation occurs frequently. Respiratory status must be monitored closely throughout the pregnancy. Corticosteroids, plasma exchange, and IVIG have been safely used during pregnancy. Magnesium sulfate, scopolamine, and large amounts of procaine are contraindicated. Care must be taken in the use of anesthesia and sedative drugs. Newborns should be observed carefully for 72 hours for neonatal myasthenia, due to passive transfer of the acetylcholine receptor antibodies from the maternal circulation. There is no contraindication to breastfeeding while using anticholinesterase drugs or prednisone.

IV. Cerebrovascular disease

A. Hemorrhagic stroke and vascular malformations: Pregnancy increases the risk of hemorrhagic stroke much higher than ischemic stroke; the greatest risk is in the early postpartum period. Causes of pregnancy-related hemorrhagic stroke include preeclampsia/eclampsia, arteriovenous malformations (AVMs), and aneurysms. Risk of aneurysmal rupture increases several fold, rising with gestational age until it peaks at 30 to 34 weeks. Mortality of pregnancy-associated aneurysmal subarachnoid hemorrhage (SAH) is 35%, with a fetal mortality of 17%; mortality can be greatly reduced by early surgery. Women with SAH should be evaluated by a neurointerventionalist, and the decision to treat should be based on the same criteria used in non-pregnant patients. Hyperventilation, hypertonic saline, hypothermia, and steroids have been safely used during pregnancy, but mannitol should be restricted. An untreated aneurysm is a relative contraindication to future pregnancies.

B. Cerebral ischemia: Pregnancy-associated ischemic stroke is rare; however, the risk of ischemic stroke is increased almost nine times during the first 6 weeks postpartum. Cardioembolism, preeclampsia/eclampsia, and cerebral venous sinus thrombosis account for most pregnancy-related ischemic stroke. The assessment of the pregnant patient with transient ischemic attacks or stroke is the same as that of stroke in a young person. Current guidelines suggest that no adverse fetal effects are associated with magnetic resonance imaging (MRI). Intravenous tissue plasminogen activator (tPA) has a short half-life and does not cross the placenta. Nevertheless, there are several concerns with its use in the pregnant population, including maternal hemorrhage, placental hemorrhage/abruption, fetal loss, and preterm delivery. At present, recombinant tissue plasminogen activator should be considered during pregnancy for all potentially disabling strokes. Mechanical thrombectomy for stroke secondary to large vessel occlusion should be considered as well. Warfarin and aspirin are both contraindicated in pregnancy.

C. Others: Sheehan syndrome of postpartum hypopituitarism is secondary to pituitary infarction (usually the anterior pituitary) due to severe shock at the time of delivery. Failure to lactate is followed by amenorrhea, hypothyroidism, and hypoadrenocorticism. Carotid cavernous sinus fistula has also been reported during the second half of pregnancy. Reversible segmental cerebral vasoconstriction is a rare syndrome presenting with headache and focal deficits, frequently in the early postpartum period.

V. Neoplasms: Excluding pituitary tumors, primary intracranial tumors do not have an increased incidence during pregnancy. Most primary brain tumors will enlarge during pregnancy and shrink again postpartum. This appears to be secondary to the intrapartum increase in intravascular volume or tumor hormone dependence. Therefore, symptoms or signs may be more apparent during the second half of pregnancy. Although slow-growing tumors can be resected postpartum, malignant gliomas and many posterior fossa tumors require prompt surgery. Choriocarcinomas frequently metastasize, and are usually hemorrhagic, to the brain.

VI. Headaches: Headaches are frequent during pregnancy. Extensive evaluation, including neuroimaging, is often required because aneurysms and AVMs may present during this period. Primary headaches account for the majority of headaches during pregnancy. Of the primary headaches, tension-type headache and migraine generally improve during pregnancy. Secondary causes of headache that are more likely to occur during pregnancy include cerebral venous thrombosis, posterior reversible encephalopathy syndrome, stroke, and pituitary apoplexy. Nondrug therapies that are safe and effective include relaxation, biofeedback, exercise, sleep hygiene, and physical therapy. Acetaminophen is the analgesic of choice for the short-term relief of mild to moderate pain and pyrexia. Aspirin and non-steroidal anti-inflammatories should be avoided in the third trimester because they are associated with premature closure of the fetal ductus arteriosus. Although opiates are safe for treatment of mild to moderate pain in pregnancy, they are inappropriate for migraine because they worsen nausea and reduce gastric motility. If prophylaxis is necessary during pregnancy, the lowest effective doses of metoprolol or propranolol are the drugs of choice.

VII. Epilepsy: Women with epilepsy contribute to an estimated 0.3% to 0.5% of all births. Pregnant women during epilepsy can be divided into two subtypes: gestational epilepsy and chronic seizure disorders.

A. Gestational epilepsy constitutes seizures occurring only during pregnancy. Only 25% have recurrent seizures during subsequent pregnancies. The seizures tend to occur in the sixth or seventh month of gestation. Most patients have no identifiable, underlying pathology. However, a small proportion will have an underlying lesion, such as tumor or vascular malformation.

B. In chronic seizure disorder, the onset of seizure is before pregnancy. Fifteen percent of these women will have an increase in seizure frequency, but most women will experience no change in seizure frequency. Less than 1% of all epileptic women experience status epilepticus during pregnancy. Multiple factors are responsible for exacerbation of seizures, including decreased antiepileptic drug (AED) levels, hormonal changes, stress, sleep deprivation, and medication noncompliance.

Pregnant women with epilepsy have been reported to be at increased risk for a number of complications such as vaginal bleeding, premature labor or delivery, abruptio placentae, fetal loss, and premature eclampsia. The rate of spontaneous abortions is comparable to that of the general population. Perinatal mortality rate is increased 1.2- to 3-fold. A convulsive seizure occurs during labor in 1% to 2% of women with epilepsy and in another 1% to 2% within 24 hours postpartum. Total AED concentration declines during pregnancy; there is an induction of AED metabolism by the high hormone levels affecting both total and unbound compartments of the circulating AED. Therefore, it is recommended to measure serum AED levels during pregnancy. Ideally, an individual therapeutic level at which the patient is doing well is documented before pregnancy. The reversal of pregnancy-induced physiologic changes postpartum may cause drug toxicity, so drug levels should be checked periodically for at least the first 2 months after delivery.

C. Epilepsy and birth defects: More than 90% of women with epilepsy who receive AEDs will deliver normal children free of birth defects. Major malformations and minor anomalies occur in a small but significant percentage of fetuses (6% to 8%) exposed in utero to AEDs. These children have been reported to be at increased risk for low birth weight, low Apgar scores, prematurity, microcephaly, prenatal and infant death, mental deficiency, development delay, and epilepsy. Risks to the fetus are probably higher when AEDs are used in combination and when there is a family history of birth defects. Dose-related risks are likely to be present with most AED intrauterine exposure. The most clearly demonstrated dose-related risk is a marked risk increase with maternal use of valproate at more than 700 mg per day. It is advisable to give folate supplementation before conception, as well as to treat with monotherapy that is adjusted to the lowest effective level to avoid unnecessary fetal exposure. Folic acid does not eliminate the risk of major congenital malformations associated with AED use.

VIII. Eclampsia: Unique to pregnancy, eclampsia is heralded by the onset of hypertension, proteinuria, and edema, occurring after 20 weeks' gestation, usually in a young primigravida. It may be complicated by oliguria or multiorgan failure. Eclampsia is also associated with chronic hypertension and renal disease. Maternal mortality rate ranges from 0% to 14%. There is now compelling scientific evidence in favor of magnesium sulfate rather than diazepam or phenytoin for treating eclamptic seizures. Hypertension control and fluid management are required. Delivery of the fetus and placenta is the definitive treatment for eclampsia occurring prepartum or intrapartum.

REFERENCES

Calhoun, A. H. (2017). Migraine treatment in pregnancy and lactation. *Curr Pain Headache Rep*, *21*(11), 46.

Feske, S., & Singhal, A. (2014). Cerebrovascular disorders complicating pregnancy. *Continuum*, *20*(1), 80–99.

PROGRESSIVE SUPRANUCLEAR PALSY

Progressive supranuclear palsy (PSP) is a type of atypical parkinsonism first described more than 50 years ago by Steele, Richardson, and Olszewski; it is the most common form of atypical parkinsonism, with an estimated annual incidence of 5 per 100,000 between age 50 and 99 years. Mean age at diagnosis is 65 years.

There are five well-established types of PSP, including:
1. Classic PSP or Richardson syndrome (RS),
2. PSP parkinsonism (PSP-P),
3. PSP corticobasal syndromes (PSP-CBS),

4. PSP with pure akinesia and gait freezing (PSP-PAGF),
5. PSP with behavioral variant of frontotemporal dementia, and two relatively new forms described as PSP with primary lateral sclerosis and PSP with cerebellar ataxia.

PATHOLOGY

Almost always a tauopathy, with abnormal tau hyper phosphorylation and deposition in the brain, with an increased 4-repeat:3-repeat tau ratio in brain. Histologic findings include tau-immunoreactive tufted astrocytes, neurofibrillary tangles, coiled bodies, and neuronal loss and gliosis. Cause is unknown, and the only established risk factor is advanced age. Genetic mutations in tau and several other genes have been reported.

DIAGNOSIS

Is primarily clinical and there are no specific biomarkers. PSP is distinguished from idiopathic Parkinson disease and from other atypical forms of parkinsonism by early onset gait/postural instability and falls, with the gait described as "drunken sailor" or "dancing bear"; unresponsiveness to levodopa (except PSP-P sub-type, which may initially be levodopa responsive); slow vertical saccades eventually leading to supranuclear palsy due to midbrain atrophy dysphagia and dysarthria, executive dysfunction. Limitation of downgaze is considered to be more sensitive than upgaze for PSP. Pseudo bulbar laughing or crying is often seen, in addition to blepharospasm and eyelid opening apraxia.

PSP subtypes show the following differences: PSP-P features early asymmetric bradykinesia, axial rigidity, and tremor resembling PD; PSP-PAGF presents with primary freezing gait mostly with initiation; PSP-CBS with asymmetric unilateral limb apraxia, alien limb phenomenon, dystonia; PSP-bvFTD with predominant behavioral and cognitive dysfunction.

The National Institute for Neurological Disorders and Stroke PSP criteria have three categories: *Possible PSP* requires the presence of a gradually progressive disorder with onset at age 40 or later, with either vertical supranuclear gaze palsy, or both slowing of vertical saccades and prominent postural instability with falls in the first year of onset, as well as no evidence of other diseases that could explain these features. *Probable PSP* requires vertical supranuclear gaze palsy, prominent postural instability, and falls in the first year of onset, as well as the other features of possible PSP. *Definite PSP* requires a history of probable or possible PSP and histopathologic evidence of typical PSP.

IMAGING

MRI may show the "hummingbird sign" on mid-sagittal section due to midbrain atrophy. Positron emission tomography with tau ligand is a promising tool for diagnosis but remains a research tool. Diffusion tension imaging may show white matter tract degeneration in the superior cerebellar peduncle, associated with RS.

TREATMENT

Treatment is supportive and should include a multidisciplinary approach with physical therapy for gait training and balance, occupational therapy for fine motor skills, and speech therapy for assistance with cognition, communication, and dysphagia. A trial of levodopa to a maximum dose of 1200 mg/day for 1 month is recommended. Dopamine agonists should be avoided due to minimum benefit and more side effects. Amantadine is recommended for gait freezing and dysphagia. Avoid anticholinergics as they worsen cognitive function. Botulinum toxin is used for blepharospasm and dystonia and cholinesterase inhibitor such as rivastigmine is used for associated dementia.

PROGNOSIS

Overall survival has an estimated median from 5 to 8 years depending on symptoms at time of diagnosis. Since PSP is uniformly fatal, consideration for end of life care and its ethical concerns is critical for clinicians to communicate in a sensitive and appropriate manner. The use of feeding tubes to prevent aspiration and pneumonia, the most common cause of death, is sometimes considered, but likely does not increase survival time, and may be considered as heroic intervention.

REFERENCES

Ling, H. (2016). Clinical approach to progressive supranuclear palsy. *J Mov Disord*, 9(1), 3–13. https://doi.org/10.14802/jmd.15060.

McFarland, N. R. (2016). Diagnostic approach to atypical Parkinsonian syndromes. *Continuum (Minneap Minn)*, 22(4), 1117–1142.

P

PSEUDOBULBAR PALSY

PSEUDOBULBAR PALSY

"Bulb" is a synonym for the medulla oblongata. As such, a lesion of medullary cranial nerve nuclei would result in a bulbar palsy. The syndrome resulting from a lesion of bilateral descending cortical tracts containing the upper motor neurons going to these nuclei is referred to as pseudobulbar palsy.

The symptoms of pseudobulbar palsy include dysphagia, dysarthria, bilateral facial weakness, and emotional lability.

Most lower brainstem nuclei are bilaterally innervated. Unilateral involvement of descending supranuclear pathways, therefore, may not produce symptoms. Bilateral involvement of corticobulbar fibers and frontal efferents subserving emotional expression, which pass through the genu of the internal capsule and the medial cerebral peduncles, results in pseudobulbar palsy. This should be distinguished from nuclear involvement (see "Bulbar Palsy"). In pseudobulbar palsy, there is decreased voluntary movement and spastic hyperreflexia of the involved muscles. Thus, gag and jaw jerk reflexes may be hyperactive, even though the patient is unable to swallow or chew. Frequently, there is a spontaneous release of emotional responses such as crying or laughing with little or no provocation (labile emotion). Frontal release signs (grasp, palmomental, suck, snout, rooting, and glabellar reflexes) may be prominent. These should be interpreted with caution, because many normal elderly persons (over age 80 years) exhibit palmomental and snout reflexes. Dementia is frequently present in patients with pseudobulbar palsy.

Although a variety of lesions (demyelinating disease, motor neuron disease) can interrupt the corticobulbar and anterior frontopontomedullary fibers, infarction is most common.

A syndrome similar to pseudobulbar palsy may occur with bilateral involvement of the opercular cortex, producing the anterior operculum syndrome (Foix-Chavany-Marie syndrome). It differs from classical pseudobulbar palsy in that emotional symptoms are rare, and there is loss of voluntary control of facial, pharyngeal, lingual, masticatory, or ocular muscles, with retention of reflexive and automatic movements in these muscle groups. This syndrome may be acquired or congenital as in Worster-Drought syndrome.

Successful treatment of pseudobulbar palsy, especially the emotional lability, has been reported with selective serotonin reuptake inhibitors (SSRIs), amitriptyline, levodopa, and amantadine.

REFERENCE

Christen, H. J., Hanefeld, F., Kruse, E., et al. (2000). Foix-Chavany-Marie (anterior operculum) syndrome in childhood: a reappraisal of Worster-Drought syndrome. *Dev Med Child Neurol, 42*, 122–132.

PSEUDOTUMOR CEREBRI

Pseudotumor cerebri, or idiopathic intracranial hypertension (IIH), is characterized by clinical signs and symptoms of increased intracranial pressure (ICP) without evidence of intracranial mass, infection, hydrocephalus, dural venous sinus thrombosis, or other apparent structural central nervous system (CNS) pathology on neuroimaging studies and cerebrospinal fluid (CSF) examination.

CLINICAL FEATURES

More than 90% of IIH patients are obese, and more than 90% are women. Mean age at diagnosis is about 30 years. Symptoms of IIH include headache (most frequent), nausea/vomiting, dizziness, pulsatile tinnitus, "sounds in head," transient visual obscurations, and changes in visual acuity that may lead to total vision loss, diplopia, and pain on eye movements. Signs include optic disk swelling, cranial nerve (CN) VI palsy, contrast sensitivity deficits, color vision loss, constricted visual fields, and visual loss late in the course. Blind spot enlargement is always present with papilledema.

ETIOLOGY

Unknown; disorders associated with IIH are obesity and hypertension. Rarely, IIH is associated with endocrinopathies, hyper/hypovitaminosis A, anemia, recent use of medications (tetracycline, indomethacin, nalidixic acid, nitrofurantoin, oral contraceptives, lithium), and prolonged use of corticosteroids. Systemic disorders linked with IIH include systemic lupus, hyperthyroidism, iron deficiency, and venous sinus thrombosis. An increased incidence of IIH is seen during pregnancy.

DIAGNOSIS

Diagnosis is made by history and exam, demonstration of increased ICP and exclusion of other causes of headache, papilledema, and increased ICP. This requires neuroimaging with magnetic resonance imaging (MRI) and lumbar puncture (LP). Dural venous sinus thrombosis must be ruled out with either CT or MR venography.

TREATMENT

Medical therapy includes acetazolamide 500 mg TID (may cause acroparesthesia) or Topamax slowly tapered up to 100 mg BID with secondary benefit of loss of weight. Lasix may also be tried. Surgical approaches may be considered in refractory cases and may include ventriculo-peritoneal shunt, lumboperitoneal drain placement, optic nerve fenestration, and gastric bypass. A more recent endovascular approach requires referral to an interventional neurologist for sinus venous stenting with evaluation with venography first to measure the pressure gradient across the area of stenosis.

REFERENCES

Levitt, M. R., Hlubek, R. J., Moon, K., et al. (2017). Incidence and predictors of dural venous sinus pressure gradient in idiopathic intracranial hypertension and non-idiopathic intracranial hypertension headache patients: results from 164 cerebral venograms. *J Neurosurg*, *126*(2), 347–353.

Sheldon, C. A., Paley, G. L., Beres, S. J., et al. (2017). Pediatric pseudotumor cerebri syndrome: diagnosis, classification, and underlying pathophysiology. *Semin Pediatr Neurol*, *24*(2), 110–115.

PTOSIS

Ptosis is the drooping of the upper eyelid and may be caused by paralysis of the third cranial nerve or dysfunction of sympathetic innervation. The differential diagnosis of ptosis is vast and includes the following:

I. Congenital ptosis
   A. Isolated
   B. With double elevator palsy
   C. Anomalous synkinesis (including Gunn jaw winking)
   D. Lid or orbital tumor (hemangioma, dermoid)
   E. Neurofibromatosis
   F. Blepharophimosis syndromes
   G. First branchial arch syndromes (Hallermann-Streiff, Treacher Collins)
   H. Neonatal myasthenia
II. Ptosis resulting from myopathy and neuromuscular junction disease
   A. Myasthenia gravis ptosis may be variable and asymmetrical; may see Cogan's lid twitch sign; improves with edrophonium
   B. Myopathy restricted to levator palpebrae superioris or including external ophthalmoplegia

C. Oculopharyngeal muscular dystrophy

D. Myotonic dystrophy

E. Polymyositis

F. Aplastic levator muscle

G. Dysthyroidism

H. Chronic progressive external ophthalmoplegia

I. Levator dehiscence-disinsertion syndrome resulting from aging, inflammation, surgery, trauma, or ocular allergy

III. Ptosis resulting from sympathetic denervation (see Horner syndrome)

IV. Ptosis resulting from third-nerve lesions

    A. Nuclear lesions involving the levator subnucleus produce severe bilateral ptosis, medial rectus weakness, skew deviation if the intravenous (IV) nerve is involved, or upgaze paresis and pupillary dilatation if entire third-nerve nucleus is involved.

    B. Peripheral third-nerve lesions produce unilateral ptosis with mydriasis and ophthalmoplegia; isolated ptosis is rare.

V. Pseudoptosis

    A. Trachoma

    B. Ptosis adiposis

    C. Blepharochalasis

    D. Plexiform neuroma

    E. Amyloid infiltration

    F. Inflammation resulting from allergy, chalazion, blepharitis, conjunctivitis

    G. Hemangioma

    H. Duane retraction syndrome

    I. Microphthalmos phthisis bulbi

    J. Enopthalmos

    K. Pathologic lid retraction on opposite side

    L. Chronic Bell palsy

    M. Hypertropia

    N. Decreased mental status

    O. Functional disorders

REFERENCE

Roy, F. H. (2012). Lids. In *Ocular differential diagnosis* (pp. 24–110). Little Rock, AR: JP Medical Ltd.

PUPIL

Pupils are examined in both light and darkness, with attention to size, shape, and reactivity to light.

Bilateral dilation (mydriasis) may be produced by the following:

I. Drugs (Table 108)

II. Emotional state

III. Thyrotoxicosis

IV. Ciliospinal reflex

TABLE 108

DRUG EFFECTS ON THE PUPILS

Miotics (Cause Constriction)	Mydriatics (Cause Dilation)

SYSTEMIC EFFECT

Narcotics	Anticholinergics
Morphine and opium alkaloids	Atropine
Meperidine	Belladonna
Methadone	Scopolamine
Propoxyphene	Propantheline
Barbiturates	Jimsonweed
Diphenoxylate	Nightshade
Chloral hydrate	Tricyclic antidepressants
Phenoxybenzamine	Trihexyphenidyl
Dibenzyline	Benztropine
Phentolamine	Antihistamines
Tolazoline	Diphenhydramine
Guanethidine	Chlorpheniramine
Bretylium	Phenothiazines
Reserpine	Glutethimide
Monoamine oxidase inhibitors	Amphetamines
Alpha-methyldopa	Cocaine
Bethanidine	Ephedrine
Thymoxamine	Epinephrine
Indoramin	Norepinephrine
Meprobamate	Ethanol
Cholinergics	Botulinum toxin
Edrophonium	Snake venom
Neostigmine	Barracuda poisoning
Pyridostigmine	Tyramine
Cholinesterase inhibitor pesticides	Hemicholinium
Phencyclidine	Magnesium compound
	(hypermagnesemia)
Thallium	Thiopental
Lidocaine and related agents	Lysergic acid diethylamide
Marijuana	Fenfluramine

LOCAL EFFECT

Pilocarpine	Phenylephrine
Carbachol	Hydroxyamphetamine
Methacholine	Epinephrine
Physostigmine	Cocaine
Neostigmine	Eucatropine
Isoflurophate	Atropine
Echothiophate	Homatropine
Demecarium	Scopolamine
Aceclidine	Cyclopentolate
Tropicamide	
Oxyphenonium	

Modified from Thurston, S. E. & Leigh, R. J. (1985). [chapter title]. In R. J. Henning & D. L. Jackson (Eds.), *Handbook of critical care neurology and neurosurgery*. New York: Praeger.

   V. Bilateral blindness resulting from severe visual system involvement anterior to the chiasm

   VI. Parinaud syndrome

   VII. Seizures

VIII. During rostrocaudal herniation caused by supratentorial mass lesions bilateral constriction (miosis) may be produced by the following:

   I. Near triad (accommodation, convergence, miosis)

   II. Old age

   III. Drugs (see Table 108)

   IV. Pontine lesions

   V. Argyll Robertson pupils

Pupillary constriction is driven by the Edinger-Westphal nucleus, which receives afferent input from the retina by way of the pretectooculomotor tract (Fig. 56).

Anisocoria, or unequal pupil size, can be an important localizing sign. A difference of less than 1 mm exists in approximately 20% of the normal population, more than 1 mm in as much as 5%. The asymmetry remains constant in light and dark. Drugs and toxins, including eye drops, may cause constriction or dilation of pupils, which is usually symmetrical unless agents are applied locally in one eye. Causes of significant anisocoria may be determined on a clinical and pharmacologic basis using Table 109.

Causes of episodic anisocoria include the following:

   I. Parasympathetic paresis (incipient uncal herniation, seizure, migraine)

   II. Parasympathetic hyperactivity (cyclic oculomotor paresis)

   III. Sympathetic paresis (cluster headache [paratrigeminal neuralgia])

   IV. Sympathetic hyperactivity (Claude-Bernard syndrome following neck trauma)

   V. Sympathetic dysfunction with alternating anisocoria (cervical spinal cord lesions)

   VI. Benign unilateral pupillary dilation (involved pupil has normal light and near responses)

Relative afferent pupillary defect (RAPD) (Fig. 57), also called Marcus Gunn pupil, results from a lesion of the optic nerve. Resting pupil sizes are normal. Both direct and consensual pupillary responses are decreased with bright illumination of the involved side, whereas both responses are normal with illumination of the normal side. When alternately stimulating each eye ("swinging flashlight test"), both pupils dilate with stimulation on the abnormal side, and both constrict with the stimulation on the normal side.

The near reflex should be tested whenever pupils react poorly to light. Have the patient fixate a distant target, then quickly fixate their own fingertip held immediately in front of their nose.

Light-near dissociation may occur in the following:

   I. Severe anterior visual dysfunction (such as severe glaucoma, bilateral optic neuropathy)

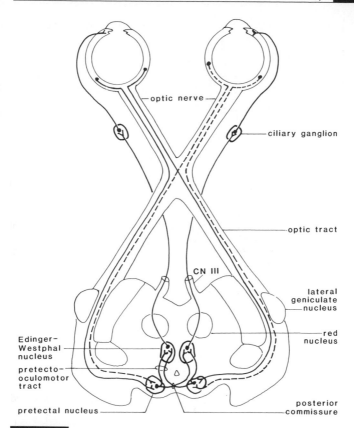

FIGURE 56

Pupillary light reflex pathways.

 II. Neurosyphilis (Argyll Robertson pupil)
III. Adie's tonic pupil: Holmes-Adie syndrome, in which nearly 90% of the people have diminished deep tendon reflexes and orthostatic hypotension. Seventy percent are females. In 80% of patients, there is unilateral involvement, although the second pupil may become involved later.
IV. Rostral dorsal midbrain syndrome (Parinaud syndrome)
 V. Aberrant III nerve regeneration
VI. Diabetes (out of proportion to any retinopathy)
VII. Amyloidosis
VIII. Myotonic dystrophy

TABLE 109

CHARACTERISTICS OF PUPILS ENCOUNTERED IN NEURO-OPHTHALMOLOGY

Condition	General Characteristics	Responses to Light and Near Stimuli	Room Condition in Which Anisocoria Is Greater	Response to Mydriatics	Response to Miotics	Response to Pharmacologic Agents
Essential anisocoria	Round, regular	Both brisk	No change	Dilates	Constricts	Normal and rarely needed
Horner syndrome	Small, round, unilateral	Both brisk	Darkness	Dilates	Constricts	Cocaine 4%, poor dilation; paredrine 1% no dilation if third-order neuron damage
Tonic pupil syndrome (Holmes-Adie syndrome)	Usually larger[a] in bright light; sector pupil palsy, vermiform movement; unilateral or, less often, bilateral	Absent to light, tonic to near; tonic redilation	Light	Dilates	Constricts	Pilocarpine 0.1% or 0.125%, constricts; mecholyl 2.5%, constricts
Argyll Robertson pupils	Small, irregular, bilateral	Poor to light, better to near	No change	Poor	Constricts	
Midbrain pupils	Mid-dilated; may be oval; bilateral	Poor to light, better to near (or fixed to both)	No change	Dilates	Constricts	
Pharmacologically dilated pupils	Very large,[b] round, unilateral	Fixed[b]	Light	Poor	No[c]	Pilocarpine 1%, does not constrict
Oculomotor palsy (nonvascular)	Mid-dilated (6–7 mm), unilateral (rarely bilateral)	Fixed	Light	Dilates	Constricts	

[a]Tonic pupil may appear smaller following prolonged near-effort or in dim illumination; affected pupil is initially large, but with passing time gradually becomes smaller.

[b]Atropinized pupils have diameters of 8 to 9 mm. No tonic, midbrain, or oculomotor palsy pupil ever is this large.

[c]Pupils may be weakly reactive, depending on interim after instillation.

From Glaser, J. S. (1989). *Neuro-ophthalmology.* Philadelphia: Lippincott.

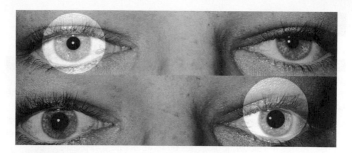

FIGURE 57

A swinging flashlight test revealing a relative afferent pupillary defect. (From Liferidge, A. What is a Marcus Gunn pupil? University of Maryland School of Medicine Department of Emergency Medicine Educational Pearls. https://umem.org/educational_pearls/1568/. Accessed October 23, 2017.)

LESIONS OF THE MIDBRAIN

Efferent pupillary defects may occur with lesions involving the oculomotor nucleus or the fascicles of the third nerve coursing ventrally to exit the brainstem. Generally, other signs of brainstem involvement or third-nerve palsy will also be apparent.

Three syndromes are clinically important:

I. Argyll Robertson pupil: Some patients have tertiary syphilis involving the CNS. Affected patients have small irregular pupils, less than approximately 2 mm, which do not react to light with normal near response (light-near dissociation) and visual acuity. Similar pupils are seen in diabetes mellitus, chronic alcoholism, and encephalitis.

II. Parinaud dorsal midbrain syndrome: This is seen in pineal tumors. Pupils are midposition with light-near dissociation. Afferent pupillary pathways in the pretectum are usually affected. Dorsal midbrain syndrome also causes paresis of conjugate upgaze (occasionally downgaze), convergence retraction nystagmus, lid lag, and Collier sign (lid retraction).

III. Pretectal afferent pupillary defects: Occasionally, a pretectal lesion will be predominantly unilateral and hence produce RAPD.

REFERENCE

Loewenfield, I. E. (1993). *The pupil: anatomy, physiology and clinical applications.* (vol 1). Ames: Iowa State University.

R

RADIAL NERVE

ANATOMY

The radial nerve is formed by axons from C5 to T1 roots and is branched off the lateral cord of the brachial plexus. Axons pass through several structures including the spiral groove of humerus, fibrous arch attachment of triceps to humerus, lateral intermuscular septum below deltoid insertion, and arcade of Frohse. Above the elbow, it branches off to innervate triceps, anconeus, brachioradialis, extensor carpi radialis longus/brevis, and posterior cutaneous nerves of the arm and forearm. At or below the elbow, branches are divided so that they come off either before or after the arcade of Frohse. Branches that come off the radial nerve before the arcade of Frohse include the superficial radial nerve, which supplies sensory innervation to dorsolateral hand and the first 3 1/2 digits, and the posterior interosseus nerve, which innervates the extensor carpi radialis brevis and supinator. Branches below the arcade of Frohse are the terminal motor branch of the posterior interosseus nerves, which innervate finger/thumb extensor, extensor carpi ulnaris, abductor pollicis longus, and articular branches to the wrist joint. Radial nerve injury is the least affected nerve among the three major nerves (median, ulnar, and radial) in the upper extremities. Radial nerve compression or injury may occur at any point along the anatomic course, ranging from proximally, involving brachial plexus, to distally, involving the radial aspect of the wrist, and may have varied causes (Table 110). The most frequent site of compression is in the proximal forearm in the area of the supinator muscle and involves the posterior interosseous branch.

TABLE 110

RADIAL NERVE LESION: LOCATION VERSUS ETIOLOGY

Location of Lesion	Etiology
Axilla	Pressure palsy; often occurs in sedated patient
Upper arm	Pressure,[a] fracture of humerus,[b] injection and neonatal
Posterior interosseus	Radial fracture, soft tissue mass, laceration, supinator syndrome[c]
Superficial radial	Rupture, synovial effusion, compression, trauma, surgery, injection, and nerve tumor

[a]Pressure on medial arm compressing against humerus; often seen in sleep paralysis (Saturday night palsy), during anesthesia, and with tourniquet.
[b]Holstein-Lewis fracture, mid-third humerus fracture.
[c]Related to repetitive pronation-supination movement. Sometimes mistakenly referred to as "resistant tennis elbow." Maximum tenderness located 4 to 5 cm distal to lateral epicondyle.

SYNDROMES

I. *Radial tunnel syndrome* is characterized by pain over the anterolateral proximal forearm in the region of the radial neck. This syndrome often appears in individuals whose work requires repetitive elbow extension or forearm rotation. It is sometimes mistakenly referred to as "resistant tennis elbow." The maximum tenderness is located 4 to 5 fingerbreadths distal to the lateral epicondyle, as compared with lateral epicondylitis (seen in tennis elbow), in which maximum tenderness is usually directly over the epicondyle. Symptoms are intensified by extending the elbow and pronating the forearm. In addition, resisted active supination and extension of the long finger cause pain. Weakness and numbness usually are not demonstrated.

II. *Posterior interosseous syndrome:* The etiology of posterior interosseous nerve syndrome is similar to that of radial tunnel syndrome. Compression is thought to occur after takeoff of the branches to the radial wrist extensors and the sensory branches. After emerging from the supinator, the nerve may be compressed before it bifurcates into medial and lateral branches, causing a complete paralysis of the digital extensors and dorsoradial deviation of the wrist secondary to paralysis of the extensor carpi ulnaris. If compression occurs after the nerve bifurcates, selective paralysis of muscles occurs, depending on which branch is involved. Compression of the medial branch causes paralysis of the extensor carpi ulnaris, extensor digiti quinti, and extensor digitorum communis. Compression of the lateral branch causes paralysis of the abductor pollicis longus, extensor pollicis brevis, extensor pollicis longus, and extensor indicis proprius. Most commonly, entrapment occurs at the proximal edge of the supinator.

III. *Wartenberg syndrome:* Patients with the diagnosis of Wartenberg syndrome complain of pain over the distal radial forearm associated with paresthesia over the dorsal radial hand. They frequently report symptom magnification with wrist movement or when tightly pinching the thumb and index digit. These individuals demonstrate a positive Tinel sign over the superficial radial sensory nerve and local tenderness. Hyperpronation of the forearm can cause a positive Tinel sign. A high percentage of these patients reveal physical examination findings consistent with De Quervain's tenosynovitis.

DIAGNOSIS

Plain x-ray can be obtained to rule out fracture, dislocation, bone tumor, and arthrosis. Magnetic resonance imaging (MRI) can be used to look for soft tissue lipoma, ganglioma, aneurysm, and synovitis. Electromyography (EMG) can also be really useful in determining the location, the timing (acute, subacute, or chronic), and the severity (demyelination or axon lost) of the nerve injury. However, EMG can be normal in the acute setting before Wallerian degeneration occurs, which usually takes about 3 to 7 days. High-resolution ultrasound evaluation of focal neuropathies may also be used in delineating nerve entrapment.

R

RADIAL NERVE

TREATMENT

A period of immobilization and anti-inflammatory medication may diminish swelling and improve symptoms. In addition, functional splints help prevent contracture and improve function as signs of nerve healing follow. Surgical approach, especially for radial tunnel syndrome, is highly controversial. However, surgical approach would be warranted if the nerve injury is caused by structure compression (i.e., bone tumor, lipoma).

REFERENCES

Hobson-Webb, L. D., & Juel, V. C. (2017). Common entrapment neuropathies. *Continuum (Minneap Minn)*, *23*, 487–511 [2, Selected Topics in Outpatient Neurology].

Peck, E., & Strakowski, J. A. (2015). Ultrasound evaluation of focal neuropathies in athletes: a clinically-focused review. *Br J Sports Med*, *49*(3), 166–175.

RADIATION INJURY

Radiation injury to the nervous system occurs either as a result of treatment of CNS tumors, when nervous tissue falls into the field of treatment of another organ system or exposure to radiation accidentally, or in warfare. Radiation can damage the cerebral cortex, spinal cord, peripheral nerves, and cerebrovascular system and induce new tumors.

CEREBRAL INJURY

I. Acute encephalopathy

Presentation and diagnosis: Occurs during the first few days of radiotherapy with headache, fever, nausea, depressed sensorium, and worsening of previous focal deficit. It is more frequent and severe in patients with large brain masses or those receiving daily dose fractions higher than 300 cGy of whole-brain irradiation. It is probably caused by an increase in preexisting cerebral edema but may not be apparent on neuroimaging.

Treatment: It responds well to increased doses of dexamethasone or pretreatment with corticosteroid 24 to 72 hours before radiotherapy in large or multiple brain tumors.

II. Early delayed encephalopathy

Presentation and diagnosis: Occurs from a few weeks up to 12 to 18 months after irradiation presenting with headache, somnolence, nausea, irritability, fever, and transient papilledema. It usually resolves after several weeks to months. Early delayed encephalopathy occurs in 50% of children who receive prophylactic whole-brain irradiation for leukemia. It is more severe in children younger than 3 years old. Magnetic resonance imaging (MRI) shows worsening edema and contrast enhancement in up to one-third of patients with gliomas within a few months after fractionated radiation therapy, and in 5% to 20% of patients following stereotactic radiosurgery for brain metastases or meningioma.

Treatment: Corticosteroids may offer symptomatic relief and hasten recovery.

III. Focal cerebral necrosis (radiation necrosis)

Presentation and diagnosis: This may develop several months to 10 years (peak onset of 15 to 18 months) after focal or whole-brain irradiation for brain tumors and head and neck cancers. It also occurs in patients who receive other forms of radiotherapy including brachytherapy, hyperfractionated radiation therapy, and stereotactic radiosurgery. Incidence is 3% to 10% after receiving 5000 cGy of daily fractionated radiation, 0% to 15% after stereotactic radiosurgery, and up to 50% of patients treated with interstitial brachytherapy. Patients usually present with a subacute space-occupying lesion. CT or MRI reveals edema and a patchy or ring-enhancing mass lesion. Positron emission tomography (PET), single photon emission computed tomography (SPECT), and several MRI techniques including MR spectroscopy, perfusion-sensitive MRI, and diffusion-weighted imaging may help to differentiate radiation necrosis from tumor recurrence and may be useful for identification of a "hot spot" for a stereotactic biopsy. Radiation necrosis occurs around the tumor and primarily involves the white matter, mostly sparing of cortex and deep gray structures, with demyelination, loss of oligodendrocytes, axonal injury, calcification, fibrillary gliosis, and mononuclear perivascular infiltrate. The most constant pathologic feature is fibrinoid vascular necrosis.

Treatment: Corticosteroids frequently provide improvement, albeit temporary. Hyperbaric oxygen treatment and high-dose vitamin E (2000 IU/day) may be of benefit in some cases. Surgical debulking of necrotic lesions may be necessary in some patients.

IV. Diffuse cerebral injury

Presentation and diagnosis: This most frequent (2% to 19%) delayed effect of radiation therapy occurs in adults with primary brain tumors receiving 4000 to 6000 cGy of whole-brain irradiation and occurs in up to 50% of children with primary brain tumors following 2500 to 4000 cGy whole-brain radiation therapy. It becomes evident as moderate to severe cortical dysfunction, progressive dementia, and gait disturbance. Initial signs include memory, attentional, and visuospatial difficulties (especially in children younger than 4 or 5 years of age), ataxia, and focal motor deficits. Children with radiation therapy and concomitant methotrexate have higher risk of developing neurocognitive impairment. MRI may show enlarged ventricles, widening sulci, areas of calcification (especially basal ganglia), and diffuse hyperintense T_2 signal abnormalities. Pathologic study shows multifocal white matter destruction, especially in the centrum semiovale and periventricular white matter, dystrophic calcification of the lenticular nuclei, and mineralizing microangiopathy.

Treatment: Methylphenidate, acetylcholinesterase inhibitors, and other psychostimulants have been used in both children and adults with attention or cognitive deficits from radiation treatment.

SPINAL CORD INJURY

I. Transient myelopathy

Presentation and diagnosis: The most common radiation-induced spinal injury, usually occurring 1 to 30 months after radiotherapy, with peak at 4 to 6 months. It occurs in 10% to 15% of patients receiving mantle field radiation therapy for Hodgkin disease. Lhermitte sign (paresthesias radiating down the spine and limbs, precipitated by neck flexion) is often present, and myelopathic signs are usually absent. CT, MRI, and myelography results are normal.

Treatment: The syndrome resolves gradually over 1 to 9 months without risk of developing delayed, severe radiation myelopathy.

II. Delayed progressive myelopathy

Presentation and diagnosis: This has a peak time of onset of 9 to 18 months after radiotherapy, with a frequency of 1% to 12%. Risk is correlated with the dose and schedule; risk is less than 5% with total doses of 4500 cGy in daily fractions of 180 cGy. Delayed progressive myelopathy usually begins with hypoesthesias or dysesthesias in lower extremities, then weakness and sphincter dysfunction. Pain is not a prominent symptom. The level of dysfunction ascends up to the area irradiated. Symptoms progress over weeks to months, with paraplegia or quadriplegia in approximately 50%. MRI may show focal or diffuse fusiform spinal cord enlargement with intrinsic cord signal abnormalities. Cerebrospinal fluid (CSF) may show high levels of protein or white blood cells. Pathologic study shows coalescing foci of demyelination, axonal degeneration, and fibrinoid vascular necrosis.

Treatment: Patients may show improvement or stabilization of symptoms spontaneously or following corticosteroids, hyperbaric oxygen, or warfarin.

III. Motor neuron syndrome

Presentation and diagnosis: Beginning 4 to 14 months after radiotherapy, this rare lower motor neuron syndrome becomes evident as subacute, diffuse leg weakness, asymmetric atrophy, fasciculations, depressed deep tendon reflexes, and flexor plantar responses without sensory or sphincter involvement. Symptoms gradually progress over several months and then stabilize without improvement. Electromyography (EMG) shows diffuse denervation in affected limb and lumbar paraspinal muscles. CSF may be normal or have increase in protein. This syndrome may result from damage to lumbosacral anterior horn cells, motor axons, or nerve roots.

Treatment: Therapy is supportive.

PERIPHERAL NERVE DAMAGE

Radiation plexopathy of the brachial or lumbosacral plexi must be distinguished from recurrent tumor in neighboring structures such as breast or lung. Radiation plexopathy tends to produce less pain but more weakness than tumor invasion. Paresthesias and edema are common. EMG may show myokymic discharges. Contrast-enhanced CT, MRI, and PET often help in differentiating radiation plexopathy from other compressive lesions.

CEREBROVASCULAR DISEASE

Extracranial carotid disease, with transient ischemic attacks or strokes, may develop 6 months to 50 years (median, 10 to 20 years) after radiation therapy for head and neck cancers. Vascular studies show disease limited to the field of radiation, including such unusual sites as proximal common carotid artery and internal carotid artery distal to the common carotid bifurcation. Occlusive disease of the intracranial arteries may follow irradiation of optic gliomas, pituitary, or suprasellar tumors (2 to 20 years later; median, 5 years). The most frequent finding on arteriography is narrowing or occlusion of the supraclinoid internal carotid artery and proximal middle cerebral artery. Vasculopathy following radiation therapy in early childhood (usually for suprasellar tumors) frequently shows a "moyamoya" pattern. Radiation-induced stenosis is better treated with stenting than open surgery.

RADIATION-INDUCED TUMORS

In order of decreasing frequency, meningiomas, gliomas, and sarcomas may occur after radiation therapy. Meningiomas have a latency of 15 to 50 years (mean, 36 years) after irradiation, and gliomas may develop approximately 10 years after irradiation.

REFERENCES

Dropcho, E. J. (2010). Neurotoxicity of radiation therapy. *Neurol Clin*, 28(1), 217–234.
Giglio, P., & Gilbert, M. R. (2010). Neurologic complications of cancer and its treatment. *Curr Oncol Rep*, 12(1), 50–59.

RADICULOPATHY

Radiculopathy is the result of any process that causes damage to or irritation of the nerve root. The spinal roots may be injured by compression (disk disease, spondylosis, hypertrophied ligaments, epidural abscess), trauma, or nondegenerative causes such as diabetes, vasculitis, tumor, infection (i.e., herpes zoster and Lyme disease), and demyelination. Cervical and lumbosacral regions are the two most commonly involved areas.

CLINICAL PRESENTATION

Radiculopathy presents as radicular pain. Radicular pain is characteristically lancinating, electrical, burning, abrupt, referred to a particular dermatome, and aggravated by maneuvers that stretch the dorsal nerve root, such as coughing or sneezing, or the Valsalva maneuver. There may be sensory changes and weakness in the affected dermatome and myotome, respectively. Exam findings comprise hypesthesia or anesthesia confined to the involved dermatome; due to overlap of cutaneous innervation, there may be little or no sensory loss on exam. Weakness may occur in the appropriate myotomal

R

RADICULOPATHY

distribution. Fasciculations may be present. Hyporeflexia or areflexia are restricted to the muscles supplied by the involved root (Table 111). Straight leg raising sign and Spurling sign (limb pain or paresthesia following extension and rotation of the neck to the side of the pain) may be present in cases of lumbar and cervical radiculopathy, respectively. Crossed straight leg raising usually indicates a larger lesion. Improvement of the radicular symptoms with shoulder abduction may also be present in cervical radiculopathy (shoulder abduction relief test). Central lumbar lesions may result in cauda equina syndrome or conus lesion (Table 112).

Although compressive radiculopathy, typically secondary to herniated intervertebral disk material, is the most common cause of radiculopathy, other mass lesions and structural abnormalities (mentioned previously) should always be considered and excluded.

EVALUATION

Magnetic resonance imaging (MRI) is currently the study of choice for most patients. Importantly, MRI with contrast should be used if there is a suspicion for nondegenerative causes of radiculopathy, such as metastatic disease or epidural abscess. Computed tomography (CT) myelography should be considered in patients with high clinical suspicion of radiculopathy whose MRI studies are normal, and when MRI is contraindicated. Plain x-rays may be indicated in trauma and when myelopathy is present. Nerve conduction studies and electromyography (EMG) may identify evidence of denervation in a root distribution, thus confirming the diagnosis of radiculopathy, and exclude entrapment neuropathies.

TREATMENT

Initial treatment of disk disease should begin conservatively with physical therapy for axial muscle strengthening exercise and nonsteroidal antiinflammatory agents, provided there are no clinical myelopathic signs. Systemic or epidural steroids may be considered in cases of severe and/or refractory pain. The majority of patients improve with time regardless of the type of intervention. Surgical decompression is indicated when symptoms are unresponsive to at least 6 to 8 weeks of optimal conservative therapy, when there is progressive weakness, or when central herniation results in myelopathy or cauda equina syndrome.

REFERENCES

Chad, D. A., & Bowley, M. P. (2016). Disorders of nerve roots and plexuses. In R. B. Daroff, J. Jankovic, J.C. Mazziotta, & S.L. Pomeroy (Eds.), *Bradley's neurology in clinical practice,* ed 7 (pp. 1766–1790). Philadelphia: Elsevier Saunders.

Snyder, L. A., Tan, L., Gerard, C., & Fessler, R. G. (2016). Spinal cord trauma. In R. B. Daroff, J. Jankovic, J. C. Mazziotta, & S. L. Pomeroy (Eds.), *Bradley's neurology in clinical practice,* ed 7 (pp. 881–902). Philadelphia: Elsevier Saunders.

TABLE 111

SIGNS AND SYMPTOMS OF RADIOCULOPATHY

Root	Pain Distribution	Sensory Abnormalities	Motor Deficits	Reflex Affected
C_5	Neck, shoulder, anterior arm	Lateral arm	Deltoid, external rotators of arm, forearm flexors	Biceps, brachioradialis
C_6	Neck, shoulder, lateral arm, dorsal forearm	Lateral forearm, lateral hand, 1st and 2nd digits	Diaphragmatic paresis if C5 fibers reach the phrenic nerve (rarely) Forearm flexion and pronation, finger and wrist extension	Biceps, brachioradialis
C_7	Neck, shoulder, dorsal forearm, 3rd digit	3rd and 4th digits	Arm extension, finger and wrist flexors and extensors	Triceps
C_8	Neck, shoulder, medial forearm and hand, 5th digit	Medial forearm and hand, 5th digit	Intrinsic hand muscles	Finger flexor
T_1	Neck, medial arm and forearm	Medial arm and forearm	Intrinsic hand muscles Ipsilateral Horner syndrome (ptosis, miosis, anhidrosis)	
L_4	Lower back, buttock, anterolateral thigh, occasionally medial lower leg	Anterior thigh (knee), occasionally medial leg	Hip adduction and flexion, knee extension	Patellar
L_5	Lower back, buttock, lateral thigh, anterolateral calf, dorsum foot, 1st toe	Lateral leg, dorsomedial foot, 1st toe	Knee flexion, foot dorsiflexion and toes	
S_1	Lower back, buttock, lateral thigh, posterior calf, lateral foot	Lateral foot, sole of foot, 5th toe	Plantar flexion of foot and toes	Achilles

R

RADICULOPATHY

TABLE 112

COMPARISON OF CAUDA EQUINA AND CONUS MEDULLARIS SYNDROME

	Cauda Equina Syndrome	Conus Medullaris Syndrome
Definition	Compression of the nerve roots below the termination of the spinal cord (between L_2 and S_1)	Compression of the terminus of the spinal cord (L_1, L_2)
Presentation	Insidious unless secondary to acute trauma Asymmetric	Sudden Symmetric
Pain	Lower back pain, radicular pain	Lower back pain
Sensory deficits	Reduced or absent sensation from saddle region and legs up to groin	Reduced or absent sensation at sacral and perineal dermatomes Sensory level at or below waist
Motor deficits	Asymmetric weakness of lower extremities Lower motor neuron involvement	Symmetric weakness of lower extremities Upper and lower motor neuron involvement
Reflexes	Absent lower extremity reflexes	Variable lower extremity reflexes
Additional findings	Sphincter dysfunction Bowel, bladder and sexual dysfunction	Early sphincter dysfunction Bowel and bladder incontinence (due to atonic anal sphincter and urinary retention, respectively)
Causes	Large lumbar disk herniation, severe spinal stenosis, acute trauma, epidural abscess, epidural hematoma, primary and metastatic neoplasms	Large lumbar disk herniation, severe spinal stenosis, acute trauma, epidural abscess, epidural hematoma, primary and metastatic neoplasms

REFLEXES

Reflexes are evaluated for latency of response, degree of activity, and duration of the contraction. Reflexes should be both observed and palpated. Relaxation is important because tendon reflexes are difficult to elicit if muscles are tense. The joint should be at approximately 90 degrees. Compare right and left sides. In general, reflexes are not pathologic if they are symmetric, unless they are absent or 4 + (Table 113). If the reflexes are difficult to elicit, try asking the patient to clench his or her teeth or to hook flexed fingers together and pull (Jendrassik maneuver).

Hyporeflexia results from dysfunction of any part of the reflex arc. Conditions include neuropathy, radiculopathy, tabes dorsalis, syringomyelia, intramedullary tumors, and spinal motor neuron dysfunction. Bilateral hyporeflexia is the hallmark of neuropathies. Isolated, unilateral absent reflexes suggest radiculopathy. Hyporeflexia may occur in late stages of primary muscle diseases because of loss of muscle mass. Areflexia with rapidly progressive weakness and only mild sensory loss is the hallmark of Guillain-Barré syndrome. Hyporeflexia is seen transiently in acute upper motor neuron lesions, such as cerebral infarction or spinal cord compression (spinal shock). Prolongation of both the contraction and relaxation times ("hung-up" reflex) is seen with hypothyroidism. This prolongation is most evident in the knee jerks. Areflexia may be a component of Adie syndrome (see Pupil; see also Hypotonic Infant).

Hyperreflexia usually results from an upper motor neuron lesion with loss of corticospinal inhibition. The extrapyramidal system may also play a role. Involvement may occur anywhere from the cortical Betz cell to just proximal to the spinal cord motor neuron. Unilateral hyperreflexia results from a unilateral lesion anywhere along the corticospinal tract, most commonly in the cerebral hemispheres or brainstem. Bilateral hyperreflexia occurs more commonly with myelopathy, but it also occurs with bilateral cerebral hemisphere or brainstem involvement. Symmetric, 3 + reflexes in the absence of clonus; Babinski, Tromner, or Hoffmann signs; or weakness and with a normal result of neurologic examination is usually benign. Reflexes are variable (usually normal) with extrapyramidal system dysfunction. Reflexes are normal, slightly decreased, or pendular with cerebellar tract dysfunction (see also Rigidity, Spasticity).

"Pathologic reflexes" (pyramidal tract reflexes) indicate upper motor neuron dysfunction. The extensor plantar response (Babinski sign) consists of dorsiflexion of the great toe and fanning of the remaining toes on stimulating the plantar surface of the foot. Hoffmann and Tromner signs are elicited by

R

REFLEXES

TABLE 113

GRADING OF MUSCLE STRETCH REFLEXES

Grade	Description
0	Absent, abnormal
1 +	Diminished, may or may not be abnormal
2 +	Normal
3 +	Increased, may or may not be abnormal
4 +	Markedly increased, abnormal; may be associated with clonus

TABLE 114

SEGMENTAL MUSCLE STRETCH AND CUTANEOUS REFLEXES

Reflex	Level	Nerve
MUSCLE STRETCH (DEEP TENDON) REFLEXES		
Jaw (masseter and temporal muscle)	CN V	Mandibular branch
Biceps	C_5, C_6	Musculocutaneous
Brachioradialis	C_5, C_6	Radial
Pectoral major	C_5, C_6, C_7	Lateral pectoral
Triceps	C_6, C_7, C_8	Radial
Finger flexors	C_8	Medial (ulnar)
Adductor	L_2, L_3, L_4	Obturator
Quadriceps (patellar knee jerks)	L_2, L_3, L_4	Femoral
Internal hamstring	L_4, L_5, S_1	Sciatic
External hamstring	L_5, S_1	Sciatic
Gastrocnemius-soleus (Achilles, ankle jerks)	L_5, S_1, S_2	Tibial
CUTANEOUS (SUPERFICIAL) REFLEXES		
Corneal	Pons	CN V (afferent) VII (efferent)
Pharyngeal gag reflex	Medulla	CN IX (afferent) X (efferent)
Upper abdominal	T_{6-9}	
Middle abdominal	T_{9-11}	
Lower abdominal	T_{11}–L_1	
Cremasteric	L_1, L_2	Femoral (afferent) genitofemoral (efferent)
Plantar	L_5, S_1, S_2	Tibial
Anal	S_3, S_4, S_5	Pudendal
Bulbocavernosus	S_3, S_4	Pudendal, pelvic autonomics

CN, cranial nerve.

"flicking" the index or middle finger down or up, respectively, producing flexion of the thumb. They may be normal if present bilaterally, especially if reflexes are 3 + and symmetric. Ankle clonus is the continuing rapid flexion and extension of the foot, elicited by forcibly and quickly dorsiflexing the foot. Pyramidal tract reflexes are normally present in infants (see Child Neurology).

Segmental muscle stretch and cutaneous reflexes are listed in Table 114.

RESPIRATORY FAILURE

Respiratory failure is the failure of the lungs and muscles of respiration to maintain adequate respiration and gas exchange.

I. Acute respiratory failure (ARF)
   A. Two main forms of acute failure are hypoxic and hypercapnic respiratory failure.
   B. Hypoxic failure (type I ARF) is the failure of the respiratory system to maintain arterial oxygenation within or greater than the predicted

normal range for a given patient's age (and ambient barometric pressure, assuming no baseline right-to-left shunting of blood)— usually arterial oxygen content at or greater than 60 mm Hg.

C. Hypercapnic failure (type II) is the failure to maintain arterial CO_2 less than 50 mm Hg (not due to respiratory compensation of metabolic alkalosis).

D. Type I ARF is usually seen in parenchymal pathologies within the lungs, such as pneumonia, pulmonary embolism, pulmonary edema, alveolar hemorrhage, or acute respiratory distress syndrome.

E. Neurologic causes constitute a prominent etiologic portion for type II ARF, including myasthenia gravis, Guillain-Barré syndrome, brainstem stroke, amyotrophic lateral sclerosis, and some myopathies (Table 115).

F. Decreased consciousness places a patient at significant risk for an inability to maintain a patent airway. Therefore, in addition to intubation of patients in ARF, patients with a Glasgow Coma Scale score less than 8 are often intubated and placed on mechanical ventilation. This will include patients with a wide variety of neurologic and neurosurgical conditions.

II. Determination of respiratory failure (clinical and laboratory)

A. Patients in ARF can develop paradoxical respiration (abdomen contracts as chest wall expands), rapid respiratory rate, and use of accessory respiratory muscles.

B. Measuring pulse oximetry will give an accurate measure of blood hypoxia, and arterial blood gas sampling will give an accurate measure of arterial CO_2 content.

TABLE 115

NEUROLOGIC CAUSES OF RESPIRATORY FAILURE

Etiology	Prominent Clinical Manifestation
Neuromuscular disease (e.g., myasthenia gravis, Guillain-Barré syndrome)	Weakness of respiratory muscles
Myopathies and neuropathies (e.g., polymyositis, critical care myopathy and neuropathy, muscular dystrophy)	Brainstem stroke
High cervical spine injury	Neuromuscular blocking agents (e.g., botulism, certain toxins or poisons)
Restrictive lung disorders (e.g. scoliosis)	Anterior horn cell disease (motor neuron disease, polio, West Nile virus)
Brainstem strokes	Inability to protect airway
Bulbar palsy	Massive ischemic or hemorrhagic strokes
Diffuse cerebral edema (from any cause)	Dysphagia/inability to clear secretions (from any cause)
Sedating medications (e.g., opiates)	Decreased drive of respiration
Brainstem injuries (ischemic stroke, hemorrhage, tumors)	Massive ischemic or hemorrhagic strokes
Central hypoventilation (Ondine curse)	

C. For patients with progressive respiratory impairment, bedside measurements of ventilatory function are useful in predicting impending respiratory failure; most commonly measured are negative inspiratory force (NIF) and the vital capacity (FVC, or simply VC). The normal NIF has an absolute value greater than 70 cm H_2O (NIF is measured as a negative pressure), and VC has a normal value of at least 60 mL/kg.

D. There is increased risk for developing respiratory failure when NIF is less than 20 cm H_2O. At a VC less than 25 mL/kg, atelectasis develops and hypoxemia may begin. At 15 mL/kg there is shunting. At 5 to 10 mL/kg hypercapnia will develop. It is recommended that patients be electively intubated at 20 mL/kg, especially if there is a risk of further compromise of respiratory drive.

E. Other laboratory tests and investigations such as a chest x-ray are useful in elucidating causes of respiratory failure. Cardiac monitoring is required in all patients with respiratory failure.

III. Treatment of respiratory failure

A. In general, treatment involves support of the respiratory system to correct hypoxia or hypercapnia.

B. This can be done through either noninvasive positive pressure ventilation or endotracheal intubation with mechanical ventilation. The appropriate use of noninvasive ventilation is currently limited.

C. Mechanical ventilation has three main modes of respiratory support: AC (assist-control), SIMV (synchronized intermittent mandatory mode of ventilation), and CPAP (continuous positive airway pressure). There are other modes used in select circumstances. In general, after endotracheal intubation with mechanical ventilation, patients are initially supported as fully as possible in their respirations, using the AC mode, to rest patients fully.

D. Recommended settings when initiating mechanical ventilation include a tidal volume of 6 mL/kg and a positive end-expiratory pressure of 5 cm H_2O.

E. The other two main modes of ventilation, SIMV and CPAP, require patient effort, and they are used as patients are weaned from mechanical ventilation. SIMV allows intubated patients to make some respiratory effort, whereas CPAP allows patients to breathe spontaneously. A 2-hour CPAP trial in intubated patients is often predictive of success in extubation.

IV. Medical aspects in patients with respiratory failure

A. Ensuring adequate nutrition

B. Prophylaxis of gastrointestinal hemorrhage

C. Prophylaxis of deep venous thrombosis

D. Monitoring of electrolytes and acid-base status

E. Prophylaxis against or treatment of ventilator-associated pneumonia (e.g., via chest physical therapy to prevent atelectasis)

F. Cardiac monitoring

REFERENCES

Brower, R. G., et al. (2004). Higher versus lower positive end-expiratory pressures in patients with the acute respiratory distress syndrome. *N Engl J Med, 351*, 327–336.

Rabinstein, A. A. (2015). Acute neuromuscular respiratory failure. *Continuum (Minneap Minn), 21*(5, Neurocritical Care), 1324–1345.

RESTLESS LEGS SYNDROME (WILLIS-EKBOM SYNDROME)

Restless legs syndrome, also known as Willis-Ekbom disease, is characterized by ill-defined, deep, "crawling" paresthesias in the lower legs, thighs, and occasionally the arms. It is usually bilateral and occurs especially while at rest or during drowsiness. It causes an unpleasant or uncomfortable urge to move the legs during periods of inactivity, especially in the evening, resulting in insomnia. It is transiently relieved by movement. It is usually intermittent and lasts from minutes to hours. There is frequently an overlap between the restless legs syndrome and periodic movements of sleep (nocturnal myoclonic movements consisting of discrete, brief, repetitive flexion at the hips, knees, and thighs during light sleep). There may be a familial predisposition. Some similarities exist between this syndrome and growing pains in children. Symptoms may be exacerbated with antihistamines (i.e., diphenhydramine), dopamine antagonists (antipsychotics and antinausea medications), or certain antidepressants (including mirtazapine, tricyclic antidepressants, and selective serotonin reuptake inhibitors [SSRIs]).

Pathophysiology: This is poorly understood. Although there are some studies that have identified a variety of central and peripheral nervous system abnormalities, there is no evidence of a neurodegenerative process.

Diagnosis Criteria: Five keys clinical features required for diagnosis published by the International Restless Legs Syndrome Study Group:

1. Urge to move legs, accompanied or caused by uncomfortable and unpleasant sensations in the legs. Sometimes the urge to move is present without the uncomfortable sensations, and sometimes the arms or other body parts are also involved.
2. Urge to move or unpleasant sensations begin or worsen during periods of rest or inactivity such as lying or sitting.
3. Urge to move or unpleasant sensations are partially or totally relieved by movement, such as walking or stretching, at least as long as the activity continues.
4. Urge to move or unpleasant sensations are worse in the evening or night or occur only in the evening or night. When symptoms are severe, the worsening at night may not be noticeable but must have been previously present.
5. Symptoms are not solely accounted for by another medical or behavioral condition, such as leg cramps or habitual foot tapping.

A variety of conditions have been described in association with restless legs syndrome. The most common implicated central nervous system alteration is reduced central iron stores. Other associated conditions include the following: low iron stores, uremia, neuropathy, spinal cord disease, multiple sclerosis, pregnancy, carcinoma, Parkinson disease, caffeine, and others.

Treatment: The treatment involves correcting the underlying condition. Iron replacement is suggested if serum ferritin is less than 75 μg/L. Dopamine agonists and alpha-2-delta calcium channel ligand are first line therapy for chronic symptoms. Dopamine agonists include pramipexole, ropinirole, and rotigotine. Alpha-2-delta calcium channel ligands include gabapentin enacarbil, pregabalin, and gabapentin. Treatments for intermittent symptoms include levodopa, benzodiazepines (clonazepam), or a low-potency opioid.

REFERENCES

Silber, M. H. (2019). Treatment of restless legs syndrome and periodic limb movement disorder in adults. UpToDate. https://www.uptodate.com/contents/treatment-of-restless-legs-syndrome-and-periodic-limb-movement-disorder-in-adults. Accessed 24.3.2019.

Ondo, W. G. (2017). *Clinical features and diagnosis of restless legs syndrome/ Willis-Ekbom disease and periodic movement disorders in adults.* UpToDate.

RETINA AND UVEAL TRACT (UVEITIS)

I. Systemic and neurologic disorders associated with retinal pigmentary degeneration
   A. *Typical retinitis pigmentosa* changes include early-onset nyctalopia, progressive visual loss, bone spicules, narrowing of retinal arterioles, and electroretinogram changes. They may be associated with the following:
      1. Myotonic dystrophy (rarely)
      2. Leber congenital amaurosis
      3. Senear-Loken disease (Leber congenital amaurosis juvenile nephronophthisis)
      4. Friedreich ataxia (may also rarely be associated with optic atrophy and deafness)
      5. Spielmeyer-Vogt disease
      6. Neonatal and childhood adrenoleukodystrophy
      7. Usher syndrome (vestibulocochlear dysfunction, mutism)
      8. Pelizaeus-Merzbacher disease (mental retardation, ataxia)
      9. Hallgren disease (mental retardation, ataxia, deafness)
   B. *Atypical central and peripheral retinal pigmentary changes occur with variable degrees of visual impairment. The presumed mechanism in storage diseases is disruption of pigment epithelial function by accumulated metabolic material with secondary retinal receptor*

degeneration. Primary rod or cone dystrophy may exist in the first four of the following syndromes:

1. Laurence-Moon-Biedl syndrome (hypogenitalism, mental retardation, polydactyly)
2. Biemond syndrome (hypogenitalism, mental retardation, iris coloboma)
3. Alström syndrome (hypogenitalism, deafness, diabetes mellitus)
4. Bassen-Kornzweig syndrome (abetalipoproteinemia, ataxia, acanthocytosis)
5. Refsum disease (polyneuropathy, ataxia)
6. Sjögren-Larsson syndrome (ichthyosis, spastic paresis, mental retardation)
7. Amalric-Dialinos syndrome (deafness)
8. Cockayne syndrome (dwarfism, neuropathy, deafness)
9. Hallervorden-Spatz syndrome (neuropathy, basal ganglia degeneration)
10. Alport syndrome (nephritis, hearing loss)
11. Hurler (mucopolysaccharidosis [MPS] I), Hunter (MPS II), Sanfilippo (MPS III), and Scheie disease (MPS V)

C. *Postinflammatory diseases*
1. Congenital and acquired syphilis
2. Congenital rubella (German measles)—"salt and pepper fundus"
3. Congenital rubeola (measles)

D. *Avitaminoses and vitamin metabolism disorders*
1. Pellagra
2. Vitamin B_{12} metabolism disorder associated with aminoaciduria

E. *Toxic*
1. Chlorpromazine
2. Thioridazine
3. Indomethacin

II. Hereditary cerebromacular dystrophies

A. *With cherry red spot of the macula*
1. Sphingolipidoses—Tay-Sachs disease, Niemann-Pick disease, Gaucher disease, metachromatic leukodystrophy (infantile form), Sandhoff disease
2. Mucolipidoses—GM1 gangliosidosis, Farber syndrome
3. Mucolipidosis I
4. Mucopolysaccharidoses—Hurler syndrome (MPS I), MPS VII
5. Goldberg disease

B. *Without cherry red spot*
1. Ceroid lipofuscinoses—Jansky-Bielschowsky disease
2. Batten-Mayou, Spielmeyer-Vogt disease
3. Kufs-Hallervorden disease

III. Central nervous system (CNS) vasculitides: All vasculitides may involve the retinal circulation with variable manifestations (arterial occlusive retinopathy, hemorrhages, retinal infiltrates).

IV. Phakomatoses
   A. *Vascular malformations of the choroid or retina and the CNS*
      1. Von Hippel-Lindau syndrome (retinal angiomas and cerebellar hemangioblastomas)
      2. Sturge-Weber syndrome (choroidal hemangioma, parieto-occipital arteriovenous malformations [AVMs])
      3. Wyburn-Mason syndrome (AVMs in the retina and brainstem)
      4. Retinal cavernous hemangioma (unclassified phakomatosis, rarely associated with intracranial AVMs)
   B. *Retinal and intracranial tumors*
      1. Tuberous sclerosis
      2. Neurofibromatosis

V. Dystrophies of the uvea
   A. *Angioid streaks (ruptures of Bruch membrane) occur in the following diseases, which may be associated with neurologic dysfunction:*
      1. Francois dyscephalic syndrome
      2. Paget disease
      3. Acromcgaly
      4. Sickle cell anemia
   B. *Gillespie syndrome (aniridia, ataxia, psychomotor retardation)*

VI. Retinovitreal syndromes and vitreal involvement
   A. Wagner vitreoretinopathy (rarely associated with encephaloceles)
   B. Dominant familial amyloidosis (diffuse vitreous opacification)

Table 116 summarizes the diseases that affect retinal and uveal tract and CNS.

REFERENCE

Grumet, P., et al. (2018). Contribution of diagnostic tests for the etiological assessment of uveitis, data from the ULISSE study (Uveitis: Clinical and medicoeconomic evaluation of a standardized strategy of the etiological diagnosis). *Autoimmun Rev, 17*(4), 331–343.

REVERSIBLE CEREBRAL VASOCONSTRICTION SYNDROME, CALL-FLEMING SYNDROME

Reversible cerebral vasoconstriction syndrome (RCVS), or Call-Fleming syndrome, is a well-recognized syndrome presenting with recurring thunderclap headaches, with or without neurologic symptoms and segmental constriction in the cerebral cortical arterial branches over a timespan of 1 to 4 weeks. The vascular changes are reversible within 3 months period.

Typical precipitants to RCVS: coughing, exercise, trauma, bathing, postpartum state, vasoactive sympathomimetic medications, and illicit

TABLE 116

DISEASES THAT MAY INVOLVE THE UVEAL TRACT AND CENTRAL NERVOUS SYSTEM

BACTERIAL INFECTIONS

Meningococcosis
Syphilis
Tuberculosis
Whipple disease
Brucellosis
Leptospirosis
Listeriosis
Lyme disease (Borrelia)

PARASITIC INFECTIONS

Trypanosomiasis
Toxoplasmosis
Ameliosis
Malaria

VIRAL INFECTIONS

Cytomegalovirus infection
Herpes simplex
Herpes zoster
Varicella
Mumps
Rubella
Rubeola
Subacute sclerosing panencephalitis
Variola

FUNGAL INFECTIONS

Aspergillosis
Candidiasis
Cryptococcosis
Histoplasmosis
Mucormycosis

GRANULOMATOUS DISEASE

Sarcoidosis
Wegener granulomatosis

COLLAGEN VASCULAR DISEASE

Systemic lupus erythematosus
Temporal arteritis
Polyarteritis

NEOPLASMS

Leukemia
Metastatic carcinoma
Reticulum cell sarcoma

OTHER

Behçet syndrome
Multiple sclerosis

Continued

R

REVERSIBLE CEREBRAL VASOCONSTRICTION SYNDROME

TABLE 116

DISEASES THAT MAY INVOLVE THE UVEAL TRACT AND CENTRAL NERVOUS SYSTEM—CONT'D

Sympathetic ophthalmia

Trauma

Uveal effusion

Vogt-Koyanagi-Harada (uveomeningoencephalitic) syndrome

Bing syndrome (chorioretinitis, ophthalmoplegia, macroglobulinemia)

Romberg syndrome (posterior uveitis, ophthalmoplegia, trigeminal neuralgia, seizures, unilateral facial atrophy)

Modified from Finelli, P. F., et al. (1977). Whipple's disease with predominantly neuroophthalmic manifestations. *Ann Neurol, 1,* 247–252.

drugs. Not infrequently, the underlying risk factor for RCS may not be found.

Brain images such as CT head and fluid-attenuated inversion recovery (FLAIR) MRI may initially show no abnormalities in spite of pervasive cerebral vasoconstriction. Brain imaging can demonstrate typical convexity subarachnoid hemorrhage (SAH) in up to 50% of cases; similar changes to posterior reversible encephalopathy syndrome may also occur with cerebral edema.

Differential Diagnosis: Migraine, SAH from aneurysm rupture or vascular malformation, arterial dissection, cerebral venous thrombus, primary or secondary central nervous system (CNS) vasculitis.

Work-up: CT scan and MRI of the brain, spinal tap for cerebrospinal fluid analysis, vascular imaging with conventional angiogram (Fig. 58).

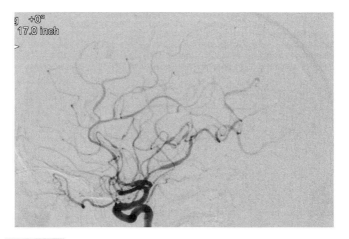

FIGURE 58

Conventional angiogram.

Treatment: Calcium channel blocker, with verapamil and magnesium, may be administered. Dantrolene and serotonin agonists have been suggested as means to reduce vasoconstriction. Short-term steroid therapy for 2 weeks may also be considered. Glucocorticoids have shown to be associated with worse outcome and have been discouraged. Fulminant cases may require intra-arterial vasodilatory therapy.

REFERENCES

Camargo, E. C. S., & Singhal, A. B. (2017). Cerebral arteriopathies, venous thrombosis, and migraine. *Semin Neurol.*, *37*(3), 339–350.

Coffino, S. W., & Fryer, R. H. (2017). Reversible cerebral vasoconstriction syndrome in pediatrics: a case series and review. *J Child Neurol.*, *32*, 614–623.

RHEUMATOID ARTHRITIS

Neurologic complications of rheumatoid arthritis (RA) usually occur in patients with moderate to severe RA and consist of neuropathy, myelopathy, myopathy, meningoencephalitis, and vasculitis.

Peripheral neuropathy is among the most frequent neurologic complications of RA and has three main types; it is primarily axonal, but demyelinating features may be present. Pure sensory neuropathy is most common, but sensorimotor neuropathy also occurs. Entrapment neuropathies, such as median mononeuropathy at the carpel tunnel, are common. Vasculitis is an uncommon cause of neuropathy that typically manifests as mononeuritis multiplex.

Compressive myelopathy of the cervical spine is also relatively common in RA. Clinical manifestations include neck pain (65%), headache, upper cervical myelopathy, brainstem signs, and occasionally vertebrobasilar insufficiency. Three patterns of upper cervical instability occur, among which atlantoaxial subluxation is most common. Upward subluxation of the odontoid process may cause compression of the upper spinal cord or lower brainstem. Subluxation of vertebrae below C_2 is the third pattern. Magnetic resonance imaging (MRI) of the cervical spinal cord is generally the best imaging modality, but plain films may reveal the underlying pathology in many cases and others may require CT myelography or vascular imaging. A minority of patients will require surgical intervention to alleviate compressive symptoms.

Neuromuscular complications include disuse atrophy, focal myositis (usually adjacent to actively involved joints), disseminated nodular myositis (nonnecrotizing lymphocytic and plasma cell perivascular infiltrates), steroid myopathy, polymyositis (rare, more malignant course), and ischemia due to vasculitis.

Inflammatory central nervous system (CNS) complications of RA are infrequent. Meningoencephalitis, manifesting as headaches, strokelike episodes, cranial neuropathies, and seizures, has been described. MRI demonstrates patchy or leptomeningeal thickening and contrast enhancement and hyperintensities on T2-weighted sequences. Cerebrospinal fluid (CSF) examination generally reveals modest monocytic pleocytosis with normal or elevated protein and occasionally low CSF glucose. High-dose glucocorticoids have been effective in case reports.

Vasculitis isolated to the CNS, or as part of a systemic involvement, rarely occurs with contemporary disease-modifying therapy and presents with protean manifestations such as acute/subacute encephalopathy, seizures, vision changes, cranial nerve deficits, and ataxia. Diagnosis is challenging, and definitive diagnosis requires biopsy. CSF is insensitive, as is conventional angiography because the small cerebral vessels are most often affected. MRI may reveal hyperintensities in the deep brain structures and periventricular white matter on T2-weighted sequences. Treatment typically consists of high-dose glucocorticoids, possibly in combination with other immunosuppression such as cyclophosphamide.

Therapeutics used to treat RA can be associated with neurologic complications as well: rituximab (small risk of PML), gold (peripheral neuropathy/cranial neuropathy, Guillain-Barré syndrome), steroids (neuropsychiatric, myopathy), antimalarials (neuropathy, myopathy, retinopathy, seizures), methotrexate/sulfasalazine (headaches), and leflunomide (headaches, peripheral neuropathy).

REFERENCE

Bhattacharyya, S., & Helfgott, S. M. (2014). Neurologic complications of systemic lupus erythematosus, Sjögren syndrome, and rheumatoid arthritis. *Semin Neurol*, *34*, 425–436.

RIGIDITY

Rigidity is a form of increased muscle tone that is present throughout the range of motion of a limb and is not dependent on velocity (compare with spasticity). Rigidity is assessed by passively flexing and extending a patient's limb. When released, the rigid limb does not spring back to its original position. Rigidity is not associated with hyperreflexia. Electromyography (EMG) reveals persistent motor unit activity during apparent relaxation.

Cogwheel rigidity is increased resistance to passive movement, with a superimposed palpable tremor. It has been described as having a ratchet-like feeling on examination. It can be observed in some extrapyramidal diseases, including parkinsonian disorders.

Lead-pipe rigidity, also called "waxy" or "plastic" rigidity, is constant resistance to movement of a limb, which may maintain its position at the end of the displacement; this may be seen in catatonia, where it is often referred to as "waxy flexibility."

There are other types of hypertonia that feel different on examination from rigidity. It is important to distinguish these from rigidity because they do not have the same clinical implications as true rigidity:

- **Paratonia** refers to increasing tone with variable resistance during passive movement. There are different forms of paratonia. To the examiner, *mitgehen* paratonia feels as if the patient is facilitating the passive movement, whereas *gegenhalten* paratonia feels like active resistance. Paratonias can be associated with dementia.
- **Clasp-knife rigidity** or clasp-knife spasticity is suggestive of an upper motor neuron lesion. It is seen when the resistive tone initially increases during the stretching of the muscle but then decreases during the movement.
- In **voluntary rigidity**, agonist-antagonist cocontraction is associated with heightened emotional states.
- **Decorticate posturing** is a slow, stereotyped flexion of arm, wrist, and fingers with adduction at the shoulder and leg extension with plantar flexion of the foot. It occurs with supratentorial processes compressing the diencephalon. **Decerebrate posturing** is pronation of the arm with adduction and internal rotation of the leg, along with plantar flexion of the foot. It occurs with more caudal compression of the midbrain and rostral pons. Extension in the arms with flexion or flaccidity in the legs is associated with lesions of the pontine tegmentum (see also Herniation).

R

RIGIDITY

ASSOCIATED CONDITIONS

Rigidity has been associated with numerous neurologic and systemic diseases, including, but not limited to: extrapyramidal disorders, Parkinson disease (PD), Wilson disease, progressive encephalomyelitis with rigidity and myoclonus, neuroleptic malignant syndrome, PLA2G6-related dystonia-parkinsonism, multisystem atrophy, TBK-1–associated frontotemporal dementia, Sjögren syndrome, manganese toxicity/accumulation in the basal ganglia, striatonigral degeneration, stiff person syndrome, progressive supranuclear palsy, 1-methyl-4-phenyl-1,2,3,5-tetrahydropyridine (MPTP) toxicity, carbon monoxide poisoning, dementia puglilistica, and vascular parkinsonism.

TREATMENT

Treatment of rigidity depends on the underlying cause. However, there are numerous medications used in the treatment of PD that can be used to address rigidity caused by other conditions and may be considered on an individualized basis.

Some of these include: levodopa-carbidopa (Sinemet), dopamine agonists such as ropinirole (Requip), pramipexole (Mirapex), rotigotine (Neupro), anticholinergics such as benztropine (Cogentin) or trihexyphenidyl (Artane), amantadine (Symmetrel), catechol-O-methyltransferase (COMT) inhibitors such as tolcapone (Tasmar) and entacapone (Comtan), and monoamine oxidase (MAO) type B inhibitors such as selegiline (Eldepryl), and rasagiline (Azilect).

In patients with mild to moderate PD, axial rigidity has been found to be related to an increased risk of falls. Rehabilitation efforts with technique such as progressive resistance exercise can be targeted towards addressing akinesia and rigidity in akinetic rigid (AR)-subtype PD patients to try to decrease the risk of falls.

Deep brain stimulation has been used for medically refractory PD by targeting the subthalamic nucleus or the globus pallidus and may help to decrease rigidity in some patients.

REFERENCES

Cano-de-la-Cuerda, R., et al. (2017). Axial rigidity is related to the risk of falls in patients with Parkinson's disease. *NeuroRehabilitation*, *40*(4), 569–577.

Członkowska, A., Litwin, T., & Chabik, G. (2017). Wilson disease: neurologic features. *Handb Clin Neurol*, *142*, 101–119.

ROMBERG SIGN

In Romberg sign, a patient's stability is tested by comparing his or her ability to stand with both feet together and eyes open, versus eyes closed. Sign is present if there is marked increase in sway. Romberg sign helps to assess a patient's vestibular and proprioceptive systems. When our eyes are open, three systems provide input to our cerebellum to help us maintain balance—vision, proprioception, and vestibular sense. We need input from two of the three to maintain balance. Closing our eyes eliminates visual input. A lesion in the vestibular or proprioceptive systems would cause loss of another input, thereby causing imbalance when the eyes are closed. Severe vestibular or proprioceptive lesions may be apparent even with eyes open, as would severe midline cerebellar lesions.

REFERENCE

Blumenfeld, H. (2010). The neurological exam as a lesson in neuroanatomy. In Blumenfeld, H. (ed): *Neuroanatomy through clinical cases* (p. 70). Sunderland: Sinauer Associates.

S

SARCOIDOSIS

DEFINITION AND EPIDEMIOLOGY

Sarcoidosis is a multisystem disorder of unknown etiology characterized by noncaseating granulomas. The pulmonary system is most often affected, but any organ system can be involved. Bilateral hilar adenopathy, pulmonary infiltrate, uveitis, and skin lesions are the most common presenting signs. In general, it affects young adults and is more common in African Americans. Isolated neurosarcoidosis is rare, with estimated incidence of less than 0.2 per 100,000. In 5% of patients, nervous system involvement is clinically apparent and sometimes can be the presenting sign. The most common neurologic symptoms are cranial nerve deficits (50%), headache (30%), and seizures (10%).

CLINICAL PRESENTATION

I. Neurologic manifestations of sarcoidosis
   A. Cranial neuropathies. The cranial nerves themselves are most commonly involved, but they can also be compressed by meningeal involvement. The facial nerve is the most commonly affected; facial motor paresis with or without dysgeusia occurs in up to 50% of those with central nervous system (CNS) sarcoidosis. The eighth nerve is the next most commonly affected, with either auditory or vestibular symptoms, which can have sudden onset. Optic nerve is affected in approximately 15% of neurosarcoidosis cases, as optic neuropathy or papilledema. Ocular motor dysfunction is seen only occasionally, as is trigeminal sensory involvement; other cranial nerves are very rarely affected.
   B. Meningitis is quite common but may be clinically inapparent. Typically it is most prominent in the basal cisterns. Meningitis manifests as cranial nerve symptoms, obstructive hydrocephalus, or rarely as mass effect on the cerebral cortex when large swellings of meninges result.
   C. Neuroendocrine dysfunction. Granulomas in the hypothalamus or pituitary area can produce secondary hypothyroidism, hypogonadism, adrenal insufficiency, syndrome of inappropriate anti-diuretic hormone (SIADH) or diabetes insipidus, or disruption of vegetative functions such as appetite or sleep.
   D. Brain parenchymal lesions present either as focal cerebral dysfunction or as hydrocephalus if occluding cerebrospinal fluid (CSF) pathways, or as diffusely raised intracranial pressure if sufficiently large. These lesions may produce a diffuse cerebral vasculitis or encephalitis, manifesting as encephalopathy or seizures. They may also mimic tumors, especially meningioma, necessitating biopsy.

E. Myelopathy. Extradural or intradural or extramedullary or intramedullary granuloma may cause cord compression and spinal block, or arachnoiditis.

F. Neuropathies. The most common sarcoid neuropathy is chronic axonal peripheral polyneuropathy; however, neuropathies can present in multiple ways, including polyradiculopathies, individual focal mononeuropathies, or mononeuritis multiplex. They can rarely mimic Guillain-Barré syndrome.

G. Myopathy, although pathologically common, is rarely clinically manifest.

H. Opportunistic infection. Because treatment is immunosuppression, important parts of the differential diagnosis of CNS involvement in a patient with known systemic sarcoidosis are the various viral, fungal, and mycobacterial infections that can result from such treatment.

II. Most common systemic manifestations

A. Pulmonary involvement is seen at some point in 90% of patients. Any combination of parenchymal inflammation and hilar lymphadenopathy may be seen.

B. Peripheral lymphadenopathy.

C. Skin. Dermal or epidermal granulomas, or erythema nodosum.

D. Eye. Inflammation of any portion of the orbit (conjunctivae, anterior chamber/iris, vitreous, or retina) can lead to visual impairment.

DIAGNOSIS

Definitive diagnosis is based on biopsy demonstration of noncaseating granulomas; otherwise, the diagnosis is based on the pattern of clinical organ involvement and imaging evidence of inflammatory involvement of typical tissues. Computed tomography (CT) or preferably magnetic resonance imaging (MRI) may be helpful in localizing lesion(s) in the CNS. Spectrum of MRI findings includes nodular or diffuse leptomeningeal enhancement (40%), periventricular white matter lesion (40%), multiple intraparenchymal lesions (35%), solitary intra-axial mass (10%), and solitary extra-axial mass (5%). CSF may show high protein level (40% to 70%), lymphocytic pleocytosis (50% to 70%), and low glucose level. High immunoglobulin G (IgG) index and oligoclonal bands may be present (70%). Serum angiotensin-converting enzyme (ACE) levels may be elevated but have a sensitivity of only 56% to 86% and very low specificity; the CSF ACE level is far less sensitive but more specific if CNS structures are involved.

High erythrocyte sedimentation rate and high calcium in serum/urine may be noted. Ophthalmologic examination, conjunctival biopsy, gallium scan, chest radiograph, and bronchoscopy may help in the diagnosis of systemic sarcoidosis.

TREATMENT

Prednisone, 0.5 to 1 mg/kg daily, is the mainstay of treatment. In acute severe cases, 1 g/day of intravenous methylprednisolone may be administered over 3 to 5 days. If steroids are not sufficient or cannot be tapered, cyclophosphamide, azathioprine, methotrexate, or cyclosporine may be added. Most patients respond to treatment, but one-third relapse when treatment is discontinued. Long-term treatment with corticosteroids is usually required, particularly in those with involvement of basal leptomeninges or diffuse parenchymal lesions. Radiation therapy with 20 Gy should be considered in medical refractory cases.

PROGNOSIS

Neurologic involvement in sarcoidosis is itself a poor prognostic sign. Peripheral nerve involvement and muscle involvement are often fairly benign. Cranial neuropathy and aseptic meningitis are the least poor prognostic central manifestations, with 90% of patients improving or recovering; those with symptomatic brain or spinal cord lesions, by contrast, very frequently have a progressive course.

REFERENCE

Fritz, D., van de Beek, D., & Brouwer, M. C. (2016). Clinical features, treatment and outcome in neurosarcoidosis: systematic review and meta-analysis. *BMC Neurol*, *16*, 220.

SCIATIC NERVE, SCIATICA

The sciatic nerve is the largest and longest single nerve in the human body. The nerve originates at the junction of the fourth and fifth lumbar nerve roots and the first three sacral nerve roots at the lumbosacral plexus. It divides into two major branches, tibial and peroneal nerves, and innervates many muscle groups, including the hamstrings, distal adductor magnus, and all the muscles of the leg and foot. It also supplies sensation to the lateral and posterior leg and to the entire foot (Fig. 59).

SCIATICA

The term "sciatica" can be misleading because it is not usually associated with a lesion of the sciatic nerve itself. Sciatica is pain that radiates down a lower extremity along the distribution of a lumbar or sacral nerve root. However, the term is widely used to describe a variety of pains in the back or lower limb. The most common cause of this condition is compression of a lumbar nerve root by a protruding disk (approximately 85% of cases). The most common levels are L_4-L_5 and L_5-S_1, with compression of the root below the corresponding disk. Other etiologies that have been implicated include spondylolisthesis, foraminal stenosis, synovial cysts, gluteal injection-site trauma, obstetrical sciatic damage by head of fetus or prolonged lithotomy position, and pelvic floor tumors.

Symptom distribution depends on the involved level. At L_4 level, the pain is in the anterolateral thigh. At L_5, the pain is typically felt in the buttock, dorsolateral thigh, lateral leg, and anterolateral foot. Compression at S_1 also

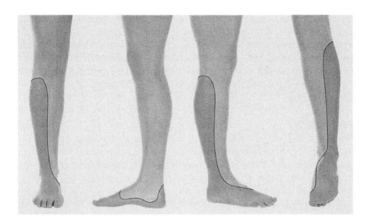

FIGURE 59
Sensory distribution of the trunk of the sciatic nerve. (From O'Brien, M. (2010). *Aids to the examination of the peripheral nervous system*, ed 5. Edinburgh: Saunders Elsevier).

causes pain at the buttock, but it radiates posteriorly and reaches the fifth toe. Other symptoms are numbness, tingling, burning, and prickling sensation. Of note, aching pain in the lower back, and its increased intensity with Valsalva maneuvers, suggest disk rupture as the cause. L_5 radiculopathy may cause foot drop, and S_1 level lesion may cause downward tilted pelvis while walking and loss of the ankle reflex. Bilateral sciatica is usually caused by compression of cauda equina roots.

TREATMENT

Usually conservative. Nonsteroidal anti-inflammatory drugs (NSAIDs) or glucocorticoids may provide some relief, but the long-term effect is controversial. Opioids are not recommended as mainstay therapy. Gabapentin, pregabalin, and muscle relaxants are used but with little supporting data. A recent trial of pregabalin failed to show efficacy. Spinal manipulation may provide short-term relief if used in conjunction with exercise. Surgery may provide relief more quickly than conservative measures, but outcomes at 1 year or longer may not differ. However, acute nerve root compression with severe symptoms does warrant surgical decompression in most cases.

REFERENCES

Longo, D. L., Ropper, A. H., & Zafonte, R. D. (2015). Sciatica. *N Engl J Med.*, *372*(13), 1240–1248. https://doi.org/10.1056/NEJMra1410151.

Mathieson, S., Maher, C. G., McLachlan, A. J., et al. (2017). Trial of pregabalin for acute and chronic sciatica. *N Engl J Med.*, *376*(12), 1111–1120. https://doi.org/10.1056/NEJMoa1614292.

SEPSIS

Sepsis is defined as life-threatening organ dysfunction caused by a dysregulated host response to infection. Patients with suspected infection may be screened with quick sequential (sepsis-related) organ failure assessment [quick sequential (sepsis-related) organ failure assessment (qSOFA)] (respiratory rate $\geq$22/min, change in mentation, systolic blood pressure [SBP] $\leq$100 mmHg); if this score is $\geq$2, these patients should be evaluated more thoroughly for organ dysfunction. Sepsis is confirmed if there is an acute change in total qSOFA score of 2 or more points.

Sepsis-associated encephalopathy (SAE) remains the most common neurologic complication of sepsis. SAE is thought to be secondary to a dysregulated host response to infection, as well as exposure to multiple toxins and medications. Clinical features of SAE include decreased level of alertness, confusion/disorientation, and inattention/restlessness. Exam findings are rather diffuse and may comprise asterixis, multifocal myoclonus, seizures, coarse tremor, and paratonia. The main differential diagnoses are primary neurologic conditions (i.e., central nervous system (CNS) infection, stroke/intracranial hemorrhage (ICH), nonconvulsive status epilepticus), alcohol or drug intoxication/withdrawal, Wernicke encephalopathy, serotonin, and neuroleptic malignant syndromes. The initial work-up usually includes neuroimaging, electroencephalography (EEG) and cerebrospinal fluid (CSF) analysis. Management consists of treatment of sepsis and treatment of reversible causes of encephalopathy (if present).

Intensive care unit–acquired weakness (ICUAW) (critical illness polyneuropathy and myopathy) is an important neuromuscular complication of sepsis. In this condition, neuropathy is a primary axonal degeneration, whereas myopathy is multifactorial and relates to impaired muscle structure and function. ICUAW affects both limb and respiratory muscles, and this diagnosis is suspected when there is difficulty in weaning from mechanical ventilation. The main risk factors are severity of illness, sepsis, multiple organ dysfunction, prolonged immobilization, and hyperglycemia. It is unclear whether steroids and neuromuscular blocking agents are risk factors for ICUAW. Exam findings include symmetric, distally pronounced weakness associated with atrophy, and fasciculations; deep tendon reflexes (DTRs) are typically absent or decreased. Electromyography/nerve conduction studies (EMG/NCS) may be pursued in select cases. Differentials include Guillain-Barré syndrome (GBS), metabolic derangements (i.e., hypophosphatemia), thyrotoxicosis, neuromuscular blockade, nutritional deficiency neuropathies, and paraneoplastic syndromes. Because there is no specific therapy for ICUAW, management involves avoidance of risk factors, early mobilization, and supportive care/rehabilitation. Most patients improve significantly over a period of months.

REFERENCES

Schmutzhard, E., & Pfausler, B. (2017). Neurologic complications of sepsis. *Handb Clin Neurol*, *141*, 675–683.

Singer, M., Deutschman, C. S., Seymour, C. W., et al. (2016). The third international consensus definitions for sepsis and septic shock (Sepsis-3). *JAMA*, *315*(8), 801–810.

SHUNTS, THIRD VENTRICULOSTOMY, VENTRICULOPERITONEAL SHUNTS

I. *Ventriculoperitoneal (VP) shunts* are used primarily for the treatment of hydrocephalus. They are favored in infants and growing children because extra tubing can be left in the peritoneal cavity, allowing for growth and extending the time between shunt revisions.

II. *Ventriculojugular (VJ)* and *ventriculoatrial shunts* are also used for the treatment of hydrocephalus and may be used after major growth is completed. Complications (thrombi, endocarditis, septic or tubing emboli, and arrhythmias) are more frequent and serious than with VP shunts, and thus these shunts are less used.

III. *Ventriculopleural (VPL) shunts* are a second line option for treatment of adult hydrocephalus cases in which VPS are unsuitable or contraindicated. VPL shunts have high revision rate, and complications include pleural effusions, pneumothorax, empyema, and overdrainage.

IV. *Endoscopic third ventriculostomy* is a newer method of approaching noncommunicating hydrocephalus that affects the third ventricle, particularly in the treatment of colloid cysts. This procedure uses an endoscope from a frontal burr hole to traverse the lateral ventricle and foramen of Monro and then enter the third ventricle to create a fistula between the third ventricle and the subarachnoid space.

V. *Lumboperitoneal shunts* are useful in communicating hydrocephalus, particularly normal-pressure hydrocephalus. Similarly, a lumbar drain can be used for temporary, constant relief of cerebrospinal fluid (CSF) pressure for the treatment of acute surgical complications. An intrathecal pump, as in the chronic administration of baclofen, can be placed in the spinal canal for more direct and efficacious treatment of spasticity.

VI. *External ventriculostomy (external ventricular drains [EVDs])* temporary shunts, placed in the lateral ventricles, are useful immediately after cranial surgical procedures when CSF protein level is very high. They are also used to measure and control intracranial pressure (ICP) in traumas or acute intracranial hemorrhage (ICH) when there is debris in the CSF.

VII. *Ventricular access devices (Ommaya reservoir)* are also available to monitor ICP, provide central nervous system (CNS) antimicrobial treatment access, and treat CNS cancers with chemotherapy. They directly access the lateral ventricle from a frontal burr hole.

Complication rates for VP shunts range from 4% to 30% in the literature, whereas endoscopic ventriculostomy yields a complication rate as high as 40%.

SHUNT MALFUNCTION

Classic symptoms of shunt dysfunction in older children and adults *are headache, lethargy, nausea,* and *vomiting.* Gradual shunt malfunction may come to medical attention as impaired school performance, irritability, or personality change. Infants may have irritability, poor feeding, vomiting, and an abnormal shrill cry. Children with repeated episodes of shunt malfunction generally come to medical attention in a similar manner with each episode.

I. *Mechanical malfunction can be due to disconnection, breakage, or obstruction,* including a ventricular catheter plugged with glia or choroid plexus, a valve plugged with high-protein CSF or debris, or a distal catheter plugged with thrombus (VJ) or omentum (VP).

Evaluation includes several steps: (1) Pump the valve. Difficulty with compression of the valve ("pumps hard") suggests distal obstruction; slow refill suggests proximal obstruction or slit ventricles. Even if the shunt pumps, it may not be working properly. (2) Palpate the shunt tubing for any interruption. (3) Obtain a shunt series. Obtain plain x-rays of the entire shunt system (reservoirs and pumps may be radiolucent) to look for interruption and a noncontrasted head computed tomography (CT) scan to assess ventricular size (old films are invaluable for comparing ventricular size). (4) Tap the shunt (Huber needle only) for CSF pressure (if obstructed proximal to reservoir, measured pressure will not be elevated) and CSF examination. More than 90% of shunt failures occur in the first 3 months. In uncomplicated shunt placements, 6- to 12-month postoperative CT should be scheduled.

II. *Shunt infection:* A shunt tap is not always necessary when a fever develops in a child with a shunt. Upper respiratory infection, otitis media, pharyngitis, urinary tract infection, and gastroenteritis are frequent causes of febrile illness in any child, including those with shunts. A tap should be performed if the child is lethargic, unusually irritable, photophobic, or has neck stiffness. A shunt tap should also be considered if there is a history of similar presentation with a previous shunt infection or if there is unexplained fever or leukocytosis. *Staphylococcus epidermidis* and *Staphylococcus aureus* are the two most common types of infective agents. Although intrathecal antibiotics may be successful, removal of an infected shunt is usually necessary for effective treatment.

III. *Other CNS complications* of shunts include meningitis, seizures, hematomas, and hygromas. Asymptomatic bilateral subdural effusions are common (30%) in VP shunts and can occur secondary to a siphoning effect of the shunt, causing excess CSF to be drained. Programmable valves lessen this complication. Peritoneal complications include ascites and cyst formation, perforation of viscus or abdominal wall, infection with obstruction of the distal end of the catheter, and peritoneal metastases from CNS tumors (e.g., medulloblastoma). Other complications include soft tissue infection along the shunt tract and pressure necrosis of the skin.

Fig. 60 shows the major components of typical shunt systems.

REFERENCE

Craven, C., Asif, H., Farrukh, A., et al. (2017). Case series of ventriculopleural shunts in adults: a single-center experience. *J Neurosurg*, *126*(6), 2010–2016.

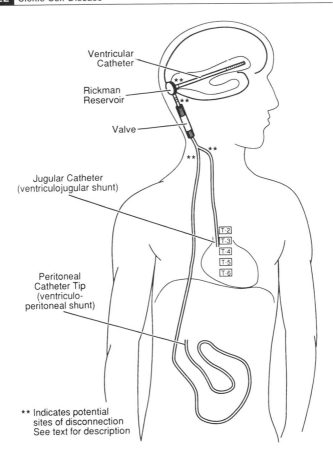

Ventricular
Catheter

Rickman
Reservoir

Valve

Jugular Catheter
(ventriculojugular shunt)

T-2
T-3
T-4
T-5
T-6

Peritoneal
Catheter Tip
(ventriculo-
peritoneal shunt)

** Indicates potential
sites of disconnection
See text for description

FIGURE 60

Typical shunt system (many variations exist).

SICKLE CELL DISEASE

Sickle cell disease (SCD) is a group of inherited red blood cell disorders characterized by the presence of two beta-globin gene mutations, at least one of which being a sickle mutation. The most common forms of SCD are sickle cell anemia (SCA) (homozygous sickle mutation; HbSS), sickle beta thalassemia (HbS/B-Th), and hemoglobin SC disease (HbSC). Conversely, sickle cell trait is defined as a carrier condition in which one beta-globin allele carries the sickle mutation and the other allele is completely normal (HbAS). In general, sickle cell trait is not symptomatic.

Sickle hemoglobin tends to polymerize when deoxygenated, resulting in damage of the red blood cells (RBC); this ultimately leads to hemolytic anemia and vascular obstruction/vasoocclusion. Virtually every organ can be affected; therefore SCD is considered a multisystem disorder. The neurologic complications of SCD include stroke (ischemic and hemorrhagic), posterior reversible encephalopathy syndrome (PRES), seizures, meningitis, headache, intracranial aneurysm, moyamoya syndrome, neurocognitive dysfunction, retinal detachment, and proliferative retinopathy.

1. Stroke (ischemic and hemorrhagic):
   a. Patients with SCD are at high risk for stroke (ischemic and hemorrhagic), especially those with SCA (HbSS) and HbS/beta^0-thalassemia.
   b. The prevalence of stroke (ischemic and hemorrhagic) in SCA is estimated as 11% by age 20, 15% by age 30, and 24% by age 45.
   c. The overall incidence is approximately 0.5 per 100 patient-years. The incidence of ischemic stroke in SCA is higher in children, adolescents, and elderly patients. Conversely, the incidence of hemorrhagic stroke is highest in individuals aged 20 to 29 years.
   d. Hemorrhagic stroke accounts for one-third of SCD-related strokes and is associated with a 25% mortality rate.
   e. The most common risk factors for ischemic stroke comprise prior transient ischemic attack (TIA), rate of and recent acute chest syndrome, high SBP, low steady state hemoglobin level, silent infarct, and high mean velocity (>200 cm/s) on transcranial Doppler (TCD).
   f. The most common risk factors for hemorrhagic stroke comprise high steady state white blood cells (WBC) and low steady state hemoglobin levels, as well as presence of aneurysm. Other suggested risk factors include recent blood transfusion and treatment with steroids or nonsteroidal anti-inflammatory drugs (NSAIDs).
   g. Most ischemic strokes are secondary to large vessel vasculopathy involving the supraclinoid internal carotid artery (ICA) and proximal middle and anterior cerebral arteries. The most common topography for cerebral infarctions includes large vessel territory, borderzone regions, and punctate lesions in the deep white matter. Silent infarcts, found in approximately one-fifth of these patients, are usually located within deep white matter.
   h. Most intracranial hemorrhages (ICHs) (intraparenchymal, subarachnoid hemorrhage (SAH), intraventricular, or a combination) do not have an identified etiology. However, when the etiology is known, it is usually SAH—often secondary to intracranial aneurysm. Other causes include hemorrhagic transformation of an ischemic infarct, cerebral venous thrombosis, and moyamoya syndrome. Importantly, the presence of ICH does not exclude the possibility of a concurrent stroke.
   i. Acute management of ischemic stroke in patients with SCD should include optimal hydration, correction of hypoxemia, correction of systemic hypotension, and blood exchange to reduce the percentage of

HbS levels to less than 30% with a target hemoglobin of approximately 10g/dL. Intravenous recombinant tissue plasminogen activator (IV r-TPA) for patients with known SCD (children and adults) and an acute ischemic stroke is not well established.

j. Acute management of ICH in patients with SCD does not differ from ICH in the general population—because there is a lack of formal evidence on the treatment of ICH in SCD.

k. Work-up should include neurovascular imaging to look for large vessel disease, aneurysm, and moyamoya syndrome. In the case of ICH, angiography should be performed if initial vascular imaging (magnetic resonance angiography/computed tomography angiography [MRA/CTA]) is unrevealing. Importantly, the use of contrast may increase the risk of stroke. Magnetic resonance venography (MRV) should be obtained if cerebral venous thrombosis (CVT) is suspected. In addition to standard stroke labs, complete blood count (CBC), reticulocyte count, percent hemoglobin S, and type and crossmatch should also be obtained. These patients should concurrently undergo thorough investigation for other possible causes of stroke (such as cardiac arrhythmia and hypercoagulability).

l. Primary and secondary ischemic stroke prevention in children with SCD involves chronic transfusion therapy. Children with SCD and high TCD velocity (>200 cm/sec) should receive chronic transfusions with a goal of reducing HbS to less than 30%. Similarly, children with SCD who have had an ischemic stroke should receive chronic transfusion therapy; these patients should also be evaluated for hematopoietic stem cell transplantation and/or hydroxyurea. Primary and secondary ischemic stroke prevention in adults has been understudied. Secondary ICH prevention relies on identifying and treating underlying causes— such as aneurysm. Cerebral revascularization may decrease the risk of recurrent stroke in patients with moyamoya syndrome.

2. PRES

a. PRES is characterized by confusion, headaches, visual symptoms, and seizures. Neuroimaging shows white matter changes predominantly in the posterior topography (occipital and parietal regions; frontal lesions may occur). This syndrome is associated with multiple conditions such as hypertension and immunosuppressive therapy, as well as SCD. Importantly, PRES can mimic stroke; differentiating these two entities is paramount and may be assisted by diffusion-weighted imaging.

3. Seizures

a. Seizures and epilepsy are 2 to 3 times more common in patients with SCD compared with nonsickle populations. Male gender and history of dactylitis are associated with a higher risk of developing epilepsy. (Dactylitis is characterized by sudden onset of severe pain associated with warmth and edema affecting the hands and/or feet. It is caused by bone marrow infarction of the carpal/tarsal bones and phalanges secondary to vascular blockage, and it is often the initial presentation in infants. An episode may last 1 to 4 weeks.) Seizures in SCD are believed to be secondary to a combination of factors including stroke/ICH and infection of the CNS, as well as other SCD-related mechanisms that potentially lead to (focal) cerebral hypoperfusion. If antiseizure medications are started, folic acid supplementation should be optimized.

4. Meningitis
   a. Patients with SCD are more susceptible to infections, especially from encapsulated bacteria—such as *Streptococcus pneumoniae*, *Haemophilus influenzae,* and *Neisseria meningitidis*—mainly due to functional asplenia caused by splenic infarction. These infections include life-threatening bacterial meningitis. Patients with SCD and suspected meningitis should undergo lumbar puncture, blood cultures should be drawn, and broad-spectrum antibiotics should be started. The latter are generally a combination of a third-generation cephalosporin and vancomycin, as well as ampicillin (if >50 years of age).

5. Headache
   a. Headache in SCD may be secondary to a variety of severe conditions including stroke, ICH, CVT, and meningitis. Headache may also be due to pain crisis or rebound cephalgia (because chronic pain medication use is common). Therefore, although benign causes of headache predominate, these patients should undergo thorough evaluation.

REFERENCES

Demaerschalk, B. M., Kleindorfer, D. O., Adeoye, O. M., et al. (2016). Scientific rationale for the inclusion and exclusion criteria for intravenous alteplase in acute ischemic stroke: a statement for healthcare professionals from the American Heart Association/American Stroke Association. *Stroke, 47*, 581–641.

Ohene-Frempong, K., Weiner, S. J., Sleeper, L. A., et al. (1998). Cerebrovascular accidents in sickle cell disease: rates and risk factors. *Blood, 91*, 288–294.

SLEEP DISORDERS

The seven major categories of sleep disorders are insomnia, sleep-related breathing disorders, central disorders of hypersomnolence, circadian rhythm sleep-wake disorders, parasomnias, sleep-related movement disorders, and other sleep disorders.

I. Insomnia is the most common sleep disorder and comes in three distinct types.
   • Short-term insomnia: This is a problem related to sleep initiation or sleep maintenance (despite adequate opportunity and circumstances for sleep) and daytime sleepiness, lasting less than 3 months. It is often associated with a stressor, and can resolve when the stressor is removed and/or adequate coping develops.
   • Chronic insomnia: This is a problem with sleep initiation or maintenance (despite adequate opportunity and circumstances for sleep) and daytime sleepiness occurring 3 times a week for 3 months or more.

S

SLEEP DISORDERS

- Other insomnia: These are insomnia that do not meet the criteria of the first two.
- Dyssomnia: This is a disorder of initiating and maintaining sleep. It is characterized by insomnia, excessive sleepiness, or abnormal circadian cycle.

II. Sleep-Related Breathing Disorders: These are abnormal respirations that occur during sleep in adults or children. They comprise four types.

- Central Sleep Apnea: This comprises: (1) with Cheyne-Stokes breathing, (2) without Cheyne-Stokes breathing, (3) high altitude periodic breathing due to medication or substance use, and (4) primary central sleep apnea.
- Obstructive Sleep Apnea (OSA): This is defined as having 15 or more respiratory events per hour, even in the absence of an associated symptom or comorbid disorders. In adults with comorbid conditions such as hypertension, coronary artery disease, atrial fibrillation, congestive heart failure, stroke, diabetes, cognitive and mood disorders; or if there are signs or symptoms including excessive sleepiness, fatigue, and/or insomnia, the diagnosis of OSA is made when there are five or more predominant obstructive respiratory events per hour.
- Sleep-related hypoventilation: Defined as elevated arterial partial pressure of carbon dioxide ($PaCO_2$). The criteria for diagnosis is $PaCO_2 > 45$ mm Hg. Examples include obesity hypoventilation, congenital central alveolar hypoventilation, late onset central hypoventilation with hypothalamic dysfunction, idiopathic, due to medication or substances, or due to a medical disorder.

III. Central Disorders of Hypersomnolence: These conditions have a primary complaint of daytime excessive sleepiness not due to another sleep disorder. Excessive sleepiness in this case is defined as daily episodes of irrepressible need to sleep or daytime lapse into sleep.

- Narcolepsy type 1: Described as having cataplexy with or without hypocretin-1 deficiency, although cerebrospinal fluid (CSF) hypocretin-1 < 110 pg/mL is diagnostic; or a mean sleep latency of ≤ 8 minutes and two sleep onset rapid eye movement periods (SOREMP) within 15 minutes of sleep onset on an MSLT (and/or the overnight polysomnogram).
- Narcolepsy type 2: Meeting the criteria of narcolepsy type 1 except for the absence of CSF hypocretin-1 level and cataplexy.
- Idiopathic hypersomnia: this is a subjective sleepiness with an MSLT < 8 min and less than 2 SOREMPs, without cataplexy and without hypocretin 1 deficiency.

Other Central Disorders of Hypersomnolence

- Kleine-Levin Syndrome
- Hypersomnia due to medical disorder
- Hypersomnia due to medication or substance use
- Hypersomnia associated with psychiatric disorder
- Insufficient sleep syndrome

IV. Circadian Rhythm Sleep-Wake Disorders: This is a group of chronic or recurrent sleep disturbances due to altered circadian system. There is a misalignment between the environmental cues and the individual sleep wake cycle. They are a common cause of excessive daytime sleepiness.
   – Time zone change (also known as "jet lag")
   – Shift work syndromes
   – Delayed/advanced sleep phase syndromes
   – Non-24 hour sleep wake rhythm disorder with fluctuating periods of insomnia and/or excessive sleepiness: caused by intrinsic circadian pacemaker out of sync with 24 hour day cycle.
   – Circadian rhythm disorders due to medical, psychiatric or neurologic disorders
   – Irregular sleep wake rhythm disorders

V. Parasomnias are abnormal undesired physiologic or behavioral events occurring at initiation of sleep, during sleep, or during arousal from sleep.
   • Non-Rapid Eye Movement (NREM)-related parasomnias: NREM-related parasomnias are arousal disorders that include sleepwalking, confusional arousals, and sleep terrors, in contrast to nightmares, which occur during rapid eye movement (REM) sleep. These episodes are recurrent, and include (1) incomplete awakening, (2) absent or inappropriate responsiveness, (3) limited or no cognition of a dream, and (4) partial or complete amnesia to the episode.
   • Rapid Eye Movement (REM) associated Parasomnias: These are associated with REM sleep and include nightmares, sleep paralysis, REM sleep behavior disorder, and sleep related painful erections.
   • Other Parasomnias:
     – sleep enuresis and bruxism
     – nocturnal paroxysmal dystonia
     – primary snoring
     – benign neonatal myoclonus
     – sleep-related abnormal swallowing
     – sleep enuresis
     – exploding head syndrome
     – parasomnia associated with medical disorders
     – parasomnia due to a medication or substance

VI. Sleep-related movement disorders: These are described as simple, stereotypic movements that disturb sleep. Dysesthesia during wakefulness is a primary symptom.
   • Restless Leg Syndrome (Willis-Ekbom Disease)—primary description is an urge to move the legs and/or presence of discomfort at rest, that is relieved with movement. There is an associated circadian component as it primarily occurs at night or in the evening, causing distress and impairment of sleep.
   • Periodic Limb Movement Disorder—diagnosed by polysomnography which notes frequent limb movements of more than 15 times per hour in adults and more than 5 in children.

- Other sleep related movement disorders include:
  - Sleep-related cramps
  - Sleep-related bruxism (teeth grinding)
  - Sleep related rhythmic movement disorder
  - Benign sleep myoclonus of infancy
  - Propriospinal myoclonus at sleep onset
  - Sleep-related movement disorder due to a medical disorder
  - Sleep-related movement disorder due to medication or substance

Treatment of Sleep Related Disorders:

- Associated medical or psychiatric conditions should be treated.
- General management of insomnia includes optimizing the patient's "sleep hygiene" as follows:
  - Behavioral therapies:
    (1) Sleep hygiene and stimulus control
    (2) Wake and sleep at the same time each day (including weekends)
    (3) Use the bed only for sleep and sex
    (4) Leave the bed if not asleep within 10 minutes of lying down in bed
    (5) Avoid heavy exercise or large meals just before bedtime
    (6) Avoid daytime napping (sleep restriction)
    (7) Make sure the bedroom is not too warm or cold
    (8) Exercise regularly, and
    (9) discontinue alcohol, caffeine, cigarettes, and psychoactive drugs.
  - Other treatments include: biofeedback, sleep restriction therapy, and cognitive behavioral therapy.
  - Approved medications include:
    - Short-acting benzodiazepines that may offer temporary adjunctive benefit, but their long-term use is not recommended.
    - Other sedatives, including melatonin agonists ramelteon, suvorexant (orexin agonist), zalephon, zolpidem, eszopiclone and diphenhydramine, may be used judiciously.
    - Antidepressants such as doxepin, amitriptyline, trazodone can be used.
    - Management of parasomnias and abnormal movements are complex and have an overarching goal to keep patient safe.
  - Work-up includes: polysomnography.
  - In Restless Leg Syndrome, labs for iron deficiency should be checked.

REFERENCES

American Academy of Sleep Medicine. (2014). In *International classification of sleep disorders*, ed 3. Darien, IL: American Academy of Sleep Medicine.
Berry, R. B., Brooks, R., Gamaldo, C. E., et al. (2017). *The AASM manual for the scoring of sleep and associated events: rules, terminology and technical specifications,* version 2.4. Darien, IL: American Academy of Sleep Medicine.

SPASTICITY

Spasticity is a velocity-dependent increase in muscle tone or tonic stretch reflex. That is, more resistance will occur with rapid stretching of a muscle than with slow stretching. The underlying mechanism is a hyperactive stretch reflex that results from damage to various descending pathways, most notably the dorsal and medial reticulospinal tract and the vestibulospinal tract. Symptoms of spasticity include clonus, dystonia, extensor or flexor spasms, abnormal reflex responses, loss of dexterity, muscle fatigue, weakness, stiffness, fibrosis, and atrophy.

TREATMENT
Pharmacological
GABA mediated agents:

I. Baclofen is a gamma-aminobutyric acid (GABA) agonist and also interferes with the release of excitatory transmitters.
   a. Starting dosage is 5 mg tid, increased by 5 mg per dose every 3 days to therapeutic effect.
   b. Maximum dosage is 80 mg/day in divided doses.
   c. Adverse effects include drowsiness, dizziness, weakness, nausea, mood changes, hallucinations, gastrointestinal symptoms, hypotension, changes in accommodation, ocular motor function, and deterioration of seizure control.
   d. Avoid abrupt withdrawal of the drug.
II. Diazepam facilitates GABA-mediated presynaptic and postsynaptic inhibition.
   a. Starting dosage is 2 mg bid, increased slowly to a maximum dosage of 40 mg/day in divided doses.
   b. Side effects are habituation and sedation.
III. Dantrolene sodium interferes with excitation-contraction coupling by decreasing the release of calcium at the sarcoplasmic reticulum.
   a. Starting dosage is 25 mg every day, increased by 25 mg every week, to a maximum dosage of 100 mg qid.
   b. Side effects are hepatotoxicity (monitor liver enzymes) and diarrhea.

Drugs that bind to α_2-adrenergic receptors and decrease sympathetic outflow, along with inhibiting afferent inputs into the spinal reflex arc, can be used to treat spasticity:

I. Tizanidine should be started at 2 mg bid and increased by 2 to 4 mg with each dose until therapeutic effect is reached. Maximum dose is 12 mg tid. It is generally well tolerated but may cause increased fatigue or sedation.
II. Clonidine 0.2 to 1 mg/day in divided doses has similar effects but may cause sedation, orthostatic hypotension, and rebound hypertension.
III. Chlorpromazine - causes α-adrenergic blockade and has been used to reduce spasticity, but sedation and fear of tardive dyskinesia have limited its use.

Other treatment includes the following:
a. Phenytoin (100 to 400 mg/day)
b. Carbamazepine (600 mg /day to 1200 mg/day)
These act on the Ia afferent muscle spindle to reduce spontaneous and stretch-evoked discharges.

Non-Pharmacological

Non-invasive neuromodulation uses weak electric current and neurochemical agents (dopaminergic and benzodiazepines) to modify and modulate synaptic properties. Electric current can be applied directly in transcranial direct current stimulation (tDCS) stimulators, or indirectly using focal magnetic fields, to induce an electric current to the brain (repetitive transcranial magnetic stimulation, rTMS). Modulating plasticity through neuronal membrane polarity is investigated for possible future clinical applications.

Surgical intervention with selective posterior rhizotomy has been used in patients with cerebral palsy and severe spasticity. Longitudinal myelotomy has been used to control severe flexor spasms. Spinal cord and cerebellar stimulation act by stimulating inhibitory pathways.

Botulinum toxin can be used to manage spasticity locally, regardless of etiology (cerebral palsy, multiple sclerosis, stroke, etc.). Side effects include flaccidity, development of neutralizing antibodies, and rare systemic weakness. Doses take effect several days after injection and may last up to 3 months.

Physical therapy, occupational therapy, and orthopedic positioning, and orthotics and instrumentation are other non-pharmacological options.

REFERENCES

Leo, A., Naro, A., Molonia, F., et al. (2017). Spasticity management: the current state of transcranial neuromodulation. *PM R*, *9*(10), 1020–1029. https://doi.org/10.1016/j.pmrj.2017.03.014.

Li, S. (2017). Spasticity, motor recovery, and neural plasticity after stroke. *Front Neurol*, *8*, 1–8. https://doi.org/10.3389/fneur.2017.00120.

SPINAL CORD

The relationships of the spinal cord segments and roots to the vertebral column are depicted in Fig. 61. Cross-sectional anatomy of the cervical cord is shown in Fig. 62. The most salient feature of the spinal cord is that it is NOT a paired structure. A very low level of suspicion must be maintained in order not to miss a potentially devastating but treatable cause of myelopathy.

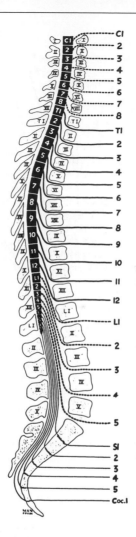

FIGURE 61

Relation of spinal segments and roots to the vertebral column. (From Haymaker, W., & Woodhall, B. (1953). *Peripheral nerve injuries: principles of diagnosis*. Philadelphia: WB Saunders).

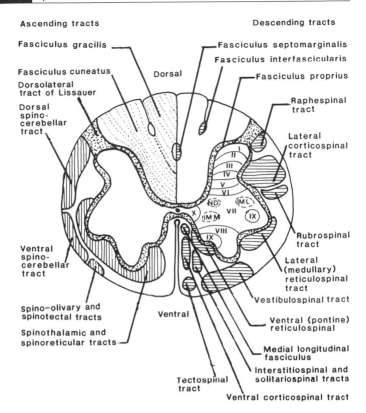

Ascending tracts | Descending tracts

- Fasciculus gracilis
- Fasciculus cuneatus
- Dorsolateral tract of Lissauer
- Dorsal spinocerebellar tract
- Ventral spinocerebellar tract
- Spino-olivary and spinotectal tracts
- Spinothalamic and spinoreticular tracts
- Dorsal
- Ventral
- Fasciculus septomarginalis
- Fasciculus interfascicularis
- Fasciculus proprius
- Raphespinal tract
- Lateral corticospinal tract
- Rubrospinal tract
- Lateral (medullary) reticulospinal tract
- Vestibulospinal tract
- Ventral (pontine) reticulospinal
- Medial longitudinal fasciculus
- Interstitiospinal and solitariospinal tracts
- Tectospinal tract
- Ventral corticospinal tract

FIGURE 62

Cervical spinal cord (cross section). Gray matter columns: *I–X*, Rexed laminae: *IML*, intermediolateral cell column; *IMM*, intermediomedial cell column; *ND*, nucleus dorsalis (Clark's column).

SPINAL CORD SYNDROMES

- *Anterior cord syndrome* is characterized by paresis and impaired pain perception; proprioception is preserved below the lesion. The syndrome is usually caused by spinal cord compression or anterior spinal artery occlusion/infarction.
- *Posterior cord syndrome* consists of pain and paresthesias out of proportion to motor impairment that are referable to the affected segments; the syndrome is commonly associated with demyelinating lesions.
- *Central cord syndrome*, often seen with hyperextension injuries in the neck, results in patchy sensory loss, urinary retention, and weakness disproportionately affecting the legs.

- *Spinal cord hemisection* produces the *"Brown-Sequard syndrome,"* consisting of (1) ipsilateral spastic paresis; (2) ipsilateral loss of touch and vibratory and joint position sense; and (3) contralateral loss of pain and temperature sensation below the level of the lesion.
- Spinal shock is seen in the acute period after a spinal cord injury. It is a syndrome of paralysis, areflexia, anesthesia, and bowel or bladder dysfunction below the level of the lesion. Spinal shock may last weeks, after which the chronic symptoms of spinal cord injury appear: spasticity, exaggerated tendon and withdrawal reflexes, and positive Babinski sign.

CAUSES OF MYELOPATHY

I. Congenital or developmental: spinal dysraphism (see Developmental Malformations), craniocervical junction abnormalities, syringomyelia, congenital cervical spinal stenosis, tethered-cord syndromes, diastematomyelia

II. Degenerative: motor neuron disease, spinocerebellar degeneration, hereditary spastic paraplegia

III. Demyelinating: multiple sclerosis, neuromyelitis optica (Devic disease)

IV. Infectious: poliomyelitis, herpes zoster, rabies, viral encephalomyelitis, bacterial meningitis, epidural or subdural abscess, syphilis, tuberculosis, typhus, spotted fever, fungal infections, trichinosis, schistosomiasis, human T-cell leukemia virus type 1 (HTLV-1), human immunodeficiency virus, cytomegalovirus

V. Inflammatory or immune response: postinfectious, postvaccination, arachnoiditis, sarcoidosis, lupus erythematosus

VI. Metabolic or nutritional: pernicious anemia (vitamin B_{12} deficiency), pellagra, chronic liver disease

VII. Neoplastic: extramedullary or intramedullary tumors, meningeal carcinomatosis, paraneoplastic syndromes

VIII. Toxic: ethanol (direct effect and through hepatic cirrhosis and portacaval shunting), arsenic, cyanide, lathyrism, clioquinol, intrathecal contrast, or chemotherapeutic agents

IX. Traumatic (see later discussion): vertebral subluxation or fracture, transection, contusion, concussion, hemorrhage, birth injury (particularly breech delivery), electrical injury, spondylosis, spondylolisthesis

X. Vascular (see later): arterial and venous infarction, hemorrhage (epidural, subdural, intraparenchymal), vasculitis, vascular malformations, aneurysms, effects of radiation therapy (see Radiation)

DEGENERATIVE JOINT DISEASE

Degenerative joint disease of the spine occurs as a result of changes in the intervertebral disks (spondylosis) with aging. Spondylosis leads to osteophyte formation, meningeal fibrosis, and disk herniation. Pain is often radicular at level of lesion.

Spondylosis in the cervical spine can cause progressive myelopathy, radiculopathy, or both. Thoracic lesions become evident mainly as paraparesis. Lumbar lesions cause radiculopathies, neurogenic claudication, or back pain syndromes.

Neurogenic claudication, like vascular claudication, causes exertional pain, but it differs from vascular claudication as follows: (1) the pain may be felt in buttock or thigh with prolonged standing or walking; (2) the pulses are normal; (3) reflexes may be decreased while at peak pain; and (4) the pain is relieved with waist flexion or rest but generally takes several minutes or more to resolve.

Syringomyelia describes a condition in which there is an abnormal cavity or cyst in the spinal cord. Syrinxes are usually cervical but may extend rostrally (syringobulbia) or caudally. They are frequently associated with developmental malformations of the craniocervical junction (Arnold-Chiari malformations, platybasia), myelomeningocele, kyphoscoliosis, intramedullary tumors, vascular malformations, or trauma. Hand numbness is the usual initial complaint with cervical syrinxes. Loss of pain and temperature sensation in a capelike (suspended) distribution with sparing of vibratory and joint position sense (dissociated sensory loss) is due to destruction of crossing pain fibers at the lesion level. Segmental weakness, atrophy, fasciculations, spasticity, incontinence, and hyperreflexia occur frequently. The course is usually slowly progressive; a sudden decline may indicate development of hematomyelia or progression of an underlying condition. Management includes cyst drainage and scrupulous hand care to prevent painless cuts and wound infections.

TRAUMA (See also SPINAL CORD TRAUMA)

Initial management of spinal cord trauma should include maintenance of airway, breathing, and circulation; immobilization (spine board, collars); bladder catheterization; nasogastric intubation; and serial neurologic examinations. Radiographic studies are directed to the area of interest but generally include cross-table lateral and anteroposterior (AP) cervical views (all seven cervical vertebrae must be seen) and films of the thoracic and lumbar spine. An open-mouth odontoid film may be obtained in conscious patients. CT is sensitive for identification of fractures. Myelography or MRI can identify acute compressive lesions such as hematomas. High-dose IV corticosteroids are commonly given, but their use is controversial. The National Acute Spinal Cord Injury Study (NASCIS) clinical trials, which have been criticized for their design flaws, fail to show conclusive evidence of the efficacy of corticosteroids in spinal cord injury. If given, methylprednisolone must be started in the first 8 hours after injury, as a bolus of 30 mg/kg, followed by an infusion of 5.4 mg/kg for 23 (first study) or 48 (second) hours.

VASCULAR SYNDROMES

I. Anterior spinal artery infarctions typically affect the midthoracic region, causing severe local, radicular, and deep pain; paraparesis; sphincter disturbance; and dissociated distal sensory loss (pain and temperature sensation more affected than vibration, touch, and joint position sense). Sacral sensation may remain intact. Causes include systemic hypotension, aortic dissection, hypotension, thrombosis, vasculitis, embolism, sickle cell disease, and extrinsic arterial compression by tumor, bone, or disk material.

II. Posterior spinal artery infarction is less common and produces pain, loss of proprioception, and variable involvement of corticospinal and spinocerebellar tracts.

III. Spinal subdural and epidural hemorrhage most commonly occurs after trauma, lumbar puncture, or spinal or epidural anesthesia. Other causes include anticoagulant use, blood dyscrasias, thrombocytopenia, neoplasm, and vascular malformation. The initial symptom is severe back pain at the level of the bleed. Myelopathy or cauda equina syndrome with symptoms dependent on lesion level develop over hours to days. MRI is especially useful in determining lesion location. Laminectomy with clot evacuation should be performed as soon as possible because prognosis for recovery is better when surgery is performed early and the preoperative deficits are not severe.

IV. Spinal subarachnoid hemorrhage is rare. Causes may include aneurysm rupture or vascular malformation hemorrhage. Other causes include aortic coarctation, spinal artery rupture, mycotic aneurysms, polyarteritis nodosa, spinal tumors, lumbar puncture, blood dyscrasias, and anticoagulants. Severe back pain followed by signs of meningeal irritation is usually the first manifestation. Multiple radiculopathies and myelopathy may develop. Headache, cranial neuropathies, and obtundation are associated with diffusion of blood above the foramen magnum. Cerebrospinal fluid (CSF) is bloody and intracranial pressure may be elevated; treatment is directed at the underlying cause.

V. Hematomyelia: Intramedullary spinal hemorrhage is rare but occurs after trauma, spinal arteriovenous malformation rupture, hemorrhage into tumor or syrinx, or venous infarction or with clotting or bleeding disorders. Emergency surgical decompression is often indicated.

See also Spinal Cord Trauma, Spinal Cord Compression, and Tumors. See also Spinal Cord Injury in the Neurologic Emergency appendix for treatment of traumatic spinal cord compression.

REFERENCES

Ahuja, C. S., et al. (2017). Traumatic spinal cord injury. *Nat Rev Dis Primers*, *3*, 17018.

Derwenskus, J., & Zaidat, O. O. (2004). In J. I. Suarez (Ed.), *Critical care neurology and neurosurgery*. Totowa, NJ: Humana Press.

Silva, N. A., et al. (2014). From basics to clinical: a comprehensive review on spinal cord injury. *Prog Neurobiol*, *114*, 25–57.

SPINAL CORD COMPRESSION (See also SPINAL CORD TRAUMA, SPINAL CORD INJURY IN NEUROLOGIC EMERGENCY APPENDIX)

CLINICAL PRESENTATION

Unlike cord trauma, spinal cord compression tends to develop more subacutely. Spinal cord compression can manifest as a result of intradural or extradural lesions. Occasionally osteoporotic compression fractures and pathologic fractures from metastatic disease can produce more acute loss of function. However, the more common causes of cord compression such as metastatic tumors, hemorrhage, and abscess tend to progress slowly over a period of days to weeks. Other causes of spinal cord compression include disc herniation and central canal stenosis. Clinically, these patients tend to present with progressive paraparesis or quadriparesis, though ataxia and altered sensory complaints may also present early depending on the location of the compressive lesion and the underlying lesion. Ventral lesions tend to produce motor symptoms early due to the ventrolateral position of the corticospinal tracts and less commonly due to involvement of the anterior spinal artery. A flaccid paralysis may occur acutely below the level of injury. More laterally placed lesions can cause the classic "crossed" sensory findings in which pain and temperature are lost below and contralateral to the lesion and vibration and proprioception are lost below and ipsilateral to the side of the lesion (the Brown-Séquard syndrome).

EVALUATION

Imaging with MRI forms the basis of diagnosis and should be obtained emergently to distinguish between demyelinating conditions and cord compression, as the outcome of compression is dependent on the time to decompression. In settings where MRI is contraindicated CT myelogram is the alternative diagnostic test to visualize a compressing lesion. The Acute Spinal Injury Association Impairment Scale is a clinical scale used to define the extent and severity of spinal cord injury (Fig. 63). The scale provides a prognostic tool for neurological recovery; as patients with complete injury (A) carry a far worse prognosis for functional recovery than incomplete injury (B through D).

TREATMENT

Rapid decompressive surgery is the definitive therapy. Administration of methylprednisolone for the treatment of acute spinal cord injury is not recommended. Metastatic compression may be treated with 10–20 mg dexamethasone followed by 6 mg given four times a day (total dose: 24 mg). Radiation therapy is another treatment option.

REFERENCES

Daroff, R. B., et al. (2015). *Bradley's neurology in clinical practice.* Elsevier Health Sciences.
Stein, D. M., & Sheth, K. N. (2015). Management of acute spinal cord injury. *Continuum (Minneap Minn)*, *21*(1 Spinal cord disorders), 159–187.

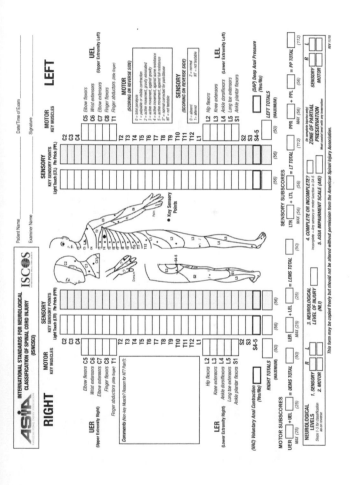

FIGURE 63
Continued

Muscle Function Grading

0 = total paralysis

1 = palpable or visible contraction

2 = active movement, full range of motion (ROM) with gravity eliminated

3 = active movement, full ROM against gravity

4 = active movement, full ROM against gravity and moderate resistance in a muscle specific position

5 = (normal) active movement, full ROM against gravity and full resistance in a functional muscle position expected from an otherwise unimpaired person

5* = (normal) active movement, full ROM against gravity and sufficient resistance to be considered normal if identified inhibiting factors (i.e. pain, disuse) were not present

NT = not testable (i.e. due to immobilization, severe pain such that the patient cannot be graded, amputation of limb, or contracture of > 50% of the normal ROM).

Sensory Grading

0 = Absent

1 = Altered, either decreased/impaired sensation or hypersensitivity

2 = Normal

NT = Not testable

When to Test Non-Key Muscles:

In a patient with an apparent AIS B classification, non-key muscle functions more than 3 levels below the motor level on each side should be tested to most accurately classify the injury (differentiate between AIS B and C).

Movement	Root level
Shoulder: Flexion, extension, abduction, adduction, internal and external rotation Elbow: Supination	C5
Elbow: Pronation Wrist: Flexion	C6
Finger: Flexion at proximal joint, extension. Thumb: Flexion, extension and abduction in plane of thumb	C7
Finger: Flexion at MCP joint Thumb: Opposition, adduction and abduction perpendicular to palm	C8
Finger: Abduction of the index finger	T1
Hip: Adduction	L2
Hip: External rotation	L3
Hip: Extension, abduction, internal rotation Knee: Flexion Ankle: Inversion and eversion Toe: MP and IP extension	L4
Hallux and Toe: DIP and PIP Flexion and abduction	L5
Hallux: Adduction	S1

ASIA Impairment Scale (AIS)

A = Complete. No sensory or motor function is preserved in the sacral segments S4-5.

B = Sensory Incomplete. Sensory but not motor function is preserved below the neurological level and includes the sacral segments S4-5 (light touch or pin prick at S4-5 or deep anal pressure) AND no motor function is preserved more than three levels below the motor level on either side of the body.

C = Motor Incomplete. Motor function is preserved at the most caudal sacral segments for voluntary anal contraction (VAC) OR the patient meets the criteria for sensory incomplete status (sensory function preserved at the most caudal sacral segments S4-S5) by LT, PP or DAP), and has some sparing of motor function more than three levels below the ipsilateral motor level on either side of the body.

(This includes key or non-key muscle functions to determine motor incomplete status.) For AIS C – less than half of key muscle functions below the single NLI have a muscle grade ≥ 3.

D = Motor Incomplete. Motor incomplete status as defined above, with at least half (half or more) of key muscle functions below the single NLI having a muscle grade ≥ 3.

E = Normal. If sensation and motor function as tested with the ISNCSCI are graded as normal in all segments, and the patient had prior deficits, then the AIS grade is E. Someone without an initial SCI does not receive an AIS grade.

Using ND: To document the sensory, motor and NLI levels, the ASIA Impairment Scale grade, and/or the zone of partial preservation (ZPP) when they are unable to be determined based on the examination results.

INTERNATIONAL STANDARDS FOR NEUROLOGICAL CLASSIFICATION OF SPINAL CORD INJURY

ISC⚬S

Steps in Classification

The following order is recommended for determining the classification of individuals with SCI.

1. Determine sensory levels for right and left sides.
The sensory level is the most caudal, intact dermatome for both pin prick and light touch sensation.

2. Determine motor levels for right and left sides.
Defined by the lowest key muscle function that has a grade of at least 3 (on supine testing), providing the key muscle functions represented by segments above that level are judged to be intact (graded as 5).
Note: in regions where there is no myotome to test, the motor level is presumed to be the same as the sensory level, if testable motor function above that level is also normal.

3. Determine the neurological level of injury (NLI)
This refers to the most caudal segment of the cord with intact sensory and antigravity (3 or more) muscle function strength, provided that there is normal (intact) sensory and motor function rostrally respectively.
The NLI is the most caudal of the sensory and motor levels determined in steps 1 and 2.

4. Determine whether the injury is Complete or Incomplete.
(i.e. absence or presence of sacral sparing)
If voluntary anal contraction = **No** AND all S4-5 sensory scores = 0 AND deep anal pressure = **No**, then injury is **Complete.**
Otherwise, injury is **Incomplete.**

5. Determine ASIA Impairment Scale (AIS) Grade.

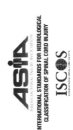

American Spinal Injury Association International Standards for Neurological Classification of Spinal Cord Injury (ISNCSCI) examination. *LEMS,* lower extremity motor score; *UEMS,* upper extremity motor score.

SPINAL CORD TRAUMA (See also SPINAL CORD COMPRESSION AND NEUROLOGIC EMERGENCIES APPENDIX)

Epidemiology: Spinal cord injury (SCI) is a leading cause of morbidity in the United States with an annual incidence of 12,000 cases per year. The most frequently affected group is young males at an average age of 31.7 years, and some 60% of cases affect males 16 to 30 years of age.

Causes: The most common causes of cord trauma are motor vehicle accident (34.5%), penetrating injuries (17.2%), falls (22%), and sports injuries (8%).

Treatment: Short-term management involves quick recognition and stabilization of the spine, along with rapid assessment for other life-threatening injuries. Prompt administration of IV methylprednisolone at 30 mg/kg over 1 hour followed by 5.4 mg/kg/hour for the next 23 hours has been shown to improve outcomes when started within 8 hours of injury. However, a 2013 revision of Guidelines for the Management of Acute Cervical Spine and Spinal Cord Injuries no longer recommends this treatment, citing risk of side effects that include gastrointestinal hemorrhage, hyperglycemia, and infections. Although controversial, some centers still use this treatment. Placement of a Foley to prevent urinary retention and initiation of deep vein thrombosis prophylaxis are also indicated. Recommended mean arterial blood pressure is between 85 to 90 mm Hg for the first 7 days following injury. Long-term care is multidisciplinary and includes spinal cord medicine physicians and nurses, neurosurgeons or orthopedic surgeons, and urologists.

Complications: Following SCI, patients can develop autonomic dysreflexia and orthostatic hypotension (in T6 or higher lesions), bone demineralization, constipation, pressure ulcers, syringomyelia, respiratory failure, neurogenic bladder, and spasticity.

Prognosis: While a devastating injury, survival is greater than 90% for isolated SCI with appropriate treatment. Overall, outcome and functionality are primarily determined by the level of injury. Initial functional independence measure (FIM) and American Spinal Injury Association scores may predict disability and outcome.

REFERENCES

Ahuja, C. S., et al. (2017). Traumatic spinal cord injury-repair and regeneration. *Neurosurgery, 80*(3S), S9–S22.

Stein, D. M., & Sheth, K. N. (2015). Management of acute spinal cord injury. *Continuum (Minneap Minn), 21*(1 Spinal Cord Disorders), 159–187.

SPINAL CORD INFARCTION

While spinal cord infarction is rare, it is often devastating and leads to significant functional impairment. The clinical presentation is usually abrupt, and the symptoms are defined by the vascular territory involved. The main clinical syndromes are anterior spinal artery (ASA) syndrome and post spinal artery (PSA) syndrome.

The most common clinical presentation of a spinal cord infarction is ASA syndrome. Patients typically present with loss of motor function and pain/temperature sensation with sparing of the vibratory and deep position sense. Pain is often present. Acutely, patients usually have flaccid weakness and loss of deep tendon reflexes; days to weeks later, spasticity and hyperreflexia usually develop. Autonomic, sexual, bowel/bladder dysfunction can also happen. Most common presentation is bilateral, however unilateral ASA syndromes are also commonly encountered.

In PSA syndrome, patients typically present with loss of vibration and deep position sensation below the level of the injury. Causes include thrombosis (sometimes secondary to hypercoagulable conditions), arterial embolism, segmental arterial occlusion, hypotension, aortic dissection or rupture, and intravascular fibrocartilaginous embolism.

In addition to the above described arterial syndromes, venous spinal cord infarction can also occur, usually in association with vascular malformations. Venous spinal cord infarcts can be non-hemorrhagic or hemorrhagic. In non-hemorrhagic infarction, venous hypertension decreases the arterial-venous pressure gradient leading to ischemia; these patients may present with acute or gradual onset of progressive symptoms.

Spinal cord infarcts can occur in children, albeit rarely. Diagnosis may be difficult as MRI may be insensitive to changes and technically difficult. Causes are varied but similar to those seen in adult patients.

The differential diagnosis of spinal cord infarction mainly includes transverse myelitis, compressive myelopathy (from abscess, hematoma, or neoplasm), and Guillain-Barré syndrome (GBS).

The diagnosis of spinal cord infarction is often suspected clinically in a patient with painful, nontraumatic spinal cord syndromes. Spinal MRI can rule out alternative diagnoses such as compressive myelopathy. The sensitivity of MRI in showing evidence of spinal cord infarct is low ($<75\%$) and diffusion-weighted imaging may be negative.

There is no specific treatment for spinal cord infarction and management focuses on rehabilitation and management of complications that can be life-threatening. These complications include neurogenic shock which is attributed to the disruption of the autonomic pathways in the spinal cord leading to reduced vascular resistance and causing symptoms of bradycardia and hypotension. Autonomic dysreflexia characterized by episodic paroxysmal hypertension, headache, bradycardia, and flushing can be life-threatening.

Prognosis depends on multiple factors that include baseline risk factors, etiology, and extent of spinal cord injury. Mortality rate can be up to 20% (the risk is highest among patients presenting with spinal cord infarction in the setting of cardiac arrest, aortic dissection or rupture). Most patients who survive make some functional improvement and independent gait can be achieved in up to 46% of patients.

REFERENCES

Nance, J. R., & Golomb, M. R. (2007). Ischemic spinal cord infarction in children without vertebral fracture. *Pediatr Neurol*, 36(4), 209–216.

Novy, J., et al. (2006). Spinal cord ischemia: clinical and imaging patterns, pathogenesis, and outcomes in 27 patients. *Arch Neurol*, 63(8), 1113–1120.

SPINAL EPIDURAL ABSCESSES

Anatomy: Below the foramen magnum there is a true epidural space in the lateral and posterior aspect of the spinal foramen that extends all the way down the length of the canal. This space is filled with fat, arteries, and venous plexus. Anterior to the cord the space is only virtual because the dura is adherent to the vertebral bodies from the foramen magnum to L1. As a result, the majority of spinal epidural abscesses (SEAs) are posterior; when anterior, they are usually below L1. Spinal dural abscesses are characterized by infectious purulent material that accumulates within the epidural space.

Infectious routes: In one third of cases no source is identified. The other two thirds are most commonly associated with skin and soft tissue infections or complications of spinal surgery and spinal procedures, including epidural catheters. The spread is usually hematogenous, but it may be contiguous from psoas, paraspinal, or retropharyngeal abscesses.

Risk factors:
- Compromised immunity: diabetes (most common), steroid or immunosuppressive therapy, malignancy, pregnancy, cirrhosis, alcoholism, and HIV infection.
- Disruption of the spinal column integrity: traumatic injury, spinal surgery, and spinal instrumentation.
- Source of infection: active urinary, respiratory, or skin infection; patients with indwelling catheters or epidural catheters; and IV drug use.

Pathogenesis: The pathogenesis is controversial. Most SEAs begin as a focal pyogenic. Inflammation and pus extend longitudinally to the epidural space, causing damage to the spinal cord at several levels by direct compression, thrombosis, and thrombophlebitis of nearby veins, interruption of arterial blood supply with ischemia, focal vasculitis, bacterial toxins, and local inflammatory process.

Microbiology: The most common is *Staphylococcus aureus* (63% to 70% of cases). The next most common is streptococcus (7% to 9% of cases). Other pathogens include gram-negative bacilli (16%), coagulase-negative staphylococci (3%), anaerobes (2%), and others (e.g. fungal, parasites, 1%). In specific settings with more subacute clinical presentation, Mycobacterium tuberculosis has been found.

Clinical presentation: The classic triad of back pain, fever, and/or neurologic deficit is seen in only 8% to 37% of cases. Usually fever appears first followed by focal and severe back pain and possibly meningismus in cervical SEA. However, sometimes fever may be absent. Root pain (shooting and electric pain) progresses over hours to days to progressive myelopathy with bladder/bowel incontinence. Once paraplegia-tetraplegia occurs, it quickly becomes irreversible.

Diagnosis: For clinically suspicious SEA, an emergent gadolinium-enhanced MRI with and without contrast of the spinal axis is ordered. CT myelography can be performed as an alternative if gadolinium-enhanced MRI is contraindicated. Initial workup also includes ESR, C-reactive protein, two sets of blood cultures, urinalysis for reflux, chest x-ray, and sputum cultures (for possible organism identification).

Differential diagnosis includes disc and bony disease, metastatic tumors, vertebral diskitis and osteomyelitis, transverse myelitis, Guillain-Barré syndrome, meningitis, and herpes zoster before the skin lesions appear.

Treatment: Early decompression and drainage and prolonged antibiotic treatment remain the cornerstone of treatment. Prompt infectious disease and neurosurgery consult is mandatory. Surgery should be performed as early as possible, within 24 to 36 hours of paralysis. Antibiotics should be started immediately. Do not wait for surgery, especially if there is significant neurological deficit or the patient is septic or critically ill. Empiric antibiotics include vancomycin (15–20 mg/kg IV every 8–12 hours; trough levels should be drawn 30 minutes prior to the next dose), PLUS either ceftriaxone 2 g IV every 12 hours or cefepime 2 g every 8 hours or ceftazidime 2 g IV every 8 hours.

Prognosis: The morbidity and mortality rates are high if untreated. The degree of recovery is related to the duration of neurologic deficits. A prompt diagnosis and the absence of neurologic symptoms for less than 24 hours conveys better outcomes.

REFERENCES

Khattar, N. K., et al. (2015). Management of spinal epidural abscess. *Contemporary Neurosurgery*, *37*(10), 1–3.

Sexton, D. J., & Sampson, J. (2017). *Spinal epidural abscess.* UpToDate. https://www.uptodate.com/contents/spinal-epidural-abscess.

SPINOCEREBELLAR ATAXIA (See also ATAXIA)

The spinocerebellar ataxias (SCAs) are a group of progressive, *autosomal dominant* ataxias that result from unstable, *nucleotide repeat expansion*. SCAs have been more recently described to result from more conventional mutations, such as gene deletion, missense, and nonsense mutation. Many of these diseases have been identified, and most are numbered from 1 to 40 (i.e., SCA1, SCA2, etc.). SCA3 is probably the most prevalent of the SCAs worldwide; it is also called Machado-Joseph disease (MJD). The episodic ataxias (EA1 through EA6) and dentatorubropallidoluysian atrophy (DRPLA) are also included in the list.

SCAs usually begin in early or middle adult life. Anticipation is more prominent with paternal transmission; age inversely correlates with the triple repeat expansion size. Clinical manifestations for patients with SCA include progressive ataxic gait, limb ataxia (dysmetria and dysdiadochokinesia), dysarthric speech, abnormal pursuit, inaccurate saccade, and nystagmus. Patients may exhibit bulbar deficit. Extrapyramidal and upper motor neuron signs can also be seen. Episodic ataxias are characterized by brief reversible episodes of ataxia. There is much clinical overlap in the syndromes, and precise genotypical diagnosis still requires molecular tests.

Phenotypic clues to specific gene mutations include upper motor signs in SCA1, 5, 7, and 8 and MJD; akinetic-rigid syndrome in MJD and SCA2; chorea in DRPLA; action tremor in SCA12 and SCA15/16; very slow saccade in SCA2 and SCA7; downbeat nystagmus in SCA6 and EA2; generalized areflexia in SCA2 and SCA4; visual loss secondary to maculopathy in SCA7; seizures in SCA 10 and early onset cases of DRPLA and SCA7; dementia in SCA12, SCA17, SCA27, and DRPLA; myoclonus in DRPLA and SCA14; intellectual disability in SCA13; SCA6 has a benign course. No effective treatment is available for SCAs. Supportive care should be provided for most patients, including physical therapy, speech therapy, and social organization. Genetic counseling is recommended for patients.

REFERENCES

Didonna, A., & Opal, P. (2016). Advances in sequencing technologies for understanding hereditary ataxias: a review. *JAMA Neurol, 73*(12), 1485–1490.

Manto, M., & Habas, C. (2016). Cerebellar disorders: clinical/radiologic findings and modern imaging tools. *Handb Clin Neurol, 135*, 479–491.

SPINOCEREBELLAR DEGENERATION (SPINOCEREBELLAR ATAXIA)

Spinocerebellar degeneration is a general term used to describe a heterogeneous group of inherited, acquired, or idiopathic disorders in which ataxia is a prominent manifestation. This group of diseases affects, to a variable extent, the cerebellar cortex, spinal cord, peripheral nerves, and variably other regions of the neuraxis (e.g. optic nerve, basal ganglia). Patients with cerebellar ataxia are typically clumsy, as the cerebellum is involved in limb coordination and control of balance. Other manifestations include ocular disturbances, speech deficits, disturbance in limb movement, deficits of posture and gait, deficits of cognitive operations, and subtle autonomic signs.

The spinocerebellar degenerations have been notably difficult to separate based purely on a clinical basis, with the notable exception of autosomal recessive Friedreich ataxia (see below). Genetic analysis has begun to clarify this situation, but has also revealed multiple genes that cause similar syndromes; it is also complicated by the occurrence of multiple phenotypes within a kindred. Up to 45 types of spinocerebellar ataxia (SCA) have been described, and many of them map to genes which had been associated with other disorders, leading to even more confusion in nomenclature.

A thorough clinical approach to these disorders requires a detailed family history with attention to multiple phenotypes within the family. Physical examination should catalog all affected parts of the neuraxis, and any associated abnormalities in other body systems. Imaging and laboratory testing to exclude other disorders affecting multiple parts of the neuraxis should be done (e.g., multiple sclerosis, neuromyelitis optica, metastatic disease, or paraneoplastic disorders). Consultation with other specialists such as ophthalmology (e.g., retinal degeneration) can help document involvement of other body systems. Genetic counseling and genetic analysis using panels designed for the most common of these syndromes can be helpful. The development of whole exome sequencing or complete DNA sequencing is likely to continue to shed light on these disorders.

I. Autosomal Dominant Progressive Degenerative Ataxias (SCA): A large and complex group of diseases affecting the cerebellum or its connections. More than 40 SCA genetic types exist. Several SCAs, including the most common ones, are due to CAG repeat expansions in the coding regions of the respective genes. SCAs may present with a "pure" cerebellar syndrome or with associated weakness, pyramidal signs, sensory loss, cranial nerve involvement, other movement disorders, dementia, epilepsy, peripheral neuropathy, optic atrophy, or retinal macular degeneration. Gait imbalance is usually the first disease manifestation. In most cases, symptoms occur in the third to fifth decade, but age of onset is variable. Neuroimaging studies show cerebellar atrophy with variable brainstem, supratentorial, and spinal cord involvement.

II. Autosomal Recessive Cerebellar Ataxias

A) Friedreich Ataxia: The most frequent autosomal recessive cerebellar ataxia. It is caused by GAA triplet expansion in the FXN gene. It is characterized by both cerebellar and proprioceptive ataxia, areflexia, and extensor plantar reflexes. Scoliosis is common and may be the first indication of disease. The initial signs occur between 7 and 25 years of age and worsen progressively. Patients generally lose independent ambulation after they have had the disease for 10–15 years. Dysarthria and dysphagia both contribute to severe disability. Two features that can aid in diagnosis are the absence of obvious cerebellar atrophy on brain MRI during the first years of the disease, and ocular "square-wave jerks." There are cardiac manifestations including left ventricular hypertrophy (LVH), palpitations, and cardiomyopathy that may require pacemakers and other cardiac interventions.

B) Ataxia Telangiectasia: Second most frequent autosomal recessive cerebellar ataxia. Hypotonia and progressive clumsiness usually develop before 5 years of age, with loss of independent ambulation by 10 years and death by 20 years of age. Cerebellar ataxia is associated with conjunctival telangiectasias, oculocephalic dissociation, chorea, dystonia, and neuropathy. Patients are prone to malignancies (lymphoma and leukemias) and recurrent infections.

REFERENCES

Anheim, M., et al. (2012). The autosomal recessive cerebellar ataxias. *NEJM*, *366*(7), 636–646.

Pandolfo, M., & Manto, M. (2013). Cerebellar and afferent ataxias. *Continuum*, *19*(5), 1312–1343.

STATUS EPILEPTICUS (See also EPILEPSY NCC AND NEUROLOGIC EMERGENCIES APPENDIX)

Status epilepticus represents one of the most common neurologic emergencies; its incidence has increased from 5 to 30 per 100,000 in recent years.

Generally, seizure activity that continues for more than 5 minutes or two or more seizures without a return to baseline mentation constitutes status epilepticus. The term status epilepticus can refer to several forms of ongoing seizure activity. The patient can be in convulsive status epilepticus, which is the classic continuous generalized tonic-clonic activity, or the patient can be in focal or partial status epilepticus, which may involve only a single part of the body such as the face or hand. Another type, which is much more difficult to diagnose, is nonconvulsive status epilepticus in which the patient is altered or comatose and has generalized seizure activity electrographically, but does not exhibit generalized tonic-clonic motor activity. Regardless of the type, all forms of status epilepticus should be treated promptly using the protocol given in the Neurologic Emergencies Appendix or some similar protocol. It has been shown that as many as 50% of cases of treated status epilepticus continue to show electrographic seizures on continuous EEG. Thus, an anticonvulsant should be IV loaded even if seizures appear to have stopped with administration of a benzodiazepine.

REFERENCE

Chen, J. W. Y., & Wasterlain, C. G. (2006). Status epilepticus: pathophysiology and management in adults. *Lancet Neurol, 5*, 246–256.

SUBDURAL HEMATOMA

A subdural hematoma (SDH) is a collection of blood that develops from the extravasation of venous blood into the subdural space underneath the dura mater surrounding the brain (and rarely, the spinal cord). SDH in infants who do not present with an obvious history of head trauma (e.g., fall or vehicular accident) needs to be investigated for child abuse (e.g., shaken baby syndrome), particularly when there is an interhemispheric SDH and retinal hemorrhages, raising suspicion of abuse.

ACUTE SUBDURAL HEMATOMA

In the majority of acute SDH, the cause is head trauma. In comatose patients with traumatic brain injuries, 20% to 25% will have an SDH. SDH is theorized to develop from injury to the bridging veins between the brain surface and adjacent dural venous sinuses or from disruption of major venous sinuses. Acceleration or deceleration injuries cause tearing or shearing of these bridging veins in the parasagittal or sylvian areas. The anatomic location of these kinds of SDH typically is along cerebral convexities, above the orbital roofs, or the temporal poles. In rare cases an acute SDH can develop following a lumbar puncture and spontaneous intracranial hypotension. On rare occasions acute SDH may develop spontaneously in patients with a bleeding diathesis. *Acute spontaneous SDH may also be seen with cerebral aneurysm or dural arteriovenous (AV) fistula.*

In acute SDH the clot tends to develop quickly, and venous bleeding may stop as the intracranial pressure rises. Typical clinical features of acute SDH include seizure, headache (usually ipsilateral to the SDH), and decreased alertness or confusion but with fluctuating mentation. Hemiparesis is usually less pronounced than a lesion within the cortical parenchyma itself. If the SDH is large enough to cause compression of the contralateral cerebral peduncle against the free edge of the tentorium (Kernohan notch), the hemiparesis may in fact be ipsilateral.

CHRONIC SUBDURAL HEMATOMA

Chronic SDH is usually noted after the fact—when patients come in for workup of nonspecific, subacute or chronic symptoms, such as headaches, lightheadedness, psychomotor slowing, apathy, drowsiness, and less commonly a seizure. Patients tend to be elderly or on anticoagulation therapy, and a history of trauma may be unclear or remote from the time of clinical presentation.

IMAGING

Head CT imaging is the first choice of a diagnostic modality for cranial SDH, with sensitivity for hematomas having a thickness greater than 5 mm exceeding 90%. Acute SDH has a hyperdense appearance on CT, consistent with the appearance of acute intracranial bleeding. The shape is often crescentic because of the spread of the SDH over the hemispheric convexities. A thin border separating the clot from the cortex is often visible. After about a week, an acute SDH changes appearance to being isodense with brain tissue. Over the succeeding 2 to 6 weeks, the SDH evolves heterogeneously toward a hypodense appearance. MRI imaging makes a similar progression over time, beginning in the acute phase as hyperintense on T_1-weighted imaging and hypointense on T_2-weighted imaging. Over time the imaging qualities show chronicity of the SDH, with hypointensity of T_1-weighted images and hyperintensity of T_2-weighted images. The chronic SDH may form a vascular capsule after several weeks, which can enhance on MRI imaging. A majority of SDHs will liquefy within the capsule (hygroma). For uncertain reasons a minority (less than half) of SDHs remain stable in size and do not liquefy. In spinal SDH the preferred modality is spinal MRI for accurate diagnosis.

TREATMENT

Neurosurgery immediate consult for large or neurologically devastating SDHs for an emergent drainage. Posterior fossa SDH carries a high risk of brainstem compression and usually requires rapid surgical evacuation. Seizure prophylaxis is recommended in patients with SDH, keeping in mind potentially worsening the underlying confusion. Such patients are appropriately admitted for observation over several days (e.g., 2 to 3 days) to observe for clot enlargement. For chronic SDHs that are large or causing neurologic deficits, burr hole drainage may suffice if the clot has liquefied sufficiently. Treatment of spinal SDH is less uniform because of its infrequency and therefore depends upon surgeon experience.

PROGNOSIS

Patients who are rapidly treated and had good surgical results may do well. Comatose patients with acute SDH uniformly tend to have poor outcomes.

REFERENCES

Nentwich, L. M., & Grimmnitz, B. (2016). Neurologic emergencies in the elderly. *Emerg Med Clin North Am, 34*(3), 575–599.

Won, S. Y., et al. (2017). A systematic review of epileptic seizures in adults with subdural haematomas. *Seizure, 45*, 28–35.

SYNCOPE

A transient loss of consciousness and postural tone that results from decreased perfusion of the cerebral cortex or reticular activating system, syncope has a number of neurologic and cardiac etiologies. This section will highlight the neurologic causes, but keep in mind that acute reduction in cardiac output secondary to cardiac arrhythmia, intrinsic heart disease, or pulmonary emboli may lead to syncope as a result of decreased cerebral blood flow and is much more common.

CLINICAL PRESENTATION

Symptoms of autonomic activation typically herald neurally mediated syncope. Sympathetic activation causes piloerection, diaphoresis, and pallor (cutaneous vasoconstriction). Pupillary vasodilation causes blurred vision. Abdominal discomfort and nausea result from vagal activation. Syncope may occur suddenly without prodrome; the "clinical rule" that the latter situation is more suggestive of an arrhythmogenic source does not preclude that an arrhythmia can also produce the prodrome described above. If cerebral hypoperfusion persists, as when the subject is held upright in a procedure chair, tonic-clonic jerks and urinary incontinence (convulsive syncope) may result. Recovery is spontaneous, and upon return to consciousness, there are no neurologic sequelae.

NEURALLY MEDIATED SYNCOPE

Neurologic causes of syncope lead to a reduction in cerebral blood flow due to failure of the autonomic reflexes that maintain systemic vascular resistance. During neurally mediated syncope, parasympathetic outflow to the sinus node of the heart increases, leading to bradycardia, and vasodilation causes blood pressure to fall. Neurogenic causes of syncope can be classified by pathophysiologic mechanism as follows:

I. Central Causes: Syncope of central origin occurs when vasodilation and bradycardia occur in response to emotions (e.g., fear or revulsion). In these cases, the stimulus most likely evokes neocortical and limbic structural activity first. Neurons in the amygdala synapse with the hypothalamic and brain stem autonomic nuclei, and these neurons may play a role in emotionally induced syncope. Emotionally induced fainting thus represents a specific autonomic response to situations of extreme fear or displeasure.

II. Reflex Causes: Occurs as the result of excessive excitation of autonomic reflexes. Carotid sinus syncope is an example of this type. Syncope has also been associated with a number of other reflexes, including micturition, defecation, and coughing. Defecating and coughing are essentially Valsalva-like maneuvers involving raised intra-abdominal and intrathoracic pressures resulting in a reduction in the venous return to the extent that cardiac output and blood pressure fall to critical levels, leading to syncope.

III. Hemodynamic Stress: The normal response to hypovolemia is vasoconstriction. However, this reflex may be abruptly inhibited, leading to vasodilation, bradycardia, and syncope. The ability to tolerate orthostatic stress before switching to a vasovagal reaction varies greatly among patients. Orthostatic stress can be countered by contraction of muscles in dependent regions that compress veins and enhance return of blood to the heart. Since syncope occurs when venous return is inadequate, individuals with relatively large blood and plasma volumes tend to have greater tolerance to orthostatic stress. The trigger mechanism for converting vasoconstriction and tachycardia to vasodilation and bradycardia remains unknown.

DIAGNOSIS

The most useful tools for evaluation of syncope are the clinical history (precipitants, body position, prodrome, prior episodes, orientation on awakening, family history, seizure risk factors, cardiac and cerebrovascular disease, autonomic and neuropathic symptoms, and medications); physical examination (orthostatic vital signs, estimate of volume status, cardiac and cervical auscultation, and peripheral nerve and autonomic examination [e.g., sinus arrhythmia on electrocardiogram (ECG)]); and ECG (always check the corrected QT interval). More sophisticated (but lower yield) evaluation can be undertaken with prolonged ambulatory ECG monitoring and head-upright tilt test (the gold standard test for diagnosis of vasovagal syncope, with an estimated specificity of 90% in the absence of provocative agents such as isoproterenol). Electroencephalogram (EEG), carotid ultrasound, magnetic resonance angiogram (MRA), and head computed tomography (CT) have low diagnostic yield with unremarkable history and examination.

TREATMENT

Treatment of vasovagal syncope may proceed in a stepwise fashion. First, patients are educated to avoid precipitants, and dietary sodium intake is liberalized. Medications that may cause or exacerbate orthostasis or volume depletion are discontinued if possible. If these measures fail, beta blockers are employed as first-line therapy. Should beta blockers fail or be contraindicated, the patient may be tried on fludrocortisone or midodrine. If pharmacologic measures fail, pacemaker placement may be considered.

REFERENCES

Cheshire, W. P. (2007). Syncope. *Continuum (Minneap Minn)*, *23*(2), 335–358.

Kapoor, W. (2000). Syncope. *NEJM*, *343*(25), 1856–1862.

SYNDROME OF INAPPROPRIATE SECRETION OF ANTIDIURETIC HORMONE (SIADH)

SIADH is due to an excess of renal water reabsorption through nonphysiologic stimulation of antidiuretic hormone (ADH) secretion, resulting in hypotonic (serum osmolality < 280 mOsm/L), hyponatremia (Na < 134 mEq/L) with concentrated urine (osmolality > 300 mmol/kg), and urine sodium excretion (>20 mEq/L).

DIAGNOSIS

Besides the clinical syndrome of hyponatremia, the diagnostic criteria include (1) euvolemia/hypervolemia; (2) normal adrenal, renal, and thyroid function; and (3) absence of an iatrogenic cause of ADH release.

ETIOLOGY

Neurologic causes include stroke, subdural hematoma, subarachnoid hemorrhage, head trauma, intracranial surgery, tumors, basal skull fractures, cerebral atrophy, acute encephalitis, tuberculous or purulent meningitis, Guillain-Barré syndrome, acute intermittent porphyria, central nervous system (CNS) lupus erythematosus, and sarcoidosis. Nonneurologic causes include bronchogenic carcinoma, tuberculosis, pulmonary aspergillosis, anemia, stress, severe pain, hypotension, acute intermittent porphyria, and drugs such as chlorpropamide, oxytocin, thiazide diuretics, oxcarbazine, and carbamazepine.

This syndrome must be differentiated from cerebral salt-wasting (CSW) syndrome, which can occur in similar intracranial disorders as SIADH. In CSW, patients are usually hypovolemic, with increased plasma albumin, blood urea nitrogen (BUN)/creatinine ratio, and high hematocrit.

Manifestations are due to the hyponatremia and include mental status changes, behavioral changes, weakness, anorexia, nausea, vomiting, muscle cramps, and extrapyramidal signs. Seizures, coma, and death may occur with severe hyponatremia.

Therapy involves identification and treatment of the underlying cause and fluid restriction to 800 to 1000 mL daily. If hyponatremia is severe or the patient is symptomatic, correction with hypertonic saline is recommended. The rate of serum sodium correction should be no faster than 0.5 mmol/hour, and should not exceed 24 mmol/72 hours, to avoid the possibility of inducing central pontine myelinolysis.

REFERENCES

Manzanares, W., Aramendi, I., Langois, P. L., & Biestro, A. (2015). Hyponatremia in the neurocritical care patient: an approach based on current evidence. *Med Intensiva*, *39*, 234–243.

Oh, J. Y., & Shin, J. I. (2015). Syndrome of inappropriate antidiuretic hormone secretion and cerebral/renal salt wasting syndrome: similarities and differences. *Front Pediatr*, *2*, 146.

SYPHILIS

Neurosyphilis results from meningeal invasion by *Treponema pallidum*; parenchymal involvement occurs in later stages (i.e., general paresis and tabes dorsalis). Symptomatic neurosyphilis develops in only 4% to 9% of patients with syphilis who do not receive treatment. Clinical syndromes include the following:

I. *Asymptomatic neurosyphilis* refers to the presence of cerebrospinal fluid (CSF) abnormalities in the absence of neurologic symptoms. The highest rate of abnormalities occurs early, 13 to 18 months after initial infection. The diagnosis is made on the basis of positive results of serum or CSF serologic tests, usually with a mildly increased level of protein, normal glucose level, and a mild lymphocytic pleocytosis. The level of CSF gamma globulins may be increased. Normal CSF 5 years after infection reduces the risk of central nervous system (CNS) syphilis to 1%. Up to 25% of patients with asymptomatic neurosyphilis who do not receive treatment become symptomatic. Lumbar puncture, therefore, should be performed in all patients in whom a diagnosis of syphilis is made beyond the primary stage, or in whom the dating of primary infection cannot be established.

II. *Acute syphilitic meningitis* usually occurs within the initial 2 years of infection and becomes evident as headache, nuchal rigidity, confusion, and cranial nerve palsies (especially CN II, III, VI, and VIII).

III. *Meningovascular syphilis* usually occurs within 4 to 7 years after initial infection and results from an endarteritis, most commonly of the middle cerebral artery. Meningovascular syphilis becomes evident as a focal ischemia that evolves acutely, or over several days, and it is often associated with a prodrome (weeks to months) of headache, dizziness, and psychiatric disturbances.

IV. *General paresis (meningoencephalitis)* usually occurs 15 years after initial infection, as a result of spirochete invasion of the cortex. Dementia is the initial manifestation. Seizures may occur. Untreated, the condition is fatal within 4 years.

V. *Tabes dorsalis* occurs 20 to 25 years after infection and results from inflammation of the posterior roots and posterior columns. Classic presentation includes triads of symptoms (lightning pain, dysuria, and ataxia) and signs (Argyll-Robertson pupils, areflexia, and proprioceptive loss). Later involvement includes visceral crises, optic atrophy, ocular motor palsies, Charcot joints, and foot ulcers. Early treatment usually arrests the progression and may reverse some of the symptoms.

VI. *Less common manifestations* include optic neuropathy, eighth nerve neuropathy, spinal neurosyphilis (e.g., meningomyelitis and meningovascular), and gumma (granulomatous mass lesions in brain or spinal cord).

VII. Patients coinfected with HIV have a higher rate of early neurosyphilis (meningitis or meningovascular) and may be at an increased risk for neurologic relapse after treatment of primary and secondary syphilis with IM benzathine penicillin.

Diagnosis depends on clinical findings, serum serologic results, and CSF examination. Serum treponemal serologic tests (venereal disease research laboratory [VDRL] and rapid plasma reagin [RPR]) become nonreactive with treatment and therefore can be used to assess therapeutic efficacy. However, their titers progressively decline, even during the course of untreated disease, becoming nonreactive in 25% of patients with late syphilis (neurosyphilis). Serum treponemal tests (fluorescent treponemal antibody absorption [FTA-ABS] and microhemagglutination assay for Treponema pallidum [MHA-TP]) are usually unaffected by treatment, their titers remaining elevated indefinitely. *Therefore, a nonreactive FTA-ABS result excludes neurosyphilis.*

CSF usually shows elevated protein level, normal glucose level, and lymphocytic pleocytosis (10 to 400 cells/mm^3). The CSF VDRL has very high specificity but low sensitivity (30% to 70%). Thus, nonreactive CSF VDRL does not exclude neurosyphilis. The CSF FTA-ABS test has a high false-positive rate, and its role is unclear. As with all CSF serologic studies, a traumatic spinal fluid sample may also give misleading results.

Treatment of neurosyphilis consists of a regimen of aqueous penicillin G, 3 to 4 million units IV q 4 hours for 10 to 14 days. An alternative treatment is penicillin G procaine, 2.4 million units IM qd with probenecid 500 mg PO qid for 10 to 14 days. In cases of penicillin allergy, treatment options include penicillin desensitization followed by standard penicillin therapy; other regimens, such as ceftriaxone 2g IV/IM daily for 10 to 14 days, or doxycycline 200 mg PO bid for 28 days, can be considered as alternative but have unproven value.

Follow-up CSF examination should be performed at 6 and 12 months. The CSF cell count is the earliest indicator of response and relapse and should normalize within 6 months. CSF protein level declines more slowly, taking as long as 2 years to normalize. CSF VDRL titers are the last to decline and may remain mildly elevated despite adequate treatment. Repeat treatment is indicated if the CSF pleocytosis persists after 6 months or is abnormal 2 years after treatment. Because CSF protein level and VDRL titers take much longer to normalize, treatment cannot be considered inadequate unless these values unequivocally increase.

REFERENCES

Drago, F., Merlo, G., Ciccarese, G., et al. (2016). Changes in neurosyphilis presentation: a survey on 286 patients. *J Eur Acad Dermatol Venereol, 30*(11), 1886–1900.

Marks, M., Jarvis, J. N., Howlett, W., et al. (2017). Neurosyphilis in Africa: a systematic review. *PLoS Negl Trop Dis, 11*(8). e0005880.

T

TASTE

Taste buds containing receptor cells are located in the anteroposterior aspect of the tongue, soft palate, pharynx, epiglottis, and proximal one third of the esophagus.

The nerves that subserve the tongue and its function:

CN VII, IX, X: (facial, glossopharyngeal, and vagus nerves)—mediate taste sensation.

CN VII: Facial nerve afferents mediate taste from the anterior two thirds of the tongue.

CN VII: (the greater superficial petrosal branch): Carries taste from the soft palate.

CN IX: The lingual, tonsillar, and pharyngeal branches of the glossopharyngeal nerve carry taste from the posterior one third of the tongue and pharynx.

CN X: The superior laryngeal branch of the vagus nerve carries taste from the esophagus and epiglottis.

All afferent taste fibers project to the solitary tract nucleus. Fibers then project to the thalamus, ventral forebrain, lateral hypothalamus, and amygdala. From the thalamus, fibers mediating taste sensation project to the insular cortex.

Ageusia or hypogeusia: loss of taste sensation due to a variety of focal and metabolic causes.

- Complete ageusia is rare.
- Loss of olfactory sensation is the most common cause of loss of "taste."
- Most common cause: aging and tobacco smoking
- Loss of salivary function (e.g., Sjögren syndrome)
- Head and neck surgery
- Postirradiation
- Amyloidosis
- Kallmann syndrome
- Vitamin B_{12} deficiency
- Inner or middle ear inflammation, viral infections of the upper respiratory tract
- Medications such as sulfa-containing drugs, calcium channel blockers, and chemotherapeutic drugs (e.g., doxorubicin) are associated with hypogeusia.

Proximal lesions of the facial nerve between the pons and facial canal where the chorda tympani joins the facial nerve, result in unilateral loss of taste.

Cerebellopontine angle tumors occasionally cause a loss of taste.

Gustatory hallucinations may occur as an aura of partial epilepsy or in delirium and are usually associated with olfactory hallucinations, typically noted more frequently in right hemispheric lesions.

Spontaneous dysgeusia or glossodynia are more complex to evaluate.

Burning mouth syndrome: persistent, severe tongue pain; some patients may have Sjögren syndrome, Vitamins B_2 or B_{12} deficiency, and many may have depressive illness.

Differential diagnosis is similar to the preceding list, but may also include entities such as diabetic neuropathy, fibromyalgia, and gastroesophageal reflux disease.

The burning tongue or burning mouth syndrome is often responsive to clonazepam, but may also respond to topical steroids, paroxetine, clotrimazole, or olanzapine.

Taste testing for the primary modalities of salty, sweet, sour, and bitter is accomplished with the use of a cotton applicator. Ideally, the patient should not speak but should point to cards with the words sweet, salty, bitter, and sour written on them. More sophisticated testing with electrogustometry or filter paper disks with progressive dilutions is sometimes clinically useful, particularly in cases of mild disease or sensory loss.

REFERENCES

Pribitkin, E., Rosenthal, M. D., & Cowart, B. J. (2003). Prevalence and causes of severe taste loss in a chemosensory clinic population. *Ann Otol Rhinol Laryngol, 112*(11), 971–978.

Ropper, A. H., Samuels, M. A., & Klein, J. P. (2014). Disorders of smell and taste. In A. H. Ropper, M. A. Samuels, & J. P. Klein (Eds.), *Adams and Victor's principles of neurology*, ed 10 (pp. 231–234).

TAUOPATHIES

The majority of neurodegenerative diseases are characterized by the deposition of insoluble protein in cells of the neurologic system. Microtubule-associated tau is a protein that has functions in healthy neurons, but forms insoluble deposits in diseases now known collectively as tauopathies. Tauopathies encompass more than 20 clinicopathological entities, including Alzheimer disease, progressive supranuclear palsy, Pick disease and corticobasal degeneration (CBD). This section will describe the important clinical features of the most prevalent tauopathies.

ALZHEIMER DISEASE

The most common cause of dementia, defined by an insidious decline in cognitive function from a previous higher level. Diagnostic criteria state that two or more cognitive domains are affected, including memory impairment and at least one of language, visuospatial function, executive function, and praxis.

Pathologically, Alzheimer disease (AD) is diagnosed by semiquantitative analysis of senile plaques, composed of extracellular Aβ-amyloid peptide deposits, and neurofibrillary tangles, composed of intraneuronal tau deposits. Tau accumulation in AD is probably a consequence of Aβ-amyloidogenic neuronal damage rather than a primary event. Progression of tau cortical involvement from entorhinal cortex to hippocampus to isocortex closely reflects the severity of cognitive dysfunction and allows for a reliable way of rating pathological and clinical severity.

PROGRESSIVE SUPRANUCLEAR PALSY

The diagnosis of progressive supranuclear palsy (PSP) requires the following: onset of disease over 40 years of age, falls within the first 12 months of disease, and vertical supranuclear palsy. Pathological diagnosis relies on the identification of tau-positive neurofibrillary tangles and neuropil threads at high densities in the pallidum, subthalamic nucleus, substantia nigra, or pons. The pathological signature of PSP is the tufted astrocyte, which is rare in other tauopathies. A proportion of patients are designated as having PSP-parkinsonism and are characterized by an asymmetric onset, tremor, and a moderate initial therapeutic response to levodopa. The factors that lead to tau accumulation and selective vulnerability of basal ganglia structures in PSP are not clear.

PICK DISEASE

Clinically characterized by the onset of behavioral changes and aphasia in the sixth or seventh decade that progress over 10 to 15 years, features of frontal lobe dysfunction include apathy, prominent and distressing social disinhibition, stereotypic behaviors, alterations in food preference, and poor self-care. There are also frontal executive dysfunctions including poor planning, forethought, reasoning, and organization. Progressive nonfluent aphasia characterized by prominent speech production deficits leading to mutism is the most common aphasia seen in this disease. Semantic dementia, defined by loss of language comprehension, and visual agnosia with preserved verbal fluency also occurs. Pathologically, Pick disease is characterized by sharply circumscribed and asymmetrical lobar atrophy of the frontal and temporal lobes with superficial spongiosis. The diagnosis can be made by identification of large numbers of tau-positive spherical cytoplasmic inclusions called Pick bodies throughout the frontal and temporal cortices and in particular the hippocampus.

CORTICOBASAL DEGENERATION

The clinical presentation of the classical, predominantly movement disorders phenotype is recognizable by the presence of asymmetric bradykinesia and rigidity with myoclonus, dystonia, and cortical sensory loss, which may ultimately lead to the alien limb syndrome. Other clinical presentations are probably more common, characterized by progressive, nonfluent aphasia, frontal lobe behavioral changes, and apraxia with levodopa nonresponsive parkinsonism. Focal cortical atrophy or hypometabolism is often seen on neuroimaging. It is defined pathologically by the presence of achromatic balloon-shaped neurons and prominent diffuse cortical glia tau pathology, including neuropil threads, coiled bodies, and astrocytic plaques.

REFERENCES

McFarland, N. R. (2016). Diagnostic approach to atypical Parkinsonian syndromes. *Continuum*, *22*(4), 1117–1142.

Williams, D. R. (2006). Tauopathies: update on neurodegenerative diseases. *Int Med J*, *36*(10), 652–660.

TEMPORAL LOBE

The temporal lobe is bordered superiorly by the sylvian fissure and merges with the parietal and occipital lobes. It consists of superior, middle, inferior, and transverse temporal gyri. The transverse temporal gyrus contains the primary auditory cortex (Brodmann area 41) and secondary auditory cortex (Brodmann area 42). The superior temporal gyrus contains *Wernicke* area on the dominant hemisphere. Other functionally important structures, such as the amygdala, hippocampus, and olfactory and entorhinal cortices, are also found within the temporal lobe. Symptoms of temporal lobe dysfunction include *partial complex seizures, memory difficulties* (especially bilateral hippocampal involvement), *Wernicke aphasia* (with dominant temporal lesion), auditory agnosias, visual field defects (superior quadrantanopias), and behavioral and emotional disturbances. *The Klüver-Bucy* syndrome of placidity, apathy, hypersexuality, hyperorality, and visual and auditory agnosia occurs with bilateral anterior temporal lobe injury, such as brain trauma, encephalitis, stroke, tumors, or degenerative dementias.

Infections, such as herpes simplex encephalitis, can target the temporal lobes. The temporal lobe is one of the most common localizations for focal epilepsy. The features of temporal lobe epilepsy can be divided into two broad categories: mesial and lateral (neocortical) onset. Many patients with temporal lobe epilepsy experience auras, a gastric rising sensation, fear, or olfactory symptoms. Dominant temporal lobe seizures cause loss of awareness and prominent automatisms. Non-dominant temporal lobe seizures have preserved awareness with oral and manual automatisms.

REFERENCES

Caciagli, L., Bernasconi, A., Wiebe, S., et al. (2017). A meta-analysis on progressive atrophy in intractable temporal lobe epilepsy: time is brain? *Neurology*, *89*(5), 506–516.

Skidmore, C. (2016). Adult focal epilepsies. *Continuum*, *22*(1), 94–115.

THYROID

Both hyperthyroidism and hypothyroidism have neurologic manifestations. Prompt recognition and treatment can result in good clinical outcomes.

HYPERTHYROIDISM

Clinically manifests as tachycardia, heat intolerance, weight loss, vomiting, diarrhea, and exophthalmic ophthalmoplegia. With profound elevations in T4 levels, thyrotoxic crisis can occur, resulting in fever and cognitive impairment. Crisis may be precipitated by infection or inadequate preparation for thyroid surgery. It is a medical emergency, as it can progress to coma and death if not treated promptly. Treatment involves thiourea agents, sodium iodide, adrenergic blockers, corticosteroids, sedatives, body cooling, and fluid/electrolyte maintenance. Prognosis can be variable; neurologic symptoms following treatment can vary from months to years until return to baseline.

  I. Steroid-responsive encephalopathy associated with autoimmune thyroiditis may occur; it is due to development of antibodies (antithyroglobulin, antithyroid microsomal and antithyroid peroxidase antibodies).
     a. Clinically, it can present with coma, encephalopathy, psychosis, seizures, stupor, and stroke-like symptoms. Often, there are electroencephalography (EEG) abnormalities (generalized slowing or frontal intermittent rhythmic delta activity [FIRDA]) and magnetic resonance imaging [MRI] abnormalities such as subcortical hyperintensities (on fluid-attenuated inversion recovery [FLAIR] images); however, both studies can be normal.
     b. Symptoms are highly responsive to corticosteroids and with achievement of a euthyroid state.
     c. Rare cases may require IgIV or plasma exchange.
 II. Psychological manifestations
     a. Apathetic hyperthyroidism is common in the elderly and may manifest as dementia with apathy and depression.
     b. Behavioral changes such as irritability and anxiety
III. Peripheral nervous system abnormalities associated with thyroid disease
     a. Chronic thyrotoxic myopathy, predominantly associated with proximal muscle weakness
         i. Increased prevalence in females compared to males
        ii. Creatine kinase is usually normal.
       iii. Electromyography (EMG) reveals short-duration polyphasic motor unit potentials. Muscle power improves as the patient becomes euthyroid.
     b. Acute thyrotoxic myopathy, associated with orofacial involvement (extraocular and bulbar muscles)
     c. Thyrotoxic periodic paralysis resembles hypokalemic periodic paralysis.

   d. Myasthenia gravis: Its development is less common in setting of hyperthyroidism. It is rare, with an estimated rate of less than 5%. Hyperthyroidism is more commonly implicated in the course of myasthenia gravis.

   e. Neuropathy is very uncommon and routine testing is not recommended.

IV. Other central nervous system (CNS) manifestations:

   a. Tremor: An accentuation of physiologic tremor, due to increased sensitivity to sympathetic input, is very common in hyperthyroid patients and involves primarily the upper extremities. Treatment consists of correcting the thyroid abnormality; propranolol is also useful.

   b. Chorea, resulting from hypersensitivity of dopaminergic receptors, responds to neuroleptics.

   c. Stroke can result from cerebral embolism in thyrotoxic atrial fibrillation. Acute anticoagulation may be appropriate.

HYPOTHYROIDISM

Hypothyroidism may present in infancy with mental retardation and growth abnormalities, resulting in *Cretinism*. Fortunately, this is now rare, because many countries have instituted neonatal screening programs.

   I. Associated signs of systemic hypothyroidism are variable. Clinical presentation includes muscle aches, fatigue, seizures, cognitive impairment, decreased deep reflexes, constipation, dry skin, and weight gain; psychosis may occur. In the elderly, hypothyroidism may present with cognitive dysfunction, sometimes confused with a primary degenerative dementia. All new-onset dementia patients should be screened for hypothyroidism. Myxedema coma occurs rarely, usually in chronic, severe, undiagnosed disease.

   a. Treatment: Emergency management consists of thyroid replacement (PO or IV); corticosteroids; treatment of hypoglycemia, fluid/electrolyte abnormalities, and hypothermia; and ventilator support as needed. Following acute treatment, patients can be managed on levothyroxine with routine monitoring of thyroid functions.

   II. Peripheral manifestations occur in a variety of forms.

   a. Myopathy: Hypothyroid myopathy consists of weakness (proximal > distal), cramps, pain, and stiffness as common complaints, but objective weakness is less common. Creatine phosphokinase is often elevated. EMG findings are nonspecific. Myoedema, a percussion-induced local mounding of contracted muscle that relaxes slowly, may be elicited, but can also occur in emaciated patients and some normal subjects. The contraction is electrically silent on EMG. Muscle hypertrophy, known as Hoffman syndrome in adults and Kocher-Debré-Semelaigne syndrome in children, is rare. Patients complain of stiffness and painful muscle cramps, and the movements are slow and weak. The muscles are large and firm. Pseudomyotonia, or delayed muscle relaxation after handshake or percussion, may be present and is differentiated from myotonia by its electrical silence on EMG.

b. Peripheral neuropathies are mostly entrapment neuropathies (carpal tunnel), resulting from mucoid infiltration of the nerve and the surrounding tissue. Eighty percent of patients complain of distal paresthesia. Polyneuropathies are less frequent.

REFERENCES

Katzberg, H. D., & Kassardjian, C. D. (2016). Toxic and endocrine myopathies. *Continuum*, 22(6), 1815–1828.

Perez, D. M., Murray, E. D., & Price, B. H. et al. (2016). Depression and psychosis in neurological practice. In R. B. Daroff, J. Jankovic, J. C. Mazziotta, & S. L. Pomeroy (Eds.), *Bradley's neurology in clinical practice*, ed 7 (pp. 92–114). Philadelphia: Elsevier.

THROMBECTOMY FOR ACUTE ISCHEMIC STROKE

BACKGROUND

Acute ischemic stroke treatment has undergone dramatic changes with steadily increasing use of intravenous tissue plasminogen activator (IV tPA) as standard of care since 1996. However, despite its proven efficacy as treatment of acute ischemic stroke in general, pharmacologic thrombolysis does not achieve high reperfusion rates in cases of large proximal vessel occlusions, mainly due to the size and composition of the thrombus. Therefore, the rationale for mechanical removal of flow obstruction has driven the evolution of thrombectomy devices and has ultimately led to a revolution in the treatment of major ischemic stroke with endovascular thrombectomy (EVT).

EVIDENCE

Multiple randomized trials were unsuccessful at proving superiority of EVT over standard medical therapy until 2015, when five well-designed randomized controlled trials (MR CLEAN, ESCAPE, SWIFT-PRIME, REVASCAT, and EXTEND-IA) finally came out with strong evidence of improved patient outcomes (number needed to treat [NNT] 2.6 to reduce modified Rankin scale by one level and NNT 3.2 to 7.1 to achieve functional independence at 90 days vs. NNT of about 11 for IV tPA within 3 hours of stroke onset, with no difference in hemorrhages and mortality). Despite some differences, these trials had many features in common: newer-generation stent-retriever devices (vs. older coil retriever devices) were used; treatment was initiated within 6 hours of onset for most patients; and patient selection was based on confirmed anterior proximal vessel occlusion and the size of ischemic core.

As a result, the American Heart Association/ American Stroke Association (AHA/ASA) issued the following EVT eligibility guidelines: (1) pre-stroke mRS score of 0 to 1; (2) causative occlusion of the internal carotid artery or middle cerebral artery (MCA) segment 1 (M1); (3) age $\geq$18 years; (4) National Institutes of Health Stroke Scale (NIHSS) score of $\geq$6; (5) Alberta Stroke Program Early CT Score (ASPECTS) of $\geq$6; and (6) treatment can be initiated (groin puncture) within 6 hours of symptom onset. The 6-hour window was further expanded when two trials proved clinical benefit of EVT up to 16 hours (DEFUSE 3) and 24 hours (DAWN) for eligible patients. In both these trials, perfusion imaging (magnetic resonance imaging [MRI] or computed tomography [CT]) was primarily used to assess the core and determine EVT eligibility. Patients having a core-penumbra mismatch or imaging-clinical mismatch would benefit the most with EVT in this extended time window.

KEY PRINCIPLES OF ENDOVASCULAR THROMBECTOMY

EVT with or without IV thrombolysis is now standard of care in eligible acute stroke patients. The currently accepted treatment window for EVT can be up to 24 hours; however, earlier treatment unequivocally leads to better outcomes in most patients. Ischemic core volume and location are very important predictors of outcome, and can be rapidly assessed by using the ASPECT score on CT head (points deducted from 10 for each key area of infarct with score of 6 to 10 indicating a small infarct core) or by CT perfusion imaging, as it can determine the degree of target mismatch (difference between ischemic core and penumbra). Vessel imaging, usually computed tomography angiography (CTA), is essential for confirming a large proximal vessel occlusion. Stent-retriever or direct contact aspiration devices are used for EVT. Reperfusion is considered successful if Thrombolysis in Cerebral Infarction score 2b-3 is achieved (at least 50% of affected arterial territory reperfused). EVT is intended to be performed in a multidisciplinary setting such as a comprehensive stroke center.

ONGOING CHALLENGES

While EVT eligibility has now expanded based on the concept of variable physiologic tissue salvageability as opposed to rigid adherence to a given timeframe, multiple clinical, imaging, and procedural challenges remain. There is clinical equipoise on EVT eligibility for strokes with a large ischemic core, distal occlusions, posterior circulation occlusions (BASICS trial ongoing), rapidly improving or mild symptoms, and very old patients. The benefit of IV tPA in addition to EVT, although suggested recently,[4] is being studied in ongoing MR CLEAN NO IV trial. Use of local anesthesia compared to general anesthesia during EVT is another important area of investigation. Multiple adjuvant therapies like neuroprotectants are being studied as well. Lastly, systemic implementation of rapid EVT to as many eligible patients as possible is an enormously complex task, requiring significant resources and a major shift in the stroke treatment paradigm worldwide.

REFERENCES

Goyal, N., Tsivgoulis, G., Frei, D., et al. (2018). Comparative safety and efficacy of combined IVT and MT with direct MT in large vessel occlusion. *Neurology*, 90(15), e1274–e1282. https://doi.org/10.1212/WNL.0000000000005299.

Powers, W. J., Rabinstein, A. A., Ackerson, T., et al. (2018). Guidelines for the early management of patients with acute ischemic stroke: a guideline for healthcare professionals from the American Heart Association/American Stroke Association. *Stroke*. 49(3),e46–e110. https://doi.org/10.1161/STR.0000000000000158.

TOURETTE SYNDROME (GILLES DE LA TOURETTE SYNDROME)

Its tics are sudden, intermittent, stereotypical involuntary movements. The syndrome is characterized by the following:

I. Multiple motor, and one or more vocal, tics have been present at some time during the illness, although not necessarily concurrently.

II. The tics may wax and wane in frequency but have persisted for more than 1 year since first tic onset.

III. Onset is before age 18 years.

IV. The disturbance is not attributable to the physiological effects of a substance (e.g., cocaine) or another medical condition (e.g., Huntington disease, postviral encephalitis).

HISTORY

Tics typically manifest after the age of 3; however, they are most commonly seen between ages 6 to 7 years. Boys are affected three to four times more than girls. Tourette syndrome typically waxes and wanes in severity. Severity may increase with age; however, many patients have a dramatic reduction of tics in their 20s. Comorbidities, such as obsessive-compulsive disorder (OCD occurs in ~20% to 40%), attention deficit hyperactivity disorder (ADHD), anxiety, and mood disturbances have a profound impact on both academic and social functions.

PHYSICAL EXAMINATION

Tics are classified as either simple or complex. Examples of simple motor tics include eye blinks or head jerks. These movements are rapid and sudden in nature. On the other hand, complex motor tics include facial gestures, grooming behaviors, jumping, or obscene gestures (copraxia). Sniffing, snorting, throat clearing, or barking are examples of simple vocal tics. They are often mistaken for other illnesses like laryngitis or asthma. Complex vocal tics include coprolalia (utterance of obscenities), echolalia, and palilalia. In contrast to public perception, coprolalia is quite rare. Tics may be exacerbated by anger or stress. They may diminish during sleep and become attenuated during some absorbing activity. Tics may be voluntarily suppressed for minutes to hours.

PATHOGENESIS

Pathogenesis is still unclear. Recent theories have focused on genetics and autoimmune causes, particularly following streptococcal infection. The term

PANDAS refers to pediatric autoimmune neuropsychiatric disorder, and this entity is somewhat controversial. Other possible risk factors include maternal caffeine, tobacco, cocaine, and alcohol use, transient perinatal hypoxia, and low Apgar scores. Other causes include side effects of medications or aftereffects of traumatic head injury.

TREATMENT

A multidisciplinary therapeutic program must be established, in close collaboration with the parents, child, and school. Treatment should be reserved for those cases in which the child's self-esteem or social interactions are affected. It is not uncommon for the parents to be more troubled about the tics than the patient. When treatment is initiated, it is often difficult to gauge efficacy because of the natural waxing and waning severity of the disorder. Thus, drastic changes in dose or medications should be avoided, especially during exacerbations, and two medications should not be started together. Clonidine, an α2-adrenergic agonist, has often been used as a first choice to delay use of neuroleptic agents. This medication is also beneficial in treating the associated hyperactivity and warrants first-line consideration based on its efficacy in controlled trials. Dopamine receptor antagonists are the mainstay in treatment. Traditionally, haloperidol and pimozide had been used for treatment, but because of side effects, transition to the "atypical" antipsychotics (fluphenazine, olanzapine, risperidone, quetiapine, and ziprasidone) has been recommended. Risperidone and olanzapine have been found to be efficacious, but their use may be limited in children because of associated weight gain. Botox can be considered if tics are severe. The associated comorbid conditions of ADHD and OCD are often more disabling and should be treated prior to treating tics since these conditions produce stress, which can often make tics worse. Stimulant medications have been accused of exacerbating tics, but this is not supported by randomized trials. These medications should be used in patients who have ADHD. OCD should be treated with selective serotonin reuptake inhibitors, such as clomipramine. Early treatment of tics does not alter the natural history. Nonpharmacologic treatments include behavioral therapy, which help with reinforcement, and techniques to aid in diminishing tics.

REFERENCES

Jankovic, J., & Lang, A. E. (2016). Diagnosis and assessment of Parkinson disease and other movement disorder. In R. B. Daroff, J. Jankovic, J. C. Mazziotta, & S. L. Pomeroy (Eds.), *Bradley's neurology in clinical practice,* ed 7 (pp. 1456–1457). Philadelphia: Elsevier.

Wu, S. V., & Gilbert, D. L. (2017). The nervous system: Gilles De La Tourette Syndrome. In E. T. Bope & R. D. Kellerman (Eds.), *Conn's current therapy* (pp. 648–650). vol. 9 (pp. 648–650). Philadelphia: Elsevier.

TRANSCRANIAL DOPPLER ULTRASOUND

Blood flow velocity is inversely related to the cross-sectional area of an artery at any given moment and can be influenced by several factors including age, gender (increased in females), pregnancy, hematocrit (increased velocity with decreasing hematocrit) and PCO_2 (increased with increasing PCO_2). Transcranial dopplers (TCDs) were introduced in 1982 as a noninvasive tool for evaluation of proximal intracranial arteries at the bedside. Specifically, TCDs measure diastolic blood flow using low emission frequency ultrasound (2 MHz). An elevated reading may signify hyperdynamic flow, stenotic arterial disease, or vasospastic reaction while the opposite may occur with low intracranial perfusion pressure, increased intracranial pressure, or brain death.

COMMON INDICATIONS

Ischemic stroke: TCD can be used to detect, among others, vascular steal, emboli, shunts, and arterial patency.

- Vascular Steal: Hypercapnia or other vasodilatory stimuli increases velocity in normal vessels, which results in a paradoxical decrease in flow velocity to ischemic areas. This is termed the Reversed Robin Hood Syndrome if the steal phenomenon results in >2- point deterioration on the NIHSS or recurrence of neurological deficit.
- Emboli: At frequency of 2 MHz, ultrasound is the gold standard for emboli detection. Microemboli may show up as HITS (high intensity transient signals) and are defined by the International Hemodynamic Society as duration <300 ms, higher intensity by 3 dB than background blood flow signal, and unidirectional. Ultrasound is often used during carotid and cardiac surgeries. Though microembolic signals (MES) are often asymptomatic, increasing frequencies can be associated with cognitive decline after cardiac or carotid surgery.
- Patent foramen ovales (PFOs) are detected in 25% to 30% of the adult population. Agitated saline is injected in the peripheral vein at the same time as patient performs the Valsalva maneuver; MES is captured on TCD if a right-to-left shunt is present. If more than 9 MES are captured with latency of <9 s, presence of a PFO is highly suggested. Studies have reported overall sensitivity of 97% and specificity of 93% for detection of right-to-left shunt with TCD compared with trans-esophageal echocardiogram (TEE). TCD may also demonstrate presence of extracardiac shunts, such as pulmonary arterio-venous malformations. The American Academy of Neurology (AAN) has labeled class II indication for both TCD and TEE for interatrial shunt detection, though only TEE may provide anatomical details of the interatrial septum.
- TCDs can be used to provide real time measurement of arterial patency to monitor recanalization and detect reocclusion in patients treated with acute reperfusion therapies.

Subarachnoid hemorrhage: Vasospasm occurs in about 70% of subarachnoid hemorrhage (SAH) patients 4 to 17 days post bleed. TCD values are well established for middle cerebral artery (MCA), but is poorly standardized or accurate for anterior cerebral artery (ACA) and posterior cerebral artery (PCA). A systematic analysis comparing TCD with angiogram has shown that a mean MCA cerebral blood flow velocity (CBFV) of >120 cm/s carries 99% specificity and 67% sensitivity for identification of angiographic vasospasm of ≥25%; velocity >200 cm/s is predictive of <1 mm residual MCA diameter.

- Lindegaard ratio is calculated using: MCA mean CBFV/extracranial internal carotid artery (ICA) mean CBFV.
- Reference range is between 1.1 and 2.3. Hyperemia may be seen if CBFV is elevated but the Lindegaard ratio is less than 3. In general, >3 indicates moderate vasospasm and >6 severe vasospasm.
- A similar equation exists to assess posterior circulation using: basilar artery CBFV/left or right vertebral artery CBFV. A value of 2.5 with basilar artery (BA) velocity higher than 85 cm/s was 86% sensitive and 97% specific for BA narrowing of more than 25%. A basilar artery/vertebral artery (BA/VA) ratio over 3.0 with BA velocities higher than 85 cm/s was 92% sensitive and 97% specific for BA narrowing of more than 50%.
- Mean CBFV increasing 50 cm/s or more within 24 hours at any time or mean CBFV increases of >65 cm/s per day from day 3 to 7 indicates high risk for delayed cerebral ischemia, which is related to adverse outcome.

Traumatic Brain Injury: During the initial 72 hours post traumatic brain injury (TBI), a reduced cerebral blood flow state, characterized by a mean MCA CBFV of less than 35 cm/s, has been associated with unfavorable outcome at 6 months as evaluated by the Glasgow Outcome Score.

Brain death: Reverberating flow patterns in MCA and BA are suggestive of circulatory arrest in brain death. Specifically, the BA and ICA or MCA of both sides are evaluated in two different studies performed at least 30 minutes apart. When specific findings are noted, this technique has been found by the AAN to have a sensitivity of 89% to 100% and a specificity of 97% to 100%.

REFERENCES

D'Andrea, A., Conte, M., Cavallaro, M., et al. (2016). Transcranial Doppler ultrasonography: from methodology to major clinical applications. *World J Cardiol*, *8*, 383–400.

Haršány, M., Tsivgoulis, G., & Alexandrov, A. V. (2016). Ultrasonography. In J. C. Grotta, G. W. Albers, J. P. Broderick, et al. (Eds.), *Stroke: pathophysiology, diagnosis, and management,* ed 6 (pp. 733–750). Elsevier.

TRANSPLANTATION

ORGAN HARVEST

Death determination prior to organ harvest is based on neurologic criteria. At present, most jurisdictions require absence of function of the entire brain (see "Brain Death").

CLINICAL SYNDROMES IN ORGAN RECIPIENTS

Following organ transplantation, 30% to 60% of patients develop neurologic complications. Various classification systems exist. Some of the syndromes are due to preexisting deficits due to underlying illness, complications during surgery, and complications after surgery. An anatomy classification distinguishes encephalopathy from peripheral nervous system complications. Others can be classified as metabolic encephalopathies, complications from neurotoxicity of immunosuppressant agents, opportunistic central nervous system (CNS) infections, secondary malignancies as a direct side effect of immunosuppression, and other specific neurologic complications seen mostly after certain organ transplantations.

Specific clinical syndromes are outlined in the following:

I. Procedure-related complications
   A. Femoral or lateral cutaneous nerve injuries after kidney transplantation
   B. Mononeuropathies after traumatic cannulation of catheters

II. Encephalopathy
   A. Post-transplantation delirium is seen in orthotopic liver transplantation (particularly for alcoholic liver disease), calcineurin inhibitors (cyclosporine and tacrolimus), opioid antagonists, beta-blockers, high-dose corticosteroids, and Wernicke encephalopathy due to total parenteral nutrition.
   B. Post-transplantation stupor or coma is seen in central pontine myelinolysis (liver transplantation), intracerebral hematoma (not uncommonly due to Aspergillus infection), hemolytic-uremic syndrome (bone marrow transplantation), acute organ rejection, bilateral cerebral or brainstem infarctions, prolonged intraoperative hypotension causing hypoxic-ischemic encephalopathy, nonconvulsive status epilepticus, and accumulation of anesthetic and sedative agents due to different pharmacokinetics in transplantation recipients.

III. Peripheral nervous system complications
   A. Peripheral Neuropathy: drugs (interferon-alfa, colchicine, tacrolimus, cyclosporine, and etoposide), critical illness neuropathy, Guillain-Barré syndrome, and chronic inflammatory demyelinating polyradiculoneuropathy (CIDP)
   B. Neuromuscular junction disorders: prolonged neuromuscular blockade, myasthenia gravis as a rare manifestation of a graft-versus-host disease
   C. Myopathy: critical illness myopathy (with IV corticosteroids), polymyositis (in bone marrow transplantation), cyclosporine, cholesterol-lowering agents, and colchicine

IV. Effect of immunosuppressant agents
   A. Calcineurin inhibitors (cyclosporine and tacrolimus)
      1. Cyclosporine can cause postural and intention tremor, headache, visual hallucination to cortical blindness, seizures, and language-motor dysfunctions.

2. Tacrolimus (FK506) produces neurologic complications that are similar to those of cyclosporine, but less frequent.

3. Risk factors for developing toxicity include high drug level, IV administration, hypomagnesemia, hyperlipidemia, high blood pressure, and concurrent high-dose steroid therapy. Magnetic resonance imaging (MRI) may show features consistent with reversible posterior leukoencephalopathy.

B. Corticosteroids can cause proximal myopathy, anxiety and dysthymia, psychosis (3%), "steroid pseudorheumatism," headache, fever, lethargy on withdrawal.

C. OKT3 monoclonal antibody may produce transient flu-like symptoms, aseptic meningitis (2% to 14%), encephalopathy (1% to 10%).

D. Busulfan can cause seizures.

E. Methotrexate can cause leukoencephalopathy.

F. Ifosfamide can cause hallucinations, mutism, and coma.

V. Opportunistic CNS infection occurs in up to 10% of recipients and carries a high mortality rate:

A. First month after transplantation: Infections are usually due to gram-negative bacteria or staphylococci from the surgical procedure itself, the hospitalization, or the presence of indwelling catheters. Bone marrow transplant patients are at risk for reactivation of a latent CNS viral infection (herpes simplex virus 1 [HSV-1], varicella zoster virus [VZV], human herpesvirus 6 [HHV-6], and Epstein-Barr virus [EBV]) in the immediate period after transplantation.

B. Two to 6 months after transplantation: Recipients are at greatest risk for the classic CNS infections associated with transplantation. Infections are mostly due to viruses (cytomegalovirus [CMV], HSV-1, HSV-2, HHV-6, VZV, and West Nile) and various opportunistic organisms (*Aspergillus spp.*, *Nocardia asteroides*, *Toxoplasma gondii*, *Candida spp.*, and *Listeria monocytogenes*).

C. Beyond 6 months after transplantation, infections are due to lingering effects of previously acquired infections.

1. Fungi: Cryptococcus is the most common pathogen, and infection usually presents after 6 months of immune suppression. Aspergillus infection often presents as vasculitis or encephalopathy. Candida causes fungemia and meningitis; it is the most common invasive fungal infection in liver transplantation patients. Neutropenia is the most significant risk factor. Rhinocerebral mucormycosis is seen in diabetic recipients.

2. Bacteria: Listeria is the most common bacterium, usually causing meningitis. Nocardia usually causes abscess. Tuberculosis is uncommon.

3. Parasites: Toxoplasmosis may result from receiving an actively infected organ or from reactivation of latent disease.

4. Viruses: Cytomegalovirus may cause chorioretinitis, meningoencephalitis, and polyradiculomyelitis. Varicella-zoster virus in a new infection may cause encephalitis with high morbidity; reactivation produces shingles, either diffusely or in dermatomal distribution. HHV-6 causes a unique syndrome of limbic encephalitis, particularly in patients with allogeneic bone marrow transplantation. HHV-6 polymerase chain reaction (PCR) in cerebrospinal fluid (CSF) is sensitive for the diagnosis. Human T-lymphotropic virus I (HTLV-1) causes myelopathy after blood transfusion in heart, bone marrow, and kidney recipients. JC virus can cause progressive multifocal leukoencephalopathy (see "Encephalitis").

VI. Post-transplant lymphoproliferative disorders are invariably EBV-driven expansions of B lymphocytes in organ transplantation patients. Intense immunosuppression has emerged as a risk factor. Two forms of post-transplant lymphoproliferative disorder are early, with onset 0.5 years after transplantation and median survival of 37 months, and late, with onset 5 years after transplantation and median survival of 1 month. MRI often shows necrotic, ring-enhancing lesion(s), resembling findings in acquired immune deficiency syndrome (AIDS)-associated primary CNS lymphoma. Treatments include modifying immunosuppressive agents and methotrexate-based chemotherapy with or without radiotherapy. Prognosis is generally poor.

VII. Other neurologic syndromes include the following:
   A. Akinetic mutism: OKT3 and cyclosporine.
   B. Cerebellar dysfunction: dysarthria, ataxia due to neurotoxicity of several immunosuppressants.
   C. Creutzfeldt-Jakob disease: increased risk for patients receiving cadaveric dura transplantation.
   D. Hearing loss: due to cyclosporine-mediated thromboembolic process or antibiotic toxicity.
   E. Language disorders: reversible, due to cyclosporine or tacrolimus neurotoxicity.
   F. Metabolic acidosis: can cause coma in kidney recipients.
   G. Migraine: in bone marrow recipients, due to cyclosporine or hypothesized defect in donor-derived platelets.
   H. Movement disorder: chorea due to cyclosporine in liver transplantation for Wilson disease; tremor in calcineurin inhibitors.
   I. Neuromyotonia: antibody-mediated channelopathy, seen in patients after bone marrow transplantation.
   J. Neurocardiogenic symptoms: angina and vasovagal syncope seen in heart recipients, presumably due to re-innervation.
   K. Pain: due to varicella-zoster virus; local effects at operative sites; musculoskeletal pain, cyclosporine effects in kidney recipients; oral mucositis in bone marrow recipients.

L. Seizures: generalized tonic-clonic seizures with a regimen of busulfan, cyclophosphamide, and cyclosporine; seen in severe cases of tacrolimus-associated neurotoxicity.

M. Sleep disorder: somnolence syndrome related to radiation in bone marrow recipient.

N. Stroke and cerebral ischemia: 44% to 59% of all neurologic complications of post-transplantation patients. Prolonged intraoperative hypotension can cause watershed infarcts. Cardioembolic sources should be considered in heart-lung transplantation. Angioinvasive fungal parasites such as Aspergillus can cause hemorrhagic infarction, particularly in liver transplantation patients.

O. Taste disturbance: in bone marrow recipients.

REFERENCES

Czartoski, T. (2006). Central Nervous System Infections in Transplant Recipients. *Continuum*, *12*(2), 95–110.

Liguori, R. (2000). Acquired neuromyotonia after bone marrow transplantation. *Neurology*, *54*, 1390–1391.

TREMORS (SEE ALSO THERAPEUTIC APPENDIX)

DEFINITION

Tremors are regular, involuntary rhythmic oscillations of any part of the body produced by alternating contraction of agonist and antagonist muscles. They usually affect the distal extremities (especially fingers and hands), head, tongue, jaw, and rarely the trunk. Tremors disappear during sleep. The frequency is usually consistent in all the affected parts, regardless of the size of muscles involved. It is important to observe the amplitude, frequency, and rhythm of the tremor, as well as the effects of physiologic (posture, limb movement, diurnal variation, and so forth) and psychological factors. It is the most common movement disorder.

Classification

I. Action or postural tremor: Presents when the limbs and trunk are held in certain positions or during active movements.

A. Physiologic tremor: Small-amplitude, high-frequency (6 to 12 Hz) tremor seen in normal individuals; exaggerated by stress, endocrine disorders (hyperthyroidism, hypoglycemia, and pheochromocytoma), drugs (such as lithium, tricyclics, phenothiazines, epinephrine, theophylline, amphetamines, thyroid hormones, isoproterenol, corticosteroids, valproate, levodopa, and butyrophenones), and toxins (such as mercury, lead, arsenic, bismuth, and carbon monoxide). Dietary factors (caffeine, monosodium glutamate, and ethanol withdrawal) may contribute.

Treatment: Management depends on the cause; relaxation methods and stress reduction may help if psychological factors are involved. Beta-blockers have been used with some success, particularly in performers with "stage fright"

B. Essential tremor: A bilateral postural tremor that often increases with action or intention. It has a frequency of 4 to 11 Hz and usually consists of flexion-extension of the fingers and hands initially, but may progress proximally; the head and neck, jaw, tongue, or voice may be involved. It is exacerbated by emotional and physical stress and diminishes with rest, relaxation, and use of ethanol. It may be familial (dominant inheritance), sporadic, or associated with other movement disorders (Parkinson disease, torsion dystonia, or torticollis).

Treatment: Propranolol is the drug of choice but is contraindicated in patients with asthma or diabetes and in older patients with h/o heart failure. Start with doses of 10 to 20 mg tid or qid, increasing the dosage if necessary. Primidone therapy is also useful, starting at 25 to 50 mg and can be increased up to 250 mg tid if tolerated. Sedation or gastrointestinal (GI) complaints may limit its use. Benzodiazepines are also useful in treating essential tremor.

C. Primary writing tremor: Occurs only during writing. Electrophysiologic studies suggest that it may be a form of dystonia.

Treatment: It may respond to anticholinergic therapy or botulinum toxin.

D. Rubral tremor: A coarse tremor is present at rest, increasing with postural maintenance and even more with movement. This tremor suggests ipsilateral cerebellar outflow lesion.

II. Rest tremors: Present when limbs are at rest.

Parkinsonian tremor has a frequency of 4 to 6 Hz with variable amplitude, sometimes asymmetrical. It occurs at rest and disappears with movement and during sleep. It is prominent in the hands, with flexion-extension or adduction-abduction of the fingers. There is also pronation-supination of the hands. Movements of the feet, jaw, and lips may be present.

Treatment consists of anticholinergic therapy or dopaminergic drugs.

III. Intention tremor.

Cerebellar tremor is a tremor of 3 to 5 Hz occurring during the performance of an exact, projected movement and worsening as the action continues. There may be tremors of the head or trunk (titubation). The oscillation begins proximally and occurs perpendicular to the line of movement. Causes include lesions of cerebellar pathways, cerebellar degeneration, MS, Wilson disease, and drugs or toxins (such as phenytoin, barbiturates, lithium, ethanol, mercury, and fluorouracil).

IV. Other tremors.
- A. Orthostatic tremor, a tremor of the legs, is present only when standing and disappears with walking. As such, it may be considered a task-specific tremor.

    Treatment: It responds to clonazepam therapy, 4 to 6 mg/day.
- B. Hysterical tremor may be a symptom of conversion disorder. The tremor is often irregular in frequency and may diminish or disappear with distraction.
- C. Dystonic tremor: Treatment is now mainly botulinum toxin (Botox).

REFERENCES

Elias, W. J., & Shah, B. B. (2014). Tremor. *JAMA, 311*(9), 948–954. https://doi.org/10.1001/jama.2014.1397.

Espay, A. J., Lang, A. E., Erro, R., et al. (2017). Essential pitfalls in "essential" tremor. *Mov Disord, 32*(3), 325–331. https://doi.org/10.1002/mds.26919.

TRIGEMINAL NEURALGIA

CLINICAL PRESENTATION

Trigeminal neuralgia is characterized by paroxysmal sharp, shooting or lancinating facial pain in a unilateral distribution. The historical term "tic douloureux" describes the reactionary tic-like grimace reaction at the onset of pain. The pain is described as brief electric shock-like pains in one or more branches of the trigeminal nerve (most commonly the maxillary or mandibular divisions). These paroxysms tend to occur in clusters and can be almost continuous. They last from a few seconds up to 2 minutes with a refractory period that can last minutes to hours. The paroxysm may be triggered by stimulation of the trigeminal nerve. The patient may experience a "lightning bolt" pain from minor stimulation such as light touch, light breeze on the face, chewing, talking, swallowing, brushing teeth, combing hair, putting on makeup, or washing one's face. Some people have multiple trigger zones and, rarely, one may have no identifiable trigger zones. The most common trigger zones include ipsilateral nasolabial fold area in the maxillary distribution, or near the commissure of the lip in the mandibular distribution. Some patients have intraoral trigger zone on teeth, mucosa, and tongue.

Onset is after age 40 years in 90% of patients and is more common in women (male-female ratio of 2:3). There is a right (61%) greater than left predominance with a very rare bilateral presentation (4%). The pain does not cross the midline. Neurologic examination may show sensory loss in up to one fourth of patients, but otherwise is unremarkable.

ETIOLOGY

There are two etiologic classifications for trigeminal neuralgia: either classic (essential or idiopathic) or symptomatic trigeminal neuralgia caused by a demonstrable structural lesion other than vascular compression. The classic trigeminal neuralgia requires the absence of a demonstrable neurologic cause. Demyelination (multiple sclerosis), compression (cerebellopontine angle tumors and schwannomas), and vascular compromise account for a small proportion of cases and should be suspected with onset before age 40. Typical finding of trigeminal sensory or motor abnormalities on examination can be found. Evaluation should also look for any other findings referable to the base of the skull or posterior fossa.

DIFFERENTIAL DIAGNOSIS

Correct diagnosis is key to treatment, and the history is of utmost importance to differentiate from trigeminal autonomic cephalalgias such as cluster headaches, short-lasting unilateral neuralgiform headache attacks with conjunctival injection and tearing, and paroxysmal hemicranias, especially in patients with first division (V1) pain. Posterior fossa mass lesions such as cerebello-pontine angle tumors (meningioma, acoustic neuroma, trigeminal neuroma), aneurysm, or arteriovenous malformations may produce trigeminal neuralgia-type symptoms.

Trigeminal neuralgia pain may be seen in multiple sclerosis, brainstem infarction, and syringobulbia. Evaluation should include magnetic resonance imaging (MRI) with gadolinium, magnetic resonance angiography (MRA), and evoked potentials for patients with sensory anomalies. The presence of a vascular loop, for example, causing trigeminal nerve compression can be detected by MRI.

TREATMENT

If trigeminal neuralgia is secondary, treatment should be focused on the underlying cause. In cases of idiopathic trigeminal neuralgia, medical treatment is pursued. In refractory cases, surgical treatment is considered.

Medications that are commonly used are as follows:

FIRST LINE
- Carbamazepine is effective in 58% to 100%. Start at 300 mg/day and increase gradually as tolerated to 2.4 g/day in divided doses.
- Oxcarbazepine 600 to 1800 mg/day

SECOND LINE
- Add on or switch to Lamotrigine 400 mg/day
- Baclofen 40 to 80 mg/day; Baclofen is started at 5 mg orally tid and increased gradually to 20 mg orally qid.
- Imipramine or amitriptyline is started at 25 to 50 mg orally at bedtime and gradually increased to 150 mg.

OTHERS: (CLASS III EVIDENCE)
    Pimozide - 4 to 12 mg/day
    Tocainide - 12 mg/day
    Tizanidine

Less evidence for the following but they have been used as there is Class IV evidence:

- – phenytoin
- – clonazepam
- – gabapentin
- – valproate

SURGERY

Surgical therapy is reserved for intractable pain unresponsive to drug treatment and includes the following:

I. Local neurolysis and nerve block runs the risk of painful anesthesia and persistent paresthesias as well as recurrence.

II. Percutaneous radiofrequency thermocoagulation of the trigeminal ganglion (gasserian ganglion [rhizotomies] can be done under local anesthesia). Painful anesthesia and recurrences are less common.

III. Microsurgical vascular decompression of the trigeminal root entry zone.

IV. Several new procedures have shown promise in patients with refractory cases. These procedures include percutaneous trigeminal nerve compression and stereotactic radiosurgery.

REFERENCES

Baad-Hansen, L., & Benoliel, R. (2017). Neuropathic orofacial pain: facts and fiction. Cephalalgia, *37*(7), 670–679.

Obermann, M. (2010). Treatment options in trigeminal neuralgia. *Ther Adv Neurol Disord*, *3*, 107–115.

TRINUCLEOTIDE REPEAT EXPANSION

Triplet repeat expansion diseases result from the amplification of CAG, CTG, CGG, CCG, or GAA motifs embedded within the coding and noncoding regions of specific genes. Expansion of triplet repeats increases in offspring of affected individuals, and this increase generally results in progressive severity of the disease or earlier age of onset, providing the molecular basis of the clinical phenomenon called "anticipation." Since the original discovery of triplet repeat expansion as the responsible mechanism for fragile X syndrome in 1991, it has proved to be a general phenomenon responsible for a growing number of neurologic disorders (Table 117).

REFERENCES

La Spada, A. R., & Taylor, J. P. (2010). Repeat expansion disease: progress and puzzles in disease pathogenesis. *Nat Rev Genet*, *11*(4), 247–258.

Paulson, H. L. (2006). Genetics of repeat expansion diseases. *Continuum*, *11*(2), 59–78.

TABLE 117

TRINUCLEOTIDE REPEAT DISORDERS

Disease	Inheritance	Gene/Chromosome	Protein	Normal No. of Repeat	No. of Repeats in Disorder Mutant Protein
Fragile X syndrome	XD	FMR1/Xq27.3	FMR1	(CGG) < 50	(CGG) > 200
Fragile XE mental retardation	X	FMR2/Xq28	FMR2	(CCG) < 35	(CCG) > 200
Myotonic dystrophy	AD	DMPK/19q13	MD protein kinase	(CTG) < 35	(CTG) > 50
Huntington disease	AD	HD/IT15/4p16	Huntingtin	(CAG) < 40	(CAG) > 40
Spinal and bulbar muscular (Kennedy disease)	XR	AR/Xq11–q12	Androgen receptor	(CAG) < 30	(CAG) > 40
SCA1	AD	SCA1/6p22–p23	Ataxin 1	(CAG) < 40	(CAG) > 40
SCA2	AD	SCA2/12q24.1	Ataxin 2	(CAG) < 30	(CAG) > 35
SCA3/MJD (Machado-Joseph disease)	AD	MJD1/SCA3/14q24.3–q31	Ataxin 3	(CAG) < 40	(CAG) > 40
SCA6	AD	CACNL1A4/19p13.1–p13.2	Voltage dependent calcium channel	(CAG) < 20	(CAG) > 20
SCA7	AD	SCA7/3p14–p21.1	Ataxin 7	(CAG) < 20	(CAG) > 40
SCA8	AD	SCA8/13q21	?	(CTG) < 40	(CTG)
Friedreich ataxia	AR	FRDA/X25/9q13	Frataxin	(GAA) < 35	(GAA) > 100
Dentatorubral-pallidoluysian atrophy (DRPLA)/Haw-River syndrome	AD	DRPLA/12p13	Atrophin 1	(CAG) < 35	(CAG) > 48
Oculopharyngeal muscular dystrophy (OPMD)	AD/AR	PABPN1 Poly(A) binding protein/14q11.2–q13	(PABPN1)	GCC < 10	GCC > 10
SCA12	AD	ERDA1/DIR1/5q32	PPP2R2B	CAG < 28	CAG > 55
SCA 17	AD	Transcription factor/6q27	TATA box binding protein	CAG < 44	CAG > 48

AD, autosomal dominant; AR, autosomal recessive; SCA, spinocerebellar atrophy; X, X-linked; XD, X-linked dominant; XR, X-linked recessive.

TUMOR EMBOLIZATION

Management of vascular head and neck tumors is challenging and might require a multimodal approach to treatment. Endovascular embolization is often employed to reduce blood loss during surgery and to increase the chance of complete tumor resection.

Vascular tumors of the head and neck that may benefit from embolization prior to surgical resection include juvenile nasopharyngeal angiofibroma, meningioma, hemangioblastoma, glomus jugular tumor, hemangiopericytoma, and metastatic lesions.

The choice of embolic material is determined by various factors that include operator preference and anatomic considerations. Commonly used materials include ethylene vinyl alcohol copolymer (onyx), N-butyl cyanoacrylate (glue), and trisacryl gelatin microspheres.

While studies have shown that tumor embolization reduced blood loss, surgery duration, and tumor recurrence, there are no randomized trials comparing surgical resection alone to embolization with surgical resection. The decision to use tumor embolization prior to surgery depends on several factors, including tumor vascularity, tumor size, ease of resection, and operator preference, among other factors. Complications of tumor embolization are classified as either procedure-related or non-procedure related. The most common procedure- related complications include cranial nerve palsy, skin and mucosal tissue necrosis, stroke, and contrast-induced nephropathy.

REFERENCE

Duffis, E. J., Gandhi, C. D., Prestigiacomo, C. J., et al. (2012). Head, neck, and brain tumor embolization guidelines. *J Neurointerv Surg*, *4*(4), 251–255.

TUMORS

The presence of tumor within the nervous system is often suspected by the development of subacute or acute progressive focal symptoms. Tumor metastases or carcinomatous meningitis may result in multifocal signs. The World Health Organization (WHO) system is the most accepted classification for primary central nervous system (CNS) tumors. Tumors are graded from I to IV, representing an estimate of malignancy (see Table 118 and Fig. 64).

BRAIN

1. Epidemiology: The annual incidence rate for malignant brain cancer for all races from 2006 to 2010 was 7.27 per 100,000 person-years and 13.77 per 100,000 person-years for primary nonmalignant brain tumors. Although primary malignant brain tumors account for only 2% of all cancers, they contribute to substantial morbidity, and prognosis is poor (sixth lowest among all type of cancers). Gliomas are the most common malignant primary brain tumors (80%). The most common nonmalignant primary tumor is meningioma.

TABLE 118

HISTOLOGIC CLASSIFICATION OF NEUROLOGIC TUMORS

Neuroepithelial tumors	Nerve sheath tumors:
Astrocytic tumors:	Schwannoma (neurilemmoma)
Diffuse astrocytoma	Neurofibroma
Astrocytoma	Neurofibrosarcoma
Anaplastic astrocytoma	Tumors of blood vessel origin:
Glioblastoma multiforme	Hemangioblastoma
Juvenile pilocytic astrocytoma	Hemangiopericytoma
Subependymal giant cell astrocytoma	Germ cell tumors:
Oligodendroglial tumors:	Germinoma
Oligodendroglioma	Embryonal carcinoma
Anaplastic oligodendroglioma	Choriocarcinoma
Ependymal tumors:	Teratoma
Ependymoma	Malignant lymphomas:
Myxopapillary ependymoma	Hodgkin disease
Anaplastic ependymoma	Non-Hodgkin lymphoma
Subependymoma	Malformative tumors:
Choroid plexus tumors:	Craniopharyngioma
Choroid plexus papilloma	Epidermoid cyst
Choroid plexus carcinoma	Dermoid cyst
Neuronal tumors:	Neuroepithelial (colloid) cyst
Ganglioglioma	Lipoma
Gangliocytoma	Regional tumors:
Primitive neuroectodermal tumors:	Chordoma
Medulloblastoma	Glomus jugulare tumor
Pineoblastoma	Chondroma
Neuroblastoma	Metastatic tumors:
Meningeal tumors:	Carcinoma
Meningioma	Sarcoma
Papillary meningioma	Lymphoma
Anaplastic meningioma	

From Cohen, M. E. (1991). Pathology and molecular genetics. In W. G. Bradley, R. B. Baroff, G. M. Fenichel & C. D. Marsden (Eds.), *Neurology in clinical practice*, Boston: Butterworth-Heinemann.

2. Clinical presentation: Symptoms and signs of CNS neoplasm may be focal as a result of tumor invasion into brain parenchyma, or by local compression from the tumor's associated edema, or hemorrhage. It can also be generalized and nonlocalizing, usually as a result of diffuse edema, hydrocephalus, or increased intracranial pressure. Brain tumors rarely cause constitutional symptoms. Symptoms are typically subacute and progressive, developing over days to weeks. Large brain tumors may produce few symptoms, reflecting the brain's ability to accommodate gradual tumor growth. Headache occurs in about half of all patients with brain tumors. Headache is usually worse in the morning and, even without treatment, resolves within a few hours. Seizures occur more often with slow-growing tumors and with tumors in the frontal and parietal lobes.

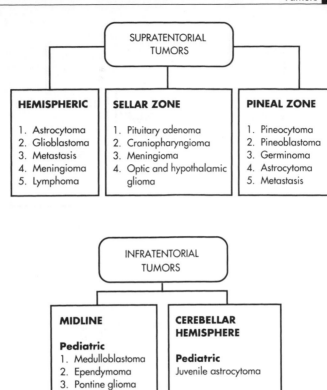

A

FIGURE 64
Continued

Vomiting occurs most consistently with posterior fossa tumors. Localizing symptoms and signs depend on tumor location. Frontal lobe masses may be silent or, if anterior and midline, may produce changes in personality and memory, sometimes mistaken for psychiatric disorders. Pineal region tumors often produce dorsal midbrain syndrome

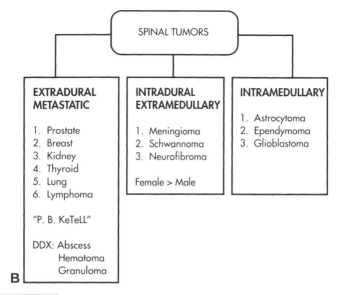

B

FIGURE 64

Tumors by location. *A*, supratentorial tumors; *B*, infratentorial tumors. (From American Academy of Neurology. Contemporary neuropathology, vol 6, Basic neurosciences, AAN Courses 1993; courtesy JC Goodman.)

(Parinaud syndrome) and aqueductal obstruction leading to hydrocephalus. Brainstem tumors produce cranial neuropathies, long-tract signs, and hydrocephalus resulting from compression of the cerebral aqueduct.

3. Diagnosis: magnetic resonance imaging (MRI) with gadolinium contrast is the imaging technique of choice. Hemorrhage occurs most often with glioblastoma multiform and metastatic tumors, especially renal cell carcinoma, melanoma, and choriocarcinoma, but the most common hemorrhagic metastases are from lung cancer. Calcification occurs more commonly with oligodendroglioma and meningioma. Skull x-rays or computed tomography (CT) with bone windows are useful in evaluating bony metastasis, while angiography helps define vascular anatomy. MR spectroscopy (elevated choline: N-acetylaspartate (NAA) ratio) and positron emission tomography (PET) scan (hypermetabolism on fluorodeoxyglucose-positron emission tomography [FDG-PET]) may be helpful in the diagnosis of some cases. In primary CNS lymphoma, ophthalmologic examination to exclude retinal involvement is indicated, and lumbar puncture for cerebrospinal fluid (CSF) cytology should be considered.

4. Treatment: Available treatment modalities include surgical resection that can improve symptoms by relieving mass effect, improving seizure control, and potentially reducing risk of recurrence and improving survival. Surgery complications incidence ranges from 5% to 30%, including hemorrhage, infarction, seizures, CSF leak or wound infection. Other modalities include radiation therapy (stereotactic radiosurgery), chemotherapy, and combinations. Adverse effects of radiation can be acute (within days), early-delayed (1–6 months), or late-delayed (months to years). Special attention should be made to *pseudoprogression* due to radiation necrosis that can be managed with corticosteroids (contrast enhancement as a result of chemoradiation therapy and not a tumor progression). The risk of leukoencephalopathy is higher with whole brain radiation, old age, vascular risk factors, and combined chemoradiation. Dexamethasone is the mainstay for symptomatic management in patients with brain tumors and is usually started at 4 mg PO/IV every 4 to 6 hours.

5. Management of CNS neoplasms

LOW-GRADE GLIOMAS

I. Biopsy to confirm diagnosis and to rule out high-grade gliomas.

II. If there are no other symptoms than well-controlled seizures, defer treatment until progression.

III. Progressive symptoms require resection with or without chemotherapy; consider radiation therapy only in refractory cases.

HIGH-GRADE GLIOMAS (ANAPLASTIC ASTROCYTOMA AND GLIOBLASTOMA MULTIFORME; WHO GRADE III OR IV)

I. Resection (better prognosis with gross total resection).

II. Radiation therapy with concurrent daily temozolomide.

III. After resection and radiation, consider adjuvant chemotherapy (e.g., Bevacizumab) or refer patients for clinical trial enrollment.

Chemotherapy options include temozolomide, nitrosoureas *(lomustine and carmustine)*, procarbazine (or PCV—procarbazine, CCNU/lomustine, vincristine), *vincristine,* and *methotrexate. Bevacizumab* is a humanized monoclonal antibody against vascular endothelial growth factor and is the only targeted therapy currently Food and Drug Administration (FDA)-approved for the treatment of glioblastoma.

PRIMARY CNS LYMPHOMA

Surgery has a limited role besides diagnosis, since primary CNS lymphoma (PCNSL) tends to be a diffuse disease. Chemotherapy is the treatment of choice with methotrexate-based regimens (the most effective single agent in PCNSL treatment). Methotrexate (MTX) combination therapy is a reasonable treatment option: MTX plus temozolomide, MTX plus cytarabine, and MTX plus procarbazine and vincristine. PCNSL is sensitive to radiation therapy but its use as an initial treatment has waned due to availability of newer chemotherapy options.

SPINAL CORD

I. Epidemiology: Cancer affects the spinal cord in 5% to 10% of all patients with cancer, either by direct tumor involvement or as a treatment complication. The majority of primary spinal cord tumors are WHO Grade I or II.

II. Location: Intradural tumors are either intramedullary (arising within the substance of the cord), most commonly ependymomas, astrocytomas, and less commonly hemangioblastoma, or extramedullary (arising from the leptomeninges or nerve roots), with meningiomas or peripheral nerve sheath tumors (schwannomas or neurofibromas) most common. Extradural cord tumors arise from the vertebral bodies and epidural tissues or are metastatic lesions to the epidural space.

III. Clinical presentation: Local back or radicular pain, myelopathy, weakness, sensory complaints, and sphincter dysfunction.

IV. Diagnosis: On plain radiographs these masses may produce widening of the interpeduncular distance or of the neural foramina, as well as scalloping of the vertebral bodies. The loss of a pedicle and signs of bone destruction are associated with malignant extradural lesions. MRI is the imaging technique of choice; myelography with CT scanning can be used if MRI is contraindicated.

V. Treatment: Treatment consists of maximal safe surgical resection or biopsy followed by observation or external beam radiation therapy. Radiation therapy is reserved for patients with high-grade tumors and those with progressive disease. Chemotherapy is used as a last resort for patients with disease progression for whom no other treatment options exist.

METASTATIC DISEASE

I. Epidemiology: Metastases to the brain parenchyma are often found at the gray-white matter junction. Up to 50% of patients with brain metastasis may present with a solitary brain lesion which may raise confusion with abscess, primary brain tumors or, rarely, tumefactive MS lesions. Metastases are typically well demarcated with a zone of surrounding edema. They are usually carcinomas rather than sarcomas or lymphomas. Diffuse involvement throughout the neuraxis is characteristic for leptomeningeal metastases (multifocal neurologic signs and symptoms). Cancers most commonly associated with metastases vary according to site as follows:

A. Skull: breast, prostate, multiple myeloma

B. Brain parenchyma: lung, breast, colorectal, renal, melanoma

C. Leptomeninges: breast, lung, melanoma, colorectal, lymphoma, leukemia

D. Epidural (spinal cord): lung, breast, prostate, lymphoma, sarcoma, renal

II. Treatment: Several factors should be considered, including performance status, age, the extent of the primary cancer and extracranial disease, and histologic subtype. With single brain lesion, or if the brain lesion is solitary (no other sites known), surgical resection or stereotactic radiosurgery (for lesions less than 3 cm) whole-brain radiation therapy is the treatment of choice. In the setting of multiple brain metastases, surgery is typically reserved for obtaining pathology or for relieving mass effect and improving symptoms from large brain metastases. For patients with poor prognosis and many brain metastases, whole-brain radiation therapy is still the initial treatment of choice for their CNS disease.

EPIDURAL SPINAL CORD COMPRESSION

I. Epidemiology: Spinal cord compression represents a neurologic emergency. The thoracic spine is the most common site for epidural metastasis (68%). The diagnosis should be suspected in anyone with a known cancer and back pain who seeks medical attention with radicular symptoms, leg weakness, or myelopathy signs. Typically, the vertebral body is affected first. Pain and weakness are the most common initial symptoms. Sensory loss may not be prominent at presentation, since these lesions are usually more ventrally located. The most common sources are breast cancer (20%), lung cancer (13%), lymphoma (11%), and prostate cancer (9%).

II. Diagnosis: Diagnosis can be suspected from the presence of bony destruction if present on plain radiographic films; confirmation should be obtained by MRI, CT myelography, or occasionally, bone scan. The entire spinal cord should be imaged to investigate the possibility of multiple lesions or multiple areas of spinal cord compression.

III. Treatment: Any patient suspected to have an epidural spinal cord compression should be treated immediately with IV dexamethasone even prior to imaging; 10 mg of dexamethasone is usually administered followed by 4 to 16 mg/day, based on severity of neurologic signs and symptoms. Once confirmed by imaging, treatment usually consists of radiotherapy and steroids. Peptic ulcer prophylaxis with H_2 blocker or proton pump inhibitors should be considered for GI prophylaxis. Chemotherapy may be of benefit in chemosensitive tumors such as lymphomas.

The decision for surgery is based on many factors, including tumor type and sensitivity to treatment, spinal deformity or stability, previous treatment, neurologic deficit, rapidity of onset, medical comorbidities, and expected longevity of the patient. Studies have generally shown similar outcomes from radiation therapy or radiation therapy plus laminectomy. Surgery of choice is vertebrectomy followed by spine stabilization.

REFERENCES

Chamberlain, M. C. (2015). Neoplastic myelopathies. *Continuum: Lifelong Learn Neurol, 21*(1, Spinal Cord Disorders), 132–145.

Daroff, R. B., Jankovic, J., Mazziotta, J. C., & Pomeroy, S. L. (Eds.) (2015). *Bradley's neurology in clinical practice,* ed. 7. Philadelphia: Elsevier Health Sciences.

ULNAR NERVE (SEE ALSO PERIPHERAL NERVE)

Entrapment at the elbow (cubital tunnel syndrome) results from compression of the ulnar nerve as it courses in the elbow joint under the aponeurosis connecting the two heads of the flexor carpi ulnaris. It may result from acute trauma, repeated movements, inflammation, nerve compression, traction, or friction (e.g., leaning on the elbow, or intraoperative malpositioning). It may result from virtually any insult leading to deformity of the elbow joint, including elbow fracture, arthritis, ganglion cysts, lipomas, and neuropathic (Charcot) joints. "Tardy ulnar palsy" is an ulnar neuropathy that evolves years after an injury to the elbow.

Symptoms of ulnar neuropathy at the elbow include elbow pain, sensory loss and paresthesias of the fifth and ulnar half of the fourth digits and ulnar aspect of the hand, and wasting of the hypothenar and intrinsic hand muscles. Marked weakness of the flexor carpi ulnaris suggests that the lesion is above the elbow. There may be claw hand deformity as well as tenderness or enlargement of the ulnar nerve (palpable in the epicondylar groove); Tinel sign may be present at the elbow.

Differential diagnosis includes C8 or T1 radiculopathy, syringomyelia, amyotrophic lateral sclerosis (ALS), lower brachial plexopathy (Pancoast syndrome), and peripheral polyneuropathy. Nerve conduction studies may show conduction block or slowing across the elbow; electromyography (EMG) may show denervation.

Treatment options include conservative measures (removing exacerbating factors, padding the elbow/armchair rests, nerve gliding exercises, splints) and surgery (decompression, nerve transposition, epicondylectomy). There is little evidence regarding choosing between conservative and operative management. Decompression and transposition appear to be equally effective; transposition, however, is associated with more wound infections. Generally, conservative measures are attempted first, and surgery is indicated if they fail or in patients with moderate-severe neuropathy (prominent weakness/sensory deficits, significant axon loss on EMG) caused by trauma or structural abnormality.

Entrapment at the wrist or hand (Guyon canal) presents with hand weakness and atrophy, and variable sensory involvement. Motor findings are the same as with more proximal lesions, except that the flexor carpi ulnaris and flexor digitorum III and IV are spared. Sensory findings depend on the location of the lesion with respect to the origin of the palmar and dorsal cutaneous branches. The most common causes are compression by ganglia from carpal joints, carpal bone fracture, repeated blunt trauma, and ulnar artery disease (i.e., aneurysm, thrombosis). Typically, EMG and nerve conduction studies demonstrate involvement of the hand ulnar motor fibers with sparing of sensory function to the dorsal hand. Treatment options include conservative measures (above-mentioned) and decompression of the ulnar tunnel (Guyon canal).

REFERENCES

Brazis, P. W., Masdeu, J. C., & Biller, J. (2011). Peripheral nerves. In *Localization in clinical neurology,* ed 6 (pp. 25–71). Philadelphia: Lippincott Williams & Wilkins.

Caliandro, P., La Torre, G., Padua, R., Giannini, F., & Padua, L. (2016). Treatment for ulnar neuropathy at the elbow. *Cochrane Database Syst Rev, 11,* CD006839.

ULTRASONOGRAPHY (SEE TRANSCRANIAL DOPPLER)

Vascular ultrasound has been used extensively for decades. Newer uses of ultrasonography include imaging of peripheral nerves, and as an aid to invasive procedures and new applications in neurotherapeutics.

The carotid and vertebral arteries and their branches can be evaluated with ultrasound—that is, sound with frequency higher than 20,000 Hz. B-mode (brightness modulation) is based on the transmission of ultrasound through tissues and reflection from tissue interfaces. This imaging technique produces a real-time two-dimensional picture of examined extracranial vessels in longitudinal or transverse view. It allows measurement of vessel diameter and reveals the presence of stenosis or occlusion. High-resolution scans can also determine plaque morphology including ulceration, calcification, or hemorrhage. In Doppler ultrasonography, the ultrasound is reflected off moving targets (erythrocytes). Increased blood flow velocity in a narrowed segment of arterial lumen (stenosis) is associated with higher frequency shift, which correlates with flow velocities. The best result in vascular ultrasonography can be obtained by combination of these two techniques in duplex ultrasonography, which combines the advantages of B-mode with exact sampling of the site, and systolic, diastolic, and mean velocities measured in Doppler mode.

Carotid duplex ultrasonography has an excellent accuracy for detection of stenotic areas compared with angiography. For arteries with more than 50% stenosis, sensitivity is approximately greater than 90%; for occlusions, sensitivity is 80% to 96% and specificity is 95%. However, these results vary considerably with the experience of the ultrasonography technician. Examination of vertebral arteries allows determination of flow direction (for example, subclavian steal syndrome), but morphologic evaluation is not always possible.

Blood flow velocities in the major intracranial arteries can be examined by transcranial Doppler (TCD). TCD has established value in detection of stenosis greater than 65% in the major basal intracranial arteries, assessing collateral flow, evaluating and monitoring vasospasm after subarachnoid hemorrhage, detecting arteriovascular malformations, and assessing patients with brain death. The accuracy of TCD also depends highly on operator skill and experience. TCD may also be used for intraoperative monitoring during carotid endarterectomy and cardiac surgery and in testing cerebrovascular reactivity and hemodynamic reserve (see section on "Transcranial Doppler").

U

ULTRASONOGRAPHY

Ultrasound is now gaining wider use in evaluation of the peripheral nervous system and musculoskeletal system. It can delineate the anatomy of nerve entrapment syndromes and detect foreign bodies impinging on nerves after penetrating trauma. Reports of intrinsic nerve lesions such as hamartomas and neuromas have been described. Ultrasound can efficiently guide biopsies, lumbar puncture, and nerve blocks, leading to more successful outcomes.

Ultrasound of cranial nerves is a developing field. Four cranial nerves can be reliably imaged—optic, facial, vagus, and spinal accessory nerves. Many reports have highlighted the detection of optic nerve anomalies and lesions with ultrasound. Another area under development is applications of ultrasound as therapy including Parkinson disease, essential tremor, and occipital neuralgia.

REFERENCES

Rangavajla, G., Mokarram, N., Masoodzadehgan, N., et al. (2014). Noninvasive imaging of peripheral nerves. *Cells Tissues Organs*, *200*, 69–77.

Tawfik, E. A., Walker, F. O., & Cartwright, M. S. (2015). Neuromuscular ultrasound of cranial nerves. *J Clin Neurol*, *11*, 109–121.

UREMIA

Uremia refers to the constellation of signs and symptoms associated with renal failure, regardless of cause. The presentation is variable, depending upon the remaining renal function and the rapidity of functional loss. Azotemia occurs when glomular filtration rate (GFR) is about 20% to 35% of normal. The likely toxins are byproducts of protein and amino acid metabolism such as urea, guanidine compounds, aliphatic amines, tyrosine, and phenylalanine.

I. Uremic encephalopathy correlates with the rate of progression of uremia, as opposed to the absolute blood urea nitrogen and creatinine levels.

   a. Clouding of consciousness may be associated with hallucinations, increased reflexes, and increased tone (may be asymmetrical). Asterixis, myoclonus and chorea, stupor, seizures, and coma are signs of terminal uremia. Encephalopathy can be complicated via other factors of chronic kidney disease, such as thiamine deficiency, electrolyte disturbances, and hypertensive encephalopathy.

   b. EEG is characterized by low voltage or slowing of the posterior background rhythm. Triphasic waves or epileptiform activity are not uncommon, and represent an underlying metabolic encephalopathy. Cerebrospinal fluid (CSF) protein level may be elevated, and aseptic meningitis may occur, accompanied by stiff neck and marked pleocytosis.

   c. Management consists of dialysis, supportive care, and antiepileptic drugs. If severe, renal transplant might be warranted in stable patients.

II. Seizures in renal failure may be focal; however, they are usually generalized. They may occur in the setting of uremic encephalopathy, hypertensive crisis, coexistent electrolyte disturbance, or drug toxicity. Purely uremic seizures often respond to dialysis. When anticonvulsants are required, dosage must be adjusted for glomerular filtration rate. Diminished renal clearance requires decreased dosages of carbamazepine, phenobarbital, and gabapentin. Changes in clearance and protein binding lead to decreased total phenytoin levels with an increased unbound fraction. These changes necessitate free-fraction monitoring for optimal control. Anticonvulsants with low protein binding affinity are sometimes preferable in patients on hemodialysis.

III. Peripheral neuropathy (distal, symmetrical sensorimotor polyneuropathy type) is common in advanced renal failure. Symptoms include reduced sensation, lower extremity hyporeflexia, and, when advanced, affect the upper extremities. Ultimately, it can result in atrophy and flaccid paralysis. It is often painful and may be associated with restless leg syndrome. Abnormal nerve conduction studies may precede clinical symptoms and signs. It is usually secondary to axonal loss, with decreased sensory and motor amplitude on electromyography (EMG). Studies have shown an association with elevated serum potassium, potentiating nerve injury in patients with renal impairment. The neuropathy stabilizes or improves with hemodialysis, and potassium levels should be normalized. The greatest improvement seems to occur with renal transplantation. Tricyclics or anticonvulsants may alleviate pain.

IV. Myopathy: Develops when GFR decreases to ~25 mL/min. Uremic myopathy is more common in patients with an underlying diagnosis of diabetes mellitus. Other contributing factors include vitamin D deficiency and hyperparathyroidism. It presents with symmetrical proximal weakness with atrophy and painful stiffness. Serum creatine kinase (CK) and aldolase levels are usually normal, but EMG shows myopathic changes, sometimes due to secondary hyperparathyroidism. Rarely, ischemic myopathy occurs with elevated levels of serum CK, severe weakness, and gangrenous skin lesions. Therapeutic options include renal transplantation and correcting metabolic derangements such as hyperparathyroidism; however, there are no specific treatments.

V. Tetany that does not respond to calcium may occur.

U

UREMIA

REFERENCES

Arnold, R., Issar, T., Krishnan, A., et al. (2016). Neurological complications in chronic kidney disease. *J R Soc Med Cardiovas Dis*, 5, 9–11.

Weissenborn, K., & Lockwood, A. (2016). Toxic and metabolic encephalitis. In R. Daroff, et al. (Eds.), *Bradley's neurology in clinical practice*, ed 7 (pp. 1217–1218). Philadelphia: Elsevier.

VASCULITIS

DEFINITION

Vasculitis refers to a clinicopathologic process characterized by inflammation of the blood vessels. Vasculitides can be primary (idiopathic) or secondary, which is related to the known cause (Table 119). Angiographic beading is common (Figure 65).

ISOLATED ANGIITIS OF THE CNS

I. Clinical presentation: This rare disease has nonspecific symptoms, including recurrent headaches, confusion, or focal signs such as hemiparesis or aphasia. Systemic symptoms are generally absent.

II. Diagnosis: Cerebrospinal fluid (CSF) shows mild lymphocytic pleocytosis and elevated protein. Erythrocyte sedimentation rate (ESR) is mildly elevated. Angiography has low sensitivity and specificity. Biopsy of the nondominant frontal or temporal pole with leptomeninges is recommended before treatment.

III. Treatment consists of high dose prednisone plus cyclophosphamide.

TEMPORAL ARTERITIS (GIANT CELL ARTERITIS)

I. Clinical presentation: Patients are older than 55 years. It mainly affects the extracranial arteries and tends to spare the intracranial vessels. The superficial temporal and the ophthalmic arteries are commonly involved. The most common symptoms are headaches and constitutional complaints. Jaw claudication is seen in 40% of the patients and is due to ischemia of the muscles. Amaurosis fugax is seen in 10% of patients and is likely to progress to blindness if left untreated. More than half of the patients with temporal arteritis have polymyalgia rheumatica.

II. Physical examination often shows erythematous, tender, tortuous, thickened, and pulseless temporal arteries.

III. Diagnosis: ESR is high in almost all cases. Angiography can demonstrate luminal irregularities and alternating stenosis and dilatation. Temporal artery biopsy should be obtained to confirm the diagnosis histologically.

IV. Treatment should be initiated immediately on the basis of the clinical suspicion with high-dose prednisone and a subsequent slow taper within 2 to 4 weeks of initiating therapy. The ESR can be used to monitor the disease activity. Methotrexate is sometimes considered as an adjunct to glucocorticoid therapy.

TAKAYASU ARTERITIS (THE PULSELESS DISEASE)

I. Clinical presentation: It affects young women (usually before age 30) of Asian and South American descent. It involves the tunica media of the aortic arch and its proximal branches. The carotids are more affected than the vertebral arteries. The intracranial arteries are typically spared.

TABLE 119

COMMON KEY MANIFESTATIONS AND EVALUATION OF VASCULITIS

Vasculitis Type	Key Clinical Feature	Diagnostic Tests
GIANT CELL ARTERITIS		
Temporal arteritis	Blindness, jaw claudication, high ESR	ESR, temporal artery biopsy
Takayasu arteritis	Pulseless disease, pulse deficit	ESR, angiography
SYSTEMIC NECROTIZING ARTERITIS		
Polyarteritis nodosa	Painful mononeuritis multiplex + kidney involvement	Inflammatory markers, angiography, and tissue biopsy
Churg-Strauss syndrome	Granuloma, eosinophilia, mononeuritis multiplex + severe asthma	Inflammatory markers and tissue biopsy
Wegener granulomatosis	Peripheral and cranial neuropathy + upper and lower respiratory tract and kidney involvement	c-ANCA-specific and sensitive, biopsy
CONNECTIVE TISSUE DISEASE VASCULITIS		
Systemic lupus erythematosus	Neuropsychiatric lupus, seizure, stroke, optic neuritis, myelitis, systemic involvement	ds- and ss-DNA, ANA titers, angiography, biopsy
Sjögren syndrome	Headaches, aseptic meningitis, myelopathy, mononeuritis + dry mouth and eyes	Schirmer test, salivary gland biopsy, inflammatory markers
Rheumatoid arthritis	Atlantoaxial subluxation with myelopathy + deforming arthritis	RF, plain x-rays, other inflammatory markers
Cogan disease	Encephalomyelitis, polyneuropathy, vestibular and auditory + interstitial keratitis	Inflammatory markers, typical clinical features, biopsy
Behçet disease	Meningitic syndrome, and multiple sclerosis-like picture + recurrent oral and genital ulcers + uveitis	Typical clinical features and inflammatory markers
HYPERSENSITIVITY VASCULITIS		
Hypocomplementemia	Encephalomyelitis + peripheral nerve involvement + systemic response	Hepatitis C, complements panel
Cryoglobulinemia	Encephalomyelitis + peripheral nerve involvement + systemic response	Hepatitis C, cryoglobulin levels

Continued

V

VASCULITIS

TABLE 119

COMMON KEY MANIFESTATIONS AND EVALUATION OF VASCULITIS—CONT'D

Vasculitis Type	Key Clinical Feature	Diagnostic Tests
INFECTIOUS VASCULITIS		
Herpes zoster	Eye and ear involvement + contralateral weakness (stroke)	Typical clinical features with viral titers, PCR
Lyme disease	Encephalomyelitis, polyradiculitis, peripheral nerve involvement + erythema migrans	Lyme titers, exposure to tick bite, CSF analysis
HIV infection	AIDS features, dementia, encephalitis, peripheral nerve involvement	Viral titers, typical clinical features, imaging findings
Drug-induced vasculitis Sympathomimetics (amphetamine, cocaine, phenylpropanolamine, pseudoephedrine)	History of exposure to drugs and cold medicine	Positive toxicology titers, negative inflammatory markers, angiogram

AIDS, acquired immune deficiency syndrome; *ANA*, anti-nuclear antibodies; *ds-DNA*, double-stranded DNA; *ESR*, Erythrocyte sedimentation rate; *HIV*, human immunodeficiency virus; *PCR*, polymerase chain reaction; *RF*, rheumatoid factor; *ss-DNA*, single-stranded DNA.

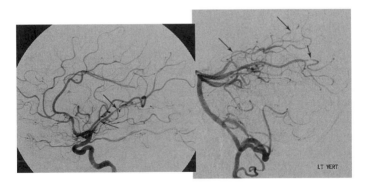

FIGURE 65

Angiographic beading.

Constitutional symptoms such as malaise, fever, weight loss, night sweats, myalgia, and arthralgia may be the presenting symptoms. Visual changes, vertigo, syncope, recurrent headache, focal neurologic deficits such as hemiparesis or aphasia, and seizures are common neurologic symptoms.

II. Physical examination reveals pulse deficits and multiple vascular bruits in most cases.

III. Diagnosis: High ESR and angiography are essential for the diagnosis.
IV. Treatment: High-dose oral steroids. If response to the steroids is poor, then methotrexate, azathioprine, or other immunosuppressive therapies can be considered. The ESR is not as reliable a parameter to follow as it is with temporal arteritis. Aggressive surgical treatment, angioplasty, or bypass grafts may improve prognosis significantly in certain cases.

POLYARTERITIS NODOSA
I. Clinical presentation: It usually develops in the fifth or sixth decade of life and affects men almost twice as often as women. This chronic disease causes patchy necrosis in the walls of medium-sized and small arteries. Kidney, heart, and liver are the most frequently affected organs. Central nervous system (CNS) involvement presents with headache, changes in mental status, seizures, visual change, or hemiparesis. The peripheral nervous system is affected in 50% to 60% of the patients. Painful mononeuritis multiplex is common, but polyneuropathies, plexopathies, and radiculopathies can also occur.
II. Diagnosis: The diagnosis is based on angiography or tissue biopsy. Many of the patients are seropositive for hepatitis B or C.
III. Treatment: Steroids combined with cyclophosphamide are the treatment of choice.

WEGENER GRANULOMATOSIS
I. Clinical presentation: Granulomatous, necrotizing vasculitis involves the small arteries and veins in the upper and lower respiratory tract, kidney (glomerulonephritis), skin or eye (50%), CNS, and peripheral nervous system (PNS). Besides the constitutional symptoms, the most common neurologic manifestations are peripheral and cranial neuropathies. Strokes and seizures are less common. The cytoplasmic antineutrophil cytoplasmic antibodies (c-ANCA) titers are sensitive and specific for active Wegener granulomatosis. ESR is usually markedly elevated.
II. Diagnosis: Biopsy of respiratory tract or renal tissues provides the diagnosis.
III. Treatment consists of prednisone combined with cyclophosphamide. Once remission has been established, it is recommended to stop these agents and instead treat with methotrexate, mycophenolate mofetil, leflunomide, or azathioprine.

CHURG-STRAUSS SYNDROME
I. Clinical presentation: Granulomatous vasculitis of the small and medium-sized arteries. Most commonly affects the lungs. There is a strong association with allergic rhinitis, severe asthma, and peripheral eosinophilia. Mononeuritis multiplex may occur, but it is not common.
II. Treatment consists of steroids, and cyclophosphamide may be added.

V

VASCULITIS

SYSTEMIC LUPUS ERYTHEMATOSUS

I. Clinical presentation: Systemic lupus erythematosus (SLE) is a disease involving multiple organs and mainly affecting women. Besides systemic symptoms, neurologic involvement in SLE is common and includes headaches, cognitive and behavioral changes, psychosis, depression, seizure, cerebral ischemia, myelitis, optic neuritis, cranial and peripheral neuropathies, and movement disorders.

II. Diagnosis: Markers, angiography, and biopsy (noninflammatory vasculopathy) provide the diagnosis.

III. Treatment: For severe CNS manifestations, high-dose IV steroids are given and then slowly tapered to an oral dosage. Cyclophosphamide or azathioprine can be used if steroids fail. Intravenous immunoglobluin (IVIG) and plasmapheresis trial was also reported in the literature.

SJÖGREN SYNDROME

I. Clinical presentation: This chronic inflammatory and autoimmune disorder affects lacrimal and salivary glands and causes dry mouth (xerostomia) and dry eyes (xerophthalmia). Neurologic symptoms include headaches, aseptic meningitis, myelopathy, mononeuritis multiplex, and focal deficits.

II. Treatment is supportive, but steroid and immunosuppressive agents are used in life-threatening conditions.

RHEUMATOID ARTHRITIS

I. Clinical presentation: Systemic arthritis can be seen in up to 25% of adult patients, but the CNS is rarely involved. Myelopathy, brainstem, or cranial nerve deficits and headache can occur due to atlantoaxial subluxation. Peripheral nerve involvement is relatively common, including distal sensory or sensorimotor neuropathy, mononeuropathy multiplex and entrapment, or compression neuropathy.

II. Treatment: High-dose steroid and cyclophosphamide. Other agents such as rituximab have been used.

COGAN DISEASE

I. This is a rare disease of the young. It presents with interstitial keratitis, vestibular and auditory dysfunction, encephalomyelitis, and polyneuropathy.

II. Treatment: Steroids are the treatment of choice. Additional immunosuppressive agents such as methotrexate may be used.

BEHÇET DISEASE

I. Clinical presentation: Recurrent oral and genital ulcers, uveitis, and nondeforming arthritis are seen. It affects mostly young patients and is more common in eastern Mediterranean countries and in Japan.

Neurologic symptoms (10%) are headache, meningitic syndrome, dementia, psychosis, and a multiple sclerosis-like picture.

II. Treatment: Uveitis and CNS involvement require high-dose prednisone in conjunction with azathioprine or cyclosporine.

HERPES ZOSTER OPHTHALMICUS HEMIPLEGIA

I. Clinical presentation: This form presents weeks or months after herpes zoster ophthalmicus in an older adult. Involvement of the ipsilateral anterior and middle cerebral arteries causes contralateral hemiparesis.

II. Treatment: Acyclovir and steroids provide treatment.

REFERENCES

Merkel, P. A. (2015). *Overview of the management of vasculitis in adults.* UpToDate https://www.uptodate.com/contents/overview-of-the-management-of-vasculitis-in-adults. Accessed 3/24/2019.

Moosig, F., Bremer, J. P., Hellmich, B., et al. (2013). A vasculitis centre based management strategy leads to improved outcome in eosinophilic granulomatosis and polyangiitis (Churg-Staruss, EGPA): monocentric experiences in 150 patients. *Ann Rheum Dis*, *72*(6), 1011–1017.

VEIN OF GALEN MALFORMATION

DEFINITION

Vein of Galen malformation (VGM) is a congenital, midline, arteriovenous fistula with aneurysmal dilatation of the vein of Galen. It comprises 30% of pediatric vascular malformations and 1% of all pediatric congenital anomalies. It may be defined as direct arteriovenous fistulas between choroidal or quadrigeminal arteries and an overlying single median venous sac. This sac could be the embryonic median prosencephalic vein of Markowski or the vein of Galen. The frequent concurrent venous abnormalities are (1) retention of fetal anatomic features and (2) frequent occlusions of the dural sinuses of the posterior fossa, especially the sigmoid sinuses. Two angiographic types of VGM have been proposed: a primary or true VGM and a secondary type, resulting from a deep arteriovenous malformation that drains into the vein of Galen.

CLINICAL PRESENTATION

The most common presenting symptoms are congestive cardiac failure, raised intracranial pressure secondary to hydrocephalus, cranial bruit, focal neurologic deficit, seizures, and hemorrhage. The most characteristic vascular supply to the midline fistula involves multiple bilateral vessels, although bilateral posterior cerebral and unilateral posterior cerebral supply are relatively common.

DIAGNOSIS

Ultrasound, magnetic resonance imaging (MRI) and magnetic resonance angiography (MRA) and angiogram provide the diagnosis.

TREATMENT

Supportive therapy consists of digoxin, diuretics, and ventilatory support. Surgical treatment involves ligation, and endovascular therapy uses coil and glue embolization. Staged therapy with medical therapy, initially followed by endovascular therapy and finally surgical therapy, may improve survival. Early overall mortality rate varies among reports in the literature and ranges between 40% and 80%. With the advance of endovascular techniques, there has been a decrease in mortality. In a contemporary largest series of 233 VGM patients treated with embolization, the reported mortality rate was 10.6% overall. Surgical and endovascular intervention does not improve mortality rate when performed early but may be better when performed after 1 month of age, or even after the first year.

REFERENCES

Brinjikji, W., Krings, T., Murad, M., et al. (2012). Endovascular treatment of vein of Galen malformations: a systematic review and meta-analysis. *AJNR Am J Neuroradiol*, *38*(12), 2308–2314.

Yan, J., Wen, J., Gopaul, R., et al. (2015). Outcome and complications of endovascular embolization for vein of Galen malformations: a systematic review and meta-analysis. *J Neurosurg*, *123*(4), 872–890.

VENOUS THROMBOSIS

CLINICAL PRESENTATION

Cerebral venous thrombosis (CVT) presents most commonly with headache, encephalopathy or coma, seizures, and focal signs. It can occur in any age group; however, 80% of those affected are <50 years of age, have a 3:1 female to male incidence, and account for 2% of all pregnancy-associated strokes. Of patients presenting with CVT in pregnancy and puerperium, 70% were primigravid, 36% were pregnant at the time of the CVT, and 64% were puerperal. Factors predisposing for CVT include dehydration, contraceptive use, hormone replacement therapy, pregnancy, puerperium, and thrombophilia (either primary or secondary to malignancy). Clots are identified in the superior sagittal sinus 70% of the time, 60% in the transverse/sigmoid sinuses, and about 60% involve multiple areas in the venous system.

EVALUATION

Contrast-enhanced CT scan may show a "negative delta" sign, with opacification of the sinus wall with noninjection of the clot inside the sinus in about 30% of cases. Sensitivity with a contrasted CT venogram is reported at 95%. MRI or MR venography may be diagnostic with asymmetry. Venous phase angiography usually shows a filling defect. Other suggestive signs include parasagittal stroke or hemorrhage; these may both be present due to thrombus propagation into surrounding cortical veins. Thrombosis may also involve the cavernous sinus (usually as a result of facial or orbital infection; characterized by facial pain, proptosis, and involvement of CN III, IV, V, and VI) or the superior petrosal sinus (as a result of otitis media; facial pain is prominent), inferior petrosal sinus (Gradenigo syndrome with retro-orbital pain and CN VI palsy), lateral petrosal sinus (increased intracranial pressure and ear pain), or internal jugular vein (as a result of catheters or pacemakers, with involvement of CN IX, X, and XI). Results of lumbar puncture, if not contraindicated by mass effect, are nonspecific and may reveal increased pressure and increased levels of protein, polymorphonuclear leukocytes (if infection is present), and red blood cells (if hemorrhage has occurred).

Causes and risk factors of venous thrombosis include the following:

I. Trauma: injury, neck surgery, indwelling IV lines
II. Infection: middle ear, sinuses, meningitis
III. Endocrine: pregnancy, oral contraceptives
IV. Volume depletion: hyperosmolar coma, inflammatory bowel disease, diarrhea, postpartum, postoperative
V. Hematologic: polycythemia vera, disseminated intravascular coagulation, sickle cell disease, cryofibrinogenemia, paroxysmal nocturnal hemoglobinuria, thrombocytosis, antithrombin III deficiency, transfusion reaction
VI. Impaired cerebral circulation: arterial occlusion, congenital heart disease, congestive heart failure, anesthesia in seated position, sagittal sinus webs
VII. Neoplasm: leukemia or lymphoma, meningeal spread, meningioma
VIII. Other: Wegener granulomatosis, polyarteritis nodosa, Behçet syndrome, Cogan syndrome, homocystinuria, idiopathic

MANAGEMENT

Central venous thrombosis is a neurological emergency and requires immediate treatment with therapeutic anticoagulation. During the first 48 hours of treatment, frequent neurological monitoring with neurological checks every 1 to 2 hours may be required, depending on the overall clot burden (major sinus involvement, numerous cortical veins) and the patient's neurological status. Therapeutic anticoagulation may be achieved with unfractionated heparin in non-pregnant patients. Enoxaparin is preferred in pregnant patients, as it does not cross the placenta or into breast milk. A 2017 meta-analysis by Ilyas et al. pooled data from 235 patients and demonstrated that endovascular mechanical thrombectomy was considered more commonly in patients that presented with encephalopathy or coma, and ultimately 76% had either complete neurological recovery or only minor neurological deficits. Ongoing clinical studies, such as the Thrombolysis of Anticoagulation for Cerebral Venous Thrombosis study, will elucidate the merits of treating severe CVT with endovascular thrombolysis. If endovascular treatment is available, it should be considered in the setting of coma, deteriorating examination despite therapeutic anticoagulation and hydration, and in cases with high clot burden. Seizures should be aggressively treated and metabolic derangements corrected while nutrition is maintained. Elevate the head of the bed to 30 degrees if not contraindicated by spinal injury. Infections should be treated with appropriate antimicrobial therapy for the suspected organism(s). Intracranial hypertension should be controlled (see also Intracranial Pressure). Standard therapy involves unfractionated heparin (although low-molecular-weight heparin may be effective, limited data is available) followed by warfarin for 3 to 6 months (or longer for underlying hypercoagulable states.) Medications associated with CVT such as oral contraceptives should be discontinued.

REFERENCES

Ilyas, A., et al. (2017). Endovascular mechanical thrombectomy for cerebral venous sinus thrombosis: a systematic review. *J Neurointerv Surg*, *9*(11), 1–8.

Qureshi, A., & Perera, A. (2017). Low molecular weight heparin versus unfractionated heparin in the management of cerebral venous thrombosis: a systematic review and meta-analysis. *Ann Med Surg (Lond)*, *17*, 22–26.

VERTEBROPLASTY/KYPHOPLASTY

Vertebral body compression fractures (VCF) are a major source of morbidity, especially in the elderly. Conservative treatment, including bed rest, bracing, and medical management, often leads to complications related to escalating narcotic and NSAID use, decreased mobility, and pulmonary compromise from bracing and progressive kyphosis. Intractable pain despite best medical management is not uncommon. Vertebroplasty and kyphoplasty offer a minimally invasive option for pain relief in this population. Both procedures involve the percutaneous injection of polymethylmethacrylate (PMMA) into the affected vertebral body under fluoroscopic guidance. The PMMA solidifies within minutes, forming an internal cast to the fracture. In kyphoplasty, a balloon is first inserted and inflated to restore the vertebral body height and sagittal alignment of the spine; the balloon is removed, and the resultant space is filled with PMMA.

Indications include painful osteoporotic VCF refractory to 3 weeks of analgesic therapy, painful vertebrae due to benign or malignant bone tumors, painful VCF with osteonecrosis, and chronic traumatic VCF with non-union. Contraindications include asymptomatic VCF, active infection, coagulopathy, good response to medical management, allergy to PMMA, and myelopathy due to canal compromise. Treatment of "pancaked" vertebral bodies (i.e., compression fractures with >75% vertebral body height loss) is controversial, although successful treatment has been reported. The initial patient evaluation should include standard spinal imaging to identify the fracture site, as well as CT or MRI to evaluate for extent of fracture, spinal canal, or neural foramen compromise by retropulsed bone or tumor, possible infections, and intactness of the posterior cortex at the involved level.

Significant pain relief occurs in 70% to 90% of patients, with little or no pain relief occurring in 5% or fewer. The effect is often immediate, although it may take 48 to 72 hours. Pain relief has been demonstrated to persist for at least 2 years. Slightly lower rates of pain relief are obtained from osteolytic fractures secondary to tumor.

Cement extravasation through the vertebral body cortex occurs in 20% to 40% of procedures. This is typically clinically insignificant, although rare symptomatic pulmonary embolization has occurred. Other complications include spinal cord or nerve root compression by either retropulsed bone fragments or cement extravasation; they rarely require surgical decompression.

REFERENCES

Burton, A. W., & Hamid, B. (2008). Kyphoplasty and vertebroplasty. *Curr Pain Headache Rep, 12*(1), 22–27.

Lieberman, I., & Reinhardt, M. K. (2003). Vertebroplasty and kyphoplasty for osteolytic vertebral collapse. *Clin Orthop Related Res, 415S*, S176–S186.

VERTIGO

DEFINITION

Vertigo is defined as perception of movement of self or surroundings, or an unpleasant distortion of orientation, with respect to gravity. Disorders causing vertigo are formulated in terms of distortion or mismatch of vestibular, visual, and somatosensory inputs. Careful history can better delineate the patient's perceptions and help differentiate vertigo from other forms of dizziness that result from disturbances of cardiovascular, visual, or motor function.

EXAMINATION

Evaluation of vertigo includes blood pressure measurement (lying and standing), hearing screen and otoscopy, general neurologic examination with special attention to past pointing, ophthalmoscopy, ocular motor examination, and characterization of nystagmus. Also noted are responses to specific maneuvers (if deemed safe), including tragal compression, rapid head turns, Valsalva maneuver, rotation in chair, hyperventilation, and postural testing (Dix-Hallpike). The latter is performed by abruptly moving the patient from a sitting to a lying position, with the head hanging 45 degrees over the end of the examining table and rotated 45 degrees to one side. This movement is repeated with the head rotated to the opposite side. The development of vertigo and the time of onset, duration, and direction of the fast phase of nystagmus are noted.

ETIOLOGY

I. Physiologic vertigo results from sensory distortion (e.g., change in refraction) or intersensory mismatch (such as motion sickness or height vertigo).

II. Pathologic vertigo is based on localization within vestibular pathways.
  A. Labyrinths: otitis media, endolymphatic hydrops, otosclerosis, cupulolithiasis, viral infection, perilymph fistula, trauma, drug toxicity (e.g., from antibiotics)
  B. Vestibular nerve and ganglia: carcinomatous meningitis, herpes zoster
  C. Cerebellopontine angle: acoustic neuroma, glomus, or other tumor; demyelination, vascular compression
  D. Brainstem and cerebellum: infarct, hemorrhage, tumor, viral infection, migraine, Arnold-Chiari malformation
  E. Hemispheric connections: temporal or parietal dysfunction (e.g., seizure)
  F. Systemic and metabolic: anemia, intoxication (such as ethanol, anticonvulsants, diuretics, and other medications), vasculitis (e.g., Cogan syndrome of deafness, interstitial keratitis, and systemic vasculitis), metabolic derangement (e.g., thyroid disease)

III. Other causes of vertigo: Psychogenic vertigo has features of rotational or linear movement rather than isolated lightheadedness. It often begins gradually, is associated with anxiety, and terminates abruptly. Forced hyperventilation may provoke vertigo. When a patient complains of severe rotational vertigo without nausea or nystagmus, a psychogenic cause is suggested.

SPECIFIC FORMS

I. Acute peripheral vestibulopathy (other terms include viral labyrinthitis, vestibular neuronitis, and peripheral vestibulopathy) is associated with spontaneous vertigo, nystagmus (fast phase away from the lesion), and nausea or vomiting, or both, lasting hours to days. The environment seems to move in the direction of the fast phase (away from the lesion). There is a subjective sense of self-motion in the direction of the fast phase. The patient may fall to the side of the lesion during Romberg testing. Past pointing is to the side of the lesion. Symptoms and signs may be brought on by hurried movement ("positioning") but not necessarily by maintaining a particular position ("positional").

Hearing is usually normal. A variable residual deficit of one peripheral vestibular system (labyrinth, nerve, or both) may persist. With a unilateral fixed deficit, central compensatory mechanisms intervene and vertigo and nystagmus decrease and may resolve. Acute peripheral vestibulopathy may recur (see below). Bacterial suppurative ear infection should be excluded.

II. Perilymph fistula is usually due to spontaneous rupture of the inner ear membranes with resultant vertigo that may be aggravated by changes in position. It is associated with a fluctuating hearing loss. The fistula may occur during strenuous activity or Valsalva maneuver. The patient may hear a "pop" in the ear at the moment of rupture. The attacks are discrete and short-lived. Therapy is bed rest. If this fails, surgery may be required.

III. Central vestibular vertigo results from lesions of the vestibular nuclei or vestibulocerebellar pathways; these patients have vertigo and nystagmus, often accompanied by diplopia, dysarthria, weakness, sensory loss, involvement of cranial nerves V and VII, and pathologic reflexes. Acoustic neuromas are usually associated with hearing loss, tinnitus, and occasionally involvement of other cranial nerves, including CN VII and V.

IV. Drug-induced vertigo is due to effects on the peripheral end-organ or nerve and may be due to aminoglycosides, furosemide, ethacrynic acid, anticonvulsants (phenytoin, phenobarbital, carbamazepine, and primidone), some anti-inflammatory agents, salicylates, and quinine. Drugs may produce only disequilibrium when the damage is bilateral but can produce vertigo when the damage is asymmetric. Some agents also produce hearing loss.

V. Meniere disease that results from endolymph hydrops is characterized by severe episodic vertigo, vomiting, fluctuating or progressive hearing loss, distortions of sound, tinnitus, and pressure or fullness in the ears. Recovery usually occurs within hours to days. The interval between attacks often ranges from weeks to months. Low-salt diet and diuretics are considered most helpful. Surgical therapy (endolymphatic drainage or vestibular nerve section) may give lasting relief but should be considered only as a last resort. Newer treatments include intratympanic injections of corticosteroids or gentamicin; the latter may be a less invasive alternative to surgery.

VI. Benign paroxysmal positional vertigo is a symptom that usually indicates benign peripheral (end-organ) disease. Vertigo and nystagmus, often with systemic symptoms such as nausea and vomiting, occur when certain positions of the head are assumed, such as lying down on the back or side. Symptoms are usually transient (<60 seconds). Latency is usually several seconds but may be as long as 30 to 45 seconds. Signs and symptoms include fatigue after onset and do not recur until there is a change in position. Nystagmus is most commonly torsional toward (upper pole) the undermost ear during positional testing. With repetitive maneuvers, signs and symptoms lessen (habituate). Therapy consists of repetitive positioning exercises to stimulate central compensation or a liberatory maneuver (Brandt-Daroff maneuvers). Elderly patients compensate more slowly. Vestibular suppressant medications generally do not help in completely alleviating symptoms.

LABORATORY STUDIES

Brain imaging (computed tomography [CT], magnetic resonance imaging [MRI]) directs attention to posterior fossa and temporal bone; MR angiography gives attention to vertebrobasilar circulation; caloric and rotational testing quantify vestibular function. Audiogram and auditory-evoked potentials detect associated cochlear or brainstem dysfunction.

MANAGEMENT

Generally, management during acute vertigo (Table 120) includes bed rest, avoiding sudden head movements, clear fluids or light diet if tolerated, and reassurance. Vestibular suppressant medications such as antihistamines and benzodiazepines (Table 121) and antiemetics may be useful in acute peripheral vestibulopathy, in acute brainstem lesions near the vestibular nuclei, and for prevention of motion sickness. These agents are of no benefit in chronic vestibulopathies. After the acute phase (approximately 1 to 3 days), a graded program of exercises hastens the adaptive recalibration of the vestibular system to provide better oculomotor and postural control and reduce vertigo.

TABLE 120

APPROACH TO PATIENT WITH VERTIGO

Do not do head maneuvers in young patient with recent trauma or possible dissection.

Do MRI and MRA in elderly patient with stroke risk factor and new vertigo.

Do the positional test and if positive for benign paroxysmal positional vertigo, go on to a particle repositioning maneuver.

Do the head impulse test in the patient and if negative, think of cerebellar infarction in a patient with a first-time attack of acute isolated spontaneous vertigo.

Order an audiogram and a caloric test and if they are normal, think of migraine rather than Meniere disease in a patient with recurrent vertigo.

Think of bilateral vestibular loss due to gentamicin, normal pressure hydrocephalus, early cerebellar ataxia, early progressive supranuclear palsy, sensory peripheral neuropathy, and orthostatic tremor in the patient who is off balance for no obvious reason.

TABLE 121

MEDICATIONS USEFUL IN TREATING SYMPTOMS OF ACUTE VERTIGO

Drug	Dosage	Route
Dimenhydrinate (Dramamine)	50–100 mg q4–6hr	PO, IM, IV, PR
Diphenhydramine (Benadryl)	25–50 mg tid to qid	PO, IM, IV
Meclizine (Antivert)	12.5–25 mg bid to qid	PO
Promethazine (Phenergan)	25 mg bid to qid	PO, IM, IV, PR
Hydroxyzine (Atarax, Vistaril)	25–100 mg tid to qid	PO, IM

REFERENCES

Edlow, J. A., & Newman-Toker, D. (2016). Using the physical examination to diagnose patients with acute dizziness and vertigo. *J Emerg Med*, *50*(4), 617–628.

Tsang, B. K. T., Chen, A. S., & Paine, M. (2017). Acute evaluation of the acute vestibular syndrome: differentiating posterior circulation stroke from acute peripheral vestibulopathies. *Intern Med J*, *47*(12), 1352–1360.

VESTIBULO-OCULAR REFLEX

The vestibulo-ocular reflex (VOR) generates eye movements that compensate for head/body movements. Head movements are sensed by the semicircular canals and otolithic organs (utricle and saccule). The reflex is mediated by fibers in the medial longitudinal fasciculus connecting the SUPERIOR vestibular nucleus and MEDIAL vestibular nucleus to the OCULOMOTOR, TROCHLEAR, and ABDUCENS nuclei, thereby linking head movements to eye movements. This allows an image to remain stable on the retina, which is key to improved visual acuity. Thus, vestibular disorders (peripheral or central) can result in eye movement abnormalities or more subtle disorders of postural control and spatial orientation. The VOR is also clinically useful when assessing eye movements in comatose patients.

After integrity of the neck is assured, rapid passive head rotation in comatose patients with a normal VOR results in compensatory contraversive eye movements. This is called the *oculocephalic reflex* or "doll's eyes" and indicates intact brainstem function. The term "doll's eyes" is confusing, since dolls with weighted or unweighted eyes were produced and this term should be avoided to avoid ambiguous clinical communication. It is clearer to say the oculocephalic reflex is present or absent. The VOR is typically suppressed in awake patients when fixating on an object. Non-suppression of the VOR (or elicitation of nystagmus) during fixation indicates cerebellar dysfunction.

Table 122 compares peripheral and central dysfunction.

REFERENCES

Blumenfeld, H. (2010). The neurological exam as a lesson in neuroanatomy. In *Neuroanatomy through clinical cases* (p. 76). Sunderland: Sinauer Associates.

Blumenfeld, H. (2010). Brainstem structures and vascular supply. In *Neuroanatomy through clinical cases* (p. 654). Sunderland: Sinauer Associates.

COMPARISON OF PERIPHERAL VERSUS CENTRAL DYSFUNCTION

Localization	Nystagmus onset/ habituation	Nystagmus direction	Associated findings
Peripheral	Delayed onset, habituates	Horizontal or rotatory, NEVER VERTICAL, does not change direction	Vertigo, hearing loss or tinnitus, no focal neurological findings, attenuates with fixation
Central	Immediate or delayed, does not habituate	Horizontal, vertical, or rotatory, can change direction	May not have vertigo, often headache, nausea, likely to have focal findings, no attenuation with fixation

VISUAL FIELDS

Vision has two main components: *central* or *macular* vision (high acuity, color perception, light-adapted) and *peripheral* or *ambulatory* vision (low acuity, poor color perception, dark-adapted). Fovea is the most sensitive part of the macula. There are several techniques for visual field examination, ranging from simple confrontation testing to sophisticated threshold static perimetry. Confrontation remains the mainstay of clinical testing.

The characteristic features of visual field deficits have high localizing value (Fig. 66). General rules of visual field interpretation:

1. Retinal nerve fiber bundle and optic nerve lesions produce an ipsilateral visual field defect.
2. Only chiasmal lesions produce bitemporal hemianopsias.
3. Optic disk lesions and retinal vascular occlusions often produce defects that respect the nasal horizontal meridian.
4. Optic nerve lesions produce monocular field defects that do not respect the vertical midline. Arcuate defects occur with segmental lesions of the optic nerve.
5. Visual acuity is not affected by unilateral lesion posterior to the chiasm.
6. Retrochiasmal lesions cause contralateral homonymous hemianopsia or quadrantanopsia, which increase in congruence as the lesions approach the occipital lobe. The visual field defects respect the vertical midline.
7. Anterior retrochiasmal lesions produce incongruent homonymous visual field defects.
8. Posterior retrochiasmal lesions produce congruent homonymous visual field defects.
9. Temporal lobe lesions give slightly incongruent homonymous hemianopsias involving the upper quadrant.

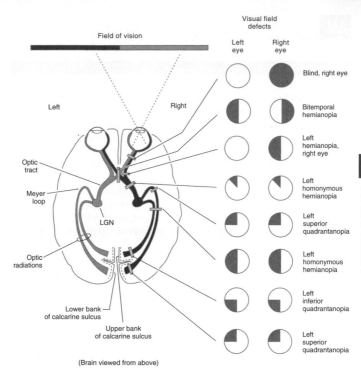

Visual field defects

Field of vision

Left eye | Right eye

Blind, right eye

Left | Right

Bitemporal hemianopia

Left hemianopia, right eye

Optic tract

Meyer loop

LGN

Left homonymous hemianopia

Left superior quadrantanopia

Optic radiations

Left homonymous hemianopia

Left inferior quadrantanopia

Lower bank of calcarine sulcus

Upper bank of calcarine sulcus

Left superior quadrantanopia

(Brain viewed from above)

V

VISUAL FIELDS

FIGURE 66

Visual field defects due to various lesions of the optic pathways. (From Chen, J., & Corbett, J. (2018). The visual system. In D. E. Haines & G. Mihailoff (Eds). *Fundamental neuroscience for basic and clinical applications*, ed 5. Philadelphia: Elsevier. Fig. 20.16).

10. A complete homonymous hemianopsia means that the lesion is retrochiasmal and contralateral to the visual field defect.
11. Homonymous hemianopsia and alexia without agraphia are caused by dominant occipital lobe lesion extending to the splenium of the corpus callosum.

REFERENCES

Daroff, R. B., Jankovic, J., Mazziotta, J. C., & Pomeroy, S. L. (Eds.). (2015). *Bradley's neurology in clinical practice,* ed 7. Philadelphia: Elsevier Health Sciences.

WADA TESTING

This test is named after John A. Wada, the neurologist who first described it. The Wada test is a physiologic and neuropsychological test whereby one part of the brain is chemically suppressed by superselectively injecting a short-acting anesthetic substance (such as sodium amobarbital, sodium methohexital, or propofol) into a specific feeding artery. Complete neuropsychological evaluation is performed prior to and after injecting the anesthetic.

The test is usually used prior to performing epilepsy surgery for language and memory lateralization testing and to guide the surgeon regarding the potential loss of language or memory after resection. In this scenario, the drug is injected selectively into the internal carotid artery. Superselective cerebral or spinal artery branch Wada testing, with or without electroencephalogram (EEG) and evoked potential testing, can also be performed during arteriovenous malformation embolization.

Functional magnetic resonance imaging (MRI) is increasingly considered a less invasive and cost-effective option for language lateralization, especially in left-lateralization, proceeding with Wada testing for atypical language dominance.

REFERENCE

Bauer, P. R., Reitsma, J. B., Houweling, B. M., Ferrier, C. H., & Ramsey, N. F. (2014). Can fMRI safely replace the Wada test for preoperative assessment of language lateralisation? A meta-analysis and systematic review. *J Neurol Neurosurg Psychiatry*, *85*(5), 581–588.

WHITE MATTER TRACT LESION IN MULTIPLE SCLEROSIS—RADIOGRAPHIC FEATURES

Magnetic resonance imaging (MRI) is the most sensitive imaging modality used for both diagnosis and surveillance in multiple sclerosis. Lesions seen on MRI represent underlying demyelination. Lesions within the brain typically involve the white matter tracts but can also involve portions of the gray matter.

Characteristic lesion locations:
- Cerebral hemispheres: periventricular, subcortical, and perpendicular to lateral ventricle
- Lesion perpendicular in a triangular shape is also referred to as Dawson fingers
- Spinal cord: The cervical cord is the most common location, but lesions can be found in other portions as well.

Lesion shape:
- Lesions are typically ovoid in shape.
- Tumefactive lesions are lesions that are greater than 2 cm in diameter and can cause mass effect.

Patterns of enhancement seen on MRI:
- FLAIR—lesions are typically hyperintense
- T1 weighted images—lesions appear hypointense
- T2 weighted images—lesions appear hyperintense
- T1 weighted + gadolinium contrast—lesions that enhance represent areas of active demyelination
  - These lesions can be ring enhancing (closed or open ring)

REFERENCES

Balashov, K. (2016). Imaging of central nervous system demyelinating disorders. *Continuum*, *22*, 1613–1633. https://doi.org/10.1212/CON.0000000000000373.

Inglese, M., Grossman, R. I., & Filippi, M. (2005). Magnetic resonance imaging monitoring of multiple sclerosis lesion evolution. *J Neuroimaging*, *15*, 22S–29S. https://doi.org/10.1177/1051228405282243.

W

WILSON DISEASE

WILSON DISEASE

DEFINITION AND PATHOPHYSIOLOGY

Wilson disease, also known as hepatolenticular degeneration, is an autosomal recessive disorder of copper metabolism and homeostasis. There is a defect of hepatic copper transport due to a loss of function mutation in the ATP7B gene on chromosome 13, leading to accumulation of copper in the liver and the central nervous system.

NEUROLOGIC PRESENTATION

Age at onset is usually between 8 and 20 years. The most common presentation, occurring in adolescence, is of movement disorders such as dystonic rigidity, chorea, and progressive tremors. Other common neurologic manifestations include dysarthria, dysgraphia, drooling, and ataxia. In a subset of patients, psychiatric symptoms may be more prominent. Behavioral or personality changes, impulsivity, irritability, or frank psychosis make the disease confounding and can delay diagnosis. These neurologic symptoms can be debilitating.

Hepatic dysfunction is identifiable in nearly all patients, and cirrhosis may be apparent early in the course before neurologic symptoms occur. Other clinical features include hemolytic anemia, joint symptoms, renal stones, cardiomyopathy, splenomegaly, pancreatic disease, and hypoparathyroidism. Kayser-Fleischer (KF) rings are present in more than 90% of patients and are virtually pathognomonic. KF rings are asymptomatic golden-brownish discoloration at the corneal limbus caused by copper deposition in Descemet membrane; this may be visible only under slit lamp examination. "Sunflower" cataracts occur due to copper deposits in the lens.

DIAGNOSIS

The diagnosis is made by observation of the KF rings, low serum level of ceruloplasmin (<20 mg/dL), elevated 24-hour urinary copper excretion, total serum copper (bound and free unbound copper), and increased level of copper in liver biopsy specimen. Serum copper measurement is often normal. Although the diagnosis may be relatively easy, Wilson disease must be suspected in children and younger adults who come to medical attention with unknown hepatic or central nervous system (CNS) syndromes, often with a psychiatric component such as psychosis. Magnetic resonance imaging (MRI) may show T2 signals in the striatum. However, there is heterogeneity in the striatal changes in terms of the location and density. These areas can show as T2 hypo- or hyperintense signals. It is important to diagnose early. A delay in diagnosis results in less favorable outcome, even after treatment. Assay of liver copper is used to confirm the diagnosis and may still be required in patients with predominantly hepatic presentation. The "panda sign" can be seen in the substantia nigra, with hyperintensity in the midbrain around the red nucleus and substantia nigra.

TREATMENT

The goal of treatment is to reverse copper overload and establish negative copper balance without resulting in copper deficiency. A common treatment is chelation with D-penicillamine. Initial dosage is 250 mg daily for children less than 100 pounds with a maximum based on their weight. For adults, dosage is 250 mg four times a day for a maximum of 1.5 g/day in divided doses. A low-copper diet to minimize acute worsening caused by mobilization of copper store is helpful. Pyridoxine, 25 mg/day, is given to counter the antimetabolite effect of penicillamine. Acute or delayed hypersensitivity reaction to penicillamine develops in up to 20% of patients receiving treatment but may be overcome in some cases with a reduced dose and concomitant administration of corticosteroids.

Trientine (a chelator) and zinc salts, which block gastrointestinal (GI) copper uptake, have been proposed as a treatment alternative to D-penicillamine. Ammonium tetrathiomolybdate has also been tried as an alternative to D-penicillamine, with variable results. Levodopa may be of some benefit in reversing neurologic symptoms not improved by chelation.

Patients with advanced disease may require orthotropic liver transplantation. Liver transplantation corrects hepatic metabolism of copper and normalizes extrahepatic copper, including in the CNS. New drugs may be developed as studies of the underlying defects in ATP7B and its suspected modifiers ATOX1 and COMMD1 continue to explore the disease's genotype-phenotype correlation. Cell-based therapy is potentially useful in that it can restore hepatic copper excretion. Human hepatocyte transplantation, allowing the hepatocyte to integrate and reconstitute in the hepatobiliary excretory system, may enhance copper excretion. In particular, use of mesenchymal stem cells that can differentiate into hepatocytes are non-immunogenic and would not require immunosuppression is being investigated (ClinicalTrials.gov). Gene therapy is a provocative approach, but further studies are needed.

REFERENCES

Clayton, P. T. (2017). Inherited disorders of transition metal metabolism: an update. *J Inherit Metab Dis*, *40*(4), 519–529. https://doi.org/10.1007/s.

Hedera, P. (2017). Update on the clinical management of Wilson's disease. *Appl Clin Genet*, *10*, 9–19.

Z

ZOSTER

ZOSTER (HERPES ZOSTER, VARICELLA-ZOSTER)

Varicella-zoster virus (VZV) is the infective organism in varicella (chickenpox) and herpes zoster (shingles). Varicella is a typical, benign, neurocutaneous disease of childhood. Complications such as meningoencephalitis, acute cerebellar ataxia, transverse myelitis, and Reye syndrome are rare and may lead to permanent deficits including paresis, seizures, and cognitive changes. In most cases, full recovery is expected.

Herpes zoster (zoster literally, "belt or girdle") is caused by a latent virus reactivation in the setting of awakened cell-mediated immunity, particularly in the elderly and the immunocompromised. Patients with lymphoma who have had radiation and splenectomy, and patients with AIDS (who usually develop disseminated disease), are at risk.

Typically, zoster presents with pain in a single or several adjacent dermatomes. The pain may precede the vesicular eruption by up to 3 weeks. Pain is described as sharp, lancinating, and associated with itching, dysesthesia, and allodynia (increased skin sensitivity). Associated findings include altered sensation in the involved dermatome; fewer than 5% have segmental weakness. The cerebrospinal fluid (CSF) may show an elevated protein and a mild lymphocytic pleocytosis. Diagnosis is often clinical and is established by typical neurocutaneous rash, Tzanck smear, direct immunofluorescence, viral culture, or comparison of acute and convalescent titers. Demonstration of the presence of VZV DNA (by polymerase chain reaction [PCR] analysis), or of antibodies in CSF to the virus, is strong evidence of infection in the appropriate clinical setting. Serum antibody analysis is of no value. Histologically, zoster is characterized by lymphocytic inflammation and vasculitis, resulting in neuronal loss in ganglia. The process may spread to leptomeninges and adjacent spinal cord.

COMPLICATIONS OF THE PERIPHERAL NERVOUS SYSTEM

- **Herpes Zoster Ophthalmicus:** VZV may become latent along the entire neuraxis. The most common sites of reactivation are thoracic and trigeminal dermatomes. When zoster affects the cranium (20% of cases), 90% of sites are in the trigeminal distribution and 60% of these will involve the first division. Complications include corneal involvement, internal or external ophthalmoplegia, iridocyclitis, and uveitis and optic neuritis (rare). The prognosis for improvement of ocular motor disturbance is excellent, whereas return of lost vision is minimal.
- **Ramsay Hunt syndrome:** Varicella zoster of the geniculate ganglion, presenting with painful vesicles on the tympanic membrane and external auditory canal, a peripheral seventh cranial nerve (CN VII) palsy, and variable CN VIII dysfunction.

- **Thoracic zoster:** May occasionally produce arm weakness (zoster paresis), whereas lumbar reactivation may be associated with leg weakness and bowel/bladder dysfunction. Rarely, the pain can occur in the absence of any rash (zoster sine herpete), leading to considerations of carcinomatous, lymphomatous, or diabetic radiculopathies.

Analysis of PCR of varicella DNA in CSF and blood mononuclear cells, and antibody titer in CSF, are usually diagnostic.

Treatment:

Acyclovir (800 mg 5 times a day for 7 days), famciclovir (500 mg tid for 7 days), or valacyclovir can be given. Pain management is essential but frequently difficult, and there may be residual pain despite multiple medications.

Postherpetic Neuralgia

Postherpetic neuralgia is characterized by persistent dysesthesias and hyperpathia, persisting beyond healing of the zoster vesicles (usually beyond 2 months).

The pain has three components:

(1) a constant, deep burning pain;
(2) paroxysms of shooting pain;
(3) sharp pains after light stimulation(allodynia).

Pathologically, it is associated with a localized small and large fiber sensory neuropathy and may result from reorganization of inputs to the second-order neurons.

Postherpetic neuralgia is rare in patients younger than 50, but it occurs in up to 50% of patients over 60 and in 75% of those over 70. It resolves within 1 month in 90% of patients and in half of the remainder by 2 months but may last up to 1 year. Only about 2% of patients have persistent pain, which may last for months or years.

Treatment:

Antiviral treatments tend to reduce incidence of the postherpetic neuralgia.

Tricyclic antidepressants: (amitriptyline/nortriptyline 25 to 75 mg PO qd);

Anticonvulsants: carbamazepine (400 to 1200 mg PO qd), phenytoin (300 to 400 mg PO qd), and gabapentin; prednisone (40 to 60 mg qd 3 to 5 days)

Topical aspirin in chloroform or capsaicin 0.75% ointment, 5 times per day for at least 4 weeks, may be used.

Topical lidocaine (ointment or skin patch) may also help.

Complications of the Central Nervous System

Occasionally, reactivation of VZV in either an immunocompetent or immunocompromised patient can cause the virus to spread into the spinal cord and brain. CNS complications of zoster include myelitis, encephalitis, large-vessel granulomatous arteritis, small-vessel encephalitis, meningitis, ventriculitis, and vasculitis. Myelitis usually occurs 1 to 2 weeks after rash development and may be confirmed by CSF PCR of varicella DNA; the illness is mostly severe in immunocompromised patients. Varicella zoster can cause encephalitis as a result of large- or small-vessel vasculopathy. Large-vessel (granulomatous) vasculitis leading to strokes is an important complication that occurs predominantly in immunocompetent patients and presents with focal deficits (strokes can be ischemic or hemorrhagic). Small-vessel encephalitis is the most common complication of CNS varicella zoster and is seen in immunocompromised patients. Deep-seated ischemic or demyelinating lesions may manifest as headache, fever, vomiting, mental status changes, seizures, and focal deficits. A few cases of ventriculitis and meningitis have occurred in immunocompromised patients. The treatment for CNS complications is with IV acyclovir; steroids are used for anti-inflammatory effects.

Treatment: Oral acyclovir accelerates cutaneous healing but has no effect on acute neuritis or postherpetic neuralgia. In the immunocompromised patient, parenteral acyclovir is more effective than vidarabine in preventing dissemination and accelerating cutaneous healing. Corticosteroids may reduce acute pain and the risk of postherpetic neuralgia, but evidence of effectiveness is inconclusive.

PREVENTION

Live attenuated zoster vaccine: Boosts VZV-specific cellular immunity in older adults. VZV zoster causes substantial morbidity. Treatments may be incompletely effective, especially as symptoms may not be caught within a 72-hour window where treatment would be of maximum benefit. The Shingles Prevention Study, a randomized, double blinded placebo-controlled trial, with 38,546 community dwelling individuals aged 60 and greater, showed that the vaccine reduced incidence of post herpetic neuralgia by 66.5%. Individuals' pain burden and functional impairment is reduced, and they experience better quality of life outcomes. The Centers of Disease Control and Prevention recommends the vaccine for immunocompetent adults 60 years or older irrespective of prior zoster exposure. The vaccine is contraindicated in patients with prior anaphylactic reactions to gelatin or neomycin, leukemia, lymphomas, other malignancies of bone marrow or lymphatic system, individuals on immunosuppressive therapy, and those on high-dose corticosteroids for more than 2 weeks.

REFERENCES

Lu, P., et al. (2016). National and state-specific shingles vaccination among adults aged ≥60 years. *Am J Prev Med*, *52*(3), 362–372. https://doi.org/10.1016/j.amepre.2016.08.031.

Nagel, M. A., et al. (2017). Varicella zoster virus vasculopathy: the expanding clinical spectrum and pathogenesis. *J Neuroimmunol*, *15*(308), 112–117.

AAN Guideline summaries appendix

EVALUATION AND PROGNOSIS OF COMA

CONFOUNDING FACTORS

Coma is a state with multiple etiologies, so it not surprising that some factors may confound the reliability of the clinical examination and ancillary tests. Major confounders could include the use or prior use of sedatives or neuromuscular blocking agents, induced hypothermia therapy, presence of organ failure (e.g., acute renal or liver failure), sensory failure (e.g., blindness, deafness), or shock (e.g., cardiogenic shock requiring pressor support). However, studies in comatose patients have not systematically addressed the role of these confounders in neurologic assessment.

COMMUNICATION WITH FAMILY AND FURTHER DECISION MAKING

The complexity of evaluation and various options of decision making require neurologic professional expertise. More than one scheduled meeting with the family is generally required to facilitate a trusting relationship. The neurologist can explain that the prognosis is largely based on clinical examination with some help from laboratory tests. In a conversation with the family, the neurologist may further articulate that the chance of error is very small. When a poor outcome is anticipated, the need for life support (mechanical ventilation, use of vasopressors or inotropic agents to hemodynamically stabilize the patient) must be discussed. Fully informed and more certain, the family or proxy is allowed to rethink resuscitation orders or even to adjust the level of care to comfort measures only. However, these decisions should be made after best interpretation of advanced directives previously voiced or written by the patient.

RECOMMENDATIONS FOR THE PROGNOSTIC VALUE OF THE CLINICAL EXAMINATION

Level of evidence	Evaluation and prognosis of coma	Study evidence
Level A	The prognosis is invariably poor in comatose patients with absent pupillary or corneal reflexes, or absent or extensor motor responses 3 days after cardiac arrest	Three class I studies, two class II studies, and five class III studies
Level B	Prognosis cannot be based on the circumstances of CPR	One class I study
	Patients with myoclonus status epilepticus within the first day after a primary circulatory arrest have a poor prognosis	Three class I studies, two class II studies, and five class III studies
	The assessment of poor prognosis can be guided by the bilateral absence of cortical somatosensory evoked potentials (SSEPs) (N20 response) within 1–3 days	One class I and seven class III studies

Continued

RECOMMENDATIONS FOR THE PROGNOSTIC VALUE OF THE CLINICAL EXAMINATION—CONT'D

Level of evidence	Evaluation and prognosis of coma	Study evidence
	Serum neuron-specific enolase (NSE) levels 33 g/L at days 1–3 post-CPR accurately predict poor outcome	One class I study, four class III studies, and one class IV study
Level C	Prognosis cannot be based on elevated body temperature alone	One class II study
	Burst suppression or generalized epileptiform discharges on electroencephalogram (EEG) predicted poor outcomes but with insufficient prognostic accuracy	One class II study and four class III studies
Level U	There are inadequate data to support or refute the prognostic value of intracranial pressure (ICP) monitoring	Two class IV studies
	There are inadequate data to support or refute whether neuroimaging is indicative of poor outcome	Ten class IV studies
	There are inadequate data to support or refute the prognostic value of other serum and cerebrospinal fluid (CSF) biochemical markers in comatose patients after CPR	

REFERENCE

Wijdicks, E. F., et al. (2006). Practice parameter: prediction of outcome in comatose survivors after cardiopulmonary resuscitation (an evidence-based review): report of the Quality Standards Subcommittee of the American Academy of Neurology. *Neurology*, 67(2), 203–210.

DIAGNOSTIC ACCURACY OF 14-3-3 PROTEIN IN SPORADIC CREUTZFELDT-JAKOB DISEASE

MODERATE EVIDENCE (LEVEL B)

For patients who have rapidly progressive dementia and are strongly suspected of having sporadic Creutzfeldt-Jakob Disease (sCJD), and for whom diagnosis remains uncertain (pretest probability ~20% to 90%), clinicians should order CSF 14-3-3 assays to reduce the uncertainty of the diagnosis.

While the 14-3-3 assay has a moderately high diagnostic accuracy, it is highly dependent on pretest probability of the disease. History, clinical presentation, and the specialist's experience or knowledge about the incidence of sCJD in a particular population should drive this probability. Further, periodic sharp wave complexes on EEG (Sn 66%, Sp 74%) and DWI/FLAIR hyperintensities in the cortical regions and basal ganglia on MRI (Sn 92%, Sp 95%) will markedly increase pretest probability. Protein assay technique should also be considered, as Western blot studies are subjective and interpreted qualitatively, and newer use of quantitative ELISA studies depend

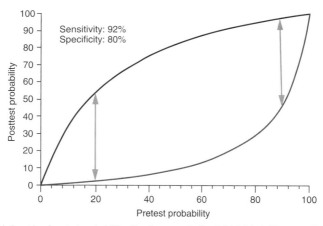

Relationship of pretest probability of having sporadic Creutzfeldt-Jakob Disease and the implications of a CSF 14-3-3 result.

on the individual lab sensitivity and specificity cutoffs. Therefore, consideration for the rarity of sCJD (incidence 1 per million per year), the practice setting (community hospital versus tertiary referral center), the patient's clinical presentation, and the results of already obtained ancillary tests will affect the diagnostic accuracy of 14-3-3 protein of diagnosing sCJD.

REFERENCES

AAN Summary of Evidence-based Guideline for clinicians. (2012). *Diagnostic accuracy of CSF 14-3-3 protein in sporadic Creutzfeldt-Jakob disease.* https://www.aan.com/Guidelines/Home/GetGuidelineContent/566. Accessed 11 June 2017.

DIAGNOSIS AND MANAGEMENT OF DEMENTIA

DEFINITION

Dementia, or neurocognitive disorder, is characterized by a decline from a previous level of function in one or more domains of cognitive criteria that is severe enough to interfere with daily function and independence. According to Diagnostic and Statistical Manual (DSM-5), the criteria for dementia now includes:

- Evidence from history and clinical assessment of significant cognitive impairment in at least one cognitive domain: learning and memory, language, executive function, complex attention, perceptual-motor function, and social cognition
- Deficits representing a decline from a previous level of functioning
- Deficits interfering with independence in everyday activities
- Deficits of insidious onset and progression
- Deficits occurring outside of delirium
- Deficits not explained by another disorder

DIAGNOSTIC APPROACH

Initial assessment of suspected dementia focuses on history provided by an informant (e.g., a family member or someone in whom cognitive disorder is not in suspicion). Adequate history of cognitive and behavioral changes includes drug history, mood disorder, malnutrition, and problems with basic and advanced activities of daily living. Identification of the underlying etiologic subtype is discussed in future chapters related to "dementia syndromes."

Evaluation and diagnosis often require serial examination necessitating follow-up visits and serial assessments of cognitive function. All patients with cognitive complaints should undergo a careful mental status evaluation with cognitive testing that may include:

- Mini-mental state examination (MMSE): A 30-point test that is corrected for education; an interpretation of 30-25 shows questionable significant impairment, 20-25 shows mild impairment, 10-20 shows clear impairment, and <10 is untestable.
- Montreal cognitive assessment: A 30-point test that is a more sensitive screening tool than MMSE for the detection of mild cognitive impairment.
- Mini-Cog: A 3-minute instrument that can increase detection of cognitive impairment in older adults that consists of a clock drawing task and an un-cued recall of three unrelated words.
- Neuropsychologic testing: Extensive evaluation of multiple cognitive domains by a trained neuropsychologist for diagnosis and management.

LABORATORY TESTING

There is no clear data to support or refute ordering "routine" laboratory studies, such as a complete blood count (CBC), complete metabolic panel (CMP), and liver function tests (LFTs). The American Academy of Neurology (AAN) recommends routine screening for B12 deficiency, hypothyroidism, depression, and structural neuroimaging with either a non-contrast head computed tomography (CT) or magnetic resonance imaging (MRI) (serial imaging is generally not informative). The AAN does not recommend genetic or neurosyphilis screening unless there is a high clinical suspicion. Patients with an atypical syndrome (e.g., younger patients (<60 years) or those with rapidly progressive dementia), may benefit from a more extensive evaluation, such as cerebrospinal fluid (CSF)-14-3-3 protein when Creutzfeldt-Jakob disease is suspected or lumbar puncture if viral encephalitis cannot be excluded.

MANAGEMENT

Having excluded reversible forms of dementia, management is principally focused upon symptom and risk management. The following medications have been shown to temporarily improve dementia symptoms (for more details, see the table below):

- Cholinesterase inhibitors: These include donepezil (Aricept), rivastigmine (Exelon), and galantamine (Razadyne) for treatment of mild to moderate dementia (MMSE 10-26). Cost, tolerance, and physician experience for efficacy appear to be similar across the drug choices. Common side effects include nausea, vomiting, diarrhea, confusion, dizziness, drowsiness, headache, insomnia, agitation, and/or hallucinations.

- Memantine (Namenda): Treatment for moderate to advanced dementia (MMSE <17). Add memantine (10 mg twice daily) to a cholinesterase inhibitor or use alone in patients who do not tolerate or benefit from a cholinesterase inhibitor. Common side effect is dizziness.
- Vitamin E: Limited mixed evidenced to support use. Some resources recommend 2000 IU daily for mild to moderate AD.
- Selegiline: Limited evidence to support use.

Drugs with unproven benefits include estrogen replacement, anti-inflammatory drugs, Ginkgo biloba, statins, and dietary supplements (e.g., vitamin B, Omega-3 fatty acids). Non-pharmacological therapies include:

- Cognitive rehabilitation: Maintain memory and higher cognitive function.
- Occupational therapy: Prevents accidents and manages behavior.
- Exercise programs: Improve physical functioning and slow the progression of functional decline.
- Modifying environment: Reduce distractions and improve structure and routine.

CHOLINESTERASE INHIBITORS AND MEMANTINE FOR THE TREATMENT OF COGNITIVE DEFICITS IN PATIENTS WITH ALZHEIMER DISEASE

Drug	Approved indication	Suggested dosage	Side effects	Additional notes/caution
CHOLINESTERASE INHIBITORS				
Donepezil (Aricept)	Mild to moderate AD Severe AD	Once daily, beginning with 5 mg/day, which can be increased to 10 mg/day (maximum dosage) after 4 weeks	AEs are mild and include nausea, vomiting, and diarrhea	Gastrointestinal-related AEs can be reduced if medication taken with food Some patients exhibit an initial increase in agitation, which subsides after first few weeks of therapy
Rivastigmine (Exelon)	Mild to moderate AD	*Oral*: Twice daily, beginning with 1.5 mg Transdermal patch: Once daily, 4.6 or 9.5 mg The target dose is 9.5 mg/24 hr per patch (a 10 cm² patch) and requires a simple one-step dose titration to	AEs include nausea, vomiting, diarrhea, weight loss, headaches, abdominal pain, fatigue, anxiety, and agitation Gastrointestinal-related AEs are less prominent with the patch: the 9.5 mg/24 hr patch provides efficacy similar to	Higher dosages are more efficacious than lower dosages No laboratory monitoring is required

Continued

CHOLINESTERASE INHIBITORS AND MEMANTINE FOR THE TREATMENT OF
COGNITIVE DEFICITS IN PATIENTS WITH ALZHEIMER DISEASE—CONT'D

Drug	Approved indication	Suggested dosage	Side effects	Additional notes/caution
		the therapeutic dose There is a higher-dose patch (20 cm^2) available, delivering 17.4 mg/ 24 hr; however, it is currently an unapproved treatment in the United States. Lack of approval was based on it having similar efficacy to the 10 cm^2 patch, but with a tolerability profile comparable to that of the capsule formulation	that of the highest dose of capsules, with 3 times fewer reports of nausea and vomiting	
Galantamine (Razadyne)	Mild to moderate AD	Twice daily, beginning with 4 mg After 4 weeks, dosage is increased to 8 mg twice daily An increase to 12 mg twice daily can be considered on an individual basis after assessment of clinical benefit and tolerability Also available in an extended-release formulation that can be taken once daily	Most common side effects are nausea, vomiting, and diarrhea	Gastrointestinal-related AEs can be minimized by titrating the dosage gradually and taking the medication with meals

Continued

CHOLINESTERASE INHIBITORS AND MEMANTINE FOR THE TREATMENT OF
COGNITIVE DEFICITS IN PATIENTS WITH ALZHEIMER DISEASE—CONT'D

Drug	Approved indication	Suggested dosage	Side effects	Additional notes/caution
NMDA ANTAGONIST				
Memantine (Namenda)	Moderate to severe AD	Twice daily, beginning with 5 mg, increasing the dose to 10 mg twice daily over 3 weeks	AEs include fatigue, pain, hypertension, headache, constipation, vomiting, back pain, somnolence, dizziness	Moderate to severe AD may respond better with memantine/donepezil combination versus donepezil alone

AD, Alzheimer disease.

- Educational programs and other support systems for caregivers: Delay time to nursing home placement.
- Risk factor control: Identify and treat risk factors for cerebrovascular disease (CVD), coronary artery disease (CAD), and dementia.

REFERENCES

Harris, M. (2017). Cognitive issues: decline, delirium, depression, dementia. *Nurs Clin North Am.*, *52*(3), 363–374.

Kolanowski, A., Boltz, M., Galik, E., Gitlin, L. N., Kales, H. C., Resnick, B., et al. (2017). Determinants of behavioral and psychological symptoms of dementia: a scoping review of the evidence. *Nurs Outlook*, *65*(5), 515–529.

CHILD NEUROLOGY: SUMMARY OF ALL GUIDELINES

AMERICAN ACADEMY OF NEUROLOGY (AAN) CHILD NEUROLOGY PRACTICE GUIDELINES; COMPLETE LIST AT https://www.aan.com/Guidelines/home/ByTopic?topicId=14

1. **CLINICAL NEUROPHYSIOLOGY/BEHAVIORAL NEUROLOGY AND NEUROPSYCHIATRY**: The Utility of EEG Theta/Beta Power Ratio in ADHD Diagnosis
2. **EPILEPSY/NEUROPHARMACOLOGY**: Efficacy and Tolerability of the New Antiepileptic Drugs I: Treatment of New-Onset Epilepsy
3. **EPILEPSY/NEUROPHARMACOLOGY**: Efficacy and Tolerability of the New Antiepileptic Drugs II: Treatment-Resistant Epilepsy
4. **EPILEPSY/NEUROSTIMULATION**: Vagus Nerve Stimulation for the Treatment of Epilepsy
5. **EPILEPSY/SEIZURES**: Diagnostic Assessment of the Child with Status Epilepticus
6. **EPILEPSY/SEIZURES**: Evaluating a First Nonfebrile Seizure in Children

CHILD NEUROLOGY SOCIETY (CNS) PRACTICE PARAMETERS;
COMPLETE LIST AT https://www.childneurologysociety.org/resources/practice-parameters

4. **HEADACHE MEDICINE**: Evaluation of Children and Adolescents with Recurrent Headaches
5. **HEADACHE MEDICINE**: Pharmacological Treatment of Migraine Headache in Children and Adolescents
6. **NEURODEVELOPMENTAL DISABILITIES/NEUROGENETICS**: Evaluation of the Child with Microcephaly
7. **NEURODEVELOPMENTAL DISABILITIES/NEUROGENETICS**: Screening and Diagnosis of Autism
8. **NEURODEVELOPMENTAL DISABILITIES/NEUROPHARMACOLOGY**: Pharmacologic Treatment of Spasticity in Children and Adolescents with Cerebral Palsy
9. **NEUROMUSCULAR DISEASES/NEUROGENETICS**: Corticosteroid Treatment of Duchenne Dystrophy

REFERENCES

American Academy of Neurology (AAN). Practice guidelines. Retrieved from https://www.aan.com/Guidelines/home/ByTopic?topicId=14.

Child Neurology Society (CNS). Practice parameters. Retrieved from https://www.childneurologysociety.org/resources/practice-parameters.

CONCUSSION: EVALUATION AND MANAGEMENT OF CONCUSSION IN SPORT

INTRODUCTION

Concussion is a constellation of transient neurologic symptoms reflecting a diffuse brain dysfunction (neurotransmitters and electrolytes abnormalities, excitotoxicity, axonal stretching, and decreased cerebral blood flow) resulting from biomechanical forces conveyed to the brain.

CLINICAL PRESENTATION AND RISK FACTORS

Symptoms of concussion tend to be maximal minutes to hours after the impact and then slowly resolve over the subsequent 7 to 10 days with complete resolution in about 85% of cases. They are nonspecific and range from cognitive symptoms (decreased attention, amnesia, slow thinking, disorientation, and loss of consciousness), physical symptoms (headache, nausea, vomiting, photophobia, phonophobia, dizziness, slurred speech, blurred vision, and incoordination), affective symptoms (emotional lability, depression, anxiety, and mania), to sleep disturbances. While age, sex, and level of competition do not increase the risk of concussion, certain sports such as American football, Australian rugby, and soccer in females carry a greater risk of concussion. Headgears may have a protective effect in sports like rugby, unlike mouth guards. In collegiate football, receivers may have a lower risk of concussion. Body mass index greater than 27 kg/m^2 and training time less than 3 hours weekly are athlete-related factors that increase the risk of concussion.

IDENTIFYING ATHLETES WITH CONCUSSION

Several tools have been developed with various sensitivity/specificity and level of training/specialization required to administer them. Among those tools, the Post-Concussion Symptom Scale and Graded Symptom Checklist, which may be administered by trained personnel, psychologists, nurses, or physicians, or be self-reported, appear to overall have the best sensitivity and specificity.

IDENTIFYING ATHLETES WITH INCREASED RISK OF SEVERE OR PROLONGED EARLY IMPAIRMENTS, NEUROLOGIC CATASTROPHE, OR CHRONIC NEUROBEHAVIORAL IMPAIRMENT

Poor performance on initial screening diagnostic tools is likely to be associated with more severe or prolonged early post-concussive cognitive impairments, although the evidence is modest. In addition, gait stability dual-tasking testing may help identify athletes with early post-concussion impairments. Ongoing clinical symptoms and prior concussion are the strongest predictors of persistent neurocognitive impairment. In addition, a history of concussion is associated with severe early post-concussion impairment. Evidence is less compelling for the role of early post-traumatic headache, fatigue/fogginess, early amnesia, alteration in mental status or disorientation, younger age, level of play, prior history of headache, dizziness, or playing the quarterback position in football. It seems that neurologic catastrophe cannot be predicted accurately based on clinical factors. Recurrent exposure, prior concussion, pre-existing learning disability, and APOE e4 genotype increase the risk of chronic neurobehavioral impairment.

MANAGEMENT/INTERVENTION TO ENHANCE RECOVERY, REDUCE THE RISK OF RECURRENT CONCUSSION, OR LONG-TERM SEQUELAE

Several lines of interventions have been proposed such as delaying the return to the field, follow up to a neurology clinic, increased water intake, increased daily caloric intake, and physical and cognitive rest. The level of evidence to support these interventions has generally remained low.

REFERENCES

Giza, C. C., et al. (2013). Summary of evidence-based guideline update: evaluation and management of concussion in sports. *Neurology*, *80*(24), 2250–2257.

WOMEN WITH EPILEPSY

Recommendations: Over 90% of women with epilepsy (WWE) can expect good pregnancy outcomes. A minority of WWE will experience a worsening of seizure control during pregnancy. A coordinated approach to the care of WWE, with contributions from a primary care provider, obstetrician, geneticist, and neurologist, is ideal. Interdisciplinary communication for counseling and management is crucial.

WOMEN WITH EPILEPSY

FOR WOMEN WITH EPILEPSY DURING AND AFTER PREGNANCY

There is strong evidence (Class I) you should:

- Optimize therapy for WWE before conception.
- Complete antiepileptic drug (AED) therapy changes at least 6 months before planned conception, if possible.
- Do not change to an alternate AED during pregnancy for the sole purpose of reducing teratogenic risk.
- Offer patients being treated with carbamazepine, divalproex sodium, or valproic acid:
  - Prenatal testing with alpha-fetoprotein levels at 14 to 16 weeks' gestation.
  - Level II (structural) ultrasound at 16 to 20 weeks' gestation; and
  - If appropriate, amniocentesis for amniotic fluid alpha-fetoprotein and acetylcholinesterase levels.
  - Counsel women that there is no substantial increased risk of cesarean delivery in WWE.
  - Counsel women that there is no significant risk of late pregnancy bleeding for WWE.
  - Educate women that there is no moderately increased risk of premature contractions or labor for WWE taking AEDs.
  - Encourage breastfeeding for WWE; monitor the neonate for sedation or feeding difficulties.

There is evidence (Class III) you should consider:

- Monitoring non-protein-bound AED levels during pregnancy. For the stable patient, levels should be ascertained before conception, at the beginning of each trimester, and in the last month of pregnancy. Additional levels should be done when clinically indicated.
- Monitor AED levels through the eighth postpartum week. If AED dosage increases have been necessary during pregnancy, subsequent dosages can probably be reduced to pre-pregnancy levels safely; this may be necessary to avoid toxicity.
- Prescribe 10 mg/day of vitamin K in the last month of pregnancy for WWE taking enzyme-inducing AEDs.

FOR WOMEN WITH EPILEPSY DURING REPRODUCTIVE YEARS

There is strong evidence (Class I) you should:

- Choose the AED most appropriate for seizure type; goal should be monotherapy.
- Counsel patients entering reproductive years about the decreased effectiveness of hormonal contraception with enzyme-inducing AEDs.
- Counsel women who are contemplating pregnancy that seizure freedom for at least 9 months prior to pregnancy is a good predictor for seizure freedom during pregnancy.

- Begin folic acid supplementation with at least 0.4 mg/day; continue through pregnancy.

There is evidence (Class III) you should:

- Recommend a formulation containing 50 μg of ethinyl estradiol or mestranol if your patient's preferred method of birth control is hormonal contraception and treatment involves an enzyme-inducing AED. The risk of contraceptive failure in this setting should be discussed with the patient and discussion documented.
  - Folic acid supplementation
  - Teratogenic potential of AEDs
  - Possible change in seizure frequency during pregnancy
  - Importance of medication compliance and AED level monitoring during pregnancy
  - Inheritance risks for seizures
  - Vitamin K supplementation last month of pregnancy
  - Pros/cons of breastfeeding

NEW ANTI-EPILEPTIC DRUGS (AED) IN THE TREATMENT OF NEWLY DIAGNOSED EPILEPSY

SUMMARY OF FDA INDICATIONS (CLASS I-III EVIDENCE) FOR AEDS IN THE TREATMENT OF NEWLY DIAGNOSED EPILEPSY

Antiepileptic drug	Monotherapy vs. adjunctive	Focal seizure	Absence	Generalized tonic clonic seizure
Gabapentin	Adjunctive	Yes	No	No
Lamotrigine	Can be used as monotherapy for partial onset seizures	Yes	No*	Yes
Levetiracetam	Adjunctive	Yes	No*	Yes
Lacosamide	Both	Yes	No	No
Oxcarbazepine	Both	Yes	No	No
Eslicarbazepine acetate	Adjunctive	Yes	No	No
Tiagabine	Adjunctive	Yes	No	No
Topiramate	Both	Yes	No	Yes
Zonisamide	Adjunctive	Yes	No*	No*
Clobazam	Adjunctive	No*	No*	No*
Parampanel	Adjunctive	Yes	No	Yes
Rufinamide	Adjunctive	Not FDA approved[†]	No	No*

*Proposed, however, not supported by class I trials.
[†]Supported in class I trials.

SUMMARY OF ADVERSE EVENTS ASSOCIATED WITH THE NEW AEDS

Drug	Mechanism of action	Half Life	Adverse Events*	
			Serious	Minor
Gabapentin	Reduces Ca^{2+} influx; binds to alpha-2-delta subunit on Ca^{2+} channels	5–7 hr	None	Weight gain, sedation, peripheral edema, behavioral changes[†]
Lamotrigine	Blocks Na^+ channels	24 hr	Rash, including Stevens-Johnson syndrome and toxic epidermal necrolysis (increased risk for children, and with use of Depakote), hypersensitivity reactions, hepatic and renal failure, disseminated intravascular coagulation (DIC), and arthritis	Tics,[†] insomnia, diplopia, nausea, vomiting, dizziness
Levetiracetam	SV2A synaptic vesicles	6–8 hr	None	Irritability/behavior change, somnolence
Lacosamide	Blocks Na^+ channels	13 hr	Cardiac arrhythmia	Fatigue, dizziness, nausea, vomiting, dizziness
Oxcarbazepine	Blocks Na^+ channels	1–4 hr	Hyponatremia (more common in elderly), rash	Diplopia, headache, fatigue, nausea, vomiting
Eslicarbazepine acetate	Blocks Na^+ channels	13–20 hr	Hyponatremia	Dizziness, rash, headache, fatigue, ataxia, blurry vision

Continued

SUMMARY OF ADVERSE EVENTS ASSOCIATED WITH THE NEW AEDS—CONT'D

Drug	Mechanism of action	Half Life	Adverse Events	
			Serious	Minor
Tiagebine	Blocks GABA reputake	7–9 hr	Stupor or spike wave stupor	Tremor, asthenia, depression, weakness
Topiramate	Augments GABA, blocks Na^+ channels, Antagonism of AMPA receptors, carbonic anhydrase inhibitor	21 hr	Nephrolithiasis, open angle glaucoma, hypohidrosis[†]	Metabolic acidosis, weight loss, language dysfunction
Zonisamide	Blocks Na^+ channels	60 hr	Rash, renal caluli, hypohidrosis[†]	Irritability; photosensitivity, weight loss
Clobazam	GABA receptor	36–42 hr	Tolerance, withdrawal seizures w/ abrupt cessation	Nystagmus, drowsiness, dysarthria
Parampanel	AMPA receptor antagonist	105 hr	Aggression, behavioral changes	Dizziness, headache, fatigue, ataxia, blurry vision
Rufinamide	Blocks Na^+ channels	6–10 hr	Shortened QT interval	Dizziness, headache, somnolence, vomiting

*Psychosis and depression are associated with epilepsy and occur in open label studies with all new AEDs. Although these side effects may appear more commonly with some drugs than with others, it is difficult to ascertain whether these relationships are causal. Consequently, these side effects have been omitted from the table.

†Predominantly children.

Note: This is not meant to be a comprehensive list, but represents the most common adverse events based on consensus of panel.

REFERENCES

Abou-Khalil, B. (2016). Antiepileptic drugs. *Epilepsy Contin Life Long Learn Neurol, 22* (1), 132–156.

Abou-Khalil, B., Gallagher, M., & McDonald, R. L. (2015). In R. B. Daroff, J. Jankovic, J. C. Mazziotta, & S. L. Pomeroy (Eds.), *Bradley's neurology in clinical practice*, ed 7 (pp. 1598–1606). Philadelphia: Elsevier.

NEW ANTI-EPILEPTIC DRUGS (AED) IN THE TREATMENT OF REFRACTORY EPILEPSY

These evidence-based guidelines were produced by a 23-member committee who performed a systematic review of the available literature published between 1987 and March 2003. As these guidelines were published in 2004, they do not include a review of more recent anti-epileptic drugs (AEDs). The column for monotherapy, in the first table, is based on a review of studies in adults. There were no published clinical trials on monotherapy of partial seizures in children.

SUMMARY OF EVIDENCE-BASED GUIDELINE RECOMMENDATIONS
FOR USE IN REFRACTORY PARTIAL EPILEPSY

AED	As adjunctive therapy in adults	As adjunctive therapy in children	As monotherapy
Gabapentin	It is appropriate to use gabapentin as add-on therapy in patients with refractory epilepsy (Level A)	Gabapentin may be used as adjunctive treatment of children with refractory partial seizures (Level A)	There is insufficient evidence to recommend gabapentin as monotherapy for refractory partial epilepsy (Level U)
Lamotrigine	It is appropriate to use lamotrigine as add-on therapy in patients with refractory epilepsy (Level A)	Lamotrigine may be used as adjunctive treatment of children with refractory partial seizures (Level A)	Lamotrigine can be used as monotherapy in patients with refractory partial epilepsy (Level B, downgraded due to dropouts)
Topiramate	It is appropriate to use topiramate as add-on therapy in patients with refractory epilepsy (Level A)	Topiramate may be used as adjunctive treatment of children with refractory partial seizures (Level A)	Topiramate can be used as monotherapy in patients with refractory partial epilepsy (Level A)
Tiagabine	It is appropriate to use Tiagabine as add-on therapy in patients with refractory epilepsy (Level A)		There is insufficient evidence to recommend tiagabine as monotherapy for refractory partial epilepsy (Level U)

Continued

SUMMARY OF EVIDENCE-BASED GUIDELINE RECOMMENDATIONS FOR USE IN REFRACTORY PARTIAL EPILEPSY—CONT'D

AED	As adjunctive therapy in adults	As adjunctive therapy in children	As monotherapy
Oxcarbazepine	It is appropriate to use Oxcarbazepine as add-on therapy in patients with refractory epilepsy (Level A)	Oxcarbazepine may be used as adjunctive treatment of children with refractory partial seizures (Level A)	Oxcarbazepine can be used as monotherapy in patients with refractory partial epilepsy (Level A)
Levetiracetam	It is appropriate to use Levetiracetam as add-on therapy in patients with refractory epilepsy (Level A)		There is insufficient evidence to recommend Levetiracetam as monotherapy for refractory partial epilepsy (Level U)
Zonisamide	It is appropriate to use Zonisamide as add-on therapy in patients with refractory epilepsy (Level A)		There is insufficient evidence to recommend Zonisamide as monotherapy for refractory partial epilepsy (Level U)

From http://tools.aan.com/professionals/practice/pdfs/clinician_ep_treatment_e.pdf.

SUMMARY OF EVIDENCE-BASED GUIDELINE RECOMMENDATIONS FOR USE IN REFRACTORY PRIMARY GENERALIZED EPILEPSY AND LENNOX-GASTAUT SYNDROME

AED	Refractory Primary Generalized Epilepsy	Lennox-Gastaut Syndrome
Gabapentin	There is insufficient evidence to recommend gabapentin for the treatment of refractory epilepsy in children (Level U)	
Lamotrigine	There is insufficient evidence to recommend lamotrigine for the treatment of refractory epilepsy in children (Level U)	Lamotrigine may be used to treat drop attacks associated with the Lennox-Gastaut syndrome in adults and children (Level A)
Topiramate	Topiramate may be used for the treatment of refractory generalized tonic-clonic seizures in adults and children (Level A)	Topiramate may be used to treat drop attacks associated with the Lennox-Gastaut syndrome in adults and children (Level A)

Continued

NEW AED IN THE TREATMENT OF REFRACTORY EPILEPSY

SUMMARY OF EVIDENCE-BASED GUIDELINE RECOMMENDATIONS FOR USE IN REFRACTORY PRIMARY GENERALIZED EPILEPSY AND LENNOX-GASTAUT SYNDROME—CONT'D

AED	Refractory Primary Generalized Epilepsy	Lennox-Gastaut Syndrome
Oxcarbazepine	There is insufficient evidence to recommend oxcarbazepine for the treatment of refractory epilepsy in children (Level U)	
Levetiracetam	There is insufficient evidence to recommend levetiracetam for the treatment of refractory epilepsy in children (Level U)	
Zonisamide	There is insufficient evidence to recommend zonisamide for the treatment of refractory epilepsy in children (Level U)	

From http://tools.aan.com/professionals/practice/pdfs/clinician_ep_treatment_e.pdf.

REFERENCES

AAN Website. http://tools.aan.com/professionals/practice/pdfs/clinician_ep_treatment_e.pdf. Accessed October 29, 2017.

French, J., Kanner, A., Bautista, J., Abou-Khalil, B., Browne, T., Harden, C., et al. (2004). Efficacy and tolerability of the new antiepileptic drugs II: treatment of refractory epilepsy: report of the Therapeutics and Technology Assessment Subcommittee and Quality Standards Subcommittee of the American Academy of Neurology and the American Epilepsy Society. *Neurology*, 62(8), 1261–1273.

PATENT FORAMEN OVALE AND STROKE

Patent foramen ovale (PFO) is a common finding with an approximate 25% prevalence in the general population. The role of PFO as a conduit for paradoxical embolism has long been suspected, and an association between PFO and embolic stroke of unknown source (ESUS) has been confirmed in multiple studies, because its prevalence in ESUS averages 40%. In addition, the presence of atrial septal aneurysm (ASA) combined with a large PFO has been found to have a particularly strong association with stroke recurrence in one study.

EVIDENCE FOR PATENT FORAMEN OVALE CLOSURE

Multiple observational studies, meta-analyses, and three prospective trials have been done in an attempt to prove efficacy and superiority of PFO closure over medical management alone in secondary stroke prevention (currently, there is no evidence to support PFO closure for primary stroke prevention for any patient population). However, the challenge has proven difficult, mainly due to the long recruitment times, inherent periprocedural risk of adverse effects, need for prolonged follow-up time, and low incidence of stroke recurrence.

The first prospective, randomized PFO closure trial was an unsuccessful CLOSURE 1 trial, in which an inferior STARFlex device was used (no longer produced due to risk of atrial fibrillation and thrombogenicity). Subsequently, the PC trial (414 patients; mean follow-up 4 years) and the RESPECT trial (980 patients; mean follow-up 2.6 years) compared the Amplatzer PFO Occluder with medical therapy alone. Again, both trials failed to reach statistical significance in recurrence of the primary outcomes between the two arms. However, the RESPECT trial did show a significant difference in the "as treated" analysis because three strokes in the device arm occurred before PFO closure.

Finally, with longer follow-up of 5.9 years, the "intention-to-treat" analysis of the RESPECT trial announced at International Stroke Conference (ISC) 2017 revealed a significant trend favoring PFO closure over medical therapy alone in preventing nonfatal ischemic strokes (hazard ratio [HR]: 0.55, 95% confidence interval [CI]: 0.305 to 0.999, log-rank $P = .046$). However, there was a higher risk of deep venous thrombosis/pulmonary embolism (DVT/PE) in the device arm. In 2017, two more trials (Gore REDUCE and CLOSE) proved superiority of PFO closure over medical therapy alone with the only exception being a small increase in mostly transient atrial fibrillation in the closure arms.

CURRENT MANAGEMENT TREND

Who can benefit from PFO closure? In general, young patients with PFO and ESUS who do not have other major stroke risk factors; in other words, those whose PFO is probably pathogenic. The well-regarded Risk of Paradoxical Embolism (RoPE) study identified patient-level variables associated with PFO status, which were then used to create a simple 11-point *RoPE score* (0 to 10). A higher score means a higher risk of PFO pathogenicity with a set of well-chosen criteria for selecting such patients based on risk stratification.

The Food and Drug Administration (FDA) approved the Amplatzer PFO Occluder on October 28, 2016 for PFO closure to reduce the risk of recurrent strokes in patients between 18 and 60 years with ESUS due to presumed paradoxical embolism, as determined by a cardiologist and a neurologist. Currently, despite the need for more research, a wise selection of an appropriate stroke population, especially with an ASA and a large right-to-left shunt, should guide clinicians toward better secondary stroke prevention in presumed PFO-related strokes. Lastly, if PFO closure is declined by the patient or is contraindicated, anticoagulation is preferred to antiplatelet therapy in the appropriately chosen population with presumed pathogenic PFO.

RISK OF PARADOXICAL EMBOLISM (ROPE) SCORE FOR
STRATIFICATION OF STROKE RISK WITH PATENT FORAMEN
OVALE (HIGHER SCORE MEANS HIGHER STROKE RISK)

Patient Characteristic	Points
No history of hypertension	+1
No history of diabetes	+1
No history of stroke or TIA	+1
Nonsmoker	+1
Cortical infarct on imaging	+1
AGE (Y)	
18–29	+5
30–39	+4
40–49	+3
50–59	+2
69–69	+1
≥70	+1
Total RoPE score	0–10

RoPE, Risk of paradoxical embolism; *TIA*, transient ischemic attack.

REFERENCES

Ntaios, G., Papavasileiou, V., Sagris, D., et al. (2018). Closure of patent foramen ovale versus medical therapy in patients with cryptogenic stroke or transient ischemic attack: updated systematic review and meta-analysis. *Stroke*, *49*(2), 412–418. https://doi.org/10.1161/STROKEAHA.117.020030.

Saver, J. L., Carroll, J. D., Thaler, D. E., et al. (2017). Long-term outcomes of patent foramen ovale closure or medical therapy after stroke. *N Engl J Med*, *377*(11), 1022–1032. https://doi.org/10.1056/NEJMoa1610057.

DIAGNOSIS OF PATIENTS WITH NEUROBORRELIOSIS

I. Diagnosis of definite nervous system Lyme disease requires all of the following criteria:
   A. Possible exposure to appropriate ticks in an area where Lyme disease occurs.
   B. One or more of the following:
      1. Erythema migrans or histopathologically proven *Borrelia* lymphocytoma or acrodermatitis
      2. Immunologic evidence of exposure to *Borrelia burgdorferi*
      3. Histopathologic, microbiologic, or polymerase chain reaction proof of the presence of *B. burgdorferi* infection
   C. Occurrence of one or more of the following neurologic disorders, after exclusion of other potential causes:
      1. Neurologic symptoms suggestive of Lyme neuroborreliosis without any other obvious reason.
      2. Cerebrospinal fluid (CSF) analysis for pleocytosis
      3. Intrathecal production of specific antibody if central nervous system (CNS) infection is suspected.

    a. Causally related neurologic disease
      i. Lymphocytic meningitis with or without cranial neuritis, painful radiculoneuritis, or both
      ii. Encephalomyelitis
      iii. Peripheral neuropathy
    b. Causally related syndrome
      i. Encephalopathy

For possible neuroborreliosis: two criteria (A, B, or C) need to be fulfilled.

II. Causal relationship asserted but highly unlikely
  A. Multiple sclerosis
  B. Amyotrophic lateral sclerosis
  C. Dementia

III. Based on a literature review and expert opinion, the following recommendations are supported as options.
  A. Localized disease is usually responsive to oral antimicrobial regimens (e.g., doxycycline or amoxicillin for 3 weeks).
  B. CNS infection probably requires parenteral antimicrobial therapy (e.g., ceftriaxone or cefotaxime or penicillin G for 2 or 4 weeks), although limited data suggest oral regimens may be efficacious in acute meningitis.

MIGRAINE DIAGNOSIS AND GENERAL TREATMENT CONSIDERATION

Migraine is a neurobiologic disorder that occurs in 18% of women and 6% of men but may be undiagnosed and often undertreated.

- Migraine is a genetically based disorder.
- It may be associated with altered sensitivity of the nervous system and activation of the trigeminal-vascular system.
- It is characterized by attacks of head pain and neurologic, gastrointestinal, and autonomic symptoms.
- It varies in frequency, duration, and disability among sufferers and between attacks.

GENERAL PRINCIPLES OF HEADACHE CARE

- Establish a diagnosis. The International Headache Society has published detailed diagnostic criteria for the headache syndromes.
- Educate migraine sufferers about their condition.
- Treatments can be divided into prophylactic and symptomatic treatment, and both have advantages and disadvantages.
  - Choose treatment based on the frequency and severity of attacks, the presence and degree of disability, and associated symptoms, such as nausea and vomiting.
  - Discuss the rationale for each particular treatment, how to use it, and what adverse events are likely.
  - Establish realistic patient expectations.

- Involve patients in managing their migraines. Encourage patients to use headache diaries to track triggers, frequency and severity of headaches, and response to treatment.
- Encourage the patient to identify and avoid triggers.
- Create a formal management plan and individualize management. Consider the patient's preference, response to, and tolerance for previously administered medications. Beware of increasing frequency of acute medications. Identify coexisting conditions (such as heart disease, gastrointestinal disease, renal impairment, pregnancy, and uncontrolled hypertension) because they may limit treatment choices.

DIAGNOSIS

- Migraine is a chronic condition with episodic manifestations; attacks vary in frequency and duration among sufferers and between attacks.
- If atypical features are present, exclude secondary headaches.
- There is insufficient evidence to recommend any diagnostic testing other than neuroimaging. Electroencephalography is not indicated in the routine evaluation of headache.
- Neuroimaging should be considered in nonacute headache patients with:
  - Unexplained abnormal neurologic examination
  - Atypical headache, headache features, or an additional risk factor, such as immune deficiency
- American Academy of Neurology guidelines suggest imaging in all headaches but do not specify timing or modality.

GOALS OF ACUTE TREATMENT

Acute care should be individualized based on the patient's symptoms and level of disability.

- Treat attacks effectively, rapidly, and consistently to minimize adverse events.
- Restore the patient's ability to function.
- Minimize the need for back-up and rescue medications.*
- Optimize self-care and reduce subsequent use of resources.

GUIDE TO ACUTE TREATMENT

- Act promptly. Failure to use an effective treatment promptly may increase pain, disability, and the impact of the headache.
- Use triptans (naratriptan, rizatriptan, sumatriptan, and zolmitriptan) and DHE in patients who have moderate or severe migraine, or whose mild-to-moderate headaches respond poorly to nonsteroidal anti-inflammatory drugs (NSAIDs) or combinations, such as aspirin plus acetaminophen plus caffeine, or other agents, such as ergotamine (see full guideline and table 1 at http://aan.com/go/practice/guidelines).

---

*A rescue medication is used at home when other treatments fail. It permits the patient to achieve relief without the discomfort and expense of a visit to the physician's office or emergency department.

- NSAIDs (oral), combination analgesics containing caffeine, and isometheptene combinations are an option for the mild-to-moderate migraine attacks or severe attacks that have been responsive in the past to similar agents.
- Select a nonoral route of administration for patients with migraine associated with severe nausea or vomiting.
- Do not restrict antiemetics only to patients who are vomiting or likely to vomit.
- Use a self-administered rescue medication for patients whose severe migraine does not respond to (or fails) other treatments.
- Limit and carefully monitor opiate- and butalbital-containing analgesics.
- Guard against medication-overuse headache ("rebound headache"). Attempt to limit acute therapy to 2 days per week (see chronic migraine criteria in the below table).

PREVENTIVE THERAPIES
Preventive therapies should be used when migraine has a substantial impact on a patient's life. Consider preventive therapies when any of the following are present:
- Frequent headaches (>2/week)
- Migraine that significantly interferes with patient's daily routines, despite acute treatment
- Contraindication to, failure, adverse effects, or overuse of acute therapies
- Patient preference
- Presence of uncommon migraine conditions, including hemiplegic migraine, basilar migraine, migraine with prolonged aura, or migrainous infarction

Goals of preventive therapies:
- Reduce attack frequency, severity, and duration.
- Improve responsiveness to acute treatment.
- Improve function and reduce disability.

Guide to preventive medication use:
- Use medication with best efficacy and fewest adverse events (see full guideline and table 2 at http://aan.com/go/practice/guidelines).
- Take coexisting conditions into account.
- Select a drug that will treat more than one condition, if possible.
- Be sure that the coexistent disease is not a contraindication to the migraine treatment.
- Be sure that the treatments used for coexistent conditions do not exacerbate migraine.
- Beware of drug interactions.
- Start low and increase dose slowly until benefits are achieved or limiting side effects occur.
- Give the drug an adequate trial at adequate dosage (2 to 3 months).
- Avoid interfering medications (e.g., overuse of acute medication).
- Consider a long-acting formulation, which may improve compliance.
- Monitor the patient's headache diary.

- Reevaluate therapy. If headache is controlled at 6 months, consider tapering or discontinuing treatment.

  Nonpharmacologic therapies:

  The following nonpharmacologic headache treatments may be used along or combined with preventive drug therapy to achieve additional clinical improvement:

- Relaxation training
- Thermal biofeedback with relaxation training
- EMG biofeedback
- Cognitive-behavioral therapy

DIAGNOSTIC CRITERIA FOR MAJOR MIGRAINE SUBTYPES

Migraine without aura	Recurrent headache disorder manifesting in attacks lasting 4–72 hr. Typical characteristics of the headache are unilateral location, pulsating quality, moderate or severe intensity, aggravation by routine physical activity and association with nausea and/or photophobia and phonophobia.
	Diagnostic criteria:
	A. At least five attacks fulfilling criteria B–D
	B. Headache attacks lasting 4–72 hr (untreated or unsuccessfully treated)
	C. Headache has at least two of the following four characteristics:
	1. unilateral location
	2. pulsating quality
	3. moderate or severe pain intensity
	4. aggravation by or causing avoidance of routine physical activity (e.g., walking or climbing stairs)
	D. During headache at least one of the following:
	1. nausea and/or vomiting
	2. photophobia and phonophobia
	E. Not better accounted for by another headache disorder
Migraine with aura	Recurrent attacks, lasting minutes, of unilateral fully reversible visual, sensory, or other central nervous system symptoms that usually develop gradually and are usually followed by headache and associated migraine symptoms.
	A. At least two attacks fulfilling criteria B and C
	B. One or more of the following fully reversible aura symptoms:
	1. visual
	2. sensory
	3. speech and/or language
	4. motor
	5. brainstem
	6. retinal

Continued

MIGRAINE DIAGNOSIS AND GENERAL TREATMENT CONSIDERATION

DIAGNOSTIC CRITERIA FOR MAJOR MIGRAINE SUBTYPES—CONT'D

	C. At least two of the following four characteristics:
	  1. at least one aura symptom spreads gradually over 5 min, and/or two or more symptoms occur in succession
	  2. each individual aura symptom lasts 5 to 60 min
	  3. at least one aura symptom is unilateral
	  4. the aura is accompanied, or followed within 60 min, by headache
	D. Not better accounted for by another headache diagnosis, and transient ischemic attack has been excluded.

Migraine with brainstem aura (basilar migraine)	Migraine with aura symptoms clearly originating from the brainstem, but no motor weakness.
	
	A. At least two attacks fulfilling criteria B–D
	B. Aura consisting of visual, sensory and/or speech/language symptoms, each fully reversible, but no or retinal symptoms
	C. At least two of the following brainstem symptoms:
	  1. dysarthria
	  2. vertigo
	  3. tinnitus
	  4. hypacusis
	  5. diplopia
	  6. ataxia
	  7. decreased level of consciousness
	D. At least two of the following four characteristics:
	  1. at least one aura symptom spreads gradually over 5 min, and/or two or more symptoms occur in succession
	  2. each individual aura symptom lasts 5 to 60 min

Hemiplegic migraine (may be familial and genetic loci have been implicated in some cases)	Migraine with aura including motor weakness.
	
	3. at least one aura symptom is unilateral
	4. the aura is accompanied, or followed within 60 min, by headache
	E. Not better accounted for by another ICHD-3 diagnosis, and transient ischemic attack has been excluded.
	A. At least two attacks fulfilling criteria B and C
	B. Aura consisting of both of the following:
	  1. fully reversible motor weakness
	  2. fully reversible visual, sensory, and/or speech/language symptoms
	C. At least two of the following four characteristics:
	  1. at least one aura symptom spreads gradually over 5 min, and/or two or more symptoms occur in succession
	  2. each individual non-motor aura symptom lasts 5–60 min, and motor symptoms last and motor symptoms last <72 hr
	  3. at least one aura symptom is unilateral
	  4. the aura is accompanied, or followed within 60 min, by headache
	D. Not better accounted for by another headache diagnosis, and transient ischemic attack and stroke are excluded

Retinal migraine	Repeated attacks of monocular visual disturbance, including scintillations, scotomata, or blindness, associated with migraine headache. A. At least two attacks fulfilling criteria B and C B. Aura consisting of fully reversible monocular positive and/or negative visual phenomena (e.g., scintillations,

Continued

MIGRAINE DIAGNOSIS AND GENERAL TREATMENT CONSIDERATION

DIAGNOSTIC CRITERIA FOR MAJOR MIGRAINE SUBTYPES—CONT'D

	scotomata or blindness) confirmed during an attack by either or both of the following: 1. clinical visual field examination 2. the patient's drawing (made after clear instruction) of a monocular field defect C. At least two of the following three characteristics: 1. the aura spreads gradually over 5 min 2. aura symptoms last 5 to 60 min 3. the aura is accompanied, or followed within 60 min, by headache D. Not better accounted for by another headache diagnosis, and other causes of amaurosis fugax have been excluded.
Chronic migraine	Headache occurring on 15 or more days per month¹ for more than 3 mo, which has the features of migraine headache on at least 8 days per month. A. Headache (tension-type-like and/or migraine-like) on 15 days per month for >3 mo and fulfilling criteria B and C B. Occurring in a patient who has had at least five attacks fulfilling criteria B-D for migraine without aura and/or criteria B and C for migraine with aura C. On 8 days per month for >3 mo, fulfilling any of the following: 1. criteria C and D for migraine without aura 2. criteria B and C for migraine with aura 3. believed by the patient to be migraine at onset and relieved by a triptan or ergot derivative D. Not better accounted for by another headache diagnosis

International Headache Society, 2013. *Cephalalgia*, 33(9), 644.

ACUTE AND PREVENTIVE THERAPY OF MIGRAINE HEADACHE IN CHILDREN AND ADOLESCENTS

SUMMARY OF RECOMMENDATIONS FOR THE ACUTE TREATMENT OF MIGRAINE IN CHILDREN AND ADOLESCENTS

Strong evidence supports:

- Ibuprofen is effective and should be considered for the acute treatment of migraine in children (class I, Level A).
- Sumatriptan nasal spray is effective and should be considered for the acute treatment of migraine in adolescents (class I, Level A).
Good evidence supports:
- Acetaminophen is probably effective and should be considered for the acute treatment of migraine in children (class I, Level B).
Evidence is insufficient to support or refute:
- There are no supporting data for the use of any oral "triptan" preparations in children or adolescents (class IV, Level U).
- There are inadequate data to make a judgment on the efficacy of subcutaneous sumatriptan (class IV, Level U).

SUMMARY OF RECOMMENDATIONS FOR PREVENTIVE THERAPY OF MIGRAINE IN CHILDREN AND ADOLESCENTS

Good evidence supports:

- Flunarizine is probably effective for preventive therapy and can be considered for this purpose, but it is not available in the United States (class I, Level B).
- Pizotifen and nimodipine (class I, Level B) and clonidine (class II, Level B) did not show efficacy and are not recommended.
Evidence is insufficient to support or refute:
- There is insufficient evidence to make any recommendations concerning the use of cyproheptadine, amitriptyline, divalproex sodium, topiramate, or levetiracetam (class IV, Level U).
- Recommendations cannot be made concerning propranolol or trazadone for preventive therapy because the evidence is conflicting (class II, Level U).

The practice parameter closes with the statement: "Failure of an agent for either the acute or preventive treatment to demonstrate efficacy to a statistically significant degree does not imply that these medications have no role in the pediatric population and their use must be based upon good clinical judgment."

SUPPORTIVE MANAGEMENT OF AMYOTROPHIC LATERAL SCLEROSIS

Amyotrophic lateral sclerosis (ALS) is a progressive neurodegenerative disease affecting principally upper and lower motor neurons. The average length of survival following diagnosis is 2 to 4 years, and pharmacologic treatment is riluzole, offering an increased survival benefit of 2 to 3 months, and edaravone, a free radical scavenger which aims to slow progression. Presently, much ALS management is devoted to symptom control to maximize physical functioning and maintain quality of life (QOL). Strength of recommendation for most treatment strategies remains weak because only a limited amount of randomized control trials specific to ALS have been conducted due to disease rarity and ethical consideration of withholding treatment among other reasons.

In general, a holistic approach involving a team of specialists can reduce and shorten hospital stays and improve QOL. Attendance at multidisciplinary clinics is associated with longer survival independent of riluzole, ventilation, or PEG tube placement.

SPECIFIC SYMPTOM MANAGEMENT:

Cramps: Quinine has long been advocated for treating cramps but can have serious cardiac and hematologic adverse events. In the United States, quinine is reserved as last resort per American Academy of Neurology (AAN) recommendation (grade B). In the United Kingdom, quinine is considered first choice, whereas European guidelines recommend the use of levetiracetam (grade C). Other options include low-dose mexiletine (grade B) to reduce cramp frequency. Placebo-controlled trials have shown that tetrahydrocannabinol and memantine are probably ineffective for the treatment of cramps (moderate-quality evidence) and vitamin E has little to no effect (low-quality evidence). No formal recommendations are available for L-threonine, gabapentin, xaliproden, riluzole, and baclofen due to the very low quality of evidence available.

Spasticity: Spasticity treatment can prevent pressure sores and contractures. Physical therapy (PT) and passive stretching are commonly used, whereas there is limited evidence for endurance-based exercise programs. Pharmaceutic options include baclofen, tizanidine or dantrolene (grade D, may worsen secretion and weakness), benzodiazepine (grade D), and intrathecal baclofen (grade C).

Pain: Pain is a common symptom that can occur in approximately 80% of patients with ALS and often increases with disease progression. There are limited ALS-specific data about this symptom in ALS patients, and the general recommendation is to follow the 1990 World Health Organization (WHO) analgesic ladder and escalate therapy as needed.

Cognitive and other neurologic deficits: Up to 50% of ALS patients show mild cognitive or behavior changes, and 10% to 15% may demonstrate behavior changes of frontotemporal dementia. Patients with dementia have a shorter survival time. Behavior treatment is symptom oriented and includes pharmacologic and nonpharmacologic approaches. There is no recommended treatment.

Dextromethorphan-quinidine can be used to treat pseudobulbar affect but may cause dizziness and somnolence and should be avoided in cardiac arrhythmia patients with QT prolongation. Selective serotonin re-uptake inhibitors (SSRI) and amitriptyline are other options (both grade C). SSRI may also be used for depression (grade D) and benzodiazepine for anxiety (grade D). Modafinil has been used to for fatigue (grade B).

Nutrition and swallowing: Malnutrition and weight loss are poor prognostic factors in ALS. Gastrostomy may offer a weak survival advantage and, if considered, should be placed before weight loss of 5%; after this threshold, irreversible metabolic changes occur and negatively affect outcome. Ethical considerations include the low likelihood of success and the invasive nature of the procedure. In general, recommendation is to have this discussion early in the disease course; gastrostomy is not recommended when nearing end of life, due to futility and complication risk, or if there is severe cognitive impairment. Techniques are dependent on degree of respiratory failure and ability to tolerate sedation. Endoscopic placement is generally reserved for those without respiratory failure and can tolerate sedation. Other options include radiologically guided gastrostomy using local sedation and peroral image guided gastrostomy via nasogastric (NG) tube with sedation while the patient is on noninvasive ventilation. Minor complications of percutaneous endoscopic gastrostomy (PEG) tube insertion range from 2% to 16%, whereas major complication such as tube failure have been reported in up to 45%. Palliative involvement is highly recommended to relieve distress over starvation, etc.

Respiratory failure: Type 2 respiratory failure is the most common cause of death in ALS. Symptoms start in rapid-eye-movement (REM) sleep, and it is recommended to monitor respiratory function at least every 3 months using objective measures such vital capacity, sniff-nasal inspiratory pressure, arterial or capillary blood gas analysis, and nocturnal oximetry. Noninvasive ventilation has been shown to provide median survival gain of 7 months and improves QOL, although the survival benefit was limited to patients with normal to moderately impaired bulbar function. Noninvasive ventilation (NIV) can be difficult to tolerate and can cause dry mouth, oropharyngeal secretions, and claustrophobia.

Secretions: For thick secretions, carbocysteine and nebulized saline with cough augmentation and suction are used. For thin secretions, hyoscine patch, amitriptyline, atropine drops, and glycopyrrolate are available options. All are recommendation grade level D. Intraglandular botulinum toxin injections can also be considered, with effect lasting up to 4 weeks, although it is generally reserved for patients with gastrostomy due to risk of worsening dysphagia.

End-of-Life Care: ALS is uniformly fatal, and ethical considerations include following living wills and power of attorney designations. Compassionate care and counseling regarding end-of-life issues are built on trust and successful doctor-patient relationships.

REFERENCES

Hobson, E. V., & McDermott, C. J. (2016). Supportive and symptomatic management of amyotrophic lateral sclerosis. *Nat Rev Neurol*, *12*, 526–538.

Ng, L., Khan, F., Young, C. A., et al. (2017). Symptomatic treatments for amyotrophic lateral sclerosis/motor neuron disease. *Cochrane Database Syst Rev*,(1). CD011776.

ALGORITHMS FOR NUTRITIONAL AND RESPIRATORY MANAGEMENT OF ALS

ALGORITHM FOR NUTRITION MANAGEMENT

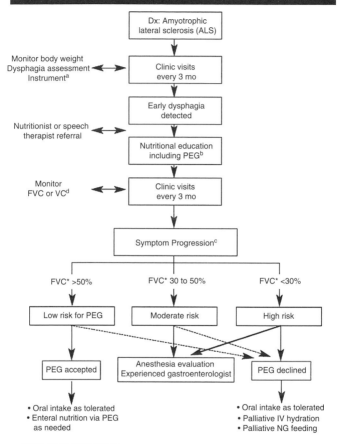

Dx: Amyotrophic lateral sclerosis (ALS)

Monitor body weight
Dysphagia assessment
Instrument[a] ⟷ Clinic visits every 3 mo

Early dysphagia detected

Nutritionist or speech therapist referral ⟷ Nutritional education including PEG[b]

Monitor FVC or VC[d] ⟷ Clinic visits every 3 mo

Symptom Progression[c]

FVC* >50% → Low risk for PEG
FVC* 30 to 50% → Moderate risk
FVC* <30% → High risk

PEG accepted
Anesthesia evaluation
Experienced gastroenterologist
PEG declined

- Oral intake as tolerated
- Enteral nutrition via PEG as needed

- Oral intake as tolerated
- Palliative IV hydration
- Palliative NG feeding

[a]Rule out contraindications

[b]Prolonged mealtime, ending meal prematurely because of fatigue, accelerated weight loss due to poor caloric intake, family concern about feeding difficulties

[c]For example, Colorado Dysphagia Disability Inventory, bulbar questions in the ALS Functional Rating Scale, or other instrument

[d]Forced vital capacity (FVC) or vital capacity (VC) can be used. VC may be more accurate in patients with bulbar dysfunction

Dx = diagnosis   PEG = percutaneous endoscopic gastrostomy

ALGORITHM FOR RESPIRATORY MANAGEMENT

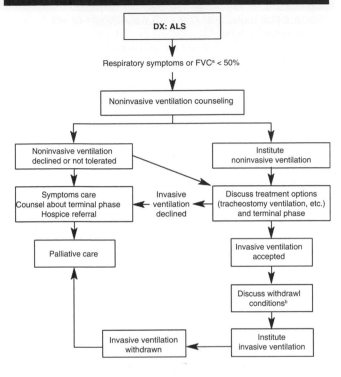

DX: ALS

Respiratory symptoms or FVC[a] < 50%

Noninvasive ventilation counseling

Noninvasive ventilation declined or not tolerated

Institute noninvasive ventilation

Symptoms care
Counsel about terminal phase
Hospice referral

Invasive ventilation declined

Discuss treatment options (tracheostomy ventilation, etc.) and terminal phase

Palliative care

Invasive ventilation accepted

Discuss withdrawl conditions[b]

Invasive ventilation withdrawn

Institute invasive ventilation

[a]Forced vital capacity (FVC) or vital capacity (VC) can be used. VC may be more accurate in patients with bulbar dysfunction

[b]Agreement needed for conditions of withdrawal prior to or concurrent with instituting invasive ventilation (e.g., locked-in state, coma, etc.)

Dx = diagnosis

Classification of management recommendations: Definitions

Standard: A principle for patient management that reflects a high degree of certainty based on class I evidence or very strong evidence from class II studies when circumstances preclude randomized trials (A)

Guideline: Recommendations for patient management reflecting moderate clinical certainty (usually class II evidence or strong consensus of class III evidence) (B)

Option: A strategy for patient management for which the evidence (class III) is inconclusive or when there is some conflicting evidence or opinion (C)

ALGORITHMS FOR NUTRITIONAL AND RESPIRATORY MANAGEMENT OF ALS

MAGNETIC RESONANCE IMAGING (MRI) IN MULTIPLE SCLEROSIS (MS) AND DIAGNOSTIC CONSIDERATION IN PATIENTS WITH WHITE MATTER LESIONS

EVIDENCE FOR USING MRI FOR EARLY DIAGNOSIS OF MS

Strong evidence supports:

1. On the basis of consistent class I, II, and III evidence, in clinically isolated demyelinating (CID) patients, the finding of three or more white matter lesions on a T_2-weighted MRI scan is a very sensitive predictor (>80%) of the subsequent development of clinically definite multiple sclerosis (CDMS) within the next 7 to 10 years (level A recommendation). It is possible that the presence of even a smaller number of white matter lesions (e.g., 1 to 3) may be equally predictive of future MS, although this relationship requires better classification.

2. The appearance of new T_2 lesions or new gadolinium (Gd) enhancement 3 or more months after a CID episode (and after a baseline MRI assessment) is highly predictive of the subsequent development of CDMS in the near term (level A recommendation).

3. The probability of making a diagnosis other than MS in CIS patients with any of the aforementioned MRI abnormalities is quite low, once alternative diagnoses that can mimic MS or the radiographic findings of MS have been excluded.

Good evidence supports:

4. The presence of two or more Gd-enhancing lesions at baseline is highly predictive of the future development of CDMS (Level B recommendation).

Evidence is insufficient to support or refute:

5. The MRI features helpful in the diagnosis of primary-progressive multiple sclerosis (PPMS) cannot be determined from the existing evidence (Level U recommendation).

DIAGNOSTIC CONSIDERATIONS IN PATIENTS WITH SUSPECTED MS OR MRI WHITE MATTER ABNORMALITIES

- Age-related white matter changes
- Acute disseminated encephalomyelitis
- Cerebral autosomal dominant arteriopathy, subcortical infarcts, and leukoencephalopathy
- Cervical spondylosis or stenosis
- Inflammatory/autoimmune: Behçet disease, sarcoid, Sjögren syndrome, vasculitis (primary central nervous system [CNS] or other), systemic lupus erythematosus, antiphospholipid antibody syndromes, and related collagen vascular disorders
- Infection: Bacterial infections (syphilis, Lyme disease), human immunodeficiency virus (HIV) infection, and human T-lymphotropic virus I/II
- Ischemic optic neuropathy (arteritic and nonarteritic)
- Leukodystrophies (e.g., adrenoleukodystrophy, metachromatic leukodystrophy)
- Neoplasms (e.g., lymphoma, glioma, meningioma)

- Migraine
- Stroke and ischemic cerebrovascular disease and spinal cord infarction
- Unidentified bright objects
- Vascular malformations
- Vitamin B_{12} deficiency

REVISED MCDONALD CRITERIA

	Number of lesions with objective clinical evidence	Additional data needed for a diagnosis of multiple sclerosis
≥2 clinical attacks	≥2	None
≥2 clinical attacks	1 (as well as clear-cut historical evidence of a previous attack involving a lesion in a distinct anatomic location)	None
≥2 clinical attacks	1	Dissemination in space demonstrated by an additional clinical attack implicating a different central nervous system (CNS) site or by magnetic resonance imaging (MRI)
1 clinical attack	≥2	Dissemination in time demonstrated by an additional clinical attack or by MRI OR demonstration of cerebrospinal fluid (CSF)-specific oligoclonal bands
1 clinical attack	1	Dissemination in space demonstrated by an additional clinical attack implicating a different CNS site or by MRI AND Dissemination in time demonstrated by an additional clinical attack or by MRI OR demonstration of CSF-specific oligoclonal bands

Thompson, A. J., Banwell, B. L., Barkhof, F., et al. (2018). Diagnosis of multiple sclerosis 2017 revisions of the McDonald criteria. *Lancet Neurol, 17*(2), 162–173.

REFERENCES

Frohman, E. M., Goodin, D. S., Calabresi, P. A., et al. The utility of MRI in suspected MS: report of the Therapeutics and Technology Assessment Subcommittee of the American Academy of Neurology. *Neurology, 61*(5), 602–611. https://doi.org/10.1212/01. WNL.0000082654.99838.EF.

Thompson, A. J., Banwell, B. L., Barkhof, F., et al. (2018). Diagnosis of multiple sclerosis: 2017 revisions of the McDonald criteria. *Lancet Neurol, 17*(2), 162–173.

MRI UTILITY IN MS AND DIAGNOSTIC CONSIDERATION

DISEASE-MODIFYING THERAPIES IN MULTIPLE SCLEROSIS

DISEASE-MODIFYING THERAPIES IN MULTIPLE SCLEROSIS

Chemical name	Route & frequency of administration (trade name)	Annual relapse rate (% relative reduction) (phase III clinical trial)	Adverse effects	Monitoring	Additional pearls
Beta-Interferon 1b (1993)	SQ QoD (Betaseron)	34% MSSG vs. placebo	Flu-like symptoms Injections-site reactions Increased liver enzymes Depression Rare: anemia, thrombocytopenia, congestive heart failure, thyroid disorders	CBC w/diff LFTs (prior to treatment, every 1, 3, 6 mo, periodically during)	Also indicated for CIS
Beta-Interferon 1a (1996, 2002)	IM QWk (Avonex) SQ TIW[a] (Rebif)	18% MSCRG vs. placebo 32% PRISMS vs. placebo	See above	See above	Drug formulations: PFS, pen
PEG Beta-Interferon 1a (2014)	SQ Q14 days (Plegridy)	35% ADVANCE vs. placebo	See above	See above	Drug formulations: PFS, pen
Glatiramer acetate (1996, 2015)	SQ daily (Copaxone 20 mg, Glatopa) SQ TIW (Copaxone 40 mg)	29% CMSSG vs. placebo 34% GALA vs. placebo	Injection-site reactions Lipoatrophy, immediate systemic reaction (palpitations, chest tightness, dyspnea), infections	None required	Also indicated for CIS

Fingolimod (2010)	PO daily (Gilenya)	54% FREEDOMS I vs. placebo	First dose bradycardia Increased blood pressure Increased LFTs Infection Lymphopenia Rare: macular edema, AV block, QTc prolongation	Prior to FDO: EKG, ophthalmic exam, CBC w/diff, LFTs, Varicella antibodies Mandatory FDO During: CBC w/diff, LFTs (periodically) 3 mo F/U: ophth exam Post therapy: CBC w/diff (×2 mo)	Contraindications: recent cardiac disease (past 6 mo),[b] Mobitz type II 2nd or 3rd degree AV block or sick sinus syndrome, baseline QTc interval ≥ 500 ms, Class Ia or III antiarrhythmics PML: rare
Dimethyl fumarate (2013)	PO BID (Tecfidera)	44% CONFIRM vs. glatiramer 20 mg vs. placebo	Flushing N/V/D, abdominal pain Infection Lymphopenia Increased LFTs	Prior to: CBC w/diff, LFTs During: CBC w/diff, LFTs (periodically)	PML: rare
Teriflunomide (2012)	PO daily (Aubagio)	31% (14 mg) TOWER vs. placebo	N/V Hair thinning Leukopenia Paresthesia Arthralgias Increased LFTs Increased blood pressure	Exclude pregnancy Prior to: TB screening, CBC w/diff, LFTs During: CBC w/diff, LFTs, blood pressure (periodically)	Contraindications: severe hepatic impairment, concomitant leflunomide, women reproductive age not using reliable contraception

Continued

DISEASE-MODIFYING THERAPIES IN MULTIPLE SCLEROSIS

DISEASE-MODIFYING THERAPIES IN MULTIPLE SCLEROSIS—CONT'D

Chemical name	Route & frequency of administration (trade name)	Annual relapse rate (% relative reduction) (phase III clinical trial)	Adverse effects	Monitoring	Additional pearls
Natalizumab (2006)	IV over 1 hr every 4 wk (**Tysabri**)	68% AFFIRM vs. placebo	Infusion reactions Fatigue Less common: hypersensitivity reactions (urticaria, dermatitis, bronchospasms) Rare: hepatic injury	*Prior to:* anti-JCV antibodies (and periodically during)	Accelerated elimination available **REMS required** *Contraindications:* PML (increased risk if: JCV positive, >2 yr natalizumab therapy, prior immunosuppressant use)
Mitoxantrone (2000)	IV Q3 months (**Novantrone**)		*Author's note:* infrequent use due to max lifetime dose associated & toxicities (cardiotoxicity, acute myeloid leukemia)		
Alemtuzumab (2014)	IV × 5 days, after 12 mo IV × 3 days (**Lemtrada**)	55% CARE-MS I vs. interferon beta-1a TIW	Rash Infusion reactions Infections (herpes virus) Autoimmune conditions (immune thrombocytopenia, anti-glomerular basement membrane disease)	*Prior to alemtuzumab:* CBC w/diff, Scr, urinalysis, TSH, skin exam *While receiving treatment & 48 mo post alemtuzumab:* Monthly: CBC w/diff, Scr,	**REMS required** *Contraindications:* HIV, concomitant antineoplastic or immunosuppressant therapies Start antiviral

| | | | Malignancies (thyroid cancer, melanoma, lymphoproliferative disorders) | urinalysis Quarterly: TSH Yearly: skin exams Exclude pregnancy | prophylaxis first day of treatment & continue at least 2 mo or until CD4 counts > 200 PML: none at this time in MS |
| Ocrelizumab (2017) | IV day 1, 15; followed by every IV 6 mo (Ocrevus) | 46% OPERA 1 vs. interferon beta-1a TIW | RRMS > 10%: URI, infusion reactions PPMS > 10%: URI, LRI, infusion reactions, skin infections Malignancies Herpes infections | Prior to: TB screening, Hepatitis B | 1st every medication approved for PPMS. Met primary & secondary study end points (ORATORIO). Contraindications: active hepatitis B infection PML: none per time of article composition in MS |

BID, Twice daily; CBC, complete blood count; CBC w/diff, complete blood count with differential; CIS, clinically isolated syndrome; EKG, electrocardiogram; FDO, first-dose observation; IM, intramuscular; IV, intravenous; JCV, JC virus; LFT, liver function test; LRI, lower respiratory infection; N/V/D, nausea/vomiting/diarrhea; PFS, prefilled syringe; PML, progressive multifocal leukoencephalopathy; PO, oral; PPMS, primary progressive multiple sclerosis; PRMS, progressive relapsing multiple sclerosis; QoD, every other day; QWK, every week; REMS, Risk Evaluation and Mitigation Strategy; RRMS, relapsing remitting multiple sclerosis; SPMS, secondary progressive multiple sclerosis; SQ, subcutaneous; TB, tuberculosis; TIW, three times weekly; TSH, thyroid stimulating hormone; ULN, upper limit of normal; URI, upper respiratory infection.

[a]Three times weekly, separated by at least 48 hr.

[b]Myocardial infarction (MI), unstable angina, stroke, transient ischemic attack (TIA), decompensated heart failure with hospitalization or classes III/IV heart failure.

DISEASE-MODIFYING THERAPIES IN MULTIPLE SCLEROSIS

REFERENCES

Aubagio package insert. http://products.sanofi.us/aubagio/aubagio.pdf. Accessed May 3, 2017.

Hauser, S. L., Bar-Or, A., Comi, G., et al. (2017). Ocrelizumab versus interferon beta-1a in relapsing multiple sclerosis. *N Engl J Med, 376*, 221–234.

SURGICAL THERAPY OF DIABETIC NEUROPATHY

USE OF SURGICAL DECOMPRESSION FOR TREATMENT OF DIABETIC NEUROPATHY

There are inadequate data concerning the efficacy of decompressive surgery for the treatment of diabetic neuropathy. Given current knowledge, this treatment is unproven (Level U).

REFERENCE

Utility of Surgical Decompression for treatment of Diabetic Neuropathy. http://tools.aan.com/professionals/practice/guidelines/surgicaldecom_clinician.pdf. Accessed April 12, 2017.

IMMUNOTHERAPY IN MANAGEMENT OF GUILLAIN-BARRÉ SYNDROME

EVIDENCE FOR IMMUNOTHERAPY IN GUILLAIN-BARRÉ SYNDROME (GBS) MANAGEMENT

	Plasma exchange (PE)	Intravenous immunoglobulin (IVIG)	Combined treatments	Corticosteroids
Strong evidence supports	PE recommended in nonambulatory patients within 4 wk of onset of neuropathic symptoms (Level A, class II)	IVIG recommended in nonambulatory patients within 2 wk of onset of neuropathic symptoms (Level A, class II)	Sequential treatment with PE followed by IVIG or vice versa does not have a greater effect than either treatment given alone (Level A, class II)	Steroids not recommended in the treatment of GBS (Level A, class I)
	PE		IVIG	
Good evidence supports	PE recommended for ambulatory patients within 2 wk of onset of neuropathic symptoms (Level B, class II) If PE started within 2 wk of onset, there are equivalent effects of PE and IVIG in patients requiring walking aids (Level B, class II) PE is a treatment option for children with severe GBS (Level B, derived from class II evidence in adults)		IVIG recommended in nonambulatory patients started within 4 wk from the onset of neuropathic symptoms (Level B, class II) If started within 2 wk of onset, IVIG has comparable efficacy to PE in patients requiring walking aids (Level B, class I) IVIG is a treatment option for children with severe GBS (Level B, derived from class II evidence in adults)	
		CEREBROSPINAL FLUID (CSF) FILTRATION	IMMUNOABSORPTION	
Evidence is insufficient to support	COMBINED TREATMENTS There is insufficient evidence to support or refute immunoabsorption treatment followed by IVIG (Level U, class IV) Insufficient evidence to combine corticosteroids with IVIG (Level U, class III)	There is insufficient evidence to support or refute the use of CSF filtration (Level U, limited class III)	The evidence is insufficient to support or refute immunoabsorption as an alternative to PE (Level U, class IV)	

TREATING PARKINSON DISEASE

RECOMMENDATIONS FOR MEDICATIONS THAT REDUCE OFF-TIME FOR PATIENTS WITH MOTOR FLUCTUATIONS

Strong Level A evidence: The following medications should be offered to reduce off-time in Parkinson disease (PD) patients with motor fluctuations:

- Entacapone
- Rasagiline

Good Level B evidence: The following medications should be considered to reduce off-time in PD patients with motor fluctuations:

- Pramipexole
- Tolcapone (should be used with caution and requires monitoring for hepatotoxicity)
- Ropinirole
- Pergolide (should be used with caution and requires monitoring for valvular fibrosis)

Weak Level C evidence: The following medications may be considered to reduce off-time in PD patients with motor fluctuations:

- Apomorphine injected subcutaneously
- Cabergoline
- Selegiline

Weak Level C evidence: The following medications may be disregarded to reduce off-time in PD patients with motor fluctuations:

- Sustained release carbidopa/levodopa and immediate-release carbidopa/levodopa
- Bromocriptine

RECOMMENDATIONS FOR THE RELATIVE EFFICACY OF MEDICATIONS THAT REDUCE OFF-TIME FOR PATIENTS WITH MOTOR FLUCTUATIONS

Weak Level C evidence: Ropinirole may be chosen over bromocriptine to reduce off-time in PD patients with motor fluctuations.

Insufficient Level U evidence: There is insufficient evidence to support or refute the use of any agent over another.

RECOMMENDATIONS FOR MEDICATIONS THAT REDUCE DYSKINESIA

Weak Level C evidence: Amantadine may be considered for patients with PD with motor fluctuations in reducing dyskinesia.

Insufficient Level U evidence: There is insufficient evidence to support or refute the efficacy of clozapine in reducing dyskinesia. Clozapine's potential toxicity, including agranulocytosis, seizures, myocarditis, and orthostatic hypotension with or without syncope, and required white blood cell count monitoring must be considered.

RECOMMENDATIONS FOR DEEP BRAIN STIMULATION (DBS)

	Recommendations for efficacy	Factors that predict improvement after DBS
DBS of the subthalamic nucleus (STN)	DBS of the STN may be considered as a treatment option in Parkinson disease (PD) patients to improve motor function and to reduce motor fluctuations, dyskinesia, and medication use (Level C). Patients need to be counseled regarding the risks and benefits of this procedure.	Based upon two class II studies, preoperative response to levodopa is probably predictive of postsurgical improvement. Preoperative response to levodopa should be considered as a factor predictive of outcome after DBS of the STN (Level B). Based on one class II study, younger age and shorter disease duration (<16 yr) are possibly predictive of greater improvement after DBS of the STN. Age and duration of PD may be considered as factors predictive of outcome after DBS of the STN. Younger patients with shorter disease duration may possibly have improvement greater than that of older patients with longer disease duration (Level C).
DBS of the globus pallidus interna (GPi)	There is insufficient evidence to make any recommendations about the effectiveness of DBS of the GPi in reducing motor complications or medication use or in improving motor function in PD patients (Level U).	There is insufficient evidence to make any recommendations about factors predictive of improvement after DBS of the GPi in PD patients (Level U).
DBS of the ventral intermediate (VIM) nucleus of the thalamus	There is insufficient evidence to make any recommendations about the effectiveness of DBS of the VIM nucleus of the thalamus in reducing motor complications or medication use or in improving motor function in PD patients (Level U).	There is insufficient evidence to make any recommendations about the effectiveness of DBS of the VIM nucleus of the thalamus in reducing motor complications or medication use or in improving motor function in PD patients (Level U).

TREATING PARKINSON DISEASE

REFERENCE

Pahwa, R., Factor, S. A., Lyons, K. E., et al. (2006). Practice Parameter: treatment of Parkinson disease with motor fluctuations and dyskinesia (an evidence-based review): report of the Quality Standards Subcommittee of the American Academy of Neurology. *Neurology, 66*(7), 983–995.

TREATING BEHAVIORAL CHANGES IN PARKINSON DISEASE

RECOMMENDATIONS FOR SCREENING FOR DEPRESSION, PSYCHOSIS, AND DEMENTIA

Depression

- The Beck Depression Inventory (BDI-I) and Hamilton Depression Rating Scale (HDRS-17) should be considered for depression screening in Parkinson disease (PD) (Level B).
- Montgomery Asberg Depression Rating Scale may be considered for screening for depression associated with PD (Level C).

Psychosis

- No recommendation is made.

Dementia

- The Mini-Mental State Examination and the Cambridge Cognitive Examination should be considered as screening tools for dementia in patients with PD (Level B).

RECOMMENDATIONS FOR TREATING DEPRESSION, PSYCHOSIS, AND DEMENTIA

Depression

- Amitriptyline may be considered in the treatment of depression associated with PD (Level C). Although the highest level of evidence is for amitriptyline, it is not necessarily the first choice for treatment of depression associated with PD.
- There is insufficient evidence to make recommendations regarding other treatments for depression in PD (Level U). Absence of literature demonstrating clear efficacy of nontricyclic antidepressants is not the same as absence of efficacy.

Psychosis

- Clozapine should be considered for patients with PD and psychosis (Level B). Clozapine use is associated with agranulocytosis and may be fatal. The absolute neutrophil count must be monitored.
- Olanzapine should not be routinely considered for patients with PD and psychosis (Level B).
- Quetiapine may be considered for patients with PD and psychosis (Level C).

Dementia

- Donepezil should be considered for the treatment of dementia in PD (Level B).
- Rivastigmine should be considered for the treatment of dementia in PD or dementia with Lewy bodies (DLB) (Level B).

STANDARDS OF TRANSCRANIAL DOPPLER APPLICATION

There are four standards for the application of transcranial Doppler (TCD):

I. TCD is able to provide information and clinical utility is established:

		Sensitivity %	Specificity %
Sickle cell disease	Screening of children aged 2– 16 yr with sickle cell disease for assessing stroke risk (type A, class I), although the optimal frequency of testing is unknown.	86	91
Angiographic vasospasm	Detection and monitoring of angiographic vasospasm after spontaneous subarachnoid hemorrhage (type A, class I–II). More data are needed to show if its use affects clinical outcomes (type U).		
	Intracranial ICA	25–30	83–91
	MCA	39–94	70–100
	ACA	13–71	65–100
	VA	44–100	42–79
	BA	77–100	42–79
	PCA	48–60	78–87

II. TCD is able to provide information, but clinical utility compared with other diagnostic tools remains to be determined:

		Sensitivity %	Specificity %
Cerebral thrombolysis	TCD is probably useful for monitoring thrombolysis of acute MCA occlusions (type B, class II–III). More data are needed to assess the frequency of monitoring for clot dissolution and enhanced recanalization and to influence therapy (type U).		
	Complete occlusion	50	100
	Partial occlusion	100	76
	Recanalization	91	93
Cerebral microembolism detection	TCD monitoring is probably useful for the detection of cerebral microembolic signals in a variety of cardiovascular/ cerebrovascular disorders/procedures (type B, class II–IV). Data do not support the use of this TCD technique for diagnosis or monitoring response to antithrombotic therapy in ischemic cerebrovascular disease (type U).		

STANDARDS OF TRANSCRANIAL DOPPLER APPLICATION

Carotid endarterectomy (CEA)	TCD monitoring is probably useful to detect hemodynamic and embolic events that may result in perioperative stroke during and after CEA in settings where monitoring is felt to be necessary (type B, class II–III).
Coronary artery bypass graft (CABG) surgery	TCD monitoring is probably useful (type B, class II–III) during CABG for detection of cerebral microemboli. TCD is possibly useful to document changes in flow velocities and CO_2 reactivity during CABG surgery (type C, class III). Data are insufficient regarding the clinical impact of this information (type U).
Vasomotor reactivity testing	TCD is probably useful (type B, class II–III) for the detection of impaired cerebral hemodynamics in patients with severe (>70%) asymptomatic extracranial ICA stenosis, symptomatic or asymptomatic extracranial ICA occlusion, and cerebral small artery disease. Whether these techniques should be used to influence therapy and improve patient outcomes remains to be determined (type U).
Vasospasm (VSP) after traumatic subarachnoid hemorrhage (SAH)	TCD is probably useful for the detection of VSP following traumatic SAH (type B, class III), but data are needed to show its accuracy and clinical impact in this setting (type U).
Transcranial color-coded sonography (TCCS)	TCCS is possibly useful (type C, class III) for the evaluation and monitoring of space-occupying ischemic MCA infarctions. More data are needed to show if it has greater value than computed tomography (CT) and magnetic resonance imaging (MRI) scanning and if its use affects clinical outcomes (type U).

III. TCD is able to provide information, but clinical utility remains to be determined:

		Sensitivity %	Specificity %
Intracranial steno-occlusive disease	TCD is probably useful (type B, class II–III) for the evaluation of occlusive lesions of intracranial arteries in the basal cisterns (especially the ICA siphon and MCA). The relative value of TCD compared with magnetic resonance (MR) angiography or CT angiography remains to be determined (type U). Data are insufficient to recommend replacement of conventional angiography with TCD (type U).		
	Anterior circulation	75–90	90–95
	Posterior circulation occlusion	50–80	80–96
	MCA	85–95	90–98
	ICA, VA, BA	55–81	96
Cerebral circulatory arrest (adjunctive test in the determination of brain death)	If needed, TCD can be used as a confirmatory test, in support of a clinical diagnosis of brain death (type A, class II).	91–100	97–100

IV. TCD is able to provide information, but other diagnostic tests are typically preferable:

		Sensitivity %	Specificity %
Right-to-left cardiac shunts	Although TCD is useful for detection of right-to-left cardiac and extracardiac shunts (type A, class II), transesophageal echocardiography is superior because it can provide direct information regarding the anatomic site and nature of the shunt.	70–100	>90
Extracranial ICA stenosis	TCD is possibly useful for the evaluation of severe extracranial ICA stenosis or occlusion (type C, class II–III), but in general, carotid duplex and MR angiography are the diagnostic tests of choice.		
	Single TCD variable	3–78	60–100
	MCA	49–95	42–100
	ACA	89	100
Contrast-enhanced TCCS (CE-TCCS)	CE-TCCS may provide information in patients with ischemic cerebrovascular disease and aneurysmal subarachnoid hemorrhage (SAH) (type B, class II–IV). Its clinical utility compared with CT scanning, conventional angiography, or nonimaging TCD is unclear (type U).		

V. Suggested vasospasm criteria based on:

	Mean cerebral blood flow velocities (MCBFVs) cm/s	Lindegaard ratio (MCA/ICA)
ICA and MCA		3–6
Mild	85–119	3–6
Moderate	120–150	>6
Severe	151–200	
Basilar Artery		Soustiel ratio (basilar artery/extracranial vertebral artery)
Mild	70–85	2–2.5
Moderate	>85	2.5–3
Severe	>85	>3

ACA, Anterior cerebral artery; BA, basilar artery; CE-TCCS, contrast enhanced transcranial color-coded sonography; CT, computed tomography; ECVA, extracranial vertebral artery; ICA, internal carotid artery; MCA, middle cerebral artery; MR, magnetic resonance; PCA, Posterior cerebral artery; SAH, subarachnoid hemorrhage; TCD, transcranial doppler ultrasound; VA, vertebral artery.

STANDARDS OF TRANSCRANIAL DOPPLER APPLICATION

REFERENCES

Csiba, L., & Baracchini, C. (Eds.), (2016). *Manual of neurosonology,* ed 1. Cambridge, UK: Cambridge University Press.

Mojadidi, M. K., et al. (2014). Accuracy of transcranial Doppler for the diagnosis of intracardiac right-to-left shunt: a bivariate meta-analysis of prospective studies. *JACC Cardiovas Imaging*, 7(3), 236–250.

STROKES GUIDELINES SUMMARY

Summary of American Heart Association/American Stroke Association (AHA/ ASA) guidelines for acute stroke management and secondary prevention

The 2015 AHA/ASA focused update of the 2013 guidelines for the early management of patients with acute ischemic stroke (AIS) regarding endovascular treatment:

Treatment with Intravenous Recombinant Tissue Plasminogen Activator (r-tPA)

- For patients who meet the eligibility guidelines, intravenous r-tPA should be administered for patients presenting within 4.5 hours of symptom onset.
- If patients who are eligible for intravenous r-tPA do not have intracranial vascular imaging as part of their initial evaluation, they should begin receiving intravenous r-tPA before being transported for additional imaging and prior to being transported for endovascular therapy.

Randomized Clinical Trials of Endovascular Treatment:

Endovascular Interventions:

- Patients eligible for intravenous r-tPA should receive it even if endovascular treatment is being considered
- Patients should receive endovascular therapy with stent retriever if they meet the following criteria
  a. Prestroke modified Rankin Scale (mRS) 0-1
  b. AIS receiving r-tPA within 4.5 hours of symptom onset.
  c. Causative occlusion of the internal carotid artery or proximal MCA (M1).
  d. Age $\geq$ 18
  e. NIHSS $\geq$ 6
  f. ASPECTS $\geq$ 6
  g. Treatment can be initiated within 6 hours of symptom onset.
- In carefully selected patients with anterior circulation occlusion who have contraindication to r-tPA, endovascular therapy with stent retrievers completed within 6 hours of stroke onset is reasonable (class IIa, Level of evidence C).
- In patients < 18, prestroke mRS > 1, NIHSS < 6, ASPECT < 6, or presenting beyond 6 hours, endovascular therapy with stent retriever may be reasonable.

Imaging:

- Emergency imaging of the brain is recommended before initiating any specific treatment for acute stroke. In most instances, CT without contrast will provide the necessary information.
- If endovascular therapy is contemplated, a noninvasive intracranial vascular imaging is strongly recommended during the initial imaging evaluation but should not delay r-tPA administration.

- The benefits of additional imaging beyond CT, and CTA or MR, and MRA such as CT perfusion, or diffusion and perfusion-weighted imaging for selecting patients for endovascular therapy are unknown.

Guidelines for the prevention of stroke in patients with stroke and transient ischemic attack:

1. **Risk factor control for all patients with TIA or ischemic stroke:**
    - Hypertension: Treatment of hypertension is possibly the most important intervention for secondary prevention of ischemic stroke. The AHA/ASA recommendations for HTN management are:
        a. Initiation of BP medication is indicated for previously untreated patients with AIS or TIA who after the first several days have an SBP ≥ 140 mm Hg or DBP ≥ 90.
        b. Goals of BP level or reduction from pretreatment baseline are uncertain, but it is reasonable to achieve SBP < 140 and DBP < 90.
        c. The available data indicate that diuretics or the combination of diuretics and an ACE inhibitor (ACEI) are useful first line BP regimen.
    - Dyslipidemia:
        a. Statin therapy with intensive lipid-lowering effects is recommended to reduce the risk of stroke and cardiovascular events among patients with AIS or TIA presumed to be due to atherosclerosis (even with LDL < 100 mg/dL) with or without evidence for other clinical ASCVD.
    - Disorders of Glucose Metabolism and DM:
        a. After a TIA or ischemic stroke, all patients should probably be screened for DM with testing of fasting plasma glucose, HbA1c, or an oral glucose tolerance test.
    - Overweight and Obesity:
        a. All patients with AIS or TIA should be screened for obesity with measurement of body mass index
    - Metabolic syndrome:
        a. The usefulness of screening patients for the metabolic syndrome following a stroke is uncertain.
    - Physical Inactivity:
        a. Patients with AIS or TIA who can engage in physical activity, at least three to four sessions per week of moderate to vigorous intensity aerobic physical exercise are reasonable to reduce stroke risk factors. Each session should last on average 40 minutes. Moderate exercise is defined as sufficient to break a sweat or increase heart rate.
        b. For patients who are able and willing to initiate increased physical activity, referral to a comprehensive program is reasonable.
        c. For individuals with disability after ischemic stroke, supervision by a healthcare professional such as a physical therapist or cardiac rehab professional may be considered.

Interventional Approaches for the Patients with Large Artery Atherosclerosis:

Extracranial carotid Disease:

Symptomatic Extracranial carotid disease:

a. Carotid endarterectomy (CEA) is recommended for patients with TIA or ischemic stroke within the past 6 months and ipsilateral (70% to 99%) carotid artery stenosis documented by noninvasive imaging.

b. CEA is recommended depending on patient's specific factors (age, sex, comorbidities, if perioperative risk < 6%) for patients with recent ischemic stroke or TIA and ipsilateral 50% to 69% carotid stenosis.

c. CEA or carotid artery stenting (CAS) are not recommended for stenosis < 50%.

d. It is reasonable to perform the revascularization procedure within 2 weeks of the index event unless there is a contraindication.

e. CAS is indicated as an alternative to CEA for symptomatic patients with > 50% stenosis and anticipated rate of per procedural stroke or death < 6%.

f. It is reasonable to choose CEA over CAS for patients older than 70 years given its association with improved outcome compared with CAS.

Extracranial Vertebrobasilar Disease Recommendations:

a. Routine preventative therapy including antiplatelet therapy, lipid lowering, BP control, and lifestyle optimization is recommended for all patients with recent symptomatic extracranial vertebral artery stenosis.

b. Endovascular stenting or open surgical procedures (vertebral endarterectomy and vertebral artery transposition) may be considered for patients who are having symptoms despite medical management.

Intracranial Atherosclerosis:

a. Plavix in addition to aspirin (ASA) might be reasonable for patients with recent stroke or TIA attributed to severe (70% to 99%) stenosis of a major intracranial artery.

b. For patients with symptomatic 50% to 99% stenosis of a major intracranial artery, achievement of SBP < 140, high-intensity statin therapy is recommended.

Medical treatment for patients with cardiogenic embolism:

a. Treatment with a vitamin K antagonist (VKA) therapy with INR target 2 to 3 for 3 months is recommended for all patients with ischemic stroke or TIA in the setting of acute MI complicated by left ventricular (LV) thrombus.

b. Treatment with VKA therapy may be considered for patents with ischemic stroke or TIA in the setting of acute anterior STEMI without LV thrombus but with anterior apical akinesis.

c. In patients with ischemic stroke or TIA in the setting of MI complicated by LV thrombus formation or anterior or apical wall–motion abnormalities with an EF < 40% who are intolerant to VKA therapy because of non-hemorrhagic adverse events, treatment with low-molecular-weight-heparin dabigatran, rivaroxaban, or apixaban for 3 months may be considered.

Cardiomyopathy:

a. In patients with ischemic stroke or TIA in the setting of LA thrombus, treatment with VKA is recommended for ≥ 3 months.

b. In patients with ischemic stroke or TIA in the setting of LVAD, treatment with VKA with INR goal 2 to 3 is reasonable.

Valvular Heart Disease:

a. For patients with ischemic stroke or TIA with rheumatic heart valve and AF, long-term therapy with VKA with INR goal 2 to 3 is recommended.

b. In patients with ischemic stroke or TIA who have rheumatic mitral valve disease without AF, long-term therapy with VKA may be considered.

c. For patients with rheumatic valve disease who have an ischemic stroke or TIA while being on adequate VKA therapy, the addition of aspirin might be considered.

d. For patients with mechanical aortic valve and history of ischemic stroke or TIA before its insertion, VKA therapy with INR 2 to 3 is recommended.

e. For patients with mechanical mitral valve and history of ischemic stroke or TIA before its insertion, VKA therapy with INR goal 2.5 to 3.5 is recommended.

f. Aspirin 75 to 100 mg is recommended in addition to VKA therapy in the previously described patients who are at low risk of bleeding.

Arterial Dissection Recommendations:

a. For patients with ischemic stroke or TIA due to extracranial dissection, either antiplatelet or anticoagulant therapy for at least 3 to 6 months is reasonable.

b. Endovascular therapy may be considered in the previously described patients when medical therapy fails.

c. Surgical treatment may be considered in the previously described patients if they are not candidates for endovascular treatment.

Patent Foramen Ovale:

a. For patients with ischemic stroke or TIA and PFO, antiplatelet therapy is recommended.

b. In the previously described patients, anticoagulation (AC) is indicated when there is a venous source of embolism.

    c. There is no evidence to support PFO closure in the setting of cryptogenic stroke or TIA and a PFO.

Sickle Cell Disease (SCD):

    a. Chronic blood transfusions are recommended for patients with SCD and prior ischemic stroke or TIA to reduce Hb S < 30%.

    b. In the previously described patients, and if blood transfusion is not available, treatment with hydroxyurea is reasonable.

Cerebral Venous Sinus Thrombosis (CVST):

    a. AC is reasonable for patients with acute CVST even in selected patients with intracerebral hemorrhage (ICH).

Guidelines for the Management of Spontaneous ICH:

Emergency Diagnosis and Assessment Recommendations:

    a. A baseline severity score should be performed as part of the initial evaluation of patients with ICH.

    b. CTA and CT with contrast may be considered to help identifying patients for risk for hematoma expansion.

Medical Treatment for ICH

    a. In patients with ICH and elevated INR due to VKA therapy, VKA therapy should be withheld; they should receive IV vitamin K and vitamin K factor–dependent replacement.

    b. In patients with ICH who are on dabigatran, rivaroxaban, or apixaban, treatment with FEIBA, other PCC, or rFVIIa might be considered.

    c. In patients with ICH and on heparin, protamine sulfate may be considered.

    d. Patients with ICH should have intermittent pneumatic compression for prevention of venous thromboembolism beginning the day of hospital admission. After documentation of cessation of bleeding, low-dose subcutaneous heparin may be considered for prevention of thromboembolism in patients with lack of mobility after 1 to 4 days from onset.

    e. In patients with ICH who are found to have deep vein thrombosis or pulmonary embolism, systemic AC or inferior vena cava filter placement is probably indicated.

Blood pressure and outcome in ICH:

    a. In patients with ICH presenting with SBP 150 to 220 mm Hg and without a contraindication to acute BP treatment, acute lowering to 140 is safe.

    b. In the previously described patients, if SBP > 220, it may be reasonable to consider aggressive reduction of BP with continuous infusion and frequent BP monitoring.

Seizures and antiseizure drugs:

    a. Continuous EEG monitoring is probably indicated in ICH patients with depressed mental status that is out of proportion to the brain injury.

    b. Prophylactic antiseizure treatment is not recommended.

ICP monitoring and treatment:

    a. Patients with Glasgow Coma Scale $\leq$ 8, those with clinical evidence of transtentorial herniation, or significant IVH or hydrocephalus might be considered for ICP monitoring and treatment.

Surgical Treatment of ICH:

    a. Patients with cerebellar hemorrhage who are deteriorating neurologically or with brainstem compression and/or hydrocephalus from ventricular obstruction should undergo surgical evacuation of the hemorrhage ASAP.

    b. The usefulness of surgery is not well established for most patients with supratentorial ICH.

    c. Decompressive craniectomy with or without hematoma evacuation might reduce mortality for patients with supratentorial ICH who are in coma, have large hematoma with significant midline shift, or have elevated ICH refractory to medical management.

Prevention of recurrent ICH:

    a. Long-term BP goal should be < 130/80 mm Hg.

    b. Avoidance of long-term AC with warfarin as the treatment of nonvalvular atrial fibrillation is probably recommended in patients with lobar ICH.

    c. In nonlobar ICH, AC and antiplatelet monotherapy after any ICH might be considered.

    d. The optimal timing to resume AC, after AC-related ICH, is uncertain. Avoidance for at least 4 weeks in patients without mechanical valves might decrease the risk of ICH recurrence.

REFERENCES

Hemphill, J. C., et al. (2015). Guidelines for the management of spontaneous intracerebral hemorrhage. *Stroke, 46*(7), 2032–2060.

Powers, W. J., et al. (2015). AHA/ASA focused update of the 2013 guidelines for the early management of patients with acute ischemic stroke regarding endovascular treatment. *Stroke*. STR-0000000000000074.

Neurologic Emergency Appendix

ACUTE ISCHEMIC STROKE

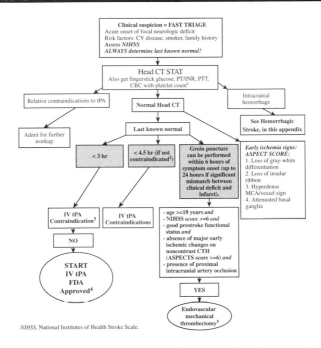

NIHSS, National Institutes of Health Stroke Scale.

1. Additional work-up is indicated, including but not limited to electrolytes with renal function studies, cardiac markers, and electrocardiogram (EKG). However, administration of tissue plasminogen activator (tPA) should not be delayed to obtain these additional tests.

2. Contraindications to intravenous recombinant tissue plasminogen activator (IV r-TPA) in the 3- to 4.5-hour window: age > 80 years, National Institutes of Health Stroke Scale (NIHSS) > 25, taking an oral anticoagulant regardless of international normalized ratio (INR), history of both diabetes, and prior ischemic stroke.

3. Relative contraindications to IV tPA: age < 18 years, systolic blood pressure (SBP) > 185 mm Hg or diastolic blood pressure (DBP) > 110 mm Hg, blood glucose (BG) < 50, INR > 1.7, platelets < 100,000/mm^3, low molecular weight heparin (LMWH) within 24 hours, novel oral anticoagulant (NOAC) use within 48 hours, active internal bleeding, previous/recent intracerebral hemorrhage (ICH), severe head trauma within 3 months, recent intracranial or intraspinal surgery (within

3 months), computed tomography (CT) showing hypodensity > 1/3 of the cerebral hemisphere.

4. IV r-tPA dose: 0.9 mg/kg (maximum dose of 90 mg); 10% as a bolus and the remainder infused over 1 hour.

5. Patients eligible for IV tPA should receive IV tPA even if endovascular treatment is being considered.

REFERENCES

Powers, W. J., Rabinstein, A. A., Ackerson, T., et al. (2018). 2018 guidelines for the early management of patients with acute ischemic stroke: a guideline for healthcare professionals from the American Heart Association/American Stroke Association. *Stroke, 49*(3), e46–e110.

Nogueira, R.G., Jadhav, A.P., Haussen, D.C., et al. (2018). Thrombectomy 6 to 24 Hours after Stroke with a Mismatch between Deficit and Infarct. *N Engl J Med, 378*, 11–21.

BACTERIAL MENINGITIS AND SEVERE ENCEPHALITIS

Treatment starts with the empiric antibiotics (ceftriaxone, vancomycin, ampicillin, metronidazole, acyclovir).

NEUROCRITICAL CARE

- In patients with a high risk of brain herniation, consider monitoring intracranial pressure and intermittent administration of osmotic diuretics (mannitol [25%] or hypertonic [3%] saline) to maintain an intracranial pressure below 15 mm Hg and a cerebral perfusion pressure of at least 60 mm Hg.
- Initiate repeated lumbar puncture, lumbar drain, or ventriculostomy in patients with acute hydrocephalus.
- Use electroencephalography (EEG) to monitor patients with a history of seizures and fluctuating scores on the Glasgow coma scale (GCS). Scores on the GCS range from 3 to 15, with 15 indicating a normal level of consciousness.

AIRWAY AND RESPIRATORY CARE

- Intubate or provide noninvasive ventilation in patients with worsening consciousness (clinical and laboratory indicators for intubation include poor cough and pooling secretions, a respiratory rate greater than 35 breaths per minute, arterial oxygen saturation below 90% or arterial partial pressure of oxygen above 60 mm Hg, and arterial partial pressure of carbon dioxide above 60 mm Hg).
- Maintain ventilatory support with intermittent mandatory ventilation, pressure-support ventilation, or continuous positive airway pressure.

CIRCULATORY CARE

- In patients with septic shock, administer low doses of corticosteroids (if there is a poor response on corticotropin testing indicating adrenocorticoid insufficiency, corticosteroids should be continued).
- Initiate inotropic agents (dopamine or milrinone) to maintain blood pressure (mean arterial pressure, 70 to 100 mm Hg).

- Initiate crystalloids or albumin (5%) to maintain adequate fluid balance.
- Consider the use of a Swan-Ganz catheter to monitor hemodynamic measurements.

GASTROINTESTINAL CARE
- Initiate nasogastric tube feeding of a standard nutrition formula.
- Initiate prophylaxis with proton-pump inhibitors.

OTHER SUPPORTIVE CARE
- Administer subcutaneous heparin as prophylaxis against deep venous thrombosis.
- Maintain normoglycemic state (serum glucose level <150 mg/dL) with the use of sliding-scale regimens of insulin or continuous intravenous administration of insulin.
- In patients with a body temperature above 40°C, use cooling by conduction or antipyretic agents.

MYASTHENIC CRISIS
OVERVIEW
- Myasthenic crisis is defined as a serious, life-threatening, rapid worsening of myasthenia gravis (MG) and potential airway compromise from ventilatory or bulbar dysfunction. It usually occurs within the first few years after disease onset and may be the presenting symptom. In the latter, the diagnosis of MG should be pursued—generally with a combination of history and examination as well as serologic and electrophysiologic studies.
- Common triggers of myasthenic crisis include infection, surgery (e.g., thymectomy), hormonal changes (e.g., pregnancy), tapering of MG medications, high doses of steroids, and use of medications that impair neuromuscular transmission (including aminoglycosides, quinolones, macrolides and, possibly, magnesium, beta-blockers, procainamide, and quinine).
- Cholinergic crises are rare but often cannot be fully excluded as a cause of clinical worsening. However, it should be assumed that the worsening is due to decompensation of MG unless there is evident overdosing of anticholinesterase medications.

MANAGEMENT
- Admit to intensive care unit
- Monitor respiratory function closely
  - Measure forced vital capacity (FVC) and negative inspiratory force (NIF) every 2 to 4 hours
  - Watch for signs and symptoms of respiratory distress (dyspnea, tachypnea, pausing during speech, use of accessory muscles of

respiration) and inability to clear secretions (severe dysphagia, weak cough, refractory hypoxia due to mucus plugging)
- Pulse oximetry and ABG abnormalities (e.g., hypercarbia and hypoxemia) are late developing signs and, therefore, insensitive measures of respiratory distress
- Noninvasive positive pressure ventilation (NIPPV, bilevel positive airway pressure [BiPAP]) may be used to prevent intubation in patients who have adequate cough and can tolerate the mask
- Consider elective intubation and mechanical ventilation if at least one of the following is present:
  - FVC < 20 mL/kg ideal body weight
  - NIF < 30 cm H_2O
  - Clinical signs of respiratory distress
  - Progressive respiratory acidosis
  - Inability to clear secretions
  - Failure to respond to NIPPV
- Regarding nonemergent intubation, ultrashort- or short-acting sedatives, hypnotics, and anesthetic agents are indicated. When rapid sequence intubation is required, either depolarizing or non-depolarizing neuromuscular blocking agents (NMBA) may be used. Importantly, in MG, depolarizing NMBA should be given at slightly higher doses (for example, succinylcholine 2 mg/kg IV), whereas non-depolarizing NMBA should be given at slightly lower doses (for example, rocuronium 0.6 mg/kg IV). The optimal mode of mechanical ventilation is unclear and should, therefore, be tailored to each patient.
- Following intubation, cholinesterase inhibitor therapy should be temporarily discontinued (to avoid excessive airway secretions) and pulmonary toilet optimized.
- Initiate immunomodulatory therapy with plasma exchange (PLEX) or IVIG
  - PLEX: five exchange treatments (3 to 5 L of plasma each) over 10 to 14 days
  - IVIG: 400 mg/kg for 5 days (total dose of 2 g/kg)
  - PLEX and IVIG are similarly effective, although PLEX may have a faster onset of action. Choosing between these two therapies depends on availability and patients' comorbidities.
- Initiate immunosuppressive therapy
  - Immunosuppressive therapy should be started concomitantly to achieve a sustained clinical response
  - Start high-dose steroids (60 to 80 mg/day)
    - If the patient is not intubated, consider delaying initiation of steroids (since high-dose steroids are associated with a transient worsening of weakness)
    - If there are contraindications to steroids, consider starting another immunosuppressant agent (e.g., azathioprine, mycophenolate)

- Treat underlying precipitant(s), discontinue/avoid medications that may impair neuromuscular transmission
- Following initiation of immunomodulatory and immunosuppressive therapies and resultant clinical improvement (FVC > 20 mL/kg and NIF < 30 cm H_2O, adequate cough and clearance of secretions), consider weaning from ventilatory support with spontaneous breathing trials

REFERENCE

Sanders, D. B., Wolfe, G. I., Benatar, M., et al. (2016). International consensus guidance for management of myasthenia gravis: executive summary. *Neurology, 87,* 419–425.

HEADACHE MANAGEMENT

APPROACH TO THE HEADACHE

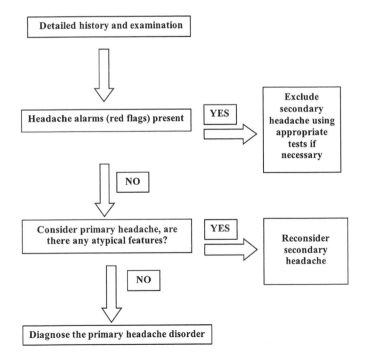

DIAGNOSIS OF HEADACHE

RED FLAGS IN THE DIAGNOSIS OF HEADACHE

Red flag	Consider	Possible investigation(s)
Sudden-onset headache	Subarachnoid hemorrhage, bleed into a mass or arteriovenous malformation (AVM), mass lesion (especially posterior fossa)	Neuroimaging, lumbar puncture (after neuroimaging evaluation)
Worsening-pattern headache	Mass lesion, subdural hematoma, medication overuse	Neuroimaging
Headache with systemic illness (fever, neck stiffness, cutaneous rash)	Meningitis, encephalitis, Lyme disease, systemic infection, collagen vascular disease, arteritis	Neuroimaging, lumbar puncture, biopsy, blood tests
Focal neurologic signs, or symptoms other than typical visual or sensory aura	Mass lesion, AVM, collagen vascular disease	Neuroimaging, collagen vascular evaluation
Papilledema	Mass lesion, pseudotumor, encephalitis, meningitis	Neuroimaging, lumbar puncture (after neuroimaging evaluation)
Triggered by cough, exertion, or Valsalva maneuver	Subarachnoid hemorrhage, mass lesion	Neuroimaging, consider lumbar puncture
Headache during pregnancy or post partum	Cortical vein/cranial sinus thrombosis, carotid dissection, pituitary apoplexy	Neuroimaging
New headache type in a patient with cancer, Lyme disease, or HIV	Metastasis, meningoencephalitis, opportunistic infection, tumor	Neuroimaging, lumbar puncture (after neuroimaging evaluation)

HEADACHE MANAGEMENT

INTERNATIONAL HEADACHE SOCIETY CLASSIFICATION OF MIGRAINE HEADACHE
1 Migraine without aura
   1.2 Migraine with aura
       1.2.1 Migraine with typical aura
       1.2.2 Migraine with prolonged aura
       1.2.3 Familial hemiplegic migraine
       1.2.4 Basilar migraine
       1.2.5 Migraine aura without headache
       1.2.6 Migraine with acute onset aura

HEMORRHAGIC STROKE, INTRACRANIAL HEMORRHAGE, SUBARACHNOID HEMORRHAGE, SEE STROKE

Hemorrhagic strokes account for about 15% of all strokes. The most commonly encountered neurological emergencies of hemorrhagic stroke are subarachnoid hemorrhage (SAH) and intracerebral hemorrhage (ICH). ICH is commonly seen with uncontrolled hypertension and located in the typical deep location such as basal ganglia, brainstem, and cerebellum. On the other hand, lobar ICH is commonly caused by amyloid angiopathy, tumor (primary or metastatic), infectious such as herpes encephalitis, and anticoagulation/coagulopathy. Common tumors that lead to hemorrhagic metastasis are lung cancer, breast cancer, renal cell carcinoma, and melanoma. The most important factor in predicting outcome following ICH is the volume of the hematoma. Estimating the ICH score that takes into account the hematoma volume, patient age, Glasgow coma scale on admission, and ICH location may help in prognostication (see "Stroke" chapter).

Spontaneous SAH is commonly caused by ruptured cerebral aneurysm and leads to prolonged hospital course and complications. The most common events following SAH are: obstructive hydrocephalus, rebleeding, seizure, sedation, dry mouth stomatitis, hyponatremia, vasospasm, and strokes. Management focuses on blood pressure (BP) control for both ICH and SAH and treating the underlying etiology (see ICH and SAH chapters).

Patient Presenting With Signs And Symptoms Suggestive of Spontaneous Hemorrhagic Stroke

STAT Head CT

Subarachnoid Hemorrhage (SAH)

Intracranial Hemorrhage (ICH)

Admit to NEURO INTENSIVE CARE UNIT
GENERAL TREATMENT

1. Intubate if Glasgow coma scale < 8
2. Hyperventilate, osmotic therapy, nonsurgical consult for impending herniation
3. Immediate blood pressure control:
   Systolic BP ~130 mm Hg
   a. Labetalol 10 mg for SAH and < 160 mm Hg for ICH IV q 10 min (hold if HR < 60), may repeat as necessary
   b. Nicardipine drip 3–5 mg/hr; titrate to goal
4. Seizure prophylaxis:
   a. Phenytoin or Levetiracetam
   b. Valproic acid, Carbamazepine
5. Pain control and analgesia
6. Nimodipine 60 mg q 4 hr for SAH
7. Start neurointerventional and neurosurgery consult if aneurysmal or vascular malformation related SAH

SAH EVALUATION
1. CT angiogram (CTA) in the emergency room
2. If CTA negative: Cerebral angiogram (DSA)
3. (See the figure in next page.)

ICH EVALUATION
1. Consider MRI in suspicious lobar and cortical cases
2. Consider conventional angiogram in patient without history of hypertension.

1. General ICU management: DVT, GI prophylaxis, nutritional support, ventilator management, infection control
2. Neuroprotective measures:
   Temperature controls
   Tight glucose controls
   Magnesium > 2.5
   Adequate CPP
3. Cerebral edema management
4. Hydrocephalus management, if present, with external ventriculostomy drainage.

HEMORRHAGIC STROKE

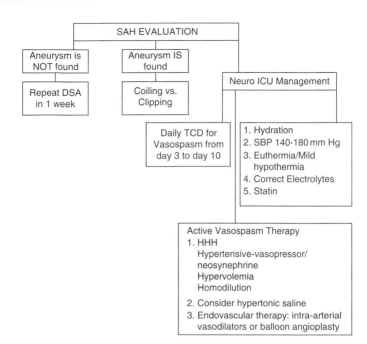

REFERENCES

Long, B., Koyfman, A., & Runyon, M. S. (2017). Subarachnoid hemorrhage: updates in diagnosis and management. *Emerg Med Clin North Am*. *35*(4), 803–824.

Zhao, Y. N., & Chen, X. L. (2016). Endoscopic treatment of hypertensive intracerebral hemorrhage: a technical review. *Chronic Dis Transl Med*. *2*(3), 140–146.

INTRACRANIAL PRESSURE MANAGEMENT

Current guidelines for the management of increased intracranial pressure (ICP) recommend maintaining an ICP <20 mm Hg as well as maintaining a cerebral perfusion pressure (CPP) between 50 and 70 mm Hg, depending on the status of cerebral pressure autoregulation. In general, patients with increased ICP should be mechanically ventilated with adequate sedation and analgesia. Ventilator settings should be adjusted to maintain normocapnia; prophylactic hyperventilation is not recommended, although brief periods of mild hyperventilation ($PaCO_2$ 30 to 35 mm Hg) can be used to treat acute neurological deterioration caused by increased ICP.

Core body temperature should be maintained at normothermia to slight hypothermia (36.5 to 37 °C). The mainstay of medical management of increased ICP is osmotic therapy, including administration of mannitol and hypertonic saline. Mannitol 20% is given as an intravenous bolus of 0.25 to1 g/kg. This can be repeated as needed for sustained elevations in ICP if serum osmolality is less than 330 milliosmoles (mOsm). Mannitol must be used cautiously, because the subsequent osmotic diuresis can lead to hypovolemia, decreased cardiac preload, and hypotension, which could compromise CPP, lead to vasodilation, and increase ICP again. Hypertonic saline may be used instead of mannitol. Dosing includes a 30-mL bolus of 23.4% solution via a central line. Alternatively, a 250-mL bolus of 3% solution (also through a central line) or 2% solution (through a peripheral line) can be given followed by a continuous infusion at the rate of 30 to 150 mL/hr. The target serum sodium is between 150 and 160 mEq/L.

An essential step of a raised ICP management is offering neurosurgical interventions if indicated. It depends on the lesion, but this includes external ventricular drain placement, which can be diagnostic and therapeutic (measures ICP and drains cerebrospinal fluid volume to reduce ICP), craniotomy, and mass lesion resection (e.g., intracranial hemorrhage or brain tumor).

The patient, or more commonly, family members, need to be informed as to course and prognosis as it develops within limits of legal disclosure and to help facilitate care planning.

INTRACRANIAL PRESSURE MANAGEMENT

Signs and symptoms of increased ICP:
Change in mental status, headache, papilledema, diplopia, or focal deficit, Cushing's triad of bradycardia, hypertension, and slowing of respiration

CT head

If Indicated

Surgical Interventions:

External ventricular drain placement

Craniotomy

Evacuation and mass resection

ICU Monitoring

Medical Therapy:

Airway management GCS<8

ICP goal <20 and CPP goal 50-70

Mild hyperventilation CO_2 30-35 mmHg

Temperature goal of 36.5–37°C

Osmotherapy (Mannitol, hypertonic saline)

Sedation and neuromuscular blockade in refractory ICP

Hypothermia and barbiturate in refractory increased ICP cases

REFERENCES

Alkhacroum, A., & De Georgia, A. (2017). General treatment of stroke in intensive care setting. In L. R. Caplan, J. Biller, & M. C. Leary, et al. (Eds.), *Primer on cerebrovascular diseases* (p. 2). San Diego: Academic Press.

Freeman, W. D. Management of intracranial pressure. *CONTINUUM Lifelong Learn Neurol. 21*(5):1299–1323.

INTOXICATION, ALCOHOL, AND ILLICIT DRUGS

Substance intoxication is a type of substance use disorder which is potentially maladaptive and impairing, but reversible, and associated with recent use. If the symptoms are severe, the term *substance intoxication delirium* is a mental health condition that occurs when the accumulation of drugs, medications, or alcohol in the bloodstream leads to a delirious, disoriented state of mind. Symptoms of substance-induced disorders run the gamut from mild anxiety and depression to full-blown mania and other psychotic reactions. Because every drug's biochemical effect interacts with a person's psychological expectations for using the drug and the social setting within which the use occurs, predication of how they respond to both intoxication and withdrawal, given the same exposure to the same substance, has its limits. The following is a brief and introductory description of the most common categories of drugs.

Most substance-induced symptoms begin to improve within hours or days after substance use has stopped. Notable exceptions to this are psychotic symptoms caused by heavy and long-term amphetamine abuse and substances directly toxic to the brain, which most commonly include alcohol, inhalants like gasoline, and amphetamines. Withdrawal symptoms for opiates, while unpleasant, are rarely fatal. In contrast, withdrawal from alcohol or benzodiazepines carries significant risk of morbidity and mortality.

INTOXICATION, ALCOHOL, AND ILLICIT DRUGS

SUBSTANCE ABUSE, EFFECTS, AND RISKS

Substances: category and name	Examples of commercial and street names	DEA schedule/ how administered	Acute effects/health risks
TOBACCO			
Nicotine	Found in cigarettes, cigars, bidis, and smokeless tobacco (snuff, spit tobacco, chew)	Not scheduled/ smoked, snorted, chewed	Increased blood pressure and heart rate/chronic lung disease; cardiovascular disease; stroke; cancers of the mouth, pharynx, larynx, esophagus, stomach, pancreas, cervix, kidney, bladder, and acute myeloid leukemia; adverse pregnancy outcomes; addiction
ALCOHOL			
Alcohol (ethyl alcohol)	Found in liquor, beer, and wine	Not scheduled/ swallowed	In low doses, euphoria, mild stimulation, relaxation, lowered inhibitions; in higher doses, drowsiness, slurred speech, nausea, emotional volatility, loss of coordination, visual distortions, impaired memory, sexual dysfunction, loss of consciousness/increased risk of injuries, violence, fetal damage (in pregnant women); depression; neurologic deficits; hypertension; liver and heart disease; addiction; fatal overdose; potentially fatal withdrawal.
CANNABINOIDS			
Marijuana	Blunt, dope, ganja, grass, herb, joint, bud, Mary Jane, pot, reefer, green, trees, smoke, sinsemilla, skunk, weed	I/smoked, swallowed	Euphoria; relaxation; slowed reaction time; distorted sensory perception; impaired balance and coordination; increased heart rate and appetite; impaired learning, memory; anxiety; panic attacks; psychosis/cough; frequent respiratory infections; possible mental health decline; addiction
Hashish	Boom, gangster, hash, hash oil, hemp	I/smoked, swallowed	

OPIOIDS

Prescription opiates	Oxycodone, oxycontin, morphine, codeine, hydromorphone, etc.	II/swallowed, snorted, injected	Euphoria; drowsiness; impaired coordination; dizziness; confusion; nausea; sedation; feeling of heaviness in the body; slowed or arrested breathing/ constipation; endocarditis; hepatitis; HIV; addiction; fatal overdose
Heroin	Diacetylmorphine: smack, horse, brown sugar, dope, H, junk, skag, skunk, white horse, China white; cheese (with OTC cold medicine and antihistamine)	I/injected, smoked, snorted	
Opium	Laudanum, paregoric: big O, black stuff, block, gum, hop	II, III, V/swallowed, smoked	

STIMULANTS

Cocaine	Cocaine hydrochloride: blow, bump, C, candy, Charlie, coke, crack, flake, rock, snow, toot	II/snorted, smoked, injected	Increased heart rate, blood pressure, body temperature, metabolism; feelings of exhilaration; increased energy, mental alertness; tremors; reduced appetite; irritability; anxiety; panic; paranoia; violent behavior; psychosis/weight loss; insomnia; cardiac or cardiovascular complications; stroke; seizures; addiction
Amphetamine	Biphetamine, Dexedrine: bennies, black beauties, crosses, hearts, LA turnaround, speed, truck drivers, uppers	II/swallowed, snorted, smoked, injected	
Methamphetamine	Desoxyn: meth, ice, crank, chalk, crystal, fire, glass, go fast, speed	II/swallowed, snorted, smoked, injected	Also, for cocaine—nasal damage from snorting Also, for methamphetamine—severe dental problems

Continued

INTOXICATION, ALCOHOL, AND ILLICIT DRUGS

SUBSTANCE ABUSE, EFFECTS, AND RISKS—CONT'D

Substances: category and name	Examples of commercial and street names	DEA schedule/ how administered	Acute effects/health risks
CLUB DRUGS			
MDMA (methylenedioxy methamphetamine)	Ecstasy, Adam, clarity, Eve, lover's speed, peace, uppers	I/swallowed, snorted, injected	*Mild hallucinogenic effects; increased tactile sensitivity, empathic feelings; lowered inhibition; anxiety; chills; sweating; teeth clenching; muscle cramping/sleep disturbances; depression; impaired memory; hyperthermia; addiction*
Flunitrazepam	Rohypnol: forget-me pill, Mexican Valium, R2, roach, Roche, roofies, roofinol, rope, rophies	IV/swallowed, snorted	*Sedation; muscle relaxation; confusion; memory loss; dizziness; impaired coordination/addiction*
GHB	Gamma-hydroxybutyrate: G, Georgia home boy, grievous bodily harm, liquid ecstasy, soap, scoop, goop, liquid X	I/swallowed	*Drowsiness; nausea; headache; disorientation; loss of coordination; memory loss/ unconsciousness; seizures; coma*
DISSOCIATIVE DRUGS			
Ketamine	Ketalar SV: cat Valium, K, Special K, vitamin K	III/injected, snorted, smoked	Feelings of being separate from one's body and environment; impaired motor function/anxiety; tremors; numbness; memory loss; nausea
PCP and analogs	Phencyclidine: angel dust, boat, hog, love boat, peace pill	I, II/swallowed, smoked, injected	Also, for ketamine—*analgesia; impaired memory; delirium; respiratory depression and arrest; death*
Salvia divinorum	Salvia, Shepherdess's Herb, Maria Pastora, magic mint, Sally-D	Not scheduled/ chewed, swallowed, smoked	Also, for PCP and analogs—*analgesia; psychosis; aggression; violence; slurred speech; loss of coordination; hallucinations*
Dextromethorphan (DXM)	Found in some cough and cold medications: Robotripping, Robo, Triple C	Not scheduled/ swallowed	Also, for DXM—*euphoria; slurred speech; confusion; dizziness; distorted visual perceptions*

HALLUCINOGENS

Drug	Names	Route	Effects
LSD	Lysergic acid diethylam de: acid, blotter, cubes, microdot, yellow sunshine, blue heaven	I/swallowed, absorbed through mouth tissues	Altered states of perception and feeling; hallucinations; nausea Also, for LSD and mescaline—*increased body temperature, heart rate, blood pressure; loss of appetite; sweating; sleeplessness; numbness; dizziness; weakness; tremors; impulsive behavior; rapid shifts in emotion* Also, for LSD—Flashbacks, Hallucinogen Persisting Perception Disorder Also, for psilocybin—*nervousness; paranoia; panic*
Mescaline	Buttons, cactus, mesc, peyote	I/swallowed, smoked	
Psilocybin	Magic mushrooms, purple passion, shrooms, little smoke	I/swallowed	

OTHER COMPOUNDS

Drug	Names	Route	Effects
Anabolic steroids	Anadrol, Oxandrin, Durabolin, Depo-Testosterone, Equipoise: roids, juice, gym candy, pumpers	III/injected, swallowed, applied to skin	Steroids—*no intoxication effects*/hypertension; blood clotting and cholesterol changes; liver cysts; hostility and aggression; acne; in adolescents—premature stoppage of growth; in males—prostate cancer, reduced sperm production, shrunken testicles, breast enlargement; in females—menstrual irregularities, development of beard and other masculine characteristics
Inhalants	Solvents (paint thinners, gasoline, glues): gases (butane, propane, aercsol propellants, nitrous oxide); nitrites (isoamyl, isobutyl, cyclohexyl): laughing gas, poppers, snappers, wr ippets	Not scheduled/ inhaled through nose or mouth	Inhalants (varies by chemical)—*stimulation; loss of inhibition; headache; nausea; cardiac and CNS toxicity; potentially fatal*

REFERENCES

Donroe, J. H., & Tetrault, J. M. (2017). Substance use, intoxication, and withdrawal in the critical care setting. *Crit Care Clin*, *33*(3), 543–558.

Ford, J. B., Sutter, M. E., Owen, K. P., & Albertson, T. E. (2014). Volatile substance misuse: an updated review of toxicity and treatment. *Clinic Rev Allerg Immunol*, *46*, 19–33.

NEUROMUSCULAR DISEASES

Suggested respiratory parameters:

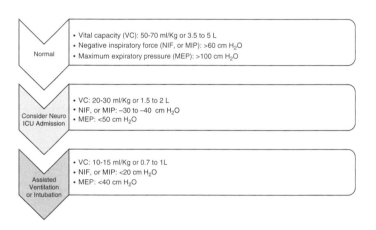

Normal
- Vital capacity (VC): 50-70 ml/Kg or 3.5 to 5 L
- Negative inspiratory force (NIF, or MIP): >60 cm H_2O
- Maximum expiratory pressure (MEP): >100 cm H_2O

Consider Neuro ICU Admission
- VC: 20-30 ml/Kg or 1.5 to 2 L
- NIF, or MIP: −30 to −40 cm H_2O
- MEP: <50 cm H_2O

Assisted Ventilation or Intubation
- VC: 10-15 ml/Kg or 0.7 to 1L
- NIF, or MIP: <20 cm H_2O
- MEP: <40 cm H_2O

NEUROPATHIC PAIN

Neuropathic pain is becoming a larger part of the medical burden regarding cost, time, and morbidity. It is imperative that neurologists be able to treat these conditions adequately.

Definition: pain arising as a direct consequence of a lesion or disease affecting the somatosensory system. This was set by the International Association for the Study of Pain special interest group on neuropathic pain (NeuPSIG) in 2008.

Epidemiology: About 10% of the population complains of neuropathic pain. It is more common in women (8% vs. 5.7%), more common >50 years old, and commonly affects the lower back, lower limbs, cervical spine, and other regions.

Etiology

Central: Cerebrovascular insult, neurodegenerative disease (e.g., Parkinson disease, Alzheimer disease), spinal cord injury, demyelinating disease, etc.

Peripheral: Diabetes mellitus, human immunodeficiency virus, auto-immune/inflammatory (e.g., Guillain-Barré), inherited channelopathies (e.g., inherited erythromelalgia), medications (e.g., chemotherapy), etc.

In either case, changes in pain signaling, ion channels, inhibitory/modulatory neurons, and mechanisms occur.

Diagnosis: Diagnosis is POSSIBLE when there is a relevant lesion or neuroanatomically plausible distribution. Diagnosis is PROBABLE when there are the above AND pain/sensory signs in the relevant distribution on exam. Diagnosis is DEFINITE when there is the above AND confirmatory testing is positive (e.g., laser-evoked potentials, quantitative sensory testing, electrophysiological testing, corneal microscopy, or skin biopsy).

There are also a multitude of validated screening tools available.

Treatment options:

Medical:

First-line therapies–tricyclic antidepressants such as amitriptyline; serotonin-noradrenalin reuptake inhibitors such as duloxetine, pregabalin, gabapentin

Second-line therapies–lidocaine patch, capsaicin patch, tramadol

Third-line therapies–opioids

Interventional: strong data are limited

Consider epidural injections for herpes zoster, steroid injections for radiculopathy, spinal cord stimulator implantation for failed back surgery syndrome or complex regional pain syndrome.

Recommend against sympathetic block for post herpetic neuralgia and radiofrequency ablation for radiculopathy.

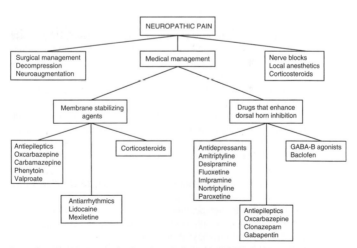

From Namaka, M., Leong, C., Grossberndt, A., et al. (2009). A treatment algorithm for neuropathic pain: an update. *Consult Pharm, 24*(12), 885–902.

REFERENCES

Colloca, L., Ludman, T., Bouhassira, D., et al. (2017). Neuropathic pain. *Nat Rev Dis Primers*, *3*, 17002.

Finnerup, N. B., Haroutounian, S., Kamerman, P., et al. (2016). Neuropathic pain: an updated grading system for research and clinical practice. *Pain*, *157*(8), 1599–1606.

NONACUTE ISCHEMIC STROKE

Nonacute ischemic stroke is discovered under various circumstances, and sometimes even completely by accident, as in patients who get brain imaging for other complaints. Patients with a recent ischemic stroke who are not eligible for acute thrombolysis/thrombectomy still need aggressive post-stroke management and evaluation. Key points for clinical approach:

- All patients with nonacute ischemic stroke need appropriate workup (unless performed recently) to ascertain its cause and risk factors for recurrence, and to begin appropriate secondary stroke prevention. Evaluation may be performed inpatient or outpatient, depending on the circumstances (size and age of stroke, hemorrhagic conversion, comorbidities, etc.). As a rule of thumb, subacute strokes need inpatient evaluation due to higher risk of stroke recurrence.
- Basic workup involves computed tomography head, magnetic resonance imaging brain, cerebrovascular imaging (computed tomography angiography, magnetic resonance angiography or/and carotid Dopplers), complete blood count, basic metabolic panel, urine drug screen, transthoracic echocardiography, fasting lipid panel and diabetes screening (Hb A1c). If a stroke is believed to be embolic from an undetermined source, outpatient Holter monitoring should be performed for at least 14 days (may be longer). Further search for etiology of stroke (transesophageal echocardiography, hypercoagulable panel, etc.) may be warranted in cases where there is no plausible explanation (e.g., young patients, genetic causes, absence of common risk factors, etc.)
- Secondary stroke prevention:
  - **Intracranial arterial stenosis**: appropriate maximal medical therapy (acetylsalicylic acid (ASA) and statin for low-density lipoprotein <70 mg/dL, management of hypertension with goal <130/90 mm Hg and diabetes with goal Hb A_{1c} <7%, smoking cessation, improved diet, and exercise). Clopidogrel may be added to ASA based on data from SAMMPRIS and CHANCE trials for up to 90 days after stroke onset.
  - **Large-vessel extracranial stenosis** and **aortic arch atherosclerosis** will require maximal medical therapy (as above) and possibly revascularization for symptomatic carotid stenosis (see "Carotid Stenosis"). Again, dual antiplatelet therapy (ASA + clopidogrel) is reasonable for up to 90 days from stroke onset.
  - **Small-vessel (lacunar) strokes** require maximal medical therapy as above (blood pressure ultimate goal <130/90 mm Hg). Dual

antiplatelet therapy is reasonable for about a week after stroke based on POINT trial results.

- **Atrial fibrillation** is usually a strong indication for anticoagulation with either warfarin or a direct oral anticoagulant, although initiation may need to be delayed for up to a few weeks for larger strokes and hemorrhagic strokes. Patients with cardiomyopathy may also be treated with antiplatelet therapy or anticoagulation (see Ischemia [Stroke]).
- **Septic embolism** requires treatment of underlying bacterial endocarditis.
- **Vasospasm**: the offending agent, if found, will need to be stopped. Inpatient admission with transcranial Doppler monitoring and calcium channel blockers may be needed if high suspicion for ongoing vasospasm.
- **Patent Foramen Ovale (PFO)**: embolic stroke patients aged 18 to 60, with PFO and no other stroke risk factors may benefit from PFO closure (see "Patent Foramen Ovale and Stroke").
- Patients with residual disability from nonacute stroke will need aggressive physical therapy and rehabilitation as tolerated.
- Strict outpatient follow-up with a stroke neurologist, adherence with appropriate medical therapy, and lifestyle modification cannot be underestimated as key to long-term success in secondary stroke prevention.

QUADRIPLEGIA

A variety of conditions must be considered in patients who present with quadriplegia (acute generalized weakness), which should always be considered a medical emergency.

DIFFERENTIAL DIAGNOSIS OF ACUTE QUADRIPLEGIA

Traumatic: Acute spinal cord injury
Autoimmune: Guillain-Barré syndrome
            Myasthenic crisis
            Transverse myelitis
Infections: Tick paralysis
         Botulism
         Diphtheria
         Tetanus
Toxins: Organophosphate toxicity
Vascular: Ischemic stroke/locked-in syndrome
Hemorrhagic spinal cord or brain stem stroke (AVM, AVF)
Electrolyte: Hypophosphatemia/calcemia/kalemia, hypermagnesemia, periodic paralysis
Hospital acquired: Critical illness Myoneuropathy
Genetic: Acute porphyria
Spinal cord injury: traumatic, rheumatologic, neoplastic, infectious, inflammatory/immunologic, vascular

    History and Physical Examination: Obtain history of possible trauma, ingestion of toxins, known history of myasthenia, tick bite, etc. Physical exam should include inspection (e.g., spinal deformity), palpation (deformity, tenderness), motor function (including sphincter function), sensory function, and deep tendon reflexes. Immediate imaging in cases of suspected acute spinal cord injury can identify the lesion(s). Magnetic resonance imaging has supplanted computed tomography and myelography, although these are sometimes necessary. Plain x-ray may identify acute vertebral fractures. For cervical spine injuries in particular, the spine must be cleared of injuries before further testing is obtained.

SPECIFIC CAUSES OF ACUTE GENERALIZED WEAKNESS
Further details may be found under chapters for the specific disease.

Guillain-Barré syndrome is a major cause of acute flaccid quadriplegia. Diagnosis is made through a combination of history and physical exam; the disease is characterized by progressive areflexic weakness. Predictors of need for mechanical ventilation include bulbar dysfunction and bilateral facial palsy, autonomic dysfunction (arrhythmias, hemodynamic instability), and short time to severe symptoms from the onset.

Myasthenia gravis can occur at any age and is characterized by weakness and fatiguability. In the acute scenario, patients can present in myasthenic or cholinergic crisis. Myasthenic crisis is usually precipitated by infection, medications, aspiration pneumonitis, upper airway obstruction, pregnancy, or surgery. Cholinergic crisis (miosis, diarrhea, increased salivation, abdominal cramps, bradycardia) is typical when patients increase their intake of anticholinergic medications. It is often difficult to differentiate them, however, on physical exam. Pupil size should be small or pinpoint in cholinergic crisis. The clinical approach should focus on predictors of mechanical ventilation, as with Guillain-Barré syndrome.

Tetanus classically presents with trismus or "lockjaw," nuchal rigidity, and dysphagia. As the disease spreads, generalized muscle spasms occur. The most common source is an infection by *Clostridium tetani* obtained through wounds or IV drug use, with risk factors being lack of immunization and diabetes. Diagnosis is solely clinical; therapy should focus on controlling respiratory function, autonomic instability, muscle spasms, and providing neutralizing agents and supportive care.

Botulism is caused by a neurotoxin of *Clostridium botulinum*, and many cases are secondary to IV drug use. Botulism in neonates may occur through tainted food. Clinical presentation is characterized by oculobulbar muscle weakness and a descending pattern of paralysis. Diagnosis is based on findings of toxin (serum, stool, wound) and electromyography (EMG). Therapy is mainly supportive with attention to respiratory status.

Periodic paralysis is a rare group of disorders, divided into two categories: hypokalemic (HypoKPP) or hyperkalemic (HyperKPP, usually presenting before adulthood). Patients are usually asymptomatic between episodes and have full recovery after the attacks. HypoKPP attacks are often precipitated by a high-carbohydrate meal and may last many hours. HyperKPP attacks are usually precipitated by fasting and tend to be short. Diagnosis is usually made by a combination of clinical evaluation and measuring serum potassium levels. For treatment of HypoKPP, oral potassium supplementation is most effective.

For HyperKPP, inhaled beta-agonists are used. In severe cases, IV calcium gluconate, insulin, and glucose are administered.

Acute intermittent porphyria is manifest by recurrent attacks of abdominal pain and neurologic complications usually precipitated by medications or infections. The neurologic manifestations include anxiety, agitation, cranial nerve palsies, muscle paralysis, seizures, and mental status changes. Diagnosis is based on detection of delta amino-levulinic acid and porphobilinogen in the urine. Therapy includes avoidance of precipitating factors and supportive treatment.

Organophosphate toxicity causes irreversible inhibition of cholinesterases often secondary to suicide attempts or accidental insecticide exposure. Nerve gas (e.g., Sarin) used in wartime or terrorist attacks is another cause of exposure. Clinical presentation is characterized by muscarinic symptoms (miosis, conjunctival hyperemia, rhinorrhea, drooling, bronchospasm, increased bronchial secretion, respiratory distress, pulmonary edema, laryngeal spasms, sweating, bradycardia, hypotension, urinary and bowel incontinence) and by nicotinic symptoms (fasciculations, paralysis). Severe intoxication ultimately leads to ataxia, dysarthria, confusion, seizures, and coma. Diagnosis is made by history of exposure, clinical picture, and serum levels of organophosphates and cholinesterase activity. Therapy consists mainly of protecting the patient from further exposure (gastric lavage, cleaning the contaminated skin or membranes) and use of atropine and pralidoxime.

Tick paralysis is caused by a paralytic toxin from the salivary glands of pregnant female ticks. Weakness begins two days post-exposure and presents with an ascending pattern with maximal evolution of symmetrical flaccid paralysis and areflexia. The tick is commonly found in the hair of the scalp and should be removed. Therapy is mainly supportive.

Critical illness myoneuropathy has been found in 33% to 44% of critically ill patients and is responsible for failure to wean from mechanical ventilation in these patients. Occurrence has been associated with sepsis and use of high-dose steroids or neuromuscular blocking agents. The diagnosis can be confirmed with EMG. Elevated serum creatine phosphokinase and muscle biopsy may be helpful in diagnosis. Therapy is supportive, and some patients eventually experience some degree of recovery.

REFERENCES

Suarez, J. I. (2004). *Critical care neurology and neurosurgery.* Totowa, NJ: Humana Press.

Torbey, M. T. (2004). Neuromuscular disorders. In A. Bhardway, M. Mirski, & J. A. Ulatowski (Eds.), *Handbook of neurocritical care.* Totowa: NJ, Humana Press.

SPINAL CORD INJURY

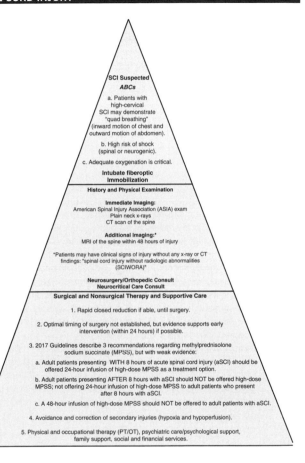

SCI Suspected

ABCs

a. Patients with high-cervical SCI may demonstrate "quad breathing" (inward motion of chest and outward motion of abdomen).

b. High risk of shock (spinal or neurogenic).

c. Adequate oxygenation is critical.

Intubate fiberoptic
Immobilization

History and Physical Examination

Immediate Imaging:
American Spinal Injury Association (ASIA) exam
Plain neck x-rays
CT scan of the spine

Additional Imaging:*
MRI of the spine within 48 hours of injury

*Patients may have clinical signs of injury without any x-ray or CT findings: "spinal cord injury without radiologic abnormalities (SCIWORA)"

Neurosurgery/Orthopedic Consult
Neurocritical Care Consult

Surgical and Nonsurgical Therapy and Supportive Care

1. Rapid closed reduction if able, until surgery.

2. Optimal timing of surgery not established, but evidence supports early intervention (within 24 hours) if possible.

3. 2017 Guidelines describe 3 recommendations regarding methylprednisolone sodium succinate (MPSS), but with weak evidence:

a. Adult patients presenting WITH 8 hours of acute spinal cord injury (aSCI) should be offered 24-hour infusion of high-dose MPSS as a treatment option.

b. Adult patients presenting AFTER 8 hours with aSCI should NOT be offered high-dose MPSS; not offering 24-hour infusion of high-dose MPSS to adult patients who present after 8 hours with aSCI.

c. A 48-hour infusion of high-dose MPSS should NOT be offered to adult patients with aSCI.

4. Avoidance and correction of secondary injuries (hypoxia and hypoperfusion).

5. Physical and occupational therapy (PT/OT), psychiatric care/psychological support, family support, social and financial services.

REFERENCES

Fehlings, M., et al. (2017). Clinical practice guideline for the management of patients with acute spinal cord injury: recommendations on the use of methylprednisolone sodium succinate. *Global Spine, 7*(3 Suppl), 203S–211S.

Rabinstein, A. (2018). Traumatic spinal cord injury. *Continuum, 24*(2), 551–556.

STATUS EPILEPTICUS, SEIZURE

TREATMENT OF CONVULSIVE STATUS EPILEPTICUS

1. Stabilization phase (0 to 5 minutes):
   a. Stabilize patient (airway, breathing, circulation), focused neurologic history (obtain time of seizure onset) and examination, focused general examination (special attention to respiratory and circulatory status, vital signs)
   b. Cardiac monitoring, pulse oximetry, frequent blood pressure checks, obtain IV access (at least two)
   c. Give oxygen via nasal cannula/mask, mechanical ventilation prn (intubation kit should be made available at bedside)
   d. Collect capillary glucose level and stat labs—electrolytes, complete blood count, Ca, Mg, P, liver function tests, toxicology screen, anti-seizure drug levels (if applicable)
   e. If glucose <60 mg/dL, give thiamine (100 to 300 mg IV) first, then glucose (50 mL of 50% dextrose solution IV). Correct metabolic derangements accordingly.
2. Initial therapy phase (5 to 20 minutes):
   a. Choose one of the following three equivalent first-line line options:
      i. IV lorazepam 0.1 mg/kg, max 4 mg/dose; may repeat dose once
      ii. IV diazepam 0.15 to 0.2 mg/kg, max 10 mg/dose; may repeat dose once
      iii. IM midazolam 10 mg for >40 kg, 5 mg for 13 to 40 kg; single dose
   b. If none of the three options are available, choose one of the following:
      i. IV phenobarbital 15 mg/kg, single dose
      ii. Rectal diazepam 0.2 to 0.5 mg/kg, max 20 mg/dose, single dose
      iii. Intranasal or buccal midazolam
   c. Proceed to next phase if seizure persists
3. Second therapy phase (20 to 40 minutes)
   a. Choose one of the following second-line options and give as single dose:
      i. IV fosphenytoin 20 mg PE/kg, max 1500 mg PE/dose, single dose
      ii. IV valproic acid 40 mg/kg, max 3000 mg/dose, single dose
      iii. IV levetiracetam 60 mg/kg, max 4500 mg/dose, single dose
      iv. If none of the options above are available, choose IV phenobarbital 15 mg/kg (if not given already)
   b. Proceed to next phase if seizure persists
4. Third phase therapy (40 to 60 minutes)
   a. There is no clear evidence to guide therapy in this phase
   b. Choices include: repeat second-line therapy or anesthetic dose of either thiopental, midazolam, pentobarbital, or propofol

    c. Continuous electroencephalogram (EEG) monitoring, intubation and mechanical ventilation (if not already performed)

    d. Consider placing arterial line; vasopressors should be made available at bedside

5. Additional scenarios and observations:

    a. Refractory status epilepticus is defined as persistence of seizures after treatment with appropriate doses of a benzodiazepine and a nonbenzodiazepine.

    b. Nonconvulsive status epilepticus: it should also be treated as soon as diagnosed. Therapeutic approach should follow the above algorithm—except for avoiding sedation (in order to prevent inducing or prolonging coma and intubation); continuous EEG is indicated in most cases.

    c. Myoclonic status epilepticus: therapeutic approach should follow the above algorithm—except for (a) preferring benzodiazepines and valproic acid, and (b) avoiding phenytoin and carbamazepine.

    d. Benzodiazepines should be avoided for the treatment of tonic status epilepticus in patients with Lennox-Gastaut syndrome.

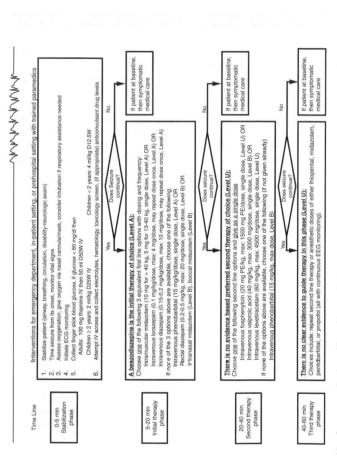

Proposed treatment algorithm for status epilepticus. (From Glauser, T., Shinnar, S., Gloss, D., et al. (2016). Evidence-based guideline: treatment of convulsive status epilepticus in children and adults: report of the guideline committee of the American Epilepsy Society. *Epilepsy Curr*, 16(1), 48–61.)

REFERENCES

Verrotti, A., Ambrosi, M., Pavone, P., et al. (2017). Pediatric status epilepticus: improved management with new drug therapies? *Expert Opin Pharmacother*, *18*(8), 789–798.

Zaccara, G., Giannasi, G., Oggioni, R., et al. (2017). Challenges in the treatment of convulsive status epilepticus. *Seizure*, *47*, 17–24.

TRAUMATIC BRAIN INJURY (TBI)

Falls and motor vehicle accidents account for most causes of traumatic brain injury (TBI). The Glasgow coma score is commonly used to classify severity: Score of 13 to 15 is considered mild, 9 to 12 is considered moderate, and 8 or less is considered severe TBI. Pathophysiology of TBI is generally divided into primary and secondary injury. Primary injury occurs at the time of trauma, and results from the combination of direct impact and acceleration/deceleration. Primary injury can cause contusions, diffuse axonal injury (DAI), petechial hemorrhage, and subarachnoid/subdural/epidural/intracerebral hemorrhage. Secondary injury occurs at the time of trauma and continues for hours or days. It results from a cascade of molecular injury mechanisms causing free radical injury, electrolyte imbalance, mitochondrial dysfunction, inflammation, and apoptosis, which could further lead to ischemia, cerebral edema, hydrocephalus, and increased intracranial pressure (ICP). TBI can also be subdivided into closed and open head injuries.

Brain computed tomography (CT) is the test of choice for emergent evaluation, while magnetic resonance imaging is more sensitive for DAI caused by shear injury with differential rotation of gray and white matter.

Acute management involves monitoring ICP in patients with severe TBI and abnormal CT showing evidence of mass effect, treating increased ICP (interventions include surgery if indicated (e.g., acute subdural hematoma), head elevation, mannitol, hyperventilation, medication-induced coma, and induced hypothermia), maintaining cerebral perfusion pressure (MAP-ICP) above 60 mm Hg in adults, and monitoring potential complications (e.g., infection, venous thromboembolism) that require additional treatment. Patients with severe TBI are often given a 7-day course of prophylactic antiepileptics (phenytoin, valproic acid or levetiracetam) since convulsions may raise ICP. Steroid and hyperbaric oxygen are not recommended. Trauma has a dose effect, and the neurological deficits of TBI varies based on the size, location, and depth of focal lesions. However, because of the susceptibility of the frontal lobes to both contusion and DAI, cognitive-behavioral impairments are the most common long-term sequelae.

The frequent occurrence of sports concussions, particularly in young athletes, has become a major public health problem. Various definitions of concussions have been used, but more recent definitions do not require the presence of loss of consciousness. Rules regarding return to play, both within a sporting event or afterwards, are being observed in order to minimize long-term sequelae of closed head injuries in athletes, using medical experts present during the sporting event. Many athletic organizations have instituted pre-season computerized cognitive testing batteries, such as IMPACT.

The identification of a concussion should result in suspending return to play and expert neuropsychological testing using in-person testing.

In mild TBI, 30% to 80% of patients experience postconcussion syndrome (PCS) starting in the first days, but often taking weeks or months to resolve. PCS symptoms include headache, dizziness, vertigo, neuropsychiatric symptoms, and cognitive impairment, especially attention and concentration problems. Imaging is often normal or nonspecific. Reassurance, bedrest, and symptomatic treatment are common approaches for PCS. A small percentage of TBI patients suffer from cranial nerve injury; symptoms include hyposmia, diplopia (injury to CN IV is most common), facial pain, and occipital neuralgia. Mild TBI is also associated with increased risk of epilepsy. Repeated concussion can cause cumulative neuropsychological deficit (e.g., chronic traumatic encephalopathy [CTE]), which is pathologically characterized by tau protein deposition, especially at the gray-white junction. CTE is commonly seen in boxers and football players or people with repetitive head injuries with multiple concussions and many subconcussive injuries. Symptoms include dementia, agitation and aggressive behavior, mood symptoms, parkinsonism, and speech and gait abnormalities. Diagnostic criteria are still being developed.

REFERENCES

Dombovy, M. L., et al. (2011). Traumatic brain injury. *Continuum*, *17*(3), 584–605.

Management of acute severe traumatic brain injury. https://www.uptodate.com/contents/management-of-acute-severe-traumatic-brain-injury?source=see_link#H22.

Mez, J., et al. (2015). Assessing clinicopathological correlation in chronic traumatic encephalopathy: rationale and methods for the UNITE study. *Alzheimers Res Ther*, *7*, 62.

Therapeutic Appendix

CHEMOTHERAPY: COMMON NEURO-ONCOLOGIC DRUGS

Agent	Mechanism	Dosage	Major side effects
Carboplatin	DNA alkylation	IV: 400 to 500mg/m^2 every 4 weeks	Myelosuppression, nausea, hypersensitivity reactions
Carmustine (BiCNU)	DNA and RNA alkylation	IV: 80 mg/m^2/day for 3 days every 8 wk for 6 cycles	Myelosuppression, nausea, pain at injection site, hypotension
Carmustine wafer (Gliadel)	Wafer implanted intracranially into the resection cavity	Implantation: 8 wafers (7.7 mg each and total dose 61.6 mg)	Seizures, cerebral edema, depression
Cisplatin	DNA alkylation	IV: 100 mg/m^2 every 3 wk	Renal toxicity, ototoxicity, hypersensitivity reactions, severe nausea
Erlotinib (Tarceva)	EGFR kinase inhibitor	Oral: 150 mg once daily	Skin rash, fatigue, diarrhea
Gefitinib (Iressa)	EGFR kinase inhibitor	Oral: 250 mg once daily	Skin reactions, diarrhea
Hydroxyurea (Droxia; Hydrea)	Antimetabolite: inhibits ribonucleoside diphosphate reductase	Oral:15 mg/kg/day	Eczema, transient myelosuppression
Imatinib (Gleevec)	c-kit and PDGFR kinase inhibitor	Oral: 400 mg twice daily	Edema, fatigue, skin rash, nausea, diarrhea
Irinotecan (Camptosar)	Topoisomerase I inhibitor	IV: 125 mg/m^2 once every 2 wk	Cholinergic syndrome, alopecia, myelosuppression, diarrhea

Drug	Mechanism	Dose	Side Effects
Lomustine (CeeNU)	DNA and RNA alkylation	Oral: PCV regimen 75 to 130 mg/m² once every 6 wk	Myelosuppression, nausea, stomatitis, pulmonary fibrosis
Methotrexate	Antimetabolite: inhibits dihydrofolate reductase	IV: 8000 mg/m² every 14 days	Arterial thrombosis, myelosuppression, hepatotoxicity
Procarbazine (Matulane)	DNA alkylation and depolymerization	Oral: 60 mg/m² (6 cycles) or 75 mg/m² (4 cycles) days 8 to 21 every 6 wk in PCV regimen	Nausea, myelosuppression, edema
13-cis-Retinoic acid (Absorica)	Inhibits cell proliferation	Oral: 160 mg/m²/day days 1 through 14 every 28 days for 6 cycles	Hypertriglyceridemia, back pain, conjunctivitis
Tamoxifen (Soltamox)	Competitively binds to estrogen receptors on tumors and decreases DNA synthesis	Oral: 20 to 40 mg daily (males and females)	Flushing, rash, hypertension
Temozolomide (Temodar)	DNA methylation	Concomitant: Oral, IV: 75 mg/m²/day for 42 days with focal radiotherapy; Maintenance: 150 mg/m²/day for 5 days of a 28-day cycle	Fatigue, peripheral edema, alopecia, myelosuppression
Vincristine (Vincasar PFS)	Inhibits RNA synthesis	IV: PCV regimen 1.4 mg/m²/dose on days 8 and 29 of a 6-wk cycle for a total of 6 cycles	Alopecia, peripheral neuropathy, constipation
Everolimus (Afinitor)	Reduces protein synthesis, cell proliferation and angiogenesis	Oral: 4.5 mg/m² daily	Pneumonitis, stomatitis, metabolic toxicity
Bevacizumab (Avastin)	Inhibits VEGF	IV: 10 mg/kg every 2 wk	Hypertension, fatigue, infections, hemorrhage

CHEMOTHERAPY: COMMON NEURO-ONCOLOGIC DRUGS

Agent	Mechanism	Dosage	Major side effects
OTHERS			
Erythropoietin alpha (Epogen; Procrit)	Erythropoiesis stimulation	SubQ: 150 units/kg 3 times a week or 40,000 units once weekly	Nausea, hypertension
Darbepoetin alfa (Aranesp)	Erythropoiesis stimulation	SubQ: 2.25 mcg/kg once weekly or 500 mcg once every 3 weeks	Hypertension, dyspnea, peripheral edema
Filgrastim (GRANIX; Neupogen)	G-CSF stimulation	SubQ, IV: 5 mcg/kg/day	Nausea, thrombocytopenia, fatigue
Pegfilgrastim (Neulasta)	G-CSF stimulation	SubQ: 6 mg once per chemotherapy cycle	Ostealgia, limb pain
Dexamethasone (Decadron)	Suppression of neutrophil migration and production of inflammatory mediators; reversal of increased capillary permeability	Cerebral edema: IV: 10 mg stat, then 4 mg IM/IV every 6 hours until response is maximized, then switch to oral regimen and gradually taper off Neoplastic epidural spinal cord compression: IV: 10 to 96 mg bolus; followed by 4 to 24 mg four times daily for 3 days and then taper over 10 days	Adrenal insufficiency, myopathy

EGFR, Epidermal growth factor receptor; *G-CSF,* granulocyte-colony stimulating factor; *PCV,* procarbazine, CeeNU, vincristine; *PDGFR,* platelet-derived growth factor receptor; *VEGF,* vascular endothelial growth factor.

CHOREA (MOVEMENT DISORDER)

Medication	Dosage	Action	Side Effects
Clozapine (Clozaril)	12.5–25 mg qh, increase by 12.5-25 mg q 3 d max 150 mg	D1 and D2 blocker, blocks serotonin type 2 (5 HT2), alpha-adrenergic, H1, and cholinergic receptors	Sedation, diarrhea, weight gain, hypotension, dose-related seizures, agranulocytosis
Haloperidol (Haldol)	Begin 0.5–1 mg and increase by 0.5 mg qw in tid dosing max 10 mg	Blocks D1 and D2 receptors in the brain	Tardive dyskinesia, acute dystonia, akathisia, swallowing, gait difficulties, parkinsonism
Perphenazine	Begin 4 mg qd, increase by 4 mg/wk tid max 24 mg	Blocks postsynaptic mesolimbic dopaminergic receptors	Tardive dyskinesia, acute dystonia, akathisia, swallowing, gait difficulties, parkinsonism
Quetiapine (Seroquel)	25 mg qh, increase by 25 mg q 3–5 d bid max 400 mg	Proposed D2 and 5-HT2 antagonist	Parkinsonism, depression, drowsiness, hypotension
Reserpine	Begin 0.1 mg, increase by 0.1 mg q 5–7 d tid or qid max 3 mg	Depletes norepinephrine and dopamine	Parkinsonism, depression, drowsiness, hypotension
Risperidone (Risperdal)	0.5–1 mg qh, increase by 0.5 mg q 3–5 d max 6 mg	Mixed D2 and 5-HT2 antagonist	Parkinsonism, depression, drowsiness, hypotension
Tetrabenazine	Begin 12.5 mg, increase q 5–7 d tid or qid max 200 mg	Presynaptic dopamine depleter, binds to central VMAT2	Parkinsonism, depression, drowsiness, hypotension
Deutetrabenazine	Begin 6 mg, increase 6 mg q 7 d bid max 96 mg	Presynaptic dopamine depleter, binds to central VMAT2	Same profile as Tetrabenazine, but milder

REFERENCES

Claassen, D. O., Carroll, B., De Boer, L. M., et al. (2017). Indirect tolerability comparison of Deutetrabenazine and Tetrabenazine for Huntington disease. *J Clin Mov Disord*, *4*(3). https://doi.org/10.1186/s40734-017-0051-5.

Dean, M., & Sung, V. W. (2018). Review of deutetrabenazine: a novel treatment for chorea associated with Huntington's disease. *Drug Des Devel Ther*, *12*, 313–319. https://doi.org/10.2147/DDDT.S138828.

DEMENTIA: PRIMARY MEDICATIONS

DEMENTIA MEDICATIONS

Medication	Donepezil (Aricept)	Galantamine (Razadyne)	Rivastigmine (Exelon)	Memantine (Namenda)
Indication	AD (Mild to Severe); PDD; DLB (Off-Label)	AD (Mild-moderate); AD (Severe; off-label); PDD, DLB (Off-label)	AD (Mild-moderate)** PDD** (Mild-moderate); DLB (Off-label);	AD (Moderate to severe); VasD (mild-moderate; off label); PDD/ DLB (off label)
Mechanism of action	AChE-I	AChE-I	AChE-I	NMDA-R antagonist
Absorption affected by food	No	Yes; take with meals	Yes; take with meals	No
Time to peak	3 hr (Extended release 23 mg tab 8 hr)	1 hr (2.5 hr with food) ER 5 hr	1 hr for tablets; Patch 8–16 hr	3–7 hr (ER 9–12 hr)
Serum t1/2	70 hr	7 hr	1.5 hr (Patch 3 hr)	60–80 hr
Metabolism	CYP-2D6 CYP-3A4	CYP-2D6 CYP-3A4	Nonhepatic	Nonhepatic
Dose: Initial	5 mg QD (ER 8 mg/day)	4mg BID (ER 8 mg QD)	1.5 mg BID (Patch 4.6 mg /24 hr)	2.5 mg BID or 5 mg QD (ER 7 mg QD)
Titration required	Yes	Yes	Yes	Yes
First effective dose:	5 mg (severe AD: 10 mg)	8 mg BID (ER 16 mg QD)	3 mg BID; 4.6 mg/24 hr patch	10 mg BID

Continued

DEMENTIA MEDICATIONS—CONT'D

Medication	Donepezil (Aricept)	Galantamine (Razadyne)	Rivastigmine (Exelon)	Memantine (Namenda)
Dose: Maximum	10 mg qd (23 mg QD)	12 mg BID (ER 24 mg QD)	6 mg BID (Patch 13.3 mg/24 hr)	10 mg BID (ER 28 mg QD)
Renal impairment adjustment	N/A	CrCl 9-59 Max dose 16 mg QD; CrCl < 9 Not recommended	None; use with caution CrCl < 50	For CrCl 15–29: max 5 mg BID (ER 14 mg QD)
Hepatic impairment	N/A	ChildPugh 7–9: Max 16 mg daily; ChildPugh 10–15: Not recommended	Max dose 4.6 mg/24 hr (applies to patch only)	N/A
Common side effects	Nausea, vomiting, diarrhea, insomnia, muscle cramps	Nausea, vomiting, diarrhea	Nausea, vomiting, diarrhea, weight loss	Dizziness, agitation, headache

AD, Alzheimer dementia; *PDD*, Parkinson disease dementia; *DLB*, Lewy body dementia; *VasD*, vascular dementia.
** Patch can be used with severe forms of AD and PDD.

DEPRESSION

SELECTED ANTIDEPRESSANTS

Generic name	Brand name	Dosage range (mg/d)	Anticholinergic effect	Sedative effect	Comments/side effects
TRICYCLICS/HETEROCYCLICS					
Amitriptyline (3)	Elavil	25–300	High	High	SE: Orthostatic hypotension, sedation, weight gain, sexual dysfunction, QT prolongation, arrhythmia, decreased seizure threshold, overdose lethal
Desipramine (2)	Norpramin	25–200	Low	Low	
Doxepin (3)	Sinequan	25–150	Moderate	Moderate	
Imipramine (3)	Tofranil	25–300	Moderate	Moderate	
Nortriptyline (2)	Aventyl, Pamelor	20–150	Low	Low	
SSRIs					
Fluoxetine	Prozac	20–60	Very low	Very low	Lexapro is effective in GAD
Sertraline	Zoloft	25–250	Very low	Very low	SE: Dry mouth, nausea, nervousness insomnia, sexual dysfunction, headache, QT prolongation (especially citalopram)
Paroxetine	Paxil	20–40	Low	Low	Paroxetine and Fluoxetine CYP2D6 inhibitors
Citalopram	Celexa	20–40	Very low	Very low	
Escitalopram	Lexapro	10–20	Very low	Very low	
SSNRIs					
Duloxetine	Cymbalta	20–60	Very low	Very low	SE: Nausea and anorexia, weight loss, nervousness, headache, insomnia, fatigue, dry mouth, constipation, sexual dysfunction, tachycardia, hyperlipidemia, diaphoresis, hypertension

Continued

DEPRESSION

SELECTED ANTIDEPRESSANTS—CONT'D

Generic name	Brand name	Dosage range (mg/d)	Anticholinergic effect	Sedative effect	Comments/side effects
Venlafaxine	Effexor	37.5–225	Very low	Low	This class is effective in treating neuropathic pain.
Desvenlafaxine	Khedezla	50	Very low	Very low	
Levomilnacipran	Fetzima	20–120	Very low	Very low	
REUPTAKE INHIBITORS AND RECEPTOR ANTAGONISTS					
Trazodone	Desyrel	50–600	Very low	High	SE: Dry mouth, nausea, dizziness
Nefazodone	Sermonette	200–600	Low	Moderate	
Mirtazapine	Remeron	15–45	Low	High (activating effect with higher doses)	Mirtazapine helpful with appetite stimulation, improved sleep, and no sexual SE.
NDRIs					
Bupropion	Wellbutrin	200–300	Very low	Very low	SE: Agitation, nausea, headache, anorexia, insomnia, hypertension, decreased seizure threshold. No sexual SE.
5-HT REUPTAKE INHIBITOR AND SELECTIVE/PARTIAL 5-HTR AGONIST					
Vilazodone	Viibryd	10–40	Very low	Very low	SE: Diarrhea, nausea, vomiting, insomnia, bleeding, suicidal ideation
Vortioxetine	Trintellix	10–20	Very low	Very low	SE: Constipation, nausea, vomiting, hyponatremia, suicidal thoughts

NDRIs, Norepinephrine and dopamine reuptake inhibitors; *SE*, side effects; *SSNRIs*, selective serotonin and norepinephrine reuptake inhibitors; *SSRIs*, selective serotonin reuptake inhibitors.

REFERENCES

Lexicomp Online. Copyright. (1978-2017). *Lexicomp, Inc.* All Rights Reserved.

Schulz, P., & Arora, G. (2015). Depression. *Continuum (Minneapolis Minn), 21*(3), 756–771.

EPILEPSY

COMMONLY PRESCRIBED ANTIEPILEPTIC DRUGS (AEDS)

AED	Best treated epilepsy type[a]	Dosage	Renal/hepatic pharmacokinetics	Adverse effects (common side effects)[b]
Carbamazepine	Partial, generalized	400 mg mg qd, increase by 200 mg mg/day at 1 wk intervals. Max 1200 mg/day	Induces CYP3A4 & CYP1A2. Primarily renal excretion.	Hyponatremia, rash, N/V, SJS, aplastic anemia, agranulocytosis
Clobazam	Lennox-Gastaut Syndrome	>30 Kg: 5 mg BID, 10 mg BID (day 7), 20 mg BID (day 14) <30 Kg: start at 2.5 mg BID with goal of 10 mg BID	CYP3A4 > CYP2C19 & CYP2B6. Primarily renal excretion.	Constipation, SJS, toxic epidermal necrolysis
Ethosuximide	Generalized (absence)	500 mg, increase by 250 mg/day at 1 wk intervals. Caution with >1.5 g/d	Induces CYP3A4 > CYP2E1. Partial renal excretion.	Anorexia, SLE-like symptoms, GI: pain, N/V/D. Skin: SJS, hirsutism, gingival hyperplasia, headache, mood changes
Eslicarbazepine	Partial	400 mg qd, increase by 400-600 mg increments to max 1600 mg/d	Induces CYP3A4 > CYP2C19. Primarily renal excretion.	N/V, diplopia, eosinophilia, transaminitis, suicidal thoughts, angioedema
Ezogabine	Partial	100 mg TID, increase by 50 mg TID at 1 wk intervals. Maint: 200-400 mg TID	No major CYP450 effects. Primarily renal excretion.	Prolonged QT interval, skin discoloration, weight gain, diplopia, retinal disorder
Gabapentin	Partial	300 mg TID. Main:: 300-600 mg TID. Max 2400 mg/day	Very slight CYP2A6 inhibition. Primarily renal excretion.	SJS, hypoglycemia, eosinophilia, mood changes, angioedema

Felbamate	Partial w/wo generalization	1200 mg/day (TID or QID); increase by 600 mg Q2wk. Max: 3600 mg/day	Substrate for CYP3A4 and CYP2E1. Inhibits CYP2C19. Primarily renal excretion.	Aplastic anemia, hepatic failure, SI
Lacosamide	Partial	100 mg BID; increase by 50 mg BID. Max: 200 mg BID	Substrate for CYP3A4, CYP2C9, CYP2C19. Primarily renal excretion.	Cardiac: atrial fibrillation/flutter, 1° AV block, prolonged PR interval; diplopia; SI; eosinophilia
Lamotrigine	Partial, Lennox-Gastaut, tonic-clonic	1st 2 wk: 25 mg Q48h. 2nd 2 wk: 25 mg Q24Hh. Increase by 25–50 mg/day Q1–2 wk to maint of 100–400 mg/day	If adding to valproate then maintenance 100–200 mg/d. Primarily renal excretion.	Ophthalmic: blurred vision, diplopia. Dysmenorrhea. Rhinitis. Derm: SJS, TEN. Liver failure. Neuromalignant syndrome.
Levetiracetam	Myoclonic associated with JME, focal, tonic-clonic	500 mg BID. Increase by 1 g/day Q2wk to Max: 3 g/day	No significant CYP activity. Primarily renal excretion.	V, decreased bone mineral density, abnormal behavior, irritability, SHS, TEN, pancytopenia, liver failure, SI
Oxcarbazepine	Partial	300 mg BID. Increase by up to 600 mg/day weekly. Max: 1200 mg/day or ER 2400 mg/day	Keto analogue of carbamazepine. Little effect on CYP450. Primarily renal excretion.	Weight gain, N/V. Derm: erythema multiforme, SJS, TEN, agranulocytosis, pancytopenia, hypersensitivity reaction, SI, angioedema
Perampanel	Partial, tonic-clonic	2 mg QHS. Increase by 2 mg/day Qwk. Maint: 8-12 mg QHS	Substrate of CYP3A4/5, CYP1A2, CYP2B6. Inhibitor of CYP2C8, CYP3A4, UGT1A9, UGT2B7. Inducer of CYP2B6, CYP3A4/5, UGT1A1, UGT1A4. Mixed excretion fecal > renal.	Various psychiatric symptoms including SI & HI; fatigue

Continued

EPILEPSY

COMMONLY PRESCRIBED ANTIEPILEPTIC DRUGS (AEDS)—CONT'D

AED	Best treated epilepsy type[a]	Dosage	Renal/hepatic pharmacokinetics	Adverse effects (common side effects)[b]
Phenobarbita	Focal and generalized seizures	50–100 mg BID or TID	CYP450 Inducer. Mostly non-renal excretion.	Megaloblastic anemia, liver damage, hallucinations, somnolence, depression, erythroderma
Phenytoin	Generalized tonic-clonic, complex partial	100 mg TID. Maint: 300–400 mg/day. Max: 600 mg/day	CYP450 Inducer. Primarily excreted in bile. Renal excretion following GI reabsorption.	Constipation, N/V, numerous dermatological and hematological symptoms, hepatotoxicity, SI
Pregabalin	Partial	75 mg BID or 50 mg TID. Max: 300 mg/day	Negligible CYP activity. Primarily renal excretion.	Peripheral edema, weight gain, constipation, xerostomia, visual disturbances, jaundice, elevated creatinine kinase, SI, angioedema
Rufinamide	Lennox-Gastaut	200–400 mg BID. Increase by 400–800 mg/day Q48H. Max: 1600 mg BID	No significant CYP activity. Primarily renal excretion.	Shortened QT interval, N/V, visual disturbances, leukopenia, SJS, SI
Tiagabine	Partial	4 mg/day. Increase by 4–8 mg Qwk in BID or QID dosing. Max: 56 mg/day	Substrate of CYP3A and possibly CYP1A2, 2D6, 2C19. Mixed excretion fecal > renal.	Pruritis, N, poor concentration, pharyngitis, SJS, SI
Topiramate	Lennox-Gastaut, partial, tonic-clonic	25–50 mg/day. Increase by 25–50 mg/day Qwk. Maint: 200 mg BID	Inducer of CYP3A4. Inhibitor of CYP2C19. Primarily renal excretion.	Flushing, weight loss, poor concentration, psychiatric disturbances including SI, SJS, TEN, hyperammonemia, hypohidrosis, metabolic acidosis, nephrolithiasis

Valproate	Absence, complex partial	15 mg/kg/day Increase 5-10 mg/kg/day Q1wk Max: 60 mg/kg/cay	Inhibitor of CYP2C9 and possibly CYP3A4. Nearly 50% renal excretion.	N, hyperammonemia, pancreatitis, myelodysplastic syndrome, thrombocytopenia, teratogenesis, hepatotoxicity
Vigabatrin	Complex partial	500 mg BID. Increase by 500 mg/cay Qwk. Max: 3 g/day	No significant CYP activity. Primarily renal excretion.	Weight gain, arthralgia, visual field/acuity defects, nystagmus, aggression, dysmenorrhea, liver failure, SI
Zonisamide	Partial	100 mg/day Increase by 100 mg/day Q2wk No benefit above 400 mg/day	No significant CYP activity. Primarily renal excretion.	Rash with sulfa-allergy, pruritis, weight loss, psychiatric disturbances, schizophrenia or disorder, agranulocytosis, SJS, TEN

[a]indications represent older terminology as indicated by FDA labeling prior to new terminology

[b]Common side effects to almost all AEDs: mental status: dizziness, drowsiness, sleepiness; cerebellar/coordination: unsteadiness, blurred vision, ataxia, tremor, nystagmus; cognitive: impaired memory, fatigue.

Side effects in bold indicate black box warning.

D, Diarrhea; *HI,* homicidal ideations; *N,* nausea; *SI,* suicidal ideations; *SJS,* Stevens-Johnson syndrome; *SLE,* systemic lupus erythematosus; *TEN,* toxic epidermal necrolysis; *V,* vomiting.

EPILEPSY

REFERENCES

Fisher, R. S., Acevedo, C., Arzimanoglou, A., et al. (2014). ILAE official report: a practical clinical definition of epilepsy. *Epilepsia*, *55*(4), 475–482.

Turner, A. L., et al. (2017). Outside the box: medications worth considering when traditional antiepileptic drugs have failed. *Seizure*, *50*, 173–185. https://doi.org/10.1016/j.seizure.2017.06.022. Epub 2017 Jun 27.

TREATMENT FOR ESSENTIAL TREMOR (MOVEMENT DISORDER)

Medication/ Procedure	Dosages	Action	Side effects
FIRST LINE			
Propanalol	60–320 mg/day BID dosing (short acting) or QD for LA	Non-Selective Beta-Adrenergic antagonist for limb and head tremor	Hypotension, bradycardia
Primidone	250 mg–750 mg/day QHS dosing (administer higher doses as BID)	GABA-A agonist for limb tremor	Sedation, Ataxia, Nystagmus
SECOND LINE			
Gabapentin	1200–3600 mg/day TID dosing	Decreases release of Calcium dependent neurotransmitters from nerve terminals, used for limb tremor	Drowsiness, Ataxia
Topiramate	150–300 mg/day BID dosing	Inhibits kainate/AMPA and sodium receptors; enhances GABA-A receptors, weak carbonic anhydrase inhibitor. It is used for limb tremor	Paresthesia, abnormal taste, word finding difficulties, and acute angle closure glaucoma
SECOND LINE, NON-MEDICAL			
Thalamic deep brain stimulation	Surgical option for limb tremor refractory to medical treatment	Direct brain action through electrical modulation	Surgery related complications, stroke, infection, failure/ recurrence
THIRD LINE, NON-MEDICAL			
Thalamotomy	Unilateral lesion as surgical option for medically refractory essential tremor of the limb	Direct brain action through lesion	Surgery related complications, stroke, infection, failure/ recurrence

REFERENCES

Connor, G. S., Edwards, K., Tarsy, D. (2008). Topiramate in essential tremor: findings from double-blind, placebo-controlled, crossover trials. *Clin Neuropharmacol*, *31*(2), 97–103.

Zesiewicz, T. A., Elble, R., Louis, E.D., et al. (2011). Evidence-based guideline update: Treatment of essential tremor. *Neurology, 77*(19), 1752–1755.

HEADACHE

TRIPTANS FOR MIGRAINE HEADACHE ABORTIVE THERAPY

Drug	Dose/route	Other considerations
Almotriptan (Axert)	6.25–12.5 mg PO, may repeat after 2 hr; max 25 mg/day	Side effects: Warm/hot sensation, tingling, chest pain/tightness, hyper/hypotension, burning, feeling of heaviness and tightness, flushing, drowsiness, malaise/fatigue, and anxiety. Precaution: All triptans should be avoided in patients with familial hemiplegic migraine, basilar migraine, ischemic stroke, ischemic heart disease, Prinzmetal angina, uncontrolled hypertension, and pregnancy. MAO inhibitors are contraindicated with triptans. Triptans should not be used within 24 hr of the use of ergotamine preparations or different other than naratriptan, Eletriptan, and Frovatriptan.
Eletriptan (Relpax)	20–40 mg PO, may repeat after 2 hr; max 80 mg/day	
Frovatriptan (Frova)	2.5 mg, may repeat after 2 hr; max 7.5 mg/day	
Naratriptan (Amerge)	1–2.5 mg PO, may repeat after 4 hr; max 5 mg/day	
Rizatriptan (Maxalt)	Tablets: 5–10 mg PO, may repeat after 2 hr; max 20 mg/day Wafers (orally disintegrating tablets): 5–10 mg PO, may repeat after 2 hr; max 20 mg/day	
Sumatriptan (Imitrex)	Oral: 25–100 mg PO, may repeat after 2 hr; max 200 mg/day SC: 1–6 mg, may repeat after 1 hr; max 12 mg/day Intranasal spray: 5–20 mg in 1 nostril, may repeat after 2 hr; max 40 mg/day Intranasal powder: 22 mg (11 mg in each nostril), may repeat after 2 hr; max 44 mg/day.	
Zolmitriptan (Zomig)	Tablets: 1.25–2.5 mg PO, may repeat after 2 hr; max 10 mg/day Wafers (orally disintegrating tablets): 2.5 mg PO, may repeat after 2 hr; max 10 mg/day Intranasal: 5 mg in 1 nostril, may repeat after 2 hr; max 10 mg/day	

HEADACHE

INSOMNIA

Good sleep practices and cognitive behavioral approach should be considered in elderly neurological patients.

MEDICATIONS USED TO TREAT INSOMNIA

Drug	Dosage range	Benefits	Side effects
FIRST-LINE PHARMACOTHERAPY (FDA APPROVED)			
Eszopiclone (Lunesta)[a,b]	1–3 mg	Short half-life provides lower risk of morning hangover effect	Rash, xerostomia, dizziness, nausea and vomiting, confusion, headache, hallucinations, nervousness, dysmenorrhea, reduced libido
Zaleplon (Sonata)[a,b]	5–10 mg (5 mg dose is largely ineffective and not routinely used)	Ultra-short half-life. Used for sleep initiation and prn for night-time awakenings (3–4 hr before rising)	Headache, drowsiness, nausea, and rash
Temazepam (Restoril)[a,b]	15–30 mg	Intermediate half-life carries a low-moderate risk of hangover effect	Headache, fatigue, nervousness, lethargy, dizziness, anxiety, and confusion
Triazolam (Halcion)[a,b]	0.125–0.5	Short half-life	Nausea, vomiting, abdominal pain, caution with depressed patients
Zolpidem (Ambien)[a,b]	10 mg (12.5 extended release)		
Ramelteon (Rozerem)[b]	8 mg	Less risk of abuse	Daytime sedation
Doxepin (Sinequan, Silenor)[b]	3–6 mg	Sleep maintenance	Hypertension, behavioral side effect
Suvorexant (Belsomra)[b]	10–20 mg		Daytime sedation

SECOND-LINE PHARMACOTHERAPY

Amitriptyline (Elavil)	10–50 mg	Longer half-life carries risk of hangover effect and cognitive impairment	Weight gain, bloating symptom, asthenia, constipation, xerostomia, dizziness, fatigue, headache, blurred vision
Trazodone (Desyrel)	25–100 mg	Shorter half-life lowers risk of hangover effect	Sweating, weight change, worsening depression, suicidal ideation

VARIABLE EVIDENCE

L-Tryptophan	500 mg–2 g	May be preferred by patient wanting a "natural medicine"	Unknown
Melatonin	1–5 mg		
Valerian root	400–900 mg		

[a]Risk of abuse.
[b]Approved by the Food and Drug Administration (FDA).

DRUGS NOT RECOMMENDED FOR TREATMENT OF INSOMNIA

Drug class	Reason
Antidepressants	Lack of evidence
Antihistamines	Excessive risk of psychomotor impairment and anticholinergic side effects
Antipsychotics (conventional)	Unacceptable risk of anticholinergic and neurologic toxicity
Antipsychotics (atypical)	Lack of evidence and unacceptable risk of metabolic toxicity
Benzodiazepines (intermediate and long-acting)	Excessive risk of daytime sedation and psychomotor impairment
Benzodiazepines (short-acting)	Unacceptable risk of memory disturbances, abnormal thinking, and psychotic behaviors
Chloral agents	Risk of tolerance, dependence, and abuse, central nervous system (CNS) and gastrointestinal (GI) effects
Muscle relaxants	Excessive risk of adverse CNS effects

REFERENCES

Lam, S., & Macina, L. O. (2017). Therapy update for insomnia in the elderly. *Consult Pharm*, *32*(10), 610–622. https://doi.org/10.4140/TCP.n.2017.610.

Matheson, E., & Hainer, B. L. (2017). Insomnia: pharmacologic therapy. *Am Fam Physician*, *96*(1), 29–35.

MULTIPLE SCLEROSIS

DISEASE-MODIFYING AGENTS

Generic Name	Recommended Dose	Comments	Side Effects
Immune Modulators			
Interferon β-1a (Avonex, Rebif)	30 μg (Avonex) IM qw self-injection	RRMS, SPMS + R	Flu-like symptoms, depression, mild anemia, impaired LFT, allergy
	44 μg (Rebif) SQ 3 q tiw self-injection		Same
Interferon β-1b (IFNb-1b, Betaseron, Extavia)	8 MIU or 250 μg SQ qod self-injection	RRMS, SPMS + R	Same + site reaction + reduced WBC
Glatiramer acetate (Copaxone, Glatopa)	20 mg SQ qd self-injection	RRMS	Local reactions, vasodilation, brief and transient panic reaction
Daclizumab (Zinbryta)	150 mg to 300 mg q4wk SC	RRMS	
Natalizumab (Tysabri) IgG monoclonal antibodies	300 mg IV over 1 hr q4wk	RRMS only in centers with TOUCH program. Approved by the FDA in June 2006	Fatal PML (? higher with other immunomodulatory and Immunosuppressant drugs), infection, hypersensitivity, increased lymphocytes, and nucleated RBC
Alemtuzumab	12 mg or 24 mg daily for 5 days in the 1st year; 3 days in the 2nd	RRMS, SPMS + R	Autoimmune disease (thrombocytopenia, thyroid, neutropenia, and Goodpasture syndrome), rash, headache, abdominal pain

Continued

MULTIPLE SCLEROSIS

Generic Name	Recommended Dose	Comments	Side Effects
Fingolimod (Gilenya)	0.5mg PO qd	RRMS, SPMS + R	PML cases reported, HSV encephalitis, cardiac arrhythmia, macular edema, hepatotoxicity, headache
Teriflunomide (AUBAGIO)	7 or 14 mg PO qd	RRMS, SPMS + R	Teratogenic, hepatotoxicity, renal disease
Dimethyl fumarate (Tecfidera)	240 mg PO BID	RRMS, SPMS + R	Cases of PML reported, leukopenia, flushing, angioedema, abdominal pains
Ocrelizumab (Ocrevus)	600 mg IV q6 months	RRMS, SPMS + R & primary progressive forms	Hepatotoxicity, infusion reaction, neutropenia, peripheral edemas
Chemotherapeutic Agents			
Mitoxantrone (Novantrone)	12 mg/m^2 IV over 15 min q 3 mo for 2–3 years	SPMS, worsening RRMS	Nausea (N) and vomiting (V), cytopenia, blue-green urine 24 hours later; infections, hair thinning, serious hepato- and Cardiotoxicity
Azathioprine (Imuran)	50–100 mg qd or bid	Same, but not FDA approved	Cytopenia, GI symptoms, N and V, impaired LFT, rash, flu-like syndrome
Cyclophosphamide (Cytoxan, Neosar)	500 mg/day 8–18 days until the total WBC ≤ 4000/mm^3 and booster doses at 700 mg/m^2 IV q 2 mo	Rapidly progressive MS, Devic syndrome, Marburg variant MS, but not FDA approved	Cytopenia, N and V, hair loss, mouth sores, sterility, renal failure, and hemorrhagic cystitis
Cyclosporine (Sandimmune)	5–7 mg/day for 1–3 years	Same	Renal failure, hypertension, PRES syndrome, cytopenia, hair thinning

Drug	Dose	Notes	Side Effects
Methotrexate (generic)	7.5 mg q w for 2–3 years	Progressive MS, but not FDA approved	Cytopenia, hair thinning, impaired LFT, N and V, stomatitis
Cladribine (Leustatin) selective lymphotoxic specificity	0.07 mg/kg/day IV for 5 days q 4 wk for 6 cycles	Progressive MS, SPMS, but not FDA approved	Bone marrow suppression and cytopenia, infection
Corticosteroids			
Methylprednisolone (Depo-Medrol, Solu-Medrol)	250 mg IV q 6 hr × 3 day with or without a taper	Acute relapses in RRMS and worsening SPMS	Electrolyte disturbances, psychiatric effect, weight gain, osteoporosis, skin changes, and infection

SUGGESTED MEDICATION FOR SPASTICITY IN MS (SLOW TITRATION)

Drug	Dose	Notes	Side Effects
Baclofen	5–20 mg PO tid	? safety in children <12 yr, possibly teratogenic	Weakness, seizure, MS changes, hypotension, hallucination, sedation, encephalopathy
Tizanidine (Zanaflex)	2–8 mg PO tid	Contraceptive pills reduce drug clearance, possibly teratogenic (Category C)	Dry mouth, urinary tract infection, impaired LFT (0, 1, 3, 6 mo monitoring), flu syndrome, dyskinesia, hypotension
Diazepam	2–10 mg PO tid	Possibly teratogenic	Sedation, ataxia, fatigue, urine retention
Dantrolene	25–50 mg PO tid	Possibly teratogenic, possible photosensitivity	Impaired LFT (more in women and those >35 years, 0, 1, 3, 6 mo monitoring), sedation, and diarrhea
Gabapentin	100–800 mg PO tid	Possibly teratogenic (Category C)	Drowsiness, ataxia, viral-like illness in children
Clonidine	0.1–0.2 mg (oral or patch)	Possibly teratogenic (Category C)	Drowsiness, hypotension, bradycardia, rebound hypertension with withdrawal

Continued

MULTIPLE SCLEROSIS

Generic Name	Recommended Dose	Comments	Side Effects
SUGGESTED MEDICATION FOR FATIGUE IN MS (SLOW TITRATION)			
Amantadine (Symmetrel)	50 or 100 PO bid	Possibly teratogenic (Category C)	Nausea, hallucination, constipation, edema, and orthostatic hypotension
Pemoline (Cylert)	18.75–75 mg PO qd	Possibly teratogenic (Category C)	Difficulty sleeping or drowsiness, dizziness, headache, nausea, anorexia
Modafinil (Provigil)	200–400 mg PO qd	Possibly teratogenic (Category C)	Headache, nervousness, rhinitis, backache, anxiety, insomnia, dizziness
Armodafinil (Nuvigil)	150–250 mg PO qd	Possibly teratogenic (Category C)	Rash, dizziness, headache, anaphylaxis
Methylphenidate (Ritalin)	10–30 mg PO in 3 divided doses	Possibly teratogenic (Category C)	Seizure, nervousness, insomnia, appetite suppression, hypersensitivity, headache, arteritis
SUGGESTED MEDICATION FOR DEPRESSION IN MS (SLOW TITRATION)			
Fluoxetine (Prozac)	20–60 mg PO qd	Anticholinergics and sedation effect—mild	Headache, anxiety, tremor, insomnia, drowsiness, fatigue, dizziness, GI complaints, excessive sweating
Bupropion (Wellbutrin)	200–300 mg daily in 2–3 divided doses	Mild anticholinergic and sedative effect	Agitation, tremor, dry mouth, insomnia, headache, N/V, constipation
Paroxetine (Paxil)	20–40 mg PO qd	Mild anticholinergic and sedative effect	N/V, insomnia, sweating, tremor, fatigue, dizziness, ejaculatory delay
Citalopram (Celexa)	20–40 mg PO qd	Mild anticholinergic and sedative effect	N/V, insomnia, somnolence, dizziness, agitation, fatigue, dry mouth

SUGGESTED MEDICATION FOR BLADDER MANAGEMENT IN MS

Oxybutynin (Ditropan XL)	5–10 mg PO qd	Anticholinergics	Dry mouth, nausea, constipation, headache, hypertension, palpitation
Tolterodine (Detrol LA)	2 mg PO qd	Anticholinergics	Dry mouth/eyes, blurred vision, headache, constipation, dizziness, drowsiness, fatigue
Mirabegron (Myrbetriq)	25–50 mg qd	B3-adrenergic receptor agonist	HTN, headache, tachycardia

SUGGESTED MANAGEMENT FOR PAIN IN MS (SLOW TITRATION) (V AND IX CN NEURALGIA, PAROXYSMAL DYSESTHETIC PAIN)

Carbamazepine	200–1600 mg in divided doses	Monitor level, slow titration	Hypersensitivity, GI side effects, SIADH
Phenytoin	300–400 mg qd	Monitor level, slow titration	Gingival hyperplasia, hypersensitivity, GI symptoms, SIADH
Lamotrigine	100–200 mg PO bid	Hypersensitivity reaction	Skin rash with Stevens-Johnson syndrome
Topiramate	15–400 mg PO qd	Cognitive side effect	Cognitive side effects, GI tolerance, weight loss
Baclofen or morphine pump, or spinal cord/deep brain stimulation		Severe pain unresponsive to conventional treatment	Infection, mechanical failure

BID, twice daily; *FDA*, Food and Drug Administration; *GI*, gastrointestinal; *HSV*, herpes simplex virus; *HTN*, hypertension; *IM*, intramuscular; *LFT*, liver function test; *MIU*, million international units; *MS*, multiple sclerosis; *PML*, progressive multifocal leukoencephalopathy; *PPMS*, primary progressive multiple sclerosis; *PRES*, posterior reversible encephalopathy syndrome; *QD*, once daily; *RBC*, red blood cell; *RRMS*, relapsing-remitting multiple sclerosis; *SIADH*, syndrome inappropriate anti-diuretic hormone; *SPMS+R*, secondary progressive *MS* with relapses; *SQ*, subcutaneous; *TID*, three times daily; *WBC*, white blood cell.

MULTIPLE SCLEROSIS

REFERENCES

Calabresi, P. (2016). *Multiple Sclerosis and demyelinating Conditions of the Central Nervous System. Shafter A, Goldman L. Goldman-Cecil Medicine* (pp. 2477–2478). Philadelphia: Elsevier.

Fabian, M., Lublin, F., & Krieger, S. (2016). *Multiple Sclerosis and Other Inflammatory Demyelinating Diseases of the Central Nervous System. Bradley's Neurology in Clinical Practice* (pp. P1176–P1183). Philadelphia: Elsevier.

MYASTHENIA GRAVIS

ACUTE MYASTHENIA GRAVIS THERAPY

Name	Time of Onset	Recommended Dose	Action	Indication	Side Effects
Plasmapheresis or plasma exchange	1–7 days (lasts for 3–4 wk)	5 exchanges every other day (3–5 L over 7–14 days)	Removes antibodies from plasma	Myasthenia crisis	Catheter complications (infection, bleeding, thrombosis), hypotension, and arrhythmias
Intravenous immunoglobulin	Less than a week (lasts for 3–6 wk)	2 g/kg over 2–5 days	Uncertain	Myasthenia crisis, refractory myasthenia, or perioperative treatment before thymectomy, or as a bridge to slower-acting immunotherapies	Headache, chills, aseptic meningitis, acute renal failure, thrombotic events, and anaphylaxis in IgA deficiency

CHRONIC MYASTHENIA GRAVIS THERAPY

Symptomatic: Acetylcholinesterase Inhibitor

Name	Time of Onset	Recommended Dose	Action	Indication	Side Effects
Pyridostigmine (Mestinon)	10–15 min	30 mg TID as a starting dose and up to 120 every 4 hr per day	Acetylcholinesterase inhibitor	Symptomatic MG management	GI: Cramps/diarrhea, increased secretions, bradycardia, and cholinergic crisis*
Pyridostigmine XR	Variable	180 mg daily	Acetylcholinesterase inhibitor	Severe weakness upon awaking	Similar to immediate release

Continued

MYASTHENIA GRAVIS

ACUTE MYASTHENIA GRAVIS THERAPY—CONT'D

Name	Time of Onset	Recommended Dose	Action	Indication	Side Effects
Immunomodulators Therapy					
Prednisone	2–3 wk	Starting dose of 20 mg daily and increase by 5 mg every 3–4 days to target 1 mg/kg/day	Inhibits T cell response	Initial therapy for MG	Acute: up to 50% transient deterioration and up to 10% respiratory failure. Chronic: hyperglycemia, hypertension, osteoporosis, fractures, gastritis, Cushing syndrome
Azathioprine (Imuran)	4–10 mo	50 mg qd and increase every 2–4 wk by 50 mg to a total dose of 2–3 mg/kg/day	Inhibits synthesis of nucleic acid and interferes with T and B cells proliferation	Chronic therapy alone (as a steroid-sparing agent) or as a combination with glucocorticoid	Flu-like symptoms, leukopenia, hepatotoxicity, pancreatitis. Get complete blood count (CBC) and LFT q 1–6 m
Mycophenolate (Cellcept)	2–4 mo	500 mg BID (twice a day), increase after 2–4 wk to 1 g BID	Blocks purine synthesis in lymphocytes and inhibits their proliferation	Chronic therapy alone (as a steroid-sparing agent) or as a combination with glucocorticoid	Nausea, diarrhea, leukopenia, hypertension, nephrotoxic. Get CBC q 1 m for the first 6 mo then less frequent

Cyclosporine	2–4 mo	2.5 mg/kg/day and up to 5 mg/kg/day	Limits the production of IL-2, inhibits T-helper cells, and T-lymphocytes dependent immune response	Chronic therapy alone (as a steroid-sparing agent) or as a combination with glucocorticoid	Hypertension, nephrotoxicity, tremor, nausea, gingival hyperplasia, flu-like symptoms, hypertrichosis, malignancy, medications interaction
Tacrolimus (FK506)	6 mo	3–5 mg/day	Similar to cyclosporine	Chronic therapy alone (as a steroid-sparing agent) or as a combination with glucocorticoid	Less nephrotoxic than cyclosporine. Hyperglycemia, hypomagnesemia, tremor, paresthesia
Rituximab	Within 2–3 wk		Monoclonal antibody against B cell membrane marker CD20	Case series support its use in refractory chronic MG, particularly effective for MuSK Ab.	Infusion reactions, progressive multifocal leukoencephalopathy
Cyclophosphamide (Cytoxan)		750 mg/m^2 every 4 wk for 6 mo	Alkylating agent that reduces proliferation of B and T cells	For refractory cases	Anorexia, nausea, vomiting, alopecia, persistent leukopenia, hemorrhagic cystitis, and increased risk of malignancies

Continued

MYASTHENIA GRAVIS

ACUTE MYASTHENIA GRAVIS THERAPY—CONT'D					
Name	Time of Onset	Recommended Dose	Action	Indication	Side Effects
Surgical Treatment					
Thymectomy	1–10 yr	NA	Thymus role in pathogenesis of MG	Indicated in patients with thymoma. It is also considered beneficial in the absence of thymoma in patients with AChR antibodies	Surgical complications

AChR, Acetylcholine receptors; *MG,* myasthenia gravis; *MuSK Ab,* muscle-specific kinase antibodies.

*AChR inhibitors side effects treatments: glycopyrrolate, Pro-Banthine, hycscyamine.

NARCOLEPSY

The following medications may be used for narcolepsy, shift worker, or OSA:

Medication	Usual Dose	Class	Major Side Effects
Dextroamphetamine (Obetrol, psychotic biphetamine)	5 mg/day–50 mg/day	Stimulant	Insomnia, restlessness, tachycardia, episodes, dizziness, diarrhea, constipation, hypertension, impotence, tolerance, and addiction
Methamphetamine (Desoxyn)	5 mg/day–15 mg/day	Stimulant	Same
Methylphenidate (Ritalin)	10 mg/day–60 mg/day	Stimulant	Nervousness, insomnia, anorexia, nausea, dizziness, hypertension, hypotension, hypersensitivity reactions, tachycardia headache, tolerance, and addiction
Mazindol (Mazanor, Sanorex)	2 mg/day–8 mg/day	Stimulant	Cardiovascular stimulation, tolerance, and addiction
Modafinil (Provigil)	100 mg/day–400 mg/day	Unknown	Headache, nausea, eosinophilia, diarrhea, dry dopamine receptor agonist mouth, and anorexia Wake-promoting agent
Armodafinil (Nuvigil)	150 mg to 250 mg/day	Unknown	Headache, nausea, dizziness, Dopamine receptor agonist xerostomia/ dry mouth, insomnia Wake-promoting agent
Sodium oxybate (Xyrem)	4.5 g/day –9 g/day	γ-Hydroxybutyrate	Nausea and headache
Selegiline (Eldepryl, Atapryl, Carbex)	20 mg/day–40 mg/day	MAO inhibitor	Nausea, dizziness, confusion, tremor, orthostatic hypotension, diet-induced hypertension
Fluoxetine (Prozac)	20 mg/day–80 mg/day	SSRI	Nausea, diarrhea, anorexia, insomnia, tremor, anxiety, somnolence
Protriptyline (Vivactil)	5 mg/day–30 mg/day	TCA	Orthostatic hypotension, hypertension, seizures, headache, anticholinergic symptoms, impotence, impaired liver function, myocardial infarction, stroke

MAO, monoamine oxidase; OSA; Obstructive sleep apnea; SSRI, selective serotonin reuptake inhibitor; TCA, tricyclic antidepressant.

NARCOLEPSY

REFERENCE

Kallweit, U., et al. (2017). Pharmacological management of narcolepsy with and without cataplexy. *Expert Opin Pharmacother*, *18*(8), 809–817. https://doi.org/10.1080/14656566.2017.1323877. Epub 2017 May 17.

NEURO-ONCOLOGY, THERAPEUTICS

There are several recommended treatment strategies for the medical and neurologic problems in patients with brain tumors. Rather than an in-depth neuro-oncology discussion, a list of treatments that can be provided to a patient with a neurologic cancer by their general neurologist is provided. Current trends have been toward emphasizing prognostic data early, and introducing palliative care at an early stage of treatment; these interventions alone have been shown to have a life-prolonging effect.

- Vasogenic Edema
  - Results from increased brain tumor permeability. It greatly increases effective tumor volume, leading to symptoms of increased intracranial pressure and more severe focal deficits. Initial therapy in a central nervous system (CNS) malignancy is reduction of edema with a steroid preparation. One exception would be when a CNS lymphoma is suspected, where steroid treatment may alter pathology findings. There are a number of options, all which can be administered intravenously or orally. Dexamethasone is usually chosen because of its low mineralocorticoid effects and long half-life. Common adverse effects include weight gain, infections, irritability, insomnia, glucose intolerance or hyperglycemia, tremor, and myopathy.
- Infections
  - Wound infections may occur days to years following craniotomy and are more common in patients who have received bevacizumab. Worsening neurologic symptoms, headache, and restricted diffusion on diffusion-weighted imaging are clues to the presence of infection. Most infections will require surgical drainage.
  - Chronic corticosteroid use in these patients increases the risk for three infections:
    - *Pneumocystis jiroveci* pneumonia
      - Patients receiving corticosteroids for >1 month should receive *Pneumocystis* prophylaxis with trimethoprim/sulfamethoxazole
    - Progressive multifocal leukoencephalopathy
    - Varicella-zoster virus
- Seizures
  - Occur in up to 70% of patients with brain tumors. They are most common in patients with low-grade gliomas. Seizure prophylaxis in patients who have brain tumors without seizures does not change subsequent seizure occurrence or patient survival; in these cases prophylactic anti-seizure medications are not recommended. Conversely, most patients with seizures in the setting of a brain tumor will need lifelong treatment.
  - For patients with brain tumors who have seizures, levetiracetam is emerging as the best first-line drug. Lamotrigine is theoretically a good choice, but requires a very long dose-escalation period. Lacosamide has received considerable interest and is used in many centers as an add-on for patients with brain tumors requiring a second drug.

Phenytoin may predispose to Stevens-Johnson syndrome in patients receiving brain radiation therapy.

- Venous Thromboembolism
  - Brain tumors carry a very high risk of venous thromboembolism. It is the second-leading cause of death in patients with cancer, and up to 30% of patients with gliomas may be affected.
  - Perioperatively, triple prophylaxis is recommended with compression stockings, pneumatic devices, and enoxaparin. However, current guidelines from the American Society of Clinical Oncology advise against the use of routine prophylaxis of venous thromboembolism in ambulatory patients with cancer.
  - Most oncologists recommend that patients with cancer who have documented venous thromboembolism should remain on lifelong anticoagulation with low-molecular-weight heparin. Placement of vena cava filters is reserved for patients who cannot be anticoagulated as there is a high risk of recurrent thrombosis.
- Arterial Thromboembolism and Hemorrhagic Stroke
  - The etiologies of stroke in patients with cancer are different from those of the noncancer stroke population. Thrombolytic agents for pulmonary embolism or ischemic stroke are contraindicated in patients with brain tumors. Choice of anticoagulation modality and duration of therapy must be weighed individually by patient clinical status, tumor type, and stroke mechanism.
- Fatigue and Mood
  - Many neuro-oncologists move directly to stimulants to improve lethargy and mood, as typical antidepressants may take too long. Methylphenidate is often used.

REFERENCE

Pruitt, A. (2015). Medical management of patients with brain tumors. *Continuum Lifelong Learn Neurol, 21*, 314–331.

OBSTRUCTIVE SLEEP APNEA-HYPOPNEA SYNDROME

Obstructive sleep apnea (OSA) is due to obstruction of the upper airway during sleep causing reduced or complete airflow interruption, leading to hypoxemia, snoring, and sleep impairment. It is a risk factor for coronary artery disease, hypertension, and cerebrovascular events.

Diagnosis: Polysomnography performed in a sleep lab is the standard method. Apnea-hypopnea index (AHI) is used to diagnose and assess severity of OSA. AHI $\geq$ 15 with or without symptoms or AHI $\geq$ 5 with symptoms is required for diagnosis. Symptoms include fatigue, insomnia, daytime sleepiness, cognitive impairment, mood disorders, or cardiovascular comorbid conditions.

Treatment	Effects	Comments
Weight loss	10% weight loss may eliminate apneic episodes by reducing the mass of the posterior airway	
Avoidance of alcohol for 4–6 hr prior to bedtime		
Sleeping on the side		
Nasal continuous positive airway pressure (CPAP)	Improves daytime sleepiness, mood, and cognitive function in people with both mild and moderate apnea. CPAP has also been shown to increase quality of life and decrease health care costs. Most effective treatment of obstructive sleep apnea Sleep study recommended to titrate pressure levels	Side effects: dry mouth, rhinitis, sinus congestion, and claustrophobia Compliance: 50% of patients use prescribed CPAP on regular basis
Apnea-hypopnea index >15	Eligible for CPAP therapy, regardless of symptomatology	
5–14.9	Indicated only if the patient has one of the following: EDS, hypertension, or cardiovascular disease	
Oral appliances	Move tongue and mandible forward, enlarge posterior airspace, better compliance	CPAP more effective at reducing apnea-hypopnea index Side effects: mucosal erosions, excess salivation, teeth loosening, TMJ pain
Surgical management		Side effects: nerve palsies, hemorrhage, difficulty swallowing, voice changes, airway stenosis
Uvulopalatopharyngoplasty	40% effectiveness	
Craniofacial reconstruction		
Geniohyoid advancement with hyoid myotomy	70% effectiveness	Uncertain long-term prognosis
Maxillomandibular osteotomy	95% effectiveness	Uncertain long-term prognosis
Tracheostomy	Definitive treatment	

OBSTRUCTIVE SLEEP APNEA-HYPOPNEA SYNDROME

REFERENCES

Qaseem, A., Dallas, P., Owens, D. K., et al. (2014). Diagnosis of obstructive sleep apnea in adults: a clinical practice guideline from the American College of Physicians. *Ann Intern Med*, *161*(3). 210–220.

Qaseem, A., Holty, J. E. C., Owens, D. K., et al. (2013). Management of obstructive sleep apnea in adults: a clinical practice guideline from the American College of Physicians. *Ann Intern Med.*, *159*(7), 471–483.

PAGET DISEASE

Medications	Dosage	Comments/Side Effects
Bisphosphonates:		Bisphosphonate tablets should be taken with 6–8 oz. of water on an empty stomach. Do not eat or lie down for 30 min after taking medication. Bisphosphonates should be avoided in patients with kidney disease.
Alendronate (Fosamax)	40 mg PO qd × 6 months. May reinstate treatment after 6 mo, if necessary.	Alendronate: The most common side effects are upper gastrointestinal symptoms.
Pamidronate (Aredia)	30–60 mg IV over 4-hr period on 2–3 consecutive days. Repeat as necessary.	Pamidronate: Transient "flu-like" syndrome of fever, myalgia, and arthralgia; rarely uveitis and acute renal failure have been reported.
Tiludronate (Skelid)	400 mg PO qd for 3 mo. Repeat as necessary.	
Risedronate (Actonel)	30 mg PO qd for 2 mo. Repeat as necessary.	Risedronate: the most common side effects are upper gastrointestinal symptoms.
Etidronate (Didronel)	5 mg/kg PO qd (if ineffective, 11–20 mg/kg PO qd for a maximum of 6 mo). Repeat as necessary.	
Calcitonin (Miacalcin injection)	200 U/mL; 100 U SC or IM once daily for 6–18 mo.	Nausea and facial flushing are common side effects of calcitonin-salmon (Calcimar)
Zoledronic Acid (Reclast)	Single 5 mg IV infusion at constant rate over >15 min.	Zoledronic acid: Patients should be appropriately hydrated prior to administration, especially if receiving diuretic therapy.
Vitamin D supplement Calcium supplement	All patients should receive 1500 mg Ca daily in divided Doses and 800 IU vitamin D daily.	

PAGET DISEASE

REFERENCES

Healy, G. M., et al. (2015). Paget's disease of bone: progress towards remission and prevention. *Ir Med J.*, *108*(10), 316–317.

Urteaga, E. M. (2012). Treatment of Paget's disease of bone. *US Pharm.*, *37*(10), 29–34.

PAIN (See also HEADACHE, AED, AND ANTIDEPRESSANTS IN AAN GUIDELINE SUMMARIES APPENDIX)

Medication Class	Medication	Dose/Ceiling Dose	Advantages	Comments/Caution/Side Effects
Nonopioid analgesic	Acetaminophen (acetyl-para-aminophenol [APAP])	PO: 650–1000 mg q4-hr, not to exceed 3,000 mg/day PR: 650 mg q4-6h; not to exceed 3,000 mg/day	Mild to moderate pain	Hepatotoxicity, usually with doses greater than 10 g/day, may occur at lower dose, within therapeutic dose in alcoholics, fasting patients, and those taking cytochrome P-450 enzyme inducing substances APAP does not have anti-inflammatory effects.
NSAIDs	Aspirin	PO: 325–1,000 mg q4-6 hr, maximum daily dose 4 g/day	Effective in various types of pain	All NSAIDs: Sodium and water retention, NSAID-induced nephrotoxicity, gastric erosions or peptic ulcers.
	Diclofenac	PO capsule: 25 mg QID PO tablet: 50 mg QID IV: 37.5 mg q6h	Narcotic sparing, some patients may respond to certain NSAIDs	Dose-dependent aspirin toxicity: Tinnitus, emesis, encephalopathy, metabolic acidosis, respiratory alkalosis, increased bleeding time
	Ketorolac	IM: 60 mg as a single dose or 30 mg every 6 hr (maximum: 120 mg/day) IV: 30 mg as a single dose or 30 mg every 6 hr (maximum: 120 mg/day)	Avoid opioid- induced respiratory depression, constipation, and nausea	Misoprostol may be effective in NSAID-induced gastric erosion or peptic ulcer, contraindicated in pregnancy Be wary of NSAID overuse or rebound headaches

Continued

PAIN

Medication Class	Medication	Dose/Ceiling Dose	Advantages	Comments/Caution/Side Effects
	Ibuprofen	PO: 400–800 mg QID, maximum daily dose 3,200 mg/day	Available over the counter	
	Naproxen	PO: 500 mg, then 250 mg q6–8h or 500 mg q12h; maximum daily dose 1,250 mg on day 1, 1,000 mg/day every subsequent day	Available over the counter	
Benzodiazepines	Alprazolam Chlordiazepoxide Diazepam Lorazepam	PO: 0.25–1.0 mg BID-TID PO: 5–10 mg TID-QID PO/IV/IM: 2–10 mg BID-QID po: 0.5–1 mg BID-TID	In patients with difficulty sleeping from pair;; BZD effective in treating anxiety and insomnia	Good as adjunctive therapy Ventilatory depression and hypotension, exacerbated by opioids, worse in COPD. Alprazolam withdrawal associated with seizures; all contraindicated in first trimester of pregnancy Caution advised in patients with liver disease
Opioid analgesics	Codeine	PO/IM: 30–60 mg q3h PRN, 30 mg Dosing changes depending on tolerance	Opioid class with mild to severe pain control, no ceiling effect with opioids	All opioids: tolerance with chronic use (1–2 wk), overdose possible with respiratory depression, nausea, vomiting, ileus, impaired gastric motility, bradycardia with fentanyl, bronchospasm with morphine Morphine is an active metabolite of codeine

	Tramadol	PO: 50–100 mg q4–6h, max 300–400 mg/day	Tramadol is effective for neuropathic pain	All opioids: tolerance with chronic use (1–2 wk), overdose possible with respiratory depression, nausea, vomiting, ileus, impaired gastric motility; serotonin syndrome with Tramadol.
	Hydrocodone Oxycodone	Vicodin 1tb PO q6 hr + aspirin or + acetaminophen, also extended-release OxyContin 10–20 mg q12h	For chronic low back pain	
	Hydromorphone	PO: 7.5 mg; IM 1.5 mg, duration 3 hr	For phantom pain	Tramadol may lower seizure threshold.
	Morphine	PO: 20–60 mg, IM: 10 mg, duration 4–6 hr	For phantom pain	Naloxone for reversal of opioid overdose
	Fentanyl	50–150 mcg patch q 72 hr, titrate slowly		Fentanyl patch onset of action may take a few days.
Antidepressants (see Antidepressants, Therapeutic Appendix)	Duloxetine (Cymbalta)	PO: 20 mg daily - BID; max 120 mg /day		Suicidal ideation; withdrawal syndrome may complicate dose reduction; needs slow titration.
	Tricyclic antidepressants	PO: 25–100 mg daily, qhs, titrate slowly	For those with trouble sleeping at night	Effective in peripheral neuropathy with insomnia or chronic pain; excessive sedation or urinary retention can be a problem due to anticholinergic effects
Antiepileptic drugs (AEDs) (see AED, Therapeutic Appendix)	Carbamazepine	PO: Initially 400 mg/day in 2–4 divided doses; increase by up to 200 mg/day on a weekly basis	Trigeminal neurologic post-stroke pain syndrome (thalamic Dejerine-Roussy syndrome)	Be wary of poor tolerance with rapid titration or SIADH; Dilantin toxicity with nausea, vomiting, ataxia, and nystagmus.

Continued

PAIN

Medication Class	Medication	Dose/Ceiling Dose	Advantages	Comments/Caution/Side Effects
	Phenytoin	PO: Maintenance doses 300–400 mg daily		Well tolerated; no active metabolites; lower dosage in renal disease
	Gabapentin (Neurontin)	PO: 1,200–3,600 mg/day in 3 divided doses	Neuropathic pain Headaches Fibromyalgia Chronic pain	Variable effectiveness Psychosis, suicidal thoughts, agitation possible
	Pregabalin	PO: Initially 150 mg/day in 2–3 divided doses, titrate up to 450 mg/day in 2–3 divided doses	Neuropathic pain Chronic headache Fibromyalgia Chronic pain	Cognitive side effect, nephrolithiasis, weight loss Do not discontinue without taper
	Topiramate	PO: 25 mg once daily initially, titrate up to 100 mg/day over 2 doses in weekly increments of 25 mg/day	Migraine prophylaxis	Tremor, hair loss, increased appetite and weight gain, hepatotoxicity
	Valproic acid	PO: 250 mg qd; doses over 1,000 mg/day show no increased benefit	Migraine prophylaxis	Post zoster/shingle infection
Others	Lidocaine patch Transcutaneous electrical nerve stimulation unit Physical therapy/ occupational therapy/ psychotherapy Local injection/ pump and surgery	5% patch	Postherpetic neuralgia	Older pumps or hardware may not be MRI compatible

IV, intravenous; *NSAID*, nonsteroidal anti-inflammatory drug; *PO*, by mouth; *QID*, 4 times a day; *SIADH*, syndrome of inappropriate antidiuretic hormone secretion

REFERENCE

Turk, D. C., Wilson, H. D., & Cahana, A. (2011). Treatment of chronic non-cancer pain. *Lancet, 377*, 2226.

PARKINSON DISEASE (MOVEMENT DISORDER)

Medication	Route	Action	Dosage	Side Effects
Levodopa/Carbidopa (IR-Sinemet; ER-Rytary)	PO	Levodopa	Levodcpa 150–1,500 mg/day divided to 3–6 times a day	N/V, sleepiness, dizzy, HA, orthostatic hypotension, confusion, motor fluctuation
Pramipexole (Mirapex)	PO	Dopamine agonist	0.125 mg TID to 1.5 mg TID	N/V, sleepiness, dizzy, HA, orthostatic hypotension, confusion, peripheral edema, impulse control disorders
Ropinirole (Requip)	PO	Dopamine agonist	0.25 mg TID to 8 mg po TID	
Rotigotine (Neupro)	Patch	Dopamine agonist	2–8 mg/day	
Apomorphine (Apokyn)	Subcu	Dopamine agonist	2–6 mg/day	
Selegiline (Emsam)	PO	MAOB inhibitor	5 mg daily to BID	N/V, confusion
Rasagiline (Azilect)	PO	MAOB inhibitor	0.5–1 mg daily	
Trihexyphenidyl (Artane)	PO	Anticholinergics	0.5 mg BID to 2 mg TID	Confusion, dry mouth, constipation, urinary retention
Benztropine (Cogentin)	PO, IM, IV	Anticholinergics	0.5–2 mg daily, or divided BID	
Amantadine	PO	Unknown, dopamine release, inhibit reuptake, stimulate receptor, NMDA antagonist	100 mg BID up to QID	Livedo reticularis, ankle edema, confusion
Tolcapone (Tasmar)	PO	COMT inhibitor	100 mg po q8h	Fatal acute fulminant liver failure, N/V, confusion, dyskinesia, orthostatic hypotension
Entacapone (Comtan)	PO	COMT inhibitor	200 mg with each dose of L-dopa, to 1,600 mg/day divided	N/V, confusion, dyskinesia, orthostatic hypotension

BID, twice daily; *COMT*, Catechol-O-Methyltransfe; *ER*, extended release; *HA*, headache; *IM*, intramuscular; *IR*, immediate release; *IV*, intravenous; *MAOB*, monoamine oxidase B; *NMDA*, N-methyl-D-aspartate; *PO*, by mouth; *TID*, three times daily.

RESTLESS LEGS SYNDROME

DRUG	DOSAGE RANGE	COMMON SIDE EFFECTS
FIRST LINE AGENTS		
Dopamine Agonist		
Pramipexole (Mirpex)	0.125 mg to 0.5 mg daily before bedtime	Orthostatic hypotension, drowsiness, nausea, dyskinesias
Ropinirole (Requip)	0.25 mg to 2 mg daily before bedtime	Orthostatic hypotension, drowsiness, nausea
Rotigotine transdermal patch(Neupro)	1 to 2 mg patch every 24 hours	Orthostatic hypotension, drowsiness, nausea
Alpha-2-delta calcium channel ligands		
Gabapentin (Neurontin)	100–900 mg TID	Dizziness, drowsiness, ataxia
Pregablin (Lyrica)	50–450 mg daily before bedtime	Dizziness, drowsiness, peripheral edema
SECOND LINE AGENTS		
Benzodiazepines		
Clonazepam (KlonoPIN)	1–2 mg before bedtime	Dizziness, drowsiness, ataxia
Opioids		
Codeine	30–180 mg before bedtime	Risk of addiction, constipation, CNS depression
Tramadol (Ultram)	50 to 100 mg before bedtime	Risk of addiction, diarrhea, CNS depression
Dopaminergic Agents		
Carbidopa/levodopa (IR)	25–100 mg (0.5 to 1 tablet) daily	Orthostatic hypotension, nausea, dizziness
Carbidopa/levodopa (CR)	25-100 mg (0.5 to 1 tablet) daily	Orthostatic hypotension, nausea, dizziness

RESTLESS LEGS SYNDROME

SEDATIVES AND PARALYTICS

Sedative Agents[a]	Induction Dose	Sedative/ Conscious sedation Dose	Infusion Dose	Mechanism of Action	Duration	Side Effects	Contraindications/ Precautions
Propofol	20–40 mg IV every 10 s until induction onset (0.5–2.5 mg/kg)	Titrate	5–50 µg/kg/min intravenous (IV) (0.3–3 mg/kg/hr)	GABA-ergic	Bolus: 3–5 min	Hypotension, pruritis, paresthesias, pain on injection	Hemodynamically unstable patients; interacts with monoamine oxidase inhibitors; abuse potential
Etomidate	0.1–0.3 mg/kg		N/A; may be potentiated by Fentany	Cl⁻ ionophore of $GABA_A$ receptor	Bolus: 3–5 min	Myoclonus, pain on injection, allergic reactions, infusion site reactions	Adrenal suppression with induction or continuous infusion
Dexmedetomidine	0.5–1 µg/kg over 10 min		0.1–0.6 µg/kg/hr	Alpha-2 agonist	Approx. 4 hr	Bradycardia, sinus arrest, hypotension	Approved only for < 24 hr continuous use; lower doses age > 65 yr
Pentobarbital	100 mg		<50 mg/min	GABA-ergic	Bolus: 5–8 min	Hypotension, respiratory depression, immunosuppression, confusion	

Midazolam	0.1–0.3 mg/kg once, over 20–30s	1–2.5 mg IV (depends on age)	0.01–0.1 mg/kg/hr; max 0.6 mg/kg	GABA-ergic	2–6 hr	Hypotension, respiratory depression	May potentiate opioid effects; not to be given by rapid IV dosing in neonates
Lorazepam		IV: 2 mg total, or 0.044 mg/kg, whichever is smaller		GABA-ergic	4–8 hr	Hypotension, respiratory depression, paradoxical agitation	Acidosis due to the solvent preparation; acute narrow angle glaucoma
Fentanyl	50–100 µg IM, 30–60 min prior to surgery.	1–2 mg/kg	25–100 µg IV/IM.	Opiate agonist	60–90 min	Bradycardia, respiratory depression	Respiratory depression; abuse potential
Remifentanil	0.5–1 µg /kg/min IV until after intubation; may give initial dose of 1 µg /kg if intubation to occur less than 8 min after start of infusion	1 µg /kg IV bolus, followed by 0.05–0.2 µg /kg/min IV	0.25–0.5 µg/kg/min IV	Opiate agonist	5–10 min	Hypotension, bradycardia, intraoperative awareness when combined with propofol	Chest wall rigidity, apnea with bolus doses

Continued

SEDATIVES AND PARALYTICS

Sedative Agents[b]	Intubation Dose	Maintenance Dose	Mechanism of Action	Duration	Side Effects	Contraindications/ Precautions
Succinylcholine	0.6 mg/kg	2.5–4.3 mg/min	Depolarizing— Acetylcholine receptor agonist	3–5 min	Slight increase in intracranial pressure	Risk for hyperkalemia and malignant hyperthermia; contraindicated if recent trauma (burns, tissue damage, etc.)
Pancuronium	0.06–0.1 mg/kg	0.04–0.1 mg/kg. 0.01 mg/kg increments	Non-depolarizing	90–120 min	Vagolytic (increased HR), weakness, respiratory depression.	Renal failure, contraindicated in neonates (contains benzyl alcohol)
Cisatracurium	0.15–0.2 mg/kg	0.03 mg/kg	Non-depolarizing	45–60 min	Bradycardia, skeletal muscle blockade, respiratory depression	contraindicated in neonates (contains benzyl alcohol)

[a]Sedative infusion can be titrated to a set sedation scale (Ramsay 3) or monitoring parameter (e.g., BIS 50–60). Remember that most agents accumulate with continuous dosing with a short redistribution half-life and a much longer elimination half-life. Continuous hemodynamic and respiratory monitoring must be used.

[b]Neuromuscular blocker infusions should generally be titrated to maintain 1 out of 4 twitches on train-of-four testing. Neuromuscular blockers should only be used with concomitant sedation to avoid an awake-paralyzed state.

These medications should be used by physicians with adequate training and skill in their use and knowledge of their actions, hazards, adverse effects, and their treatments.

SPASTICITY (MOVEMENT DISORDER)

Medication	Dosage	Action	Side Effects
Tizanidine (Zanaflex)	2–8 mg q8h	Alpha 2 agonist	Hypotension, sedation
Gabapentin (Neurontin)	300 mg TID	Unknown	Dizziness, sedation, leg swelling
Baclofen (Lioresal)	5 mg TID, max 20 mg QID	GABA-B agonist	Dizziness, sedation
Dantrolene (Dantrium)	25 mg daily to TID, max 100 mg QID	Ca channel inhibition	Hepatotoxicity, weakness, N/V
Clonazepam (Klonopin)	0.25 mg daily up to 1 mg BID	GABA-A agonist	Dizziness, sedation
Botulinum toxin type a (Botox)	Dose varies	Neuromuscular blocker	Weakness
Physical and occupational therapy			

BID, twice a day; *TID*, three times a day; *QID*, four times a day.

STROKE

STROKE MEDICAL THERAPY AND RISK FACTORS MANAGEMENT

Generic name	Trade name	Dosage	Indications	Side Effects
Aspirin		50–325 mg/day	Reduce recurrent stroke risk Reduce risk of stroke in certain high-risk conditions (e.g., nonvalvular atrial fibrillation)	Bleeding
Alteplase	Activase	0.9 mg/kg (10% given as bolus and remainder infused over 1 hr; max dose 90 mg)	Acute ischemic stroke within 3 hr of onset	Bleeding Anaphylaxis Hypotension
Clopidogrel	Plavix	75 mg/day	Reduction in atherosclerotic events in patients with stroke, coronary artery disease, and peripheral arterial disease	GI bleeding Diarrhea Rash GI symptoms
Aspirin/ extended release dipyridamole	Aggrenox	1 cap bid (25 mg aspirin/ 200 mg extended release dipyridamole per cap)	Reduce risk of stroke in patients with transient ischemic attack or completed ischemic stroke	Dizziness Headache GI effects Hypotension
Heparin		Varies	Varies	Hemorrhage Urticaria Thrombocytopenia Skin necrosis Anaphylactoid reactions Gangrene Priapism

Ticlopidine	Ticlid	250 mg PO bid with food	Reduce risk of thrombotic stroke in patients intolerant to aspirin	GI symptoms Neutropenia Purpura Abnormal liver function tests
Ticagrelor	Brilinta	90 mg PO BID	Reduce risk of stroke in patients with acute coronary syndrome/myocardial infarction	Shortness of breath, headache, bleeding
Warfarin	Coumadin	Varies; goal pt-inr varies by indication	Prophylaxis or treatment of thromboembolic complications associated with atrial fibrillation and cardiac valve replacement	Hemorrhage from *any* tissue or organ Priapism
Nimodipine	Nimotop	60 mg PO q4h for 21 days (initiate within 96 hr)	Improvement in neurologic outcome in Hunt and Hess grades i–iii subarachnoid hemorrhage	Purple toes syndrome Hypotension, edema Diarrhea Rash, acne Depression Muscle pain and cramps

MANAGEMENT OF STROKE RISK FACTORS

Risk Factor	Goal	Recommendations
Hypertension	Stage 1: Systolic between 130–139 or diastolic between 80–89 should be treated in patient with history of stroke or transient ischemic stroke but not in the acute phase.	Lifestyle modification and antihypertensive medications.
Smoking	Cessation	Strongly encourage patient and family to stop smoking. Provide counseling, nicotine replacement, and formal programs.
Diabetes mellitus	Glucose < 126 mg/dL (6.99 mmol/L)	Diet, oral hypoglycemics, insulin.
Lipids	LDL < 100 mg/dL (2.59 mmol/L) HDL > 35 mg/dL (0.91 mmol/L) TC < 200 mg/dL (5.18 mmol/L) TG < 200 mg/dL (2.26 mmol/L)	Start AHA step ii diet: ≤ 30% fat, < 7% saturated fat, < 200 mg/day cho esterol, and emphasize weight management and physical activity. If target goal not achieved with these measures, add drug therapy (e.g., statin agent) if LDL > 130 mg/dL (3.37 mmol/L) and consider drug therapy if LDL 100–130 mg/dL (2.59–3.37 mmol/L).
Alcohol	Patients with ischemic stroke or TIA who are heavy drinkers should eliminate or reduce their consumption of alcohol (Class 1, Level of Evidence C).	Strongly encourage patient and family to stop excessive drinking or provide formal alcohol cessation program.
Physical activity	30–60 min of activity at least 3–4 times/wk	Moderate exercise (e.g., brisk walking, jogging, cycling, or other aerobic activity). Medically supervised programs for high-risk patients (e.g., cardiac disease) and adaptive programs depending on neurological deficits are recommended.
Weight	≤120% of ideal body weight for height	Diet and exercise.

AHA, American Heart Association; *DBP*, diastolic blood pressure; *HDL*, high-density lipoproteins; *LDL*, low density lipoprotein; *SBP*, systolic blood pressure; *TC*, total cholesterol; *TG*, triglycerides.

REFERENCE

Whelton, P. K., Carey, R. M., Aronow, W. S., et al. 2017. ACC/AHA/AAPA/ABC/ACPM/ AGS/APhA/ASH/ASPC/NMA/PCNA Guideline for the Prevention, Detection, Evaluation, and Management of High Blood Pressure in Adults: Executive Summary: A Report of the American College of Cardiology/American Heart Association Task Force on Clinical Practice Guidelines. *Circulation*, *138*(17), e426–e483.

TICS (MOVEMENT DISORDER)

MEDICATIONS FOR TICS*

Medication	Dosage	Side Effects
Tetrabenazine (Xenazine)	12.5–50 mg qd	Sedation, fatigue, nausea, insomnia, akathisia, parkinsonism, depression
Clonidine (Catapres)	0.05–0.4 mg qd (pediatric dose)	Drowsiness, dry mouth, itchy eyes, postural hypotension, headache
Guanfacine (Tenex)	0.05–0.12 mg/kg/day (pediatric dose)	Somnolence, headache, dizziness, xerostomia, syncope
Haloperidol (Haldol)	0.5–20 mg qd po	Rigidity, parkinsonism, involuntary movements, weight gain, sedation,
Fluphenazine	0.5–40 mg qd (not recommended in children)	Rigidity, parkinsonism, involuntary movements, weight gain, sedation, hyperprolactinemia, constipation
Risperidone (Risperdal)	0.5–6 mg qd	Sedation, depression, drowsiness, hypotension, weight gain, hyperprolactinemia, constipation
Pimozide (Orap)	0.5–10 mg qd	Rigidity, parkinsonism, involuntary movements, weight gain, sedation, hyperprolactinemia, constipation
Olanzapine (Zyprexa)	2.5–20 mg qd	Sedation, weight gain, transient hypoglycemia, orthostasis
Aripiprazole (Abilify)	5–30 mg qd	Weight gain, headache, sedation, sleep problems
Clonazepam (Klonopin)	0.5–4 mg qd	Drowsiness
Ropinirole (Requip)	0.5–3 mg qd	Very well tolerated at very low doses
Botulinum toxin injections		Local injection to focal areas

*Many of these medications are off label for this indication.

Scales Appendix

CHALFONT SEIZURE SEVERITY SCALE

The Chalfont seizure severity scale was first introduced by Duncan and Sander in 1991, to quantitatively assess the severity of seizures. It has since been revised, and the revised form is known as the National Hospital Seizure Severity Scale. The scale is both patient-based and observer-based. It can be completed by the physician in an interview with the patient or by the eyewitness of the seizure. The scoring system is based on several major aspects of the seizure, with a higher score meant to represent a more severe seizure. Points are given for loss of awareness, warning sign, dropping/spilling a held object, falling to the ground, having an injury including tongue-biting, bruising and laceration, incontinence (urine and/or feces), automatism (e.g., chewing, repeated swallowing, fiddling with objects), convulsion, duration of the seizure, and time to return to normal from onset. If the seizures occur in sleep, the total score is divided by 2. A score of 1 is added if the total score is otherwise 0 (e.g., a simple partial seizure with an aura that lasts less than 10 seconds). For example, a patient with generalized tonic-clonic seizure, with no warning sign, drops an object and falls to the ground with a tongue bite and urinary incontinence, no automatism, with a convulsion of 4 minutes and returns to normal in 2 hours. The seizure severity score is 103. Based on the score, physicians can determine the efficacy of medical and surgical treatments of the seizures. It is important to note that the scale does not measure the overall life quality of the patient as the result of the seizure. Higher scores do not correlate with increased seizure frequency. Results need to be interpreted cautiously in a clinical context.

CHALFONT SEIZURE SEVERITY SCALE

Classification of Seizure Type	Seizures		
	Type 1	Type 2	Type 3
Loss of awareness. No = 0, Yes = 1			
Warning (if loss of awareness). No = 1, Yes = 0			
Drop/spill a held object. No = 0, Yes = 4			
Fall to ground. No = 0, Yes = 4			
Injury. No = 0, Yes = 20			
Incontinent. No = 0, Yes = 8			

Continued

CHALFONT SEIZURE SEVERITY SCALE—CONT'D

	Seizures		
Classification of Seizure Type	Type 1	Type 2	Type 3
Automatism.			
No = 0			
Mild (chew, swallow, fiddle) = 4,			
Severe (shout, undress, run, hit) = 12			
Convulsion.			
No = 0, Yes = 12			
Duration of seizure.			
< 10 s $= 0$, 10 s^{-1} min $= 1$			
1–10 min $= 4$, > 10 min $= 16$			
Time to return to normal from onset.			
< 1 min $= 0$, 1–10 min $= 5$, 10–30 min $= 20$			
30–60 min $= 30$, 1–3 hr $= 50$, > 3 hr $= 100$			
IF FPII FPTIC EVENT (EG. BRIEF AURA)			
WITH TOTAL SCORE $= 0$, THEN ADD 1.			
DIVIDE SCORE BY 2 IF ONLY IN SLEEP			
TOTAL			

From Duncan, J. S. & Sander, J. W. (1991). The Chalfont seizure severity scale. *J Neurol Neurosurg Psychiatry, 54*(10), 873–876.

REFERENCES

Aghaei-Lasboo, A., & Fisher, R. S. (2016). Methods for measuring seizure frequency and severity. *Neurol Clin, 34*(2), 383–394.

Cramer, J. A. (2001). Assessing the severity of seizures and epilepsy: which scales are valid? *Curr Opin Neurol, 14*, 225–229.

EPWORTH SLEEPINESS SCALE

Situation	Would Never Doze	Slight Chance of Dozing	Moderate Chance of Dozing	High Chance of Dozing
1. Sitting and reading	0	1	2	3
2. Watching TV	0	1	2	3
3. Sitting and inactive in public place (theater or a meeting)	0	1	2	3
4. As a passenger in a car for an hour without a break	0	1	2	3
5. Lying down to rest in the afternoon when circumstances permit	0	1	2	3
6. Sitting and talking to someone	0	1	2	3
7. Sitting quietly after lunch (without alcohol)	0	1	2	3

8. In a car, while stopped for a few minutes in traffic	0	1	2	3

Score: Add up scores for items 1–8 for total score (range 0–24).

<10 = normal awakeness.

10–18 = moderately sleepy.

>18 = very sleepy.

FISHER SCALE

The Fisher scale assesses the amount of subarachnoid hemorrhage (SAH) based on the head CT scan:

1: No blood, SAH diagnosed by lumbar puncture (LP)

2: Less than 1 mm layering of SAH in the cisterns

3: More than 1 mm layering of SAH in the cisterns

4: Intraventricular or intracerebral hematoma, loculated hematoma

GLASGOW COMA SCALE

The best guide to the severity of head injury is the conscious state.

The Glasgow coma scale (GCS) allows quantitation of conscious state.

GCS 3 to 8: Severe head injury

GCS 9 to 12: Moderate head injury

GCS 13 to 15: Mild head injury

Assessment	Score	Infants	Children and Adults
Eye opening	4	Spontaneous	Spontaneous
	3	To shout	To verbal command
	2	To pain	To pain
	1	No response	No response
Best motor response	6	Norm/spontaneous movement	Follows commands
	5	Withdraws to touch	Localizes pain
	4	Withdraws to pain	Withdraws to pain
	3	Flexion to pain	Flexion to pain
	2	Extension to pain	Extension to pain
	1	No response	No response
Best verbal response	5	Coos and babbles	Orientated
	4	Irritable cry	Confused
	3	Cries to pain	Inappropriate words
	2	Moans to pain	Sounds
	1	No response	No response

Notes:

1. The GCS should be scored on the patient's best responses.

2. The GCS may be falsely low if one of the following is present: shock, hypoxia, hypothermia, intoxication, postictal state, sedative drug administration.

3. The GCS may be impossible to evaluate accurately if the patient is agitated, uncooperative, dysphasic, or intubated or has significant facial or spinal cord injuries.

GLASGOW COMA SCALE

GLASGOW OUTCOME RATING SCALE

The Glasgow outcome rating scale is used mainly to assess traumatic head injury but can also be used for stroke and other neurologic diseases.

Score	Description
1	**Dead**
2	**Vegetative state**
	Unable to interact with environment; unresponsive
3	**Severe disability**
	Able to follow commands/unable to live independently
4	**Moderate disability**
	Able to live independently; unable to return to work or school
5	**Good recovery**
	Able to return to work or school

HUNT AND HESS CLINICAL SEVERITY SCALE FOR SUBARACHNOID HEMORRHAGE

1. Asymptomatic or mild headache
2. Moderate or severe headache, nuchal rigidity, can have oculomotor palsy
3. Confusion, drowsiness, or mild focal signs
4. Stupor or hemiparesis
5. Comatose or extensor posturing

KURTZKE EXPANDED DISABILITY STATUS SCALE (EDSS)

Rating	Functional Status
0	Normal neurologic examination
1.0	No disability, minimal symptoms
1.5	No disability, minimal signs in more than one area
2.0	Slightly more disability in one area
2.5	Slightly greater disability in two areas
3.0	Moderate disability in one area but still walking independently
3.5	Walking independently but with moderate disability in one area and more than minimal disability in several others
4.0	Walking without aid, self-sufficient, up and about some 12 hr a day despite relatively severe disability; able to walk 500 m without aid or rest
4.5	Walking without aid, up and about much of the day, able to work a full day, may have some limitation of full activity or require some help, relatively severe disability but able to walk 300 m without aid or rest
5.0	Walking without aid or rest for about 200 m, disability severe enough to impair full daily activities, can work a full day without special provisions
5.5	Ambulatory without aid or rest for about 100 m; disability severe enough to prevent full daily activities
6.0	Intermittent or unilateral constant assistance (cane, crutch, brace) required to walk about 100 m with or without resting
6.5	Needs canes, crutches, braces to walk for 20 m without resting
7.0	Unable to walk beyond 5 m even with aid; mostly confined to a wheelchair; wheels self in standard wheelchair and transfers alone; up and about in wheelchair some 12 hr a day

Rating	Functional Status
7.5	Unable to take more than a few steps; restricted to wheelchair; may need aid in transfer; wheels self but cannot carry on in standard wheelchair a full day; may require motorized wheelchair
8.0	Essentially restricted to bed, chair, or wheelchair, but may be out of bed itself much of the day; retains many self-care functions; generally has effective use of arms
8.5	Essentially restricted to bed much of day; has some effective use of arms; retains some self-care functions
9.0	Helpless bed patient; can communicate and eat
9.5	Totally helpless bed patient; unable to communicate effectively or eat/swallow
10.0	Death due to MS

REFERENCE

Kurtzke, J. F. (1983). Rating neurologic impairment in multiple sclerosis: an expanded disability status scale (EDSS). *Neurology, 33*(11), 1444–1452.

KURTZKE FUNCTIONAL SYSTEMS SCORES (FSS)

- Pyramidal functions
  - 0: Normal
  - 1: Abnormal signs without disability
  - 2: Minimal disability
  - 3: Mild to moderate paraparesis or hemiparesis (detectable weakness but most function sustained for short periods, fatigue a problem); severe monoparesis (almost no function)
  - 4: Marked paraparesis or hemiparesis (function is difficult), moderate quadriparesis (function is decreased but can be sustained for short periods); or monoplegia
  - 5: Paraplegia, hemiplegia, or marked quadriparesis
  - 6: Quadriplegia
  - 9: Unknown
- Cerebellar functions
  - 0: Normal
  - 1: Abnormal signs without disability
  - 2: Mild ataxia (tremor or clumsy movements easily seen, minor interference with function)
  - 3: Moderate truncal or limb ataxia (tremor or clumsy movements interfere with function in all spheres)
  - 4: Severe ataxia in all limbs (most function is very difficult)
  - 5: Unable to perform coordinated movements because of ataxia
  - 9: Unknown

  (Record #1 in small box when weakness [grade 3 or worse on pyramidal] interferes with testing.)
- Brainstem functions
  - 0: Normal
  - 1: Signs only

    2: Moderate nystagmus or other mild disability

    3: Severe nystagmus, marked extraocular weakness, or moderate disability of other cranial nerves

    4: Marked dysarthria or other marked disability

    5: Inability to swallow or speak

    9: Unknown

- Sensory function

    0: Normal

    1: Vibration or figure-writing decrease only in one or two limbs

    2: Mild decrease in touch or pain or position sense, or moderate decrease in vibration in one or two limbs (vibratory can be substituted with decreased figure writing, virabroty alone in three or four limbs)

    3: Moderate decrease in touch or pain or position sense, or essentially lost vibration in one or two limbs; or mild decrease in touch or pain or moderate decrease in all proprioceptive tests in three or four limbs

    4: Marked decrease in touch or pain or loss of proprioception, alone or combined, in one or two limbs; or moderate decrease in touch or pain or severe proprioceptive decrease in more than two limbs

    5: Loss (essentially) of sensation in one or two limbs; or moderate decrease in touch or pain or loss of proprioception for most of the body below the head

    6: Sensation essentially lost below the head

    9: Unknown

- Bowel and bladder function (rate on the basis of the worse function, either bowel or bladder)

    0: Normal

    1: Mild urinary hesitance, urgency, or retention

    2: Moderate hesitance, urgency, retention of bowel or bladder, or rare urinary incontinence (intermittent self-catheterization, manual compression to evacuate bladder, or finger evacuation of stool)

    3: Frequent urinary incontinence

    4: In need of almost constant catheterization (and constant use of measures to evacuate stool)

    5: Loss of bladder function

    6: Loss of bowel and bladder function

    9: Unknown

- Visual function

    0: Normal

    1: Scotoma with visual acuity (corrected) better than 20/30

    2: Worse eye with scotoma with maximal visual acuity (corrected) of 20/30 to 20/59

    3: Worse eye with large scotoma, or moderate decrease in fields, but with maximal visual acuity (corrected) of 20/60 to 20/99

    4: Worse eye with marked decrease of fields and maximal visual acuity (corrected) of 20/100 to 20/200; grade 3 plus maximal acuity of better eye of 20/60 or less

5: Worse eye with maximal visual acuity (corrected) less than 20/200; grade 4 plus maximal acuity of better eye of 20/60 or less

6: Grade 5 plus maximal visual acuity of better eye of 20/60 or less

9: Unknown

(Record #1 in small box for presence of temporal pallor.)

- Cerebral (or mental) functions

0: Normal

1: Mood alteration only (does not affect EDSS)

2: Mild decrease in mentation

3: Moderate decrease in mentation

4: Marked decrease in mentation (chronic brain syndrome, moderate)

5: Dementia or chronic brain syndrome, severe or incompetent

9: Unknown

REFERENCE

Kurtzke, J. F. (1983). Rating neurologic impairment in multiple sclerosis: an expanded disability status scale (EDSS). *Neurology*, *33*(11), 1444–1452.

MINI-MENTAL STATE EXAMINATION (MMSE)

- The MMSE is one of the most widely used brief omnibus mental status tests.
- The MMSE is a 30-point standardized screening tool for assessing orientation (10 points), attention (5 points), short-term memory (retention and recall) (6 points), naming (2 points), repetition (1 point), simple verbal and written commands (4 points), writing (1 point), and construction (1 point).
- The questions should be asked in the order listed and scored immediately; the test is not timed. The MMSE may be administered in 5 to 10 minutes, and the test is available in many different languages.
- Importantly, demographic variables (such as age and education) have been shown to influence the MMSE. The validity of the test is unclear for people with less than 8 grades of formal education. Another prominent limitation of the test is the ceiling effect; people of varying cognitive ability may get the maximum 30 point score, so its resolving power in those with subjective cognitive impairment or very early mild cognitive impairment is limited; thus detailed neuropsychological testing is often advisable in this situation. Therefore, these parameters should always be taken into consideration when interpreting MMSE scores.

Another important issue is accurate scoring and the use of alternative questions on the test. Training for administering the MMSE should emphasize the need for consistent scoring, and pitfalls such as scoring after an early mistake in serial 7s or spelling "WORLD" backwards such that a single mistake does not result in losing multiple points. Orientation to place is also problematic, as multiple levels of accuracy, and multiple names for the same place may exist. Thus, a person may be correct in saying they are in "Brooklyn," "New York City," or the neighborhood where the test is being given. Serial 7s are more difficult than spelling WORLD backwards, resulting in different scores for the same test. Similarly, seasons are not determined by weather at the time of the test, and some leeway around change in seasons (± 1 week) is appropriate. The intersecting pentagons are only correct if the two pentagons form a four-sided figure.

The MMSE is also not sensitive to change in individuals with Alzheimer disease. The test–retest variability is about 2 points, and annual decline rates of about 3 points are average.

Mini-Mental State Examination (MMSE)	Name: DOB: Hospital Number:		
One point for each answer DATE:			
ORIENTATION			
Year Season Month Date Time	....../ 5	....../ 5	....../ 5
Country Town District Hospital Ward/Floor	....../ 5	....../ 5	....../ 5
REGISTRATION			
Examiner names three objects (e.g., apple, table, penny) and asks the patient to repeat (1 point for each correct. THEN the patient learns the 3 names repeating until correct).	....../ 3	....../ 3	....../ 3
ATTENTION AND CALCULATION			
Subtract 7 from 100, then repeat from result. Continue five times: 100, 93, 86, 79, 65. (Alternative: spell "WORLD" backwards: DLROW).	....../ 5	....../ 5	....../ 5
RECALL			
Ask for the names of the three objects learned earlier.	....../ 3	....../ 3	....../ 3
LANGUAGE			
Name two objects (e.g., pen, watch)	....../ 2	....../ 2	....../ 2
Repeat "No ifs, ands, or buts."	....../ 1	....../ 1	....../ 1
Give a three-stage command. Score 1 for each stage. (E.g., "Place index finger of right hand on your nose and then on your left ear.")	....../ 3	....../ 3	....../ 3
Ask the patient to read and obey a written command on a piece of paper. The written instruction is: "Close your eyes."	....../ 1	....../ 1	....../ 1
Ask the patient to write a sentence. Score 1 if it is sensible and has a subject and a verb.	....../ 1	....../ 1	....../ 1

COPYING

Ask the patient to copy a pair of intersecting pentagons.

...... / 3 ...... / 3 ...... / 3

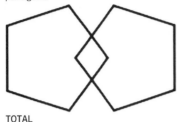

TOTAL   ...... / 3 ...... / 3 ...... / 3

MMSE Scoring
24–30: no cognitive impairment
18–23: mild cognitive impairment
0–17: severe cognitive impairment
From "Mini-Mental State Examination (MMSE)." *Oxford Medical Education.* www.
oxfordmedicaleducation.com/geriatrics/mini-mental-state-examination-mmse/. Accessed
15 April 2016.

REFERENCE

Folstein, M. F., Folstein, S. E., & McHugh, P. R. (1975). "Mini-mental state". A practical method for grading the cognitive state of patients for the clinician. *J Psychiatr Res*, *12*(3), 189–198.

MODIFIED RANKIN CLINICAL DISABILITY SCALE

0: No symptoms at all (used often in stroke patients)
1: No significant disability despite symptoms; able to carry out all usual duties and activities
2: Slight disability; unable to carry out all previous activities but able to look after own affairs without assistance
3: Moderate disability requiring some help, but able to walk without assistance
4: Moderate-severe disability; unable to walk without assistance and unable to attend to own bodily needs without assistance
5: Severe disability; bedridden, incontinent, and requiring constant nursing care and attention
6: Death

NIH STROKE SEVERITY SCALE (NIHSSS)

Items to be tested	Points to be scored
Level of consciousness	
• Alert, keenly responsive	0
• Obeys, answers, or responds to minor stimulation	1

Continued

Items to be tested	Points to be scored
• Responds only to repeated stimulation or painful stimulation (excludes reflex response)	2
• Responds only with reflex motor or totally unresponsive	3

Ask the month and patient's age; answer must be exactly right

• Answers both correctly	0
• Answers one correctly or patient unable to speak because of any reason other than aphasia or coma	1
• Answers neither correctly, or too stuporous or aphasic	2

Ask patient to open and close eyes and then grip and release nonparetic hand

• Performs both tasks correctly	0
• Performs 1 task correctly	1
• Performs neither task correctly	2

Best gaze: only horizontal movements tested; oculocephalic reflex use is ok, but not calorics

• Normal	0
• Partial gaze palsy	1
• Forced deviation or total gaze paresis not overcome by oculocephalic maneuver	2

Visual fields tested by confrontation

• No visual loss	0
• Partial hemianopia	1
• Complete hemianopia	2
• Bilateral hemianopia (blind from any cause including cortical blindness)	3

Facial palsy: encourage patient to smile and close eyes or grimace; check symmetry

• Normal symmetrical movement	0
• Minor paralysis (flattened nasolabial fold, asymmetry on smiling)	1
• Partial paralysis (total or near total lower face paralysis)	2
• Complete paralysis (absence of facial movement upper/lower face)	3

Right arm motor: extend right arm palm down at 90 degrees (sitting) or 45 degrees (supine)

• No drift, holds for full 10 seconds	0
• Drifts down before 10 seconds but does not hit bed/support	1
• Some effort against gravity, but cannot get up to 90 (or 45 if supine) degrees	2
• No effort against gravity, limb falls	3
• No movement	4

Left arm motor: extend left arm palm down at 90 degrees (sitting) or 45 degrees (supine)

• No drift, holds for full 10 seconds	0
• Drifts down before 10 seconds but does not hit bed/support	1
• Some effort against gravity, but cannot get up to 90 (or 45 if supine) degrees	2

Items to be tested	Points to be scored
• No effort against gravity, limb falls	3
• No movement	4

Right leg motor: extend right leg and flex at hip to 30 degrees

• No drift, holds for full 5 seconds	0
• Drifts down before 5 seconds but does not hit bed/support	1
• Some effort against gravity	2
• No effort against gravity, limb falls	3
• No movement	4

Left leg motor: extend left leg and flex at hip to 30 degrees

• No drift, holds for full 5 seconds	0
• Drifts down before 5 seconds but does not hit bed/support	1
• Some effort against gravity	2
• No effort against gravity, limb falls	3
• No movement	4

Limb ataxia: finger/nose and heel/shin done on both sides (Not ataxia if hemiplegic or unable to comprehend. Ataxia must be out of proportion to any weakness present.)

• Absent	0
• Present in 1 limb	1
• Present in two limbs	2

Sensory to pinprick

• Normal	0
• Pinprick less sharp or dull on affected side	1
• Severe to total sensory loss; patient unaware of being touched	2

Best language using pictures, naming items, and reading short sentences

• No aphasia	0
• Some loss of fluency or comprehension	1
• Severe aphasia—fragmentary communication, listener carries burden of communication	2
• Mute, global aphasia, no usable speech or auditory comprehension	3

Dysarthria: if not obviously present, have patient read

• Normal	0
• Slurs some words	1
• So slurred as to be unintelligible, or mute	2

Extinction/inattention

• No abnormality	0
• Inattention to any sensory modality or extinction to bilateral simultaneous stimulation in one sensory modality	1
• Profound hemi-inattention or hemi-inattention to more than one modality; does not recognize own hand	2

NIH STROKE SEVERITY SCALE (NIHSSS)

PARKINSON DISEASE RATING SCALES

HOEHN AND YAHR STAGING OF PARKINSON DISEASE

1. Stage One
   a. Signs and symptoms on one side only
   b. Symptoms mild
   c. Symptoms inconvenient but not disabling
   d. Usually presents with tremor of one limb
   e. Friends have noticed changes in posture, locomotion, and facial expression
2. Stage Two
   a. Symptoms are bilateral
   b. Minimal disability
   c. Posture and gait affected
3. Stage Three
   a. Significant slowing of body movements
   b. Early impairment of equilibrium on walking or standing
   c. Generalized dysfunction that is moderately severe
4. Stage Four
   a. Severe symptoms
   b. Can still walk to a limited extent
   c. Rigidity and bradykinesia
   d. No longer able to live alone
   e. Tremor may be less than earlier stages
5. Stage Five
   a. Cachectic stage
   b. Invalidism complete
   c. Cannot stand or walk
   d. Requires constant nursing care

UNIFIED PARKINSON DISEASE RATING SCALE (UPDRS)

The UPDRS is a rating tool to follow the longitudinal course of Parkinson disease. It is made up of the (1) Mentation, Behavior, and Mood, (2) Activities of daily living (ADL), and (3) Motor sections. These are evaluated by interview. Some sections require multiple grades assigned to each extremity. A total of 199 points are possible, with 199 representing the worst (total) disability, and 0 representing no disability.

I. Mentation, Behavior, Mood
   - Intellectual Impairment
     0: None
     1: Mild (consistent forgetfulness with partial recollection of events with no other difficulties)
     2: Moderate memory loss with disorientation and moderate difficulty handling complex problems
     3: Severe memory loss with disorientation to time and often place, severe impairment with problems
     4: Severe memory loss with orientation only to person, unable to make judgments or solve problems

- Thought Disorder
  - 0: None
  - 1: Vivid dreaming
  - 2: "Benign" hallucination with insight retained
  - 3: Occasional to frequent hallucination or delusions without insight, could interfere with daily activities
  - 4: Persistent hallucination, delusions, or florid psychosis.
- Depression
  - 0: Not present
  - 1: Periods of sadness or guilt greater than normal, never sustained for more than a few days or a week
  - 2: Sustained depression for >1 week
  - 3: Vegetative symptoms (insomnia, anorexia, abulia, weight loss)
  - 4: Vegetative symptoms with suicidality
- Motivation/Initiative
  - 0: Normal
  - 1: Less of assertive, more passive
  - 2: Loss of initiative or disinterest in elective activities
  - 3: Loss of initiative or disinterest in day-to-day (routine) activities
  - 4: Withdrawn, complete loss of motivation

II. Activities of Daily Living
- Speech
  - 0: Normal
  - 1: Mildly affected, no difficulty being understood
  - 2: Moderately affected, may be asked to repeat
  - 3: Severely affected, frequently asked to repeat
  - 4: Unintelligible most of time
- Salivation
  - 0: Normal
  - 1: Slight but noticeable increase, may have nighttime drooling
  - 2: Moderately excessive saliva, minimal drooling
  - 3: Marked drooling
- Swallowing
  - 0: Normal
  - 1: Rare choking
  - 2: Occasional choking
  - 3: Requires soft food
  - 4: Requires NG tube or G tube
- Handwriting
  - 0: Normal
  - 1: Slightly small or slow
  - 2: All words small but legible
  - 3: Severely affected, not all words legible
  - 4: Majority illegible
- Cutting Food/Handing Utensils
  - 0: Normal

    1: Somewhat slow and clumsy but no help needed
    2: Can cut most foods, some help needed
    3: Food must be cut, but can feed self
    4: Needs to be fed

- Dressing
  - 0: Normal
  - 1: Somewhat slow, no help needed
  - 2: Occasional help with buttons or arms in sleeves
  - 3: Considerable help required but can do some things alone
  - 4: Helpless
- Hygiene
  - 0: Normal
  - 1: Somewhat slow but no help needed
  - 2: Needs help with shower or bath or very slow in hygienic care
  - 3: Requires assistance for washing, brushing teeth, going to bathroom
  - 4: Helpless
- Turning in Bed/Adjusting Bed Clothes
  - 0: Normal
  - 1: Somewhat slow, no help needed
  - 2: Can turn alone or adjust sheets but with great difficulty
  - 3: Can initiate but not turn or adjust alone
  - 4: Helpless
- Falling Unrelated to Freezing
  - 0: None
  - 1: Rare falls
  - 2: Occasional, less than one per day
  - 3: Average of once per day
  - 4: >1 per day
- Freezing When Walking
  - 0: Normal
  - 1: Rare, may have start hesitation
  - 2: Occasional falls from freezing
  - 3: Frequent freezing, occasional falls
  - 4: Frequent falls from freezing
- Walking
  - 0: Normal
  - 1: Mild difficulty, may drag legs or decrease arm swing
  - 2: Moderate difficultly requires no assist
  - 3: Severe disturbance requires assistance
  - 4: Cannot walk at all even with assist
- Tremor
  - 0: Absent
  - 1: Slight and infrequent, not bothersome to patient
  - 2: Moderate, bothersome to patient
  - 3: Severe, interferes with many activities
  - 4: Marked, interferes with many activities

- Sensory Complaints Related to Parkinsonism
  - 0: None
  - 1: Occasionally has numbness, tingling, and mild aching
  - 2: Frequent, but not distressing
  - 3: Frequent painful sensation
  - 4: Excruciating pain

III. Motor Exam
  - Speech
    - 0: Normal
    - 1: Slight loss of expression, diction, volume
    - 2: Monotone, slurred but understandable, moderately impaired
    - 3: Marked impairment, difficult to understand
    - 4: Unintelligible
  - Facial Expression
    - 0: Normal
    - 1: Slight hypomimia, could be poker face
    - 2: Slight but definite abnormal diminution in expression
    - 3: Moderate hypomimia, lips parted some of time
    - 4: Masked or fixed face, lips parted 1/4 inch or more with complete loss of expression
  - Tremor at Rest
    - A. Face
      - 0: Absent
      - 1: Alight and infrequent
      - 2: Mild and present most of time
      - 3: Moderate and present most of time
      - 4: Marked and present most of time
    - B. Right Upper Extremity (RUE)
      - 0: Absent
      - 1: Slight and infrequent
      - 2: Mild and present most of time
      - 3: Moderate and present most of time
      - 4: Marked and present most of time
    - C. Left Upper Extremity (LUE)
      - 0: Absent
      - 1: Slight and infrequent
      - 2: Mild and present most of time
      - 3: Moderate and present most of time
      - 4: Marked and present most of time
    - D. Right Lower Extremity (RLE)
      - 0: Absent
      - 1: Slight and infrequent
      - 2: Mild and present most of time
      - 3: Moderate and present most of time
      - 4: Marked and present most of time

PARKINSON DISEASE RATING SCALES

    E. Left Lower Extremity (LLE)
- 0: Absent
- 1: Slight and infrequent
- 2: Mild and present most of time
- 3: Moderate and present most of time
- 4: Marked and present most of time

- Action or Postural Tremor
  - A. RUE
    - 0: Absent
    - 1: Slight, present with action
    - 2: Moderate, present with action
    - 3: Moderate, present with action and posture holding
    - 4: Marked, interferes with feeding
  - B. LUE
    - 0: Absent
    - 1: Slight, present with action
    - 2: Moderate, present with action
    - 3: Moderate, present with action and posture holding
    - 4: Marked, interferes with feeding
- Rigidity
  - A. Neck
    - 0: Absent
    - 1: Slight or only with activation
    - 2: Mild/moderate
    - 3: Marked, full range of motion
    - 4: Severe
  - B. RUE
    - 0: Absent
    - 1: Slight or only with activation
    - 2: Mild/moderate
    - 3: Marked, full range of motion
    - 4: Severe
  - C. LUE
    - 0: Absent
    - 1: Slight or only with activation
    - 2: Mild/moderate
    - 3: Marked, full range of motion
    - 4: Severe
  - D. RLE
    - 0: Absent
    - 1: Slight or only with activation
    - 2: Mild/moderate
    - 3: Marked, full range of motion
    - 4: Severe
  - E. LLE
    - 0: Absent
    - 1: Slight or only with activation
    - 2: Mild/moderate

       3: Marked, full range of motion

       4: Severe

- Finger Taps
  - A. Right
    - 0: Normal
    - 1: Mild slowing and/or reduction in amplitude
    - 2: Moderately impaired, definite and early fatiguing, may have occasional arrests
    - 3: Severely impaired, frequent hesitations and arrests
    - 4: Can barely perform
  - B. Left
    - 0: Normal
    - 1: Mild slowing, and/or reduction in amplitude
    - 2: Moderately impaired, definite and early fatiguing, may have occasional arrests
    - 3: Severely impaired, frequent hesitations and arrests
    - 4: Can barely perform
- Hand Movements (open and close hands in rapid succession)
  - A. Right
    - 0: Normal
    - 1: Mild slowing and/or reduction in amplitude
    - 2: Moderately impaired, definite and early fatiguing, may have occasional arrests
    - 3: Severely impaired, frequent hesitations and arrests
    - 4: Can barely perform
  - B. Left
    - 0: Normal
    - 1: Mild slowing and/or reduction in amplitude
    - 2: Moderately impaired, definite and early fatiguing, may have occasional arrests
    - 3: Severely impaired, frequent hesitations and arrests
    - 4: Can barely perform
- Rapid Alternating Movements (pronate and supinate hands)
  - A. Right
    - 1: Normal
    - 0: Mild slowing and/or reduction in amplitude
    - 2: Moderately impaired, definite and early fatiguing, may have occasional arrests
    - 3: Severely impaired, frequent hesitations and arrests
    - 4: Can barely perform
  - B. Left
    - 0: Normal
    - 1: Mild slowing and/or reduction in amplitude
    - 2: Moderately impaired, definite and early fatiguing, may have occasional arrests
    - 3: Severely impaired, frequent hesitations and arrests
    - 4: Can barely perform

- Leg Agility (tap heel on ground, amplitude should be 3 inches)
  - A: Right
    - 1: Normal
    - 0: Mild slowing and/or reduction in amplitude
    - 2: Moderately impaired, definite and early fatiguing, may have occasional arrests
    - 3: Severely impaired, frequent hesitations and arrests
    - 4: Can barely perform
  - B: Left
    - 0: Normal
    - 1: Mild slowing and/or reduction in amplitude
    - 2: Moderately impaired, definite and early fatiguing, may have occasional arrests
    - 3: Severely impaired, frequent hesitations and arrests
    - 4: Can barely perform
- Arising from Chair (patient arises with arms folded across chest)
  - 0: Normal
  - 1: Slow, may need more than one attempt
  - 2: Pushes self up from arms or seat
  - 3: Tends to fall back, may need multiple tries but can arise without assistance
  - 4: Unable to arise without help
- Posture
  - 0: Normal erect
  - 1: Slightly stooped, could be normal for older person
  - 2: Definitely abnormal, moderately stooped, may lean to one side
  - 3: Severely stooped with kyphosis
  - 4: Marked flexion with extreme abnormality of posture
- Gait
  - 0: Normal
  - 1: Walks slowly, may shuffle with short steps, no festination or propulsion
  - 2: Walks with difficulty, little or no assistance, some festination, short steps or propulsion
  - 3: Severe disturbance, frequent assistance
  - 4: Cannot walk
- Postural Stability (retropulsion test)
  - 0: Normal
  - 1: Recovers unaided
  - 2: Would fall if not caught
  - 3: Falls spontaneously
  - 4: Unable to stand
- Body Bradykinesia/Hypokinesia
  - 0: None
  - 1: Minimal slowness, could be normal, deliberate character

2: Mild slowness and poverty of movement, definitely abnormal, or decreased amplitude of movement

3: Moderate slowness, poverty, or small amplitude

4: Marked slowness, poverty, or amplitude

Schwab and England Activities of Daily Living

Rating can be assigned by rater or by patient.

- 100%: Completely independent. Able to do all chores without slowness, difficulty, or impairment.
- 90%: Completely independent. Able to do all chores with some slowness, difficulty, or impairment. May take twice as long.
- 80%: Independent in most chores. Takes twice as long. Conscious of difficulty and slowing.
- 70%: Not completely independent. More difficulty with chores. 3 to 4 times along on chores for some. May take large part of day for chores.
- 60%: Some dependency. Can do most chores, but very slowly and with much effort. Errors, some impossible.
- 50%: More dependent. Needs help with half of chores. Difficulty with everything.
- 40%: Very dependent. Can assist with all chores but few alone.
- 30%: With effort, now and then does a few chores alone or begins alone. Much help needed.
- 20%: Nothing alone. Can do some slight help with some chores.
- Severe invalid.
- 10%: Totally dependent, helpless.
- 0%: Vegetative functions such as swallowing, bladder, and bowel function are not functioning. Bedridden.

SPETZLER-MARTIN SCALE FOR ARTERIOVENOUS MALFORMATION

	Score
Size of arteriovenous malformation (AVM)	
Small (<3 cm)	1
Medium (3–6 cm)	2
Large (>6 cm)	3
Eloquence of adjacent brain	
Noneloquent	0
Eloquent	1
Pattern of venous drainage	
Superficial only	0
Deep	1

Score: Grade the AVM by adding the scores on each feature (range 1–5).

Index

Note: Page numbers followed by *f* indicate figures and *t* indicate tables.